To Jay,

Good luck to you in our

profesion.

Best Regards

Terry R. Yoch

ESSENTIALS OF SKELETAL RADIOLOGY

Volume One

ESSENTIALS OF SKELETAL RADIOLOGY

Volume One

TERRY R. YOCHUM
B.S., D.C., D.A.C.B.R., F.C.C.R.(C), F.I.C.C.
Adjunct Professor of Radiology, Los Angeles College of Chiropractic
Whittier, California
Director, Rocky Mountain Chiropractic Radiological Center
Denver, Colorado

Formerly:
Senior Lecturer, Department of Diagnostic Sciences
Division Head, Department of Radiology
Phillip Institute of Technology—School of Chiropractic
Melbourne, Australia

Professor and Chairman, Department of Radiology
Logan College of Chiropractic
St. Louis, Missouri

Assistant Professor of Radiology, National College of Chiropractic
Lombard, Illinois

LINDSAY J. ROWE
B.App.Sc.(Chiro), D.A.C.B.R., F.C.C.R.(C)
Private Radiology and Clinical Practice
Sydney, Australia

Formerly:
Associate Professor and Chairman, Radiology Department
Northwestern College of Chiropractic
Minneapolis, Minnesota

Professor and Chairman, Department of Radiology
Canadian Memorial Chiropractic College
Toronto, Ontario, Canada

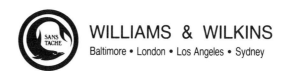

WILLIAMS & WILKINS
Baltimore • London • Los Angeles • Sydney

Editor: Jonathan W. Pine, Jr.
Associate Editor: Victoria M. Vaughn
Copy Editor: S. Minton
Design: JoAnne Janowiak
Illustration Planning: Asterisk Group/Alice Sellers/Wayne Hubbel
Production: Raymond E. Reter

Printed in the United States of America

Library of Congress Cataloging-in-Publication Data

Essentials of Skeletal Radiology.

   Includes bibliographies and index.
   1. Skeleton—Diseases—Diagnosis. 2. Skeleton—Radiography. I. Yochum, Terry
R. II. Rowe, Lindsay J. [DNLM: 1. Bone and Bones—radiography. WE 225 E78]
RC930.5.E85 1987   616.7'107572   86-5469
ISBN 0-683-09329-0

87 88 89 90 91
10 9 8 7 6 5 4 3 2

Dedication

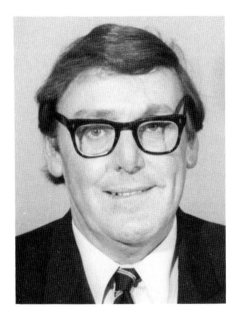

Within a lifetime, a few select individuals will significantly affect the life of another. For both of us, Bryan Hartley, M.D., was one of those individuals. He was a person who seemed to achieve whatever he wanted in life: an extraordinary professional career, diversified personal interests, and close ties with family and friends. Bryan was born at Aldershot, England, in 1926 and studied medicine at Guy's Hospital Medical School in London. He was appointed house surgeon at the Royal Infirmary, Edinburgh, in 1950, following which he emigrated to Australia. He became a flight lieutenant in the R.A.A.F. medical branch and was a Fulbright traveling scholar. He was appointed medical officer in the Northern Territory Medical Services and continued his medical training at the Royal Perth Hospital in Western Australia and was a resident medical officer at General Hospital in Tasmania.

Bryan Hartley's early postgraduate training appointments alternated between the fields of surgery and radiology. He held appointments in surgery at the Union Memorial Hospital in Baltimore, Maryland; Launceston General Hospital in Tasmania; the Royal Children's Hospital in Melbourne, Victoria; and as Surgeon Superintendent at the Lyell District Hospital, Tasmania. His appointments in radiology were at the Launceston General Hospital, St. Vincent's Hospital, Melbourne, and the Royal Hobart Hospital in Tasmania. After a short appointment in Rome as a radiologist for the Department of Immigration, Bryan returned to Melbourne to become the director of the Department of Radiology at the Repatriation General Hospital and held this position until 1981. At that time, he accepted a position as staff radiologist in the Department of Radiology at the Austin Hospital also in Melbourne, the post he occupied until his death.

In his chosen career of medicine, Bryan Hartley excelled in both surgery and radiology, holding specialist qualifications in both fields. This interest in surgery was of considerable advantage to him in radiology, as it enabled him to see a diagnostic problem in its proper clinical perspective. A unique combination of clinical understanding, experience, and aptitude for clear expression made Bryan an outstanding teacher for his many students, residents, and colleagues. His boundless enthusiasm and wry humor provided for stimulating and informative discussions on almost any topic. His opinions were highly valued, particularly in patient evaluation and treatment.

For both of us, it was Bryan who, by example, provided the stimulus for developing our knowledge and abilities and advancing the standards of our profession. His influence on our careers is reflected not only in the use of his personal case material in this text, but more importantly in the knowledge, expertise, and teaching methods he so freely shared with us. His untimely death in 1984 now deprives us and others of the opportunity of sharing his special gifts. He is survived by his wife, Beverley, and their children, Lynne and John.

In gratitude we dedicate this book to Bryan Hartley, M.D.

Terry R. Yochum
Lindsay J. Rowe

Foreword

Although there are a number of excellent books dealing with skeletal radiology, the addition of these volumes to the literature is more than welcome. The unique format and the approach taken by Drs. Yochum and Rowe should make this book particularly valuable as a reference source. Happily, the material is also very readable and should serve as an excellent textbook. As an educator I am especially pleased to have the chapter dealing with *principles of radiological interpretation* included since this material in detail is not found elsewhere.

The compilation of this material indeed represents a monumental effort. Contributions of case material from doctors of various disciplines worldwide not only augments the extensive material Drs. Yochum and Rowe and the other authors have compiled but also speaks to the esteem in which the authors are held and the increasing cooperation among the several healing arts.

The ultimate reward for a teacher is to see his students excell. As Dr. Yochum's chief I take pride in his accomplishments and those of Dr. Rowe, his former student. The results of their efforts in compiling this work will stand as a tribute to unceasing dedication and excellence in their chosen field. I deem it a privilege to be a contributor to this work. I expect that *Essentials of Skeletal Radiology* will be the benchmark for publications by doctors of chiropractic and will find a place among the standard works in skeletal radiology.

Joseph W. Howe, D.C., D.A.C.B.R., F.I.C.C.

Professor and Chairman
Radiology Department
Los Angeles College of Chiropractic

Foreword

I have known Drs. Yochum and Rowe for many years. When they visited Dr. William E. Litterer in Elizabeth, New Jersey, it was not uncommon for us to spend many hours in front of the viewboxes viewing and sharing interesting cases, many of which now appear in this text.

Both authors possess a unique quality that I refer to as a passion for knowledge. It is because of this thirst for knowledge and a willingness to share information that this book has become a reality.

Essentials of Skeletal Radiology is an excellent book that can serve as both a core textbook and a reference text. Although originally written for the chiropractic profession, I would recommend this book to anyone interested in skeletal radiology.

I congratulate Drs. Yochum and Rowe for a job well done.

Steven P. Brownstein, M.D.

Chief of Computed Tomography Section
East Orange Veterans Administration Hospital
East Orange, New Jersey
Associate Attending Professor of Radiology
University Hospital
Newark, New Jersey
Clinical Assistant Professor of Radiology
New Jersey University Medical and Dental School
Newark, New Jersey

Foreword

Radiology is such a dynamic medical specialty. We students of the field have amassed a wealth of information since the first x-rays were taken in the nineteenth century. Those of us who have been around radiology for more than a few years have seen tremendous improvements in our imaging departments. We have not only many ways to produce an image but also many ways to capture and view the image we want. And we can do it with less radiation to the patient or no radiation at all. This delightful growth in radiology parallels the careers of the two accomplished doctors who are the authors of this fine text. I have had the privilege of watching these two charming and interesting fellows as their careers began to bloom and focus on radiology. They possess an insatiable thirst for radiology and a special propensity for skeletal radiology. They have studied and traveled around the globe not only to improve their knowledge, but also, as I now see, to share their expertise with fellow students and radiologists.

This book represents a tremendous compilation of material. Terry and Lindsay say it all in a rare flow of concise reading, fine charts, and excellent radiographs. This is a gem, a quality jewel of a book that we all will enjoy using and telling friends, students, practitioners and fellow radiologists, "Pick up Yochum and Rowe's *Essentials of Skeletal Radiology.*"

M. Bruce Farkas, D.O.

Professor of Radiology
Chicago College of Osteopathic Medicine
Chicago, Illinois

Preface

The conception of this textbook, *Essentials of Skeletal Radiology*, began in 1980 in Melbourne, Australia. A set of unique circumstances brought an American radiology professor (TRY) and an Australian radiology resident (LJR) together. Both felt the frustration of utilizing multiple texts from which to teach and to learn about disorders that afflict the human skeleton. A tentative table of contents and a sample chapter were submitted to Williams & Wilkins for review. In 1982, at the November Radiological Society of North America (RSNA) meeting in Chicago, a formal contract to create this textbook was agreed upon. We ventured into this project essentially not knowing how much time and effort would actually be required. We began with enthusiasm and optimism in different countries, Dr. Yochum in Australia and Dr. Rowe in Canada, and later joined forces in the United States.

The initial tasks were to catalogue the photographed case material we already had and to seek out from diverse sources that which we did not have but felt should be included in a comprehensive text. The magnitude of this aspect alone is represented by the final selection of some 2500 illustrative cases from a collective pool of more than 7000. All of this without a single word yet written!

After the accumulation of the resource material, the creation of the text, beginning in January 1984, was another journey into the unknown. Every word was initially handwritten, amassing some 10,000 pages of raw manuscript. At completion we filled 30 computer discs and gained a unique appreciation for the amazing properties of word processing. We sympathize with authors who have compiled even larger and more complex texts in years past without such technology available to them. Thorough review of the copy edited manuscript was followed by proofreading the voluminous galleys and page proofs and compiling the comprehensive index.

An explanation of the title, *Essentials of Skeletal Radiology*, may help to clarify the book's purpose and scope. The word "essentials" was selected as the fundamental guiding concept throughout the compilation of this work. From the vast and overwhelming body of knowledge of skeletal disorders we have extracted the core facts and brought them together into a single unique source. It is the desire and intent of the authors that through this endeavor the process of learning and understanding the radiology of skeletal disorders will become somewhat easier for all, from the student of radiology to the experienced clinician. We have combined these "essentials" with our own personal observations sometimes interpreted as experience. Our intent for this work is that it perform as a textbook. A textbook, as defined by Webster, is "a book containing the principles of a subject, used as a basis for instruction." Practically interpreted, a textbook serves as a foundation and provides the framework upon which one should add his or her own "experience."

To serve this purpose the book has been carefully constructed around a clear and concise mode of presentation. The subject of each chapter was thoughtfully selected and placed in a logical sequence, beginning with the technology of producing diagnostic skeletal radiographs and interpreting the depicted normal radiographic anatomy. Following this, the many diverse congenital anomalies and normal skeletal variants are presented both in text and pictorial atlas format. Then follow the radiographic measurements and the biomechanically related disorders of the musculoskeletal system: scoliosis, spondylolisthesis and spinal stenosis. These precede an introductory chapter into the principles of radiographic interpretation of the more complex pathological entities. This chapter is a keystone to comprehending the basic principles of radiographic diagnosis of the skeleton. The chapters that follow deal with the seven categories of bone disease: skeletal dysplasias, trauma, arthritic disorders, tumor and tumor-like processes, infection, vascular and hematological disorders, and nutritional, metabolic and endocrine disorders. This forms the nucleus of the pathological aspect of this text. The last three chapters cover often-neglected aspects of skeletal radiology: report writing, radiographic artifacts, and a pictorial atlas of vertebral names.

The methodology of presentation we have chosen is to break down the subject material into logical headings. Initially a discussion of *general* and occasionally *historical considerations* of each disorder is given. Under the next heading of *clinical features* we have accurately outlined the physical and laboratory abnormalities demonstrated with each condition. Specific details have been included that relate to clinical presentation, incidence, age, sex, location and any distinctive physical characteristics. The *pathological features* offer a fundamental presentation covering etiology, pathogenesis and histopathological abnormalities basic to the radiographic signs. The *radiological features* have formed the major emphasis of discussion for each disorder, and the essential roentgenographic signs are stressed. The understanding of these signs is augmented by photographic reproductions of many actual radiographs, as well as illustrative line drawings. Wherever possible, *treatment* and *prognosis* have been discussed. A highlight of the text is an outline of the core material of the chapter in a concise *capsule summary*. The summaries are distinguished by a different typeface and by their placement within shaded blocks. Their purpose is to provide a quick and easy reference source.

A comprehensive bibliography from many health disciplines has been integrated within the text to substantiate the facts presented and to provide resources to stimulate further investigation.

The large number of case studies and illustrations reflects our desire to depict visually the essential roentgenographic signs of even the most complex skeletal disorders. The captions describe details to be noted in the illustrations. Aspects of particular importance are indicated by arrows on the figures. Additionally, important facts are reinforced with a *comment* section at the conclusion of the caption.

The comprehensive index was compiled with considerable thought and effort. The page numbers of the primary discussion of the selected disorder are printed in bold type to facilitate the reader's search.

In conclusion, this text is meant to be read from cover to cover and also to be used as a reference source. Use this book as it is intended—to help you master the knowledge and perfect the skill of interpreting skeletal radiographs so that you might better evaluate, understand and treat your patients.

Terry R. Yochum
Lindsay J. Rowe

Acknowledgments

To complete a task of this magnitude, many people have been involved in various ways. They deserve our heartfelt thanks for their help and inspiration, for without them our path would have been significantly more difficult.

Because of our known intense interests in skeletal radiology, we have been privileged to receive many cases from all over the world, and some of these have been included within the text. The contributors represent a wide diversity of health disciplines, as is evidenced by the varied qualifications they have attained. For this reason, we have included a glossary of abbreviations for attained degrees listed.

A special thank you to those physicians who have graciously provided the forewords for this text: Steven P. Brownstein, MD; M. Bruce Farkas, DO; and Joseph W. Howe, DC, DACBR.

We are indebted to and extend a special thanks to our contributing authors—Gary M. Guebert, DC, DACBR; Bryan Hartley, MD; Joseph W. Howe, DC, DACBR; Margaret A. Seron, DC, DACBR; and David P. Thomas, MD—for the incorporation of their expertise in four chapters of this text.

Distinctively there have been a few contributors—Steven P. Brownstein, MD; Bryan Hartley, MD; William E. Litterer, DC, DACBR; and David P. Thomas, MD—who unselfishly gave of their own unique and extraordinary case materials. We thank the many other contributors of case material and have duly acknowledged them where their cases are presented in the text. Our thanks also extend to those contributors whose cases were not chosen for this first edition.

The unenviable task of interpreting and typing our manuscripts rested with Pamela J. Morgenthaler, whose skill as a typist is only exceeded by her dedication to this textbook. We marveled at her technical abilities, her eagerness to take on more and more work, her good humor and also her apparent resistance to pain. It was she who sorted the way through the maze of computer jargon, relieving us of a considerable additional burden that we could not have otherwise overcome. Feelings of gratitude are also extended to Diann Albers, who provided additional typing.

Many people have been involved in the editorial process and have given unsparingly of their time and knowledge. In particular we thank Marshall N. Deltoff, DC for his untiring efforts in lending his expertise during the final stages of editing. The circumstances that allowed this to happen were created through the kind consideration and cooperation of the administrative staff of the Los Angeles College of Chiropractic, Joseph W. Howe, DC, DACBR, and the following radiology residents: Gary L. Bustin, DC; Tracy C. Matsumoto, DC; Gary D. Schultz, DC; Phillip J. Shanks, DC; and Lawrence H. Wyatt, Jr., DC. We acknowledge them in gratitude. We would like to express special and deep appreciation to John K. Hyland, DC and Jeffrey R. Thompson, DC, DACBR for giving unselfishly of their time, their professional expertise and their literary talents. We also wish to thank the following friends and associates who volunteered their time and energies to the editorial process: Philip S. Bolton, DC; Peter Clark, MD; Donald E. Freuden, DC, FACO, FICC; Lynton G. F. Giles, MSc, DC; Gary M. Guebert, DC, DACBR; Philip C. Lening, DC; Daniel M. Martello, DC; Reed B. Phillips, DC, DACBR, MSCM, PhD; Edward J. Wheeler, DC; and John H. Wilson, JP, MA, AAIM.

We sincerely appreciate the time and expert review given on Chapter 5, The Natural History of Spondylolysis and Spondylolisthesis, by the following noted authorities: Stanley J. Bigos, MD; J. David Cassidy, DC, FCCS(C); Hugo A. Keim, MD; William H. Kirkaldy-Willis MD; Alf L. Nachemson, MD; Reed B. Phillips, DC, DACBR, MSCM, PhD; and Leon L. Wiltse, MD.

To the staff of Williams & Wilkins in general and to our outstanding editor, Jonathan W. Pine, Jr., we are most grateful for bringing our manuscript to publication.

The high technical quality of the photo reproductions is due to the efforts of several individuals to whom we extend our sincere thanks. In the tedious initial step of the actual photography of the case material we were assisted by Jeffrey R. Thompson, DC, DACBR, with contributions by Vinton L. Albers, DC, DACBR. Our gratitude goes to Ian Troup of Latrobe Studios, Melbourne, Australia for doing much of the initial production of proof sheets and negatives. Additional thanks to Duane Turner and his staff at Professional Color Services in Minneapolis, Minnesota for their creation of the actual prints. To Paul W. Thielen, DC a special word of thanks for his many hours radiographing the various bony specimens utilized primarily in Chapter 1 and throughout the text. We also wish to acknowledge Karl E. Anderson, DC, who served as the model for the radiographic positioning section of Chapter 1. General assistance was plentiful in the photocopying of the photographs that was necessary for arrow placement, and for this service we thank Daniel M. Martello, DC; Pat G. Napoli, DC; Laurie A. Reiner, DC; and Paul W. Thielen, DC. Our gratitude is also extended to Phillip J. Shanks, DC, and Stephen M. Foreman, DC for their photographic assistance covering a significant portion of the photos in Chapter 6. We appreciate the cooperation of Williams & Wilkins and Jack Edeiken, MD for granting permission to utilize two previously published cases and additional unpublished cases.

The majority of the illustrations were provided by the artistic expertise of Robert Bonawitz. Additional illustrations were created by Inge Yochum, and in Chapter 6 by Marshall N. Deltoff, DC. The design and layout for the cover of the text were provided by Inge Yochum.

In finding and obtaining the many references for each topic a few people gave generously of their time to assist in this tedious task. Thanks to Cheryl A. Bjerke, MLS, whose expertise and patience with the computer searches time and again quickly and efficiently uncovered the essential reference material. Frances E. Portine, BA cheerfully and openly doubled her work load with our pursuits to obtain "just another article." Carole E. Jones, BA and Jan L. Adams, BA unselfishly gave of their time and energies as we repetitively disrupted their busy schedules. Additional reference materials were obtained through the efforts of Norman W. Kettner, DC, DACBR for Chapter 11 and Paul W. Thielen, DC for Chapters 2 and 3.

During the entire time period in which this work was being compiled, many people had their own schedules and personal interests infringed upon. In this regard to all of those students, residents, friends, clinicians and administrators, our thanks and admiration for remaining tolerant and, more importantly, completely supportive throughout.

Finally, our gratitude is expressed to Bryan Hartley, MD, in our Dedication.

Terry R. Yochum
Lindsay J. Rowe

It is with my deepest gratitude and love that I thank my mother Cecelia Yochum, and my father Kenneth E. Yochum, DC for their love and never ending support and guidance throughout my career. My father has been a model for me, not only in the pursuit of personal growth and integrity but also in the endeavor to attain professional excellence. I thank my sister, Kay Annette, and her family for always lending a receptive ear and showing their sincere interest in this project. To my wife, Inge, words cannot express how much I appreciate the love, understanding and support that she gave me through this arduous task. My love and appreciation go to my children, Kimberley Ann, Philip Andrew and Alicia Marie for their patience and their tolerance of my frequent absences. A special thank you to my wife's aunt, Mrs. Franzi Valny, for helping Inge with the care of our children and household and for being there when my time would not permit.

I am indebted to the late Joseph Janse, DC for the environment he helped create at the National College of Chiropractic so that I and many others could receive resident training in radiology. On a more personal level Dr. Janse was a great inspiration to me, always exemplary in the striving for academic, professional and personal excellence. Special thanks are conveyed to my original professors of radiology, the late Donald B. Tomkins, DC, DACBR and James F. Winterstein, DC, DACBR. My gratitude is extended to my good friend Bruce Farkas, DO for the training he provided me during my residency program. His guidance and encouragement have continued through the years and for that I am most appreciative. It has been a comfort to have the reliable support and encouragement of my close friend John F. Beckman, EdD. He has worked with zeal in the planning of my lectures and I thank him for his understanding when frequently the writing of this book took valuable time away from our seminar programs.

It is an honor and privilege to have been a student and resident under the direction of Joseph W. Howe, DC, DACBR, FICC. He has been my mentor. Our early student-professor relationship has grown into the close friendship we now share. I admire his unmatched unselfishness with his knowledge and time, since in many ways this has paved my path throughout my career. I am grateful for his wisdom, his encouragement and his friendship.

A special word of thanks is conveyed to my immediate professional associates and close friends, Donald E. Freuden, DC, FACO, FICC, and Donald M. Kuppe, DC and the staff at the North Suburban Chiropractic Clinic for the support and patience they displayed throughout this project. My gratitude is extended also to Connie Jones, RT, who unceasingly showed her understanding and to Jerry Collyer, RT. Together they efficiently carried on with the daily tasks of my radiology practice. I am deeply indebted to Pamela J. Morgenthaler for her untiring commitment and unmatched perfectionism in the typing and finalization of the manuscript.

The inspiration to write this text came from my many students and teachers and I thank them for providing the ongoing stimulus to tackle this task and to bring it to its completion.

Finally, to one of my most outstanding residents, coauthor and close friend, Lindsay J. Rowe, BApp Sc(Chiro),

DACBR, FCCR(C), I offer a special thanks for his support and contribution in the production of this textbook.

Terry R. Yochum

The most truly enjoyable part of assembling the material for this text has always been derived from the communication with and encouragement of many long-time friends and the many newly acquired ones. My sincere appreciation and gratitude to these same people is second only to their friendship.

I will always be indebted to my close friends, Geoffry Rymer, DC and his wife Pauline, for being my personal confidants and supporters when I most needed them throughout the early years of my training and later away from my homeland. Their wise counsel, encouragement and friendship have provided the stimulus to strive for excellence academically, clinically and personally.

My close colleague, Peter Rissis, DC, I value for his insight, support and friendship no matter where I am in the world at any time of day. I have been privileged to be influenced by James R. Brandt, DC, FACO, a leader in health care. I thank him for his example of the pursuit of excellence and appreciate his intuitive guidance. I have been enthused and supported by Donald E. Freuden, DC, FACO, FICC and Donald M. Kuppe, DC, who have given unselfishly of their time and busy schedules to raise my spirits and spur me on to completion. The influence of Kenneth E. Yochum, DC since our first meeting has been profound and extends into my writings in this book. I have appreciated his guidance, insights and perspectives that have made my contributions take on a more meaningful direction. To Joseph W. Howe, DC, DACBR, FICC, who always has given so freely of his time, expertise and friendship, I am deeply grateful.

Numerous friends have provided the necessary encouragement and enthusiasm over the last five years to complete this project: Veronica Gerber, Pat Masanz, John Zappetillo, Wyn Lee, David and Toni Mathieson, Robyn Cunningham, John and Lynne Broadrick, Connie Jones, RT, Frances Portine, BA, Carol Jones, BA and Cheryl Bjerke, MLS. I look to them with admiration and respect for their patience, tolerance and most importantly their continued friendship. To Pamela Morgenthaler, our typist and friend, I extend my heartfelt thanks for applying her superb technical abilities and unique character to see this project through to its fruition.

For my coauthor, Terry R. Yochum, DC, DACBR, FICC, FCCR(C), I find few words to describe the deep admiration and respect I have for him. Since our relationship began in 1977, I remain humbled by his efforts and in awe of his prowess as an instructor, author and radiologist. It is a rare privilege to be sharing this book with my professor, mentor and friend. I convey my deepest gratitude to his wife, Inge, for being so understanding of the long hours of attention directed to this project that allowed Terry and me to channel our energies toward completion.

To my parents, Robert and Dorothy Rowe, my sister Robyn, brother Graham and their families, I am forever grateful for their love, support and understanding while in the pursuit of this book away from their proximity. Their continued encouragement throughout has been a constant source of inspiration. For their unselfish sacrifices and understanding, I am and always will be, indebted.

Lindsay J. Rowe

Contributing Authors

GARY M. GUEBERT, B.S., D.C., D.A.C.B.R.
Private Radiology Practice
St. Louis, Missouri
formerly:
Assistant Professor and Chairman, Radiology Department
Texas Chiropractic College
Pasadena, Texas

BRYAN HARTLEY, M.D. (deceased)
Staff Radiologist
Austin Hospital
Melbourne, Australia
formerly:
Head, Department of Radiology
Heidelberg Repatriation Hospital
Melbourne, Australia

JOSEPH W. HOWE, D.C., D.A.C.B.R., F.C.C.R.(C), F.I.C.C.
Professor and Chairman, Radiology Department
Los Angeles College of Chiropractic
Whittier, California
Associated Radiological Consulting Group
Whittier, California
formerly:
Professor and Chairman, Department of Roentgenology and Clinical Science Division
National College of Chiropractic
Lombard, Illinois
Director of Radiology and Research
Associates Diagnostic and Research Center
Tallmadge, Ohio

MARGARET A. SERON, D.C., D.A.C.B.R.
Postgraduate Faculty Member
Los Angeles College of Chiropractic
Private Radiology Practice
Denver, Colorado
formerly:
Assistant Professor of Radiology
Los Angeles College of Chiropractic
Whittier, California

DAVID P. THOMAS, M.D.
Head, Department of Radiology
Austin Hospital
Melbourne, Australia

Contents

Abbreviations of Attained Degrees

B. App. Sc. (Chiro)   Bachelor of Applied Science (Chiropractic)
This is the chiropractic qualification issued by the Phillip Institute of Technology-School of Chiropractic, Melbourne, Australia.

D.C.   Doctor of Chiropractic

*D.A.C.B.R.   Diplomate of the American Chiropractic Board of Radiology

D.A.C.B.R.(Hon)   Honorary Diplomate of the American Chiropractic Board of Radiology

*D.O.   Doctor of Osteopathy

D.P.M.   Doctor of Podiatric Medicine

Ed.D   Doctor of Education

F.A.C.O.   Fellow of the Academy of Chiropractic Orthopedists

F.C.C.R.(C)   Fellow Chiropractic College of Roentgenologists (Canada)

F.I.C.C.   Fellow of the International College of Chiropractors

*M.D.   Doctor of Medicine

M.I.R.   Member of the Institute of Radiography

M.Sc. or M.S.   Master of Science

M.S.C.M.   Master of Science in Community Medicine

Ph.D.   Doctor of Philosophy

*Physicians referred to in this text holding these degrees are radiologists.

Skeletal Radiology: A Historical Perspective

All disciplines within the health sciences have undergone radical changes as new technologies have evolved, and radiology is no exception. In less than 100 years since the discovery of x-rays, the first crude pieces of equipment and vague shadows have been replaced by sophisticated machines that produce exquisitely detailed images. So explosive have the technological gains been that radiology is no longer limited to utilizing x-rays for the diagnosis of disease. Advancements in technology have expanded the scope of diagnostic radiology to include the imaging capabilities of ultrasonic waves, radioisotopes, computers, and magnetic fields.

The history of the development of radiology is long and intricate. As with so many other significant advancements in science, x-rays were discovered accidentally. In 1895, Wilhelm Conrad Roentgen, a professor at the University of Würzburg in Germany, was working on experiments in his laboratory. He was investigating the properties of an early cathode ray tube, called a Crookes' tube, which accelerated electrons in a manner similar to today's x-ray apparatus. While conducting a stream of electrons from the cathode through the evacuated tube, he noticed that a plate covered with barium platinocyanide located at some distance away began to fluoresce. Not knowing what to call these invisible rays from the Crookes' tube that induced fluorescence he named them "x-rays," X standing for the unknown quantity. Roentgen then feverishly began experimenting and defining their characteristics, and in little more than a month he had described all the major properties of the x-ray as they are recognized today. Professor Roentgen produced the first clinical radiograph, an image of his wife's hand, on November 8, 1895, (Fig. A) and first reported his findings on December 8, 1895, to the Würzburg Physico-Medical Society. In recognition of his discovery he received the first Nobel Prize for Physics in 1901. Others soon recognized the potential role of the x-ray in industry and the health care professions. Examples of the earliest diagnostic x-rays are those made in 1896 by Pupin of a hand imbedded with multiple shotgun pellets, those made by Frost of a fractured wrist, and a case of osteosarcoma imaged by Manell.

Thereafter, a global technological revolution began. Pupin developed the first intensifying screen, and Edison, the first fluoroscope, to mention only two developments. In 1921, Potter and Bucky introduced a moving grid mechanism. Sausser, a chiropractor, in 1935, was the first to produce a single exposure, anteroposterior full spine radiograph. The cumulative result of all of these refinements was the production of diagnostic images of improved quality, which depicted abnormalities directing more effective treatment. (Figs. B–D)

These early advancements were not without cost, however. Before the harmful effects of radiation were recognized, many severe and often fatal injuries occurred to

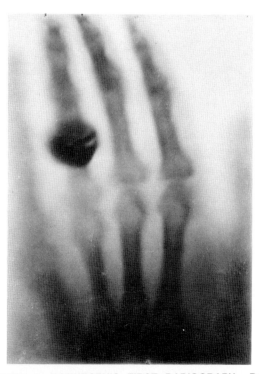

FIGURE A. ROENTGEN'S FIRST RADIOGRAPH. Professor Roentgen's historic first radiograph of his wife's hand taken November 8, 1895, in Würzburg, Germany. (Courtesy of Deutsches Rontgen-Museum, Remscheid-Lennep, West Germany)

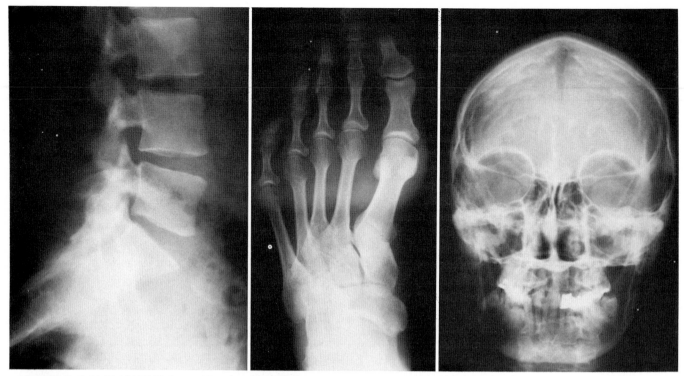

FIGURE B. (left) PLAIN FILM. Lateral Lumbar Skeletal Radiograph.
FIGURE C. (center) PLAIN FILM. Dorsoplantar View of the Foot. Observe the filtration of the forefoot and toes used to obtain a uniform exposure.
FIGURE D. (right) PLAIN FILM. Posteroanterior Skull Radiograph.

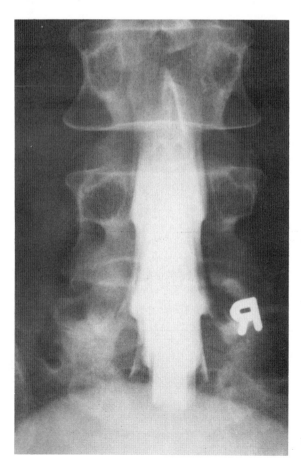

FIGURE E. METRIZAMIDE LUMBAR MYELOGRAM. Demonstrates the normal anatomical details of the cauda equina.

those who pioneered the research in radiology. As a result, the use of the x-ray came under close bureaucratic scrutiny and control. Despite these complications and in the face of increasingly poor publicity, the usefulness of this new diagnostic tool could not be ignored, and innovations in imaging technology continued.

The use of radiopaque contrast media within hollow organs and body spaces improved the diagnostic evaluations. Introduction of radiopaque substances into the subarachnoid space of the spine (myelography) provided information not previously available, especially in regard to intraspinal and intervertebral disc lesions. (Fig. E) In the skeletal system, an opaque medium placed into the joint space (arthrography) allowed demonstration of cartilage, synovium, and ligamentous structures. The inherent lack of sensitivity of conventional radiography was countered by the administration of selective radioisotopes (nuclear medicine) that seek out specific tissues and areas of cellular activity. In skeletal disorders the administration of isotopes such as technetium—99m and gallium provided information on bone activity not recognizable with conventional procedures. (Fig. F) This has been particularly important in the early detection of many skeletal disorders.

In the early 1970's, computed tomograms (CT scans, CAT scans) were first produced combining the technology of the computer with the advances in x-ray technology. With refinements in machine and computer technology, exquisite sectional images are now produced in almost every anatomical plane. Computed tomograms have had a particular impact on the evaluation of spinal and neurological diseases. (Figs. G and H) More recently images totally revolutionary to the field of diagnosis have been produced using strong magnetic fields (Magnetic Resonance Imaging, MRI). (Figs. I and J)

In spite of all these technological advances, many fundamental principles of imaging remain unchanged. The

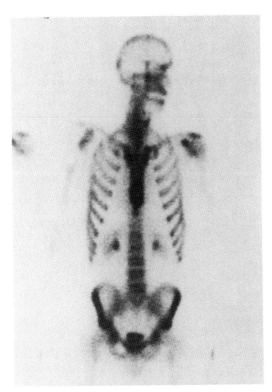

FIGURE F. FULL BODY BONE SCAN. Demonstrates the normal uptake of radioactive isotope in metabolically active areas of the skeleton. (Courtesy of Nuclear Medicine Department, M.D. Anderson Hospital, Houston, Texas)

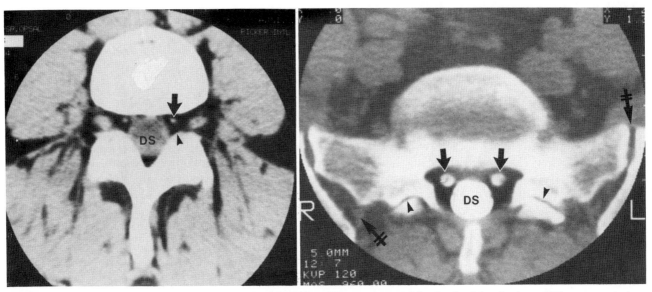

FIGURE G. (left) COMPUTED TOMOGRAM OF THE L4 LEVEL.   Observe the exquisite details of the dural sac (DS), nerve roots (arrow), perineural fat (arrowhead), paravertebral musculature and bony confines.
FIGURE H. (right) CONTRAST ENHANCED (MYELOGRAM) COMPUTED TOMOGRAM OF THE S1 LEVEL.   The dural sac (DS) and the S1 spinal nerve roots (arrows) are accurately depicted. Additionally the lumbosacral (arrowheads) and sacroiliac (crossed arrows) articulations are demonstrated.

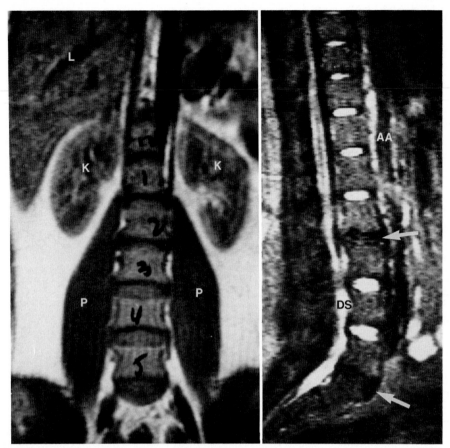

FIGURE I. (left) ANTEROPOSTERIOR MAGNETIC RESONANCE IMAGE (MRI) OF THE ABDOMEN AND INTERVERTEBRAL DISCS.   This view clearly shows the liver (L), kidneys (K), and psoas muscles (P).

FIGURE J. (right) LATERAL MAGNETIC RESONANCE IMAGE OF THE LUMBAR SPINE.   This projection shows a lack of signal intensity at the L2 and L5 disc levels (arrows) due to decreased water content from degenerative disc disease. The dural sac (DS) and the abdominal aorta (AA) are also visible.

plain film radiograph still forms the foundation for a large portion of the diagnostic investigations in clinical practice, especially in the evaluation of skeletal disorders.

This is demonstrated by a recent chance encounter with an example from the past. (Fig. K) The depicted radiograph was taken in 1897 at the John Sealy Hospital in Galveston, Texas, just 2 years after Roentgen's discovery of x-rays. In 1976 the patient, Mrs. Minne Powell Bowers, consulted a chiropractor in Conroe, Texas, for evaluation of a low back complaint. When questioned about prior x-rays, she stated that she had fallen at the age of 14 and her father, a medical doctor, had decided to transport her from Willis, Texas, to Galveston in a horse drawn wagon to have her hip pain evaluated with this new "x-ray"

procedure. Mrs. Bowers brought on her next visit to the chiropractor the radiograph pictured in Figure K. Although the radiograph has aged and lacks technical clarity, careful observation of the image reveals an acute angular deformity of the femoral neck due to a displaced fracture. Even today, some 90 years later, the initial diagnostic examination of choice for a similar case is still the same: *the plain film radiograph.*

For examinations of the skeleton, there is no modality to match the time and cost effectiveness of the plain film radiograph. It is from this "plain film" perspective that *Essentials of Skeletal Radiology* has been written and supplemented with examples of more complex sophisticated imaging technologies.

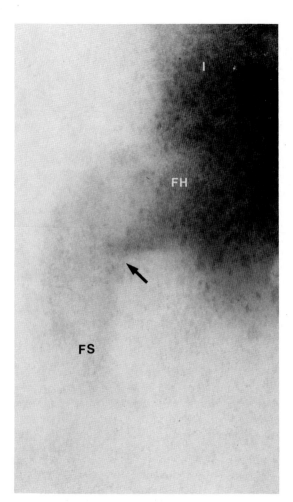

FIGURE K. RADIOGRAPHIC ANTIQUE: A FRACTURED FEMUR FROM 1897. Despite the crude radiographic image observe the ilium (I), femoral head (FH), and femoral shaft (FS). Careful observation reveals an acute angular deformity of the femoral neck due to a fracture (arrow). (Courtesy of Michael L. Davis, DC, Conroe, Texas)

1

Radiographic Positioning and Normal Anatomy

LINDSAY J. ROWE
TERRY R. YOCHUM

Introduction

Since the discovery of the "X" ray by Wilhelm Conrad Roentgen in 1895, attempts to accurately depict the skeleton have undergone little change. (1) What was true in 1895 in terms of positioning and anatomy remains true today, with only the technical aspects undergoing significant modification. (2,3)

The purpose of this first chapter is to provide a foundation for the chapters that follow. It is comprised of two parts—radiographic positioning and normal anatomy. These are combined in a synthesis fashion to allow the reader to be able to perform the examination and comprehend the normal anatomy demonstrated on the obtained radiograph. For each projection a concise description of the positioning parameters is given, supplemented with photographs demonstrating the actual position. In addition, the resulting radiograph is shown and labelled, along with relevant anatomical and radiographic specimens, to augment understanding.

More detailed and specialized texts should be consulted for views not included in this chapter. (4–7)

In radiology, as in other clinical disciplines, to understand and recognize the abnormal a thorough knowledge and familiarity with normal is mandatory. Of equal importance is the technological process involved in producing the radiograph, since it is the quality of the image upon which the accuracy of the interpretation is largely based. To produce radiographs of inadequate technical quality is to handicap the interpretation, which ultimately compromises patient care. It is for these reasons that the student of radiology and health care practitioner who utilizes skeletal radiographic procedures must master these two aspects of the discipline.

RADIOGRAPHIC POSITIONING

Format of Presentation

Each projection to follow is described in a standard format for simplicity and easy reference. The various parameters for each projection are concisely provided under various headings.

Basic Projections. List of routine views.

Optional Projections.   List of nonroutine views.

Demonstrates.   The structures shown on the projection are listed.

Measure.   The point which is measured for calculating the exposure factors. This is usually through the central ray.

kVp.   The optimum kVp and range is stated for the body part being examined. (Table 1.1) kVp values are recommended throughout this chapter for the purpose of creating a diagnostic radiograph of adequate contrast and should be applicable to most current film-screen combinations. Those readers utilizing detail (extremity) rare earth screens may experience underexposed radiographs if values less than 55 kVp are routinely used, due to diminished light output of the crystals at this relatively low energy level. For these practitioners a kVp value of 55 or greater should be used for the production of those radiographs.

Film Size.   As a guide, the film size is given; however, clinical discretion should be applied according to the size of the body part under examination.

Grid.   Extremities measuring under 10 cm, lateral, flexion/extension, and oblique cervicals, and chest films may all be done without a grid. All other projections should use a grid. A minimum grid ratio of 10:1 is recommended, while a 12:1 ratio is considered optimal.

Tube-Film Distance (TFD).   Distance between the tube and film. While a 40-inch TFD is traditionally offered, faster film/screen combinations make it practical to use 60–80 inches for some exposures, which then reduces exposure to the patient due to an increase in the ratio of entrance dose to exit dose.

Tube Tilt.   The angulation of the tube in relation to the head (cephalad) and feet (caudad).

Patient Position.   The postural attitude of the patient (upright, recumbent, seated, etc.).

Part Position.   The position of the body part which is being radiographed (flexion, extension, supination, etc.).

Central Ray (CR).   The theoretical center of the radiographic beam as defined by the position of the light localizer crosshairs from the collimator.

Collimation.   Limiting the irradiated film size is a practical decision based on the patient and film size. However, the smallest size compatible with the body component should be obtained and **never** should exceed the film size.

Side Marker.   Appropriate side markers should be placed, preferably in the corner of the radiographic field, so as not to obstruct any anatomical details.

Breathing Instructions.   The patient is told either to stop breathing (arrested respiration), take a deep breath in and hold it (suspended deep inspiration), or let the breath out and hold it (suspended expiration). These respirations may be partial or complete. Occasionally, a breathing technique is utilized to intentionally blur obscuring overlying anatomy.

Special Considerations.   Any special detail as it relates to the positioning or anatomy is briefly listed.

Positioning Terminology

Equipment-Related Factors.   The equipment described in this chapter will only be dealt with briefly, such that the positioning can be described succinctly and accurately.

Radiographic Series.   In any body location a minimum of two views perpendicular to each other must be performed on initial evaluation. A series is the set of radiographs obtained on a particular body area. A "scout" radiograph is a single view taken for the sole purpose of obtaining a general, nonspecific overview of the body part, which is later followed by more specific projections.

Spot Projections.   These are isolated, closely collimated views of a particular region, to more closely evaluate an area which is not well seen on routine views or which may be abnormal.

Film Identification.   Each film **must** be identified with the patient's name, date of exposure, and clinic where taken.

Bucky.   This is virtually synonomous with the surface the patient lies on or stands up against during the exposure. In actual fact, the bucky is a mechanism for housing and moving the grid, to eliminate scatter radiation from reaching the film. An exposure time of less than 0.2 seconds may "freeze" the grid and create grid lines. The bucky is used on thicker body parts to improve image quality.

On thinner body parts less than 10 cm, the chest, and cervical spine (except for APLC and APOM) a bucky need not be used, since the scatter radiation generated is relatively small.

Table 1.1.
Optimum Kilovolts Peak (kVp)

Region	kVp
Skull	85
Sinuses	85
Cervical Spine	80
Thoracic Spine	90
Lumbar Spine	
Anteroposterior	85
Lateral	90
Pelvis	80
Sacrum	80
Coccyx	80
Full Spine	90
Hip	80
Knee	60
Ankle	55
Foot	55
Toes	55
Shoulder	75
Clavicle	70
Acromioclavicular	70
Elbow	55
Wrist	55
Hand	55
Fingers	55
Thumb	55
Ribs	80
Chest	110
Abdomen	
Soft tissue	100
Calcific densities	70

Grid. When x-rays penetrate and enter the body, they interact with atoms by ejecting orbital electrons, displacing orbital electrons to another shell or altering the electrical charge of the atomic nucleus. The net result is an alteration of the electrical charge of the atom ("ionizing radiation"). Following any of these interactions, x-rays of lower energy are produced which have an altered path ("scattered radiation"). These create an overall decrease in image quality by graying the densities (fog). (8)

A grid functions to eliminate this scattered radiation and prevent its reaching the film. The structure of a grid consists of lead strips separated by a radiolucent material. The scattered rays tend to be multidirectional and do not easily pass between the lead strips as do the primary (undiverted) rays. The end result is that there is an overall decrease in film fog, which increases film contrast and image quality. (8)

Utilizing a grid necessarily increases patient dose and need not be used for body parts less than 10 cm in thickness and for air-gap techniques such as lateral cervical views.

Tube. This is the apparatus where the x-rays are produced and emitted toward the patient.

Tube Tilt. The angle of the beam is occasionally altered to better depict certain anatomical details. A general rule with tube tilt is for every 5 degrees of angulation move the tube 1 inch closer to the patient; otherwise, the film will be underexposed.

Tube/Film Distance (TFD). This is the measured distance between the tube and film.

Collimator. This is a cube-shaped structure on the outside of the x-ray tube which can be manipulated to reduce the field size of the emitted radiation. Placed inside the collimator is a light source which produces a light beam which accurately simulates the exiting radiation. On this light beam intersecting lines which represent the center of the emission can be easily identified.

kVp (Kilovolts Peak). This is the potential difference created between the cathode (filament) and anode during the exposure. It is responsible for the speed that electrons will have when they interact at the anode. This determines the "strength" of the emitted x-rays, which translates into the ability to pass through the body (penetration). Therefore, kVp is the main determinant of beam quality and alters the film's scale of contrast (gray scale). (8,9) As body thickness increases, generally, so does the kVp. In this chapter, optimum kVp's are given for each body region.

mAs (Milliampere Seconds). This is the number of electrons generated per second and determines the density (film blackness) of the image. A linear relationship exists between film density and mAs which allows simpler computation when presented with performing a retake of an over- or underexposed radiograph. (8,9)

Lead Blockers. These are usually used to block off part of a cassette during an exposure, to protect that portion of film from scatter radiation so that it can be used for multiple projections on the same film. This is commonly used in examinations of the extremities on the same piece of film.

Markers. (Fig. 1.1A–C) The general rule with markers is to always mark the side closest to the film, on oblique and lateral views, and to place it in an area which will not obstruct important structures. Many types of markers are available. At a minimum, on anteroposterior views the right or left side should be identified, and on laterals and obliques the side closest to the film is marked. Specialized projections, such as stress studies of the spine, can be identified with the addition of an arrow to show the direction of patient motion. Upright and recumbent studies can be identified by the appropriate word, arrow, or a mercury ball inside the marker.

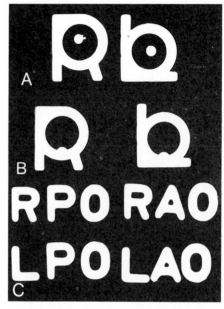

Figure 1.1. EXAMPLES OF RADIOGRAPHIC MARKERS. A. Recumbent Mitchell Right (R) and Left (L) Side Markers. Note the central position of the mercury ball, indicating the horizontal plane of the marker. **B. Upright Mitchell Right (R) and Left (L) Side Markers.** The mercury ball has now gravitated inferior, indicating the vertical plane of the marker. **C. Oblique Markers. RPO:** Right posterior oblique; **LPO:** Left posterior oblique; **RAO:** Right anterior oblique; **LAO:** Left anterior oblique.

Filtration. (Fig. 1.2A–E) The placement of aluminum and/or aluminum-copper filters (added filtration) at the collimator considerably reduces the amount of low-energy x-rays reaching the patient. In addition to reducing patient radiation dose, filters (sectional filtration) can be used to compensate for varying body thicknesses. This is especially the case in the thoracic and lumbar spine. The effect is to eliminate overexposure of thinner body parts, creating a more homogeneous density radiograph. (8,10)

Relative Exposure. Radiographs are assessed according to film density (film blackness). Assuming an optimal kVp, an overexposed film will appear exceedingly dark, due to too much mAs, while an underexposed film will be too light due to too little mAs.

Object Density. If an area on a radiograph appears black, it is termed radiolucent; if it appears to be whiter, then it is called radiopaque.

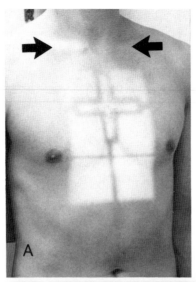

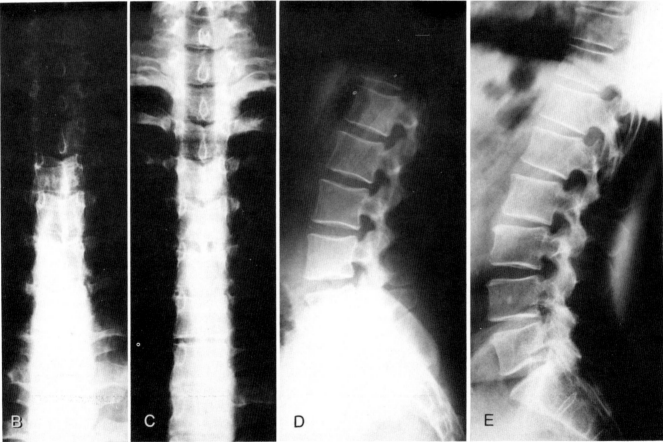

Figure 1.2. THE EFFECTS OF DENSITY EQUALIZING FILTRATION. A. Anteroposterior Thoracic Spine: With Filtration. Demonstrates the filtered region (arrows), the filter being located on the collimator. **B. Anteroposterior Thoracic Spine Radiograph: Without Filtration.** Observe the overexposed (dark) upper thoracic spine and underexposed (light) lower thoracic spine. **C. Anteroposterior Thoracic Spine Radiograph: With Filtration.** The radiographic density of the thoracic spine has been made more uniform with the use of a filter over the upper thoracic spine. **D. Lateral Lumbar Spine Radiograph: Without Filtration.** Distinct differences in radiographic density are evident. The lumbosacral area is severely underexposed (light), while the thoracolumbar area is overexposed (dark). **E. Lateral Lumbar Radiograph: With Filtration.** Numerous filters have been used to produce this uniformly exposed radiograph—one for the lower lung fields, one from the iliac crests upward, and one for the spinous processes. (Courtesy of Felix G. Bauer, DC, DACBR (Hon), Sydney, Australia)

Patient-Related Factors.

Patient Position. (Fig. 1.3) Various terms are commonly used to describe the patient's body position in relation to the x-ray beam.

1. Posteroanterior (PA). The x-ray beam enters the posterior surface and exits the anterior surface.

2. Anteroposterior (AP). The x-ray beam enters the anterior surface and exits the posterior surface.

3. Lateral (L). Right lateral (RL) indicates that the right side of the patient is in contact with the film. Left lateral (LL) indicates the left side of the patient is in contact with the film.

4. Right anterior oblique (RAO). The right anterolateral surface of the body is closest to the film.

5. Left anterior oblique (LAO). The left anterolateral surface of the body is closest to the film.

6. Right posterior oblique (RPO). The right posterolateral surface of the body is closest to the film.

7. Left posterior oblique (LPO). The left posterolateral surface of the body is closest to the film.

8. Upright (erect). The patient stands for the film.

9. Recumbent. The patient lies down for the film.

10. Lateral decubitis. The patient lies on one side, with the beam passing through horizontally.

11. Seated. Sitting on a chair, with the unaffected body parts placed outside the path of the x-ray beam.

Patient Variability. Various differences in body type, position, and bone density alter certain aspects of the technology involved in producing optimum radiographs.

1. *Obese patients.* Although the overall dimensions of the body part may be increased, fat is of relatively low radiodensity and may cause inadvertent overexposure. For this reason, recumbent projections will compress the body tissues and provide a better radiographic exposure. A reduction in kVp will help to improve film contrast.

2. *Muscular patients.* As muscle mass increases, this can be compensated for by an increase in kVp of approximately 10 from the original optimum kVp settings.

3. *Pediatric patients.* To ensure a proper exposure, younger patients must be appropriately immobilized. In the extremities routine bilateral views for comparison are discouraged. They should only be performed when specifically indicated.

4. *Upright and recumbent projections.* The body thickness alters with changes in postural position. A measurement obtained in the upright position will not be accurate for determining exposure factors in the recumbent position due to tissue compression.

5. *Bone density changes.* Decreased bone density (osteopenia) is frequently associated with various disorders. Under these conditions, and with increasing age (senile osteoporosis), a reduction in the mAs of approximately 25 percent may avoid overexposure. Conversely, in disorders of increased bone density the mAs should be increased by approximately 25 percent.

6. *Traumatized patient.* Under no circumstances should optimal patient positioning be preferred (mandated) without regard to patient safety. Attempts to position the truly injured patient may exacerbate the injury, with potentially catastrophic results in some instances.

Motion. Causes of motion include inadequate stabilization of the respective body part, misinstruction of the patient, long exposure time, and patient discomfort. All such factors should be controlled as much as possible.

Patient Protection. In general, an attempt is always made to remove all unrelated body parts at the site of study from the x-ray beam. To reduce patient exposure to primary radiation, collimation to film size (or smaller) must be performed. A pregnant woman should not be irradiated unless the clinical circumstances are life threatening. The risk of irradiating an early stage developing fetus can be reduced by appropriate patient questioning and application of the 10-day rule. (11)

Gonadal Shielding. In general, every attempt to reduce gonadal radiation must be made. Various methods for gonadal shielding have been devised which require accurate placement. In examinations of the hips or pelvis, especially in females, shields should not be used if the suspected pathology would be obscured. Female patients following *complete* hysterectomy or who are postmenopausal do not require gonadal shielding.

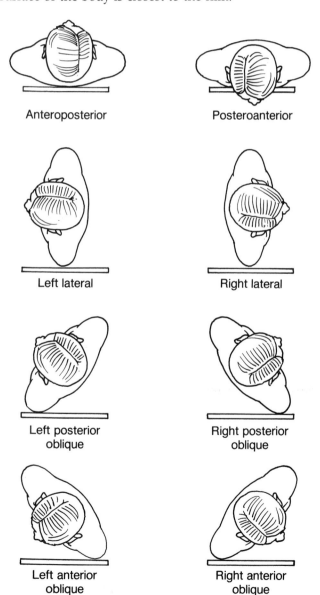

Anteroposterior

Posteroanterior

Left lateral

Right lateral

Left posterior oblique

Right posterior oblique

Left anterior oblique

Right anterior oblique

Figure 1.3. Nomenclature of the various radiographic positions.

The Bureau of Radiological Health recommends that gonadal shielding be used in three particular instances: 1) when gonads lie within the primary x-ray field or within close proximity (about 5 cm); 2) if the clinical objective of the examination will not be compromised; and 3) if the patient has a reasonable reproductive potential. (12)

Measurement.   Measuring calipers are used to determine the thickness of the body part, usually through the central ray. On the basis of this measurement, the exposure may then be calculated.

Relationship Terms.
Cephalad.   Towards the head.
Caudad.   Towards the feet.
Proximal.   Towards the center of the body.
Distal.   Toward the periphery of the body.
Lateral.   Toward the outside of the body.
Medial.   Toward the middle of the body.
Flexion.   The angle between body parts is decreased.
Extension.   The angle between body parts is increased.
Abduction.   Movement of the body part away from the midline.
Adduction.   Movement of the body part toward the midline.
Eversion.   Outward movement of the foot or ankle.
Inversion.   Inward movement of the foot or ankle.
Supination.   Palm up.
Pronation.   Palm down.
Patient Preparation.   Before examination of a particular body part, various steps should be performed as follows.
1. Removal of all clothing and putting on a gown, if necessary.
2. Removal of all metallic objects or dental appliances within the radiographic field. (Table 1.2)
3. Evacuation of the bowel or bladder, if the abdomen, sacrum, or coccyx is being examined.

Breathing Instructions.   In most projections respiration is transiently halted to prevent motion of the body part (arrested respiration). On occasion breathing may assist in blurring out overlying structures, such as the ribs on a lateral thoracic spine study. Suspended deep inspiration is used for chest and thoracic exposures to depress the diaphragm, while suspended expiration is used in abdominal films to elevate the diaphragm.

RADIOGRAPHIC ANATOMY

In radiographic evaluations of the skeleton the major structures demonstrated are the bones, joints, and surrounding soft tissues (muscle, viscera, skin). A more in-depth discussion of these features is to be found in Chapter 7. The basic background details related to this chapter will be presented.

Skeletal Anatomy

Osteology.   Osteology is the study of bones. (6,7,13) There are a total of 206 separate bones, divided into the axial and appendicular skeleton. (Table 1.3) The axial skeleton consists of 80 bones, which includes the skull, vertebral column, ribs, and sternum. The appendicular skeleton consists of 126 bones, which includes the upper and lower extremities, as well as the shoulder and pelvic girdles.

These bones are frequently referred to according to their shape—long, short, flat, or irregular.

Long Bones.   These bones are located in the appendicular skeleton. Typical examples include the femur, tibia, humerus, and radius.

Each long bone can be divided into five components—the epiphysis, physis, metaphysis, diaphysis, apophysis, and periosteum.

1. *Epiphysis.* This is the expanded end of a long bone, which is covered by articular cartilage and contains artic-

Table 1.2.
Common Artifacts of Various Body Regions

SKULL	Hairpins, wigs, false teeth, eyeglasses, necklaces, earrings, bizarre hair styles.
CERVICAL SPINE	Hairpins, wigs, false teeth, eyeglasses, necklaces, earrings, bizarre hair styles, clothing.
THORACIC SPINE	Necklaces, brassieres, clothing.
LUMBAR SPINE	Orthopedic supports, brassieres, underwear, pants with objects in the pockets.
PELVIS, HIPS, AND SHOULDERS	Orthopedic supports, brassieres, underwear, pants with objects in the pockets.
WRIST AND HAND	Watches, rings, bracelets, orthopedic supports.
ANKLE AND FOOT	Shoes, socks, orthopedic supports.

Table 1.3.
Total Number of Bones by Region

Axial Skeleton		Appendicular Skeleton	
SKULL		SHOULDER GIRDLES	
Cranium	8	Clavicle	2
Facial bones	14	Scapula	2
HYOID	1	UPPER EXTREMITIES	
AUDITORY OSSICLES	6	Humerus	2
VERTEBRAL COLUMN		Ulna	2
Cervical	7	Radius	2
Thoracic	12	Carpals	16
Lumbar	5	Metacarpals	10
Sacrum	1	Phalanges	28
Coccyx	1	PELVIC GIRDLE	
THORAX		Innominate	2
Sternum	1	LOWER EXTREMITIES	
Ribs	24	Femur	2
Total	80	Tibia	2
		Fibula	2
		Patella	2
		Tarsals	14
		Metatarsals	10
		Phalanges	28
		Total	126

ular cortex and underlying supporting bone. Its prime function is related to supporting joint movement.

2. *Physis* (growth plate). In growing, immature bones this region is cartilaginous and is responsible for enchondral bone growth. Radiographically, the physis will appear as a radiolucent band at the base of the epiphysis.

3. *Metaphysis.* The expanded area beneath the growth plate which tapers into the normal caliber of the shaft is called the metaphysis. It is the greatest metabolic region of bone and is responsible for forming the long bone shape during growth.

4. *Diaphysis* (shaft). This is the narrowest and longest portion of the bone. Its main function is mechanical support and housing for the bone marrow.

5. *Apophysis* (greater tuberosity, lesser trochanter, etc.). An apophysis is a bony attachment for ligaments or tendons and is usually seen as a protuberance beyond the bone contour.

6. *Periosteum.* This is a soft tissue envelope around and attached to the entire diameter of the bone. Notably, it is not located within the joint. Its function is to maintain the caliber of the bone by appositional bone growth. Radiographically, the periosteum is not visible unless it is mechanically elevated or chemically irritated, which will result in external periosteal new bone formation.

In addition to these divisions, the structure of a long bone is classified according to bone density, of which there are two—compact and cancellous. Compact bone is recognized on the radiograph as a thick, white outer bone shell which is called the cortex. The cortex has two divisions—an outer cortex and the inner cortex, often referred to as the endosteum. Notably, cortical thickness is greatest in the middle portion of the bone and gradually tapers toward the end of the bone. At the metaphysis the cortex is sharply attenuated from a thick band to a thin line. Internal to the cortex lies the medullary cavity, which is traversed by thin trabeculae (spongy bone).

Short Bones. These are small, cube-shaped bones; e.g., the wrist and ankle.

Flat Bones. These are rich in marrow and are characterized by their broad surfaces. The cortical thickness is relatively large and the medullary space is interposed. In the skull the cortices are called tables, and the medullary space the diploe.

Irregular Bones. Bones which do not conform to any particular shape are massed together in this category. These include bones of the cranial base and the vertebrae.

Arthrology. Arthrology is the study of joints (articulations). (6,7,13) Articulations can be categorized by two classifications—joint motion or articular histology.

Joint Motion. Three types are recognized—synarthroses, amphiarthroses, and diarthroses.

1. Synarthroses. Fixed, immobile joints. Examples include the skull sutures and growth plates.

2. Amphiarthroses. Slightly movable joints. Examples include intervertebral discs and symphysis pubis.

3. Diarthroses. Freely movable joints. Examples include the hips and shoulder joints.

Articular Histology. This classification emphasizes the tissue type found in the joint space and is especially useful in understanding joint disease. Three histologic types of joints are identified—fibrous, cartilaginous, and synovial. Essentially, these are equivalent to the joint motion classification, with fibrous tissue being present in synarthroses, cartilage within amphiarthroses, and synovial tissue within diarthroses.

Radiogical Features. A joint is readily identified by a smooth, regular lucent articular space and opposing parallel bony surfaces. For a joint to be adequately demonstrated, the x-ray beam must pass through the same plane as the joint surfaces.

Basic
***Lateral (right and left)**
Posteroanterior Caldwell
Anteroposterior Towne's

Skull

Lateral Projection Positioning
(Figure 1.4A and B)

Optional
Vertex

Demonstrates: Lateral cranial structures closest to the bucky (temporal, parietal), sella turcica, sphenoid sinus, occipitocervical junction, and calvarium. (1–5)
Measure: At the central ray.
kVp: 85 (80–90).
Film Size: 10 x 12 inches (24 x 30 cm).
Grid: Yes.
TFD: 40 inches (102 cm).
Tube Tilt: None.
Patient Position: Semiprone.
Part Position: Head is in true lateral position against the bucky. The infraorbital meatal line is parallel with the long edge of the cassette, and the interpupillary line is perpendicular.
CR: Passes ¾ inch superior and ¾ inch anterior to the external auditory meatus.
Collimation: To the patient's skull size.
Side Marker: Side closest to the film placed in film corner.
Breathing Instructions: Suspended expiration.
Special Considerations: Both right and left laterals should be performed routinely. (4) A well-positioned lateral should show superimposition of the mandibular rami, orbital roofs, and sella turcica.

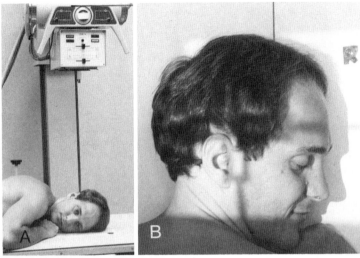

Figure 1.4A. Patient positioning.
Figure 1.4B. Collimation and central ray.

Normal Anatomy (Figure 1.4C)

1. Frontal bone.
2. Parietal bone.
3. Occipital bone.
4. Squamous portion, temporal bone.
5. Petrous portion, temporal bone.
6. Middle meningeal artery.
7. Frontal sinus.
8. Ethmoid sinus.
9. Maxillary sinus.
10. Sphenoid sinus.
11. Mastoid air cells.
12. Transverse venous sinus.
13. Sella turcica.
14. Internal occipital protuberance (IOP)
15. External occipital protuberance (EOP)
16. Inner table.
17. Diploe.
18. Outer table.
19. Parietal star (diploic venous confluence).
20. Pinna of the ear.
21. Internal auditory meatus.
22. Temporomandibular joint.
23. Nasopharynx.
24. Hard palate.
25. Orbit.
26. Odontoid.

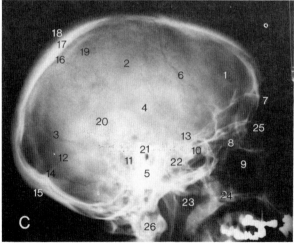

Figure 1.4C. Lateral skull radiograph.

Basic
Lateral (right and left)
*Posteroanterior Caldwell
Anteroposterior Towne's

Skull
**Posteroanterior Caldwell Projection
Positioning**
(Figure 1.5A and B)

Demonstrates: Frontal bone, frontal sinus, ethmoid sinus, orbits, sphenoid wings, petrous ridges, internal auditory canals. (1–5)
Measure: Through the central ray.
kVp: 85 (80–90).
Film Size: 10 x 12 inches (24 x 30 cm).
Grid: Yes.
TFD: 40 inches (102 cm) (must correct for tube tilt).
Tube Tilt: 15 degrees caudad.
Patient Position: Prone or upright.
Part Position: Frontal bone in contact with the bucky. Remove all head tilt and rotation. The orbitomeatal line should be perpendicular to the cassette.
CR: Exits through the nasion.
Collimation: To skull size.
Side Marker: In open space above the cranium.
Breathing Instructions: Suspended expiration.
Special Considerations: Done upright, this is a useful projection in the evaluation of sinus disease. Orbital detail is superior in this projection in comparison to the straight posteroanterior view without tube tilt.

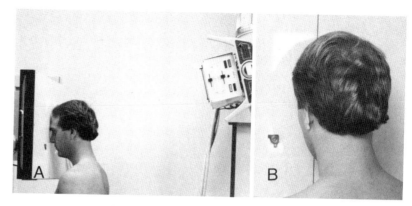

Figure 1.5A. Patient positioning.
Figure 1.5B. Collimation and central ray.

Normal Anatomy (Figure 1.5C)

1. Frontal bone.
2. Frontal sinus.
3. Ethmoid sinus.
4. Maxillary sinus.
5. Nasal septum.
6. Petrous ridge.
7. Greater wing of sphenoid.
8. Infraorbital rim.
9. Supraorbital rim.
10. Nasal turbinates.
11. Mandible.

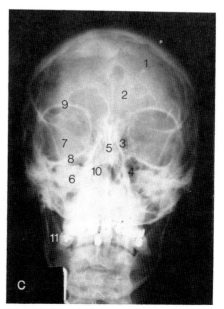

Figure 1.5C. Posteroanterior Caldwell skull radiograph.

Skull
Anteroposterior Towne's Projection
Positioning
(Figure 1.6A and B)

Demonstrates: Occipital bone, petrous pyramids, posterior foramen magnum, dorsum sellae, posterior clinoids, zygomatic arches, and mandibular condyle. (1–5)

Measure: Through the central ray.

kVp: 85 (80–90).

Film Size: 10 x 12 inches (24 x 30 cm).

Grid: Yes.

TFD: 40 inches (must correct for tube tilt).

Tube Tilt: 35 degrees caudad.

Patient Position: Supine or upright.

Part Position: Centered, with removal of head tilt and rotation. Infraorbital meatal line is perpendicular to the cassette.

CR: Passes through the midline at the external auditory meatus.

Collimation: To skull size.

Side Marker: In open space at film corner.

Breathing Instructions: Suspended expiration.

Special Considerations: The dorsum sellae and posterior clinoid processes should project into the anterior portions of the foramen magnum.

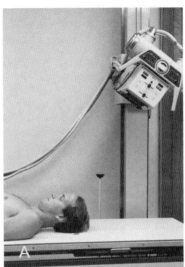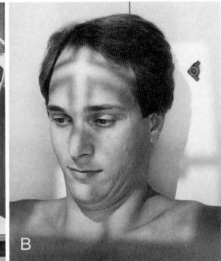

Figure 1.6A. Patient positioning.
Figure 1.6B. Collimation and central ray.

Normal Anatomy (Figure 1.6C)

1. Occipital bone.
2. Parietal bone.
3. Lambdoidal suture.
4. Sagittal suture.
5. Internal occipital protuberance.
6. Transverse venous sinus.
7. Petrous pyramids.
8. Mastoid air cells.
9. Foramen magnum.
10. Dorsum sellae.
11. Mandibular condyle.
12. Zygomatic arch.
13. Cervical pillar.

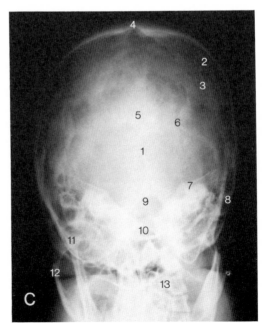

Figure 1.6C. Anteroposterior Towne's skull radiograph.

Paranasal Sinuses
Lateral Sinus and Facial Bones
(Figure 1.7A)

Demonstrates: Maxilla, hard palate, maxillary sinus, ethmoid sinus, sphenoid sinus, frontal sinus, and orbits. (1–4)

Measure: Between left and right lateral canthus.

kVp: 85 (80–90).

Film Size: 8 x 10 inches (18 x 24 cm).

Grid: Yes.

TFD: 40 inches (102 cm).

Tube Tilt: None.

Patient Position: Semiprone or upright, with head turned to lateral position.

Part Position: Head is turned to a true lateral position. The midsagittal plane is parallel to the cassette, and the interpupillary line is perpendicular.

CR: At the lateral canthus of the eye.

Collimation: To the film.

Side Marker: Side closest to the film, near a corner.

Breathing Instructions: Suspended expiration.

Special Considerations: Upright films are preferred to demonstrate fluid levels within the sinuses.

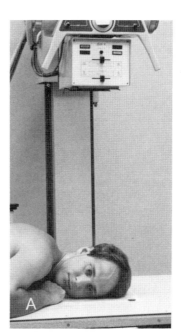

Figure 1.7A. Patient positioning.

Normal Anatomy (Figure 1.7B)

1. Vascular impression of middle meningeal artery.
2. Orbital plate, frontal bone.
3. Frontal bone.
4. Tuberculum sellae and anterior clinoids.
5. Posterior clinoids.
6. Sella turcica.
7. Clivus (dorsum sellae)
8. Sphenoid sinus.
9. Ethmoid sinus.
10. Maxillary sinus.
11. Frontal sinus.
12. Frontal process, zygoma.
13. Hard palate.
14. Soft palate.
15. Posterior wall, maxillary sinus.
16. Petrous portion, temporal bone.

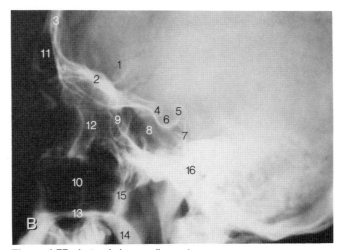

Figure 1.7B. Lateral sinus radiograph.

Basic
Lateral
***Waters**

Paranasal Sinuses

Water's Projection
(Figure 1.8A and B)

Optional
Submentovertical

Demonstrates: Maxillary sinuses, ethmoid sinuses, frontal sinuses, orbits, zygomatic arches. (1–4)
Measure: Through the central ray.
kVp: 85 (80–90).
Film Size: 8 x 10 inches (18 x 24 cm).
Grid: Yes.
TFD: 40 inches (102 cm).
Tube Tilt: None.
Patient Position: Prone or upright (posteroanterior).
Part Position: Midline, with no head tilt or rotation. The head is extended such that the canthomeatal line is elevated 37 degrees relative to the central ray.
CR: Should exit just below the nares.
Collimation: To film size.
Side Marker: In open space.
Breathing Instructions: Suspended expiration.
Special Considerations: Can be done with the mouth open, to visualize the sphenoid sinus, or closed. Upright positioning is preferred to demonstrate fluid levels within the sinuses.

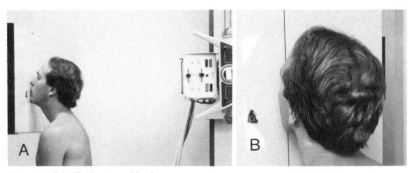

Figure 1.8A. Patient positioning.
Figure 1.8B. Collimation and central ray.

Normal Anatomy (Figure 1.8C)

1. Frontal sinus.
2. Ethmoid sinus.
3. Maxillary sinus (antrum).
4. Supraorbital fissure.
5. Frontal process, zygoma.
6. Inferior turbinate.
7. Greater wing of sphenoid.
8. Lesser wing of sphenoid.
9. Nasal septum.
10. Infraorbital foramen.
11. Coronoid process, mandible.
12. Top incisors.
13. Zygomatic arch.
14. Frontal bone.

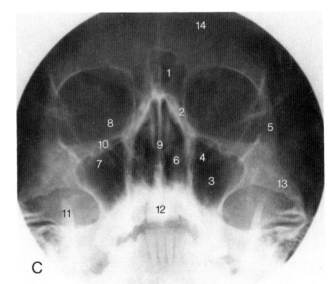

Figure 1.8C. Water's projection of the paranasal sinuses.

Cervical Spine
Anteroposterior Lower Cervical
(Figure 1.9A and B)

Demonstrates: Lower five cervical vertebrae (especially vertebral bodies, von Luschka joints, and spinous processes), the upper two or three thoracic vertebrae and ribs, medial border of the clavicles, lung apices, trachea, and neck muscles. (1–4)

Measure: At C4 level (apex of thyroid cartilage)

kVp: 80 (75–85).

Film Size: 8 x 10 inches (18 x 24 cm), or 10 x 12 inches (24 x 30 cm).

Grid: Yes.

TFD: 40 inches (must correct for tube tilt).

Tube Tilt: 15 degrees cephalad, dependent on lordosis.

Patient Position: Upright or supine.

Part Position: Center cervical spine to the midline of the bucky. Extend head so that a line from the lower edge of the chin to the base of the occiput is perpendicular to the film.

CR: Thyroid cartilage (C4).

Collimation: To film size, with an 8-inch wide collimation used so that the lung apices are included. Exclude the mandible.

Side Marker: Indicate left or right lateral to the midportion of the neck.

Breathing Instructions: Suspended expiration.

Special Considerations: If the cervical lordosis is reduced, the cephalad tube angulation should also be decreased to allow the rays to pass through the intervertebral disc spaces. It may be helpful to expose and develop the lateral radiograph first, to better approximate the angle of the lower disc spaces.

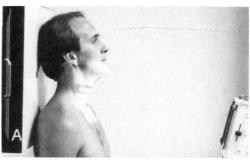
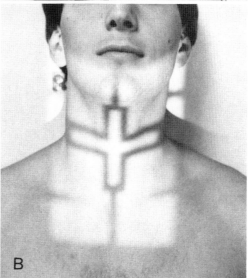

Figure 1.9A. Patient positioning.
Figure 1.9B. Collimation and central ray.

Normal Anatomy (Figure 1.9C–E)

1. C7 spinous process.
2. C7 lamina.
3. C7 pedicle.
4. C7 transverse process.
5. C6 articular pillar.
6. C5-C6 von Luschka joint (uncinate process and fossa)
7. T1 spinous process.
8. T1 lamina.
9. T1 pedicle.
10. T1 transverse process.
11. First costotransverse joint.
12. First rib.
13. Second costotransverse joint.
14. Medial clavicle.
15. Trachea.
16. Mastoid process.
17. Angle of mandible.
18. C5 intervertebral foramen.
19. Lung apex.

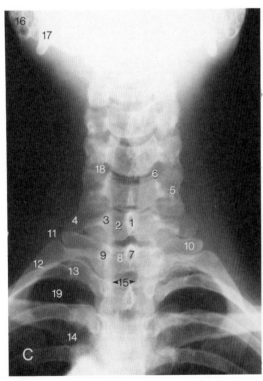

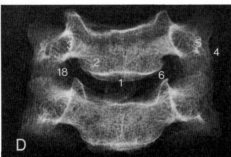

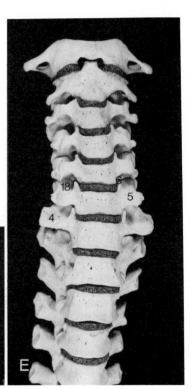

Figure 1.9C. Anteroposterior lower cervical radiograph.
Figure 1.9D. Specimen radiograph.
Figure 1.9E. Anatomic specimen.

Cervical Spine
Anteroposterior Open Mouth
(Figure 1.10A and B)

Demonstrates: Upper two cervical verte-brae and occipital condyles. (5,6)

Measure: At C4 level.

kVp: 80 (75–85).

Film Size: 8 x 10 inches (18 x 24 cm).

Grid: Yes.

TFD: 40 inches (102 cm).

Patient Position: Upright or supine.

Part Position: Center cervical spine to the midline of the bucky. The head is positioned so that the lower border of the upper inci-sors and the tips of the mastoid processes are in the same plane perpendicular to the film. The patient's mouth is opened as wide as possible.

CR: Directed to the midpoint of the open mouth, through the uvula.

Collimation: Below patient's eyes, in-clude mastoid processes laterally and ex-clude the symphysis menti.

Side Marker: Place appropriate marker inferior to mastoid process at film edge.

Breathing Instructions: Suspended res-piration.

Special Considerations: Due to close col-limation, it is suggested that the mAs be increased by at least 50 percent, and, occa-sionally, a doubling of the mAs may be necessary to ensure adequate exposure. Dental applicances should be removed for this projection. A combination open mouth and lower cervical projection can be ob-tained with an extended exposure time, while moving the jaw and providing appro-priate head stabilization (Ottenello's projec-tion). (7,8)

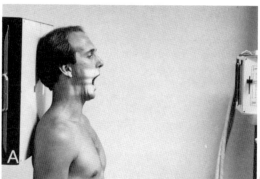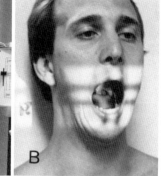

Figure 1.10A. Patient positioning.
Figure 1.10B. Collimation and central ray.

Normal Anatomy (Figure 1.10C and D)

1. Atlas lateral mass.
2. Atlas anterior arch.
3. Atlas posterior arch.
4. Atlas transverse foramen.
5. Atlas transverse process.
6. Atlanto-occipital joint.
7. Mastoid process.
8. Odontoid process.
9. Axis pedicle.
10. Axis lamina.
11. Axis spinous process.
12. Axis transverse foramen.
13. Axis transverse process.
14. Mandible.
15. Tongue.
16. Styloid process.

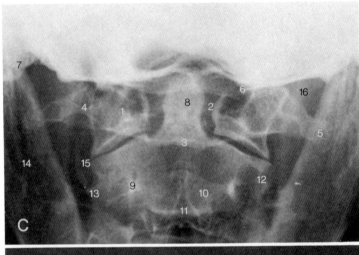

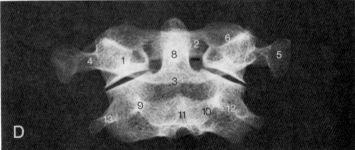

Figure 1.10C. Anteroposterior open mouth radiograph.
Figure 1.10D. Specimen radiograph.

Cervical Spine
Neutral Lateral Cervical
(Figure 1.11A and B)

Demonstrates: Cervical spine, soft tissues of the neck and the base of the skull. (1–4,9,10)

Measure: At C6 level (base of neck).

kVp: 80 (75–85).

Film Size: 8 x 10 inches (18 x 24 cm), or 10 x 12 inches (24 x 30 cm).

Grid: No. Use vertical cassette holder.

TFD: 72 inches (183 cm).

Tube Tilt: None.

Patient Position: Upright lateral, either standing or sitting. Place the convex side of a scoliosis next to the film.

Part Position: Shoulder in contact with cassette holder. Head and neck in true lateral position. Relax and drop shoulders as much as possible (patient may hold weights).

CR: C4. Center film to CR.

Collimation: Superior to inferior collimation to the top of the ear and tip of the shoulder.

Side Marker: Side closest to the bucky is marked, just below the mandible.

Breathing Instructions: Suspended full expiration.

Special Considerations: If the C7 vertebra is not visualized because of the overlying density of the shoulders, this can be overcome by (1) increasing the exposure and doing a spot projection, (2) having the patient hold weights during the exposure, or (3) performing a "swimmer's" lateral of the cervicothoracic junction. Occasionally, tomography will be the only means of demonstrating the C7 vertebra.

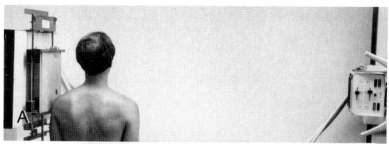

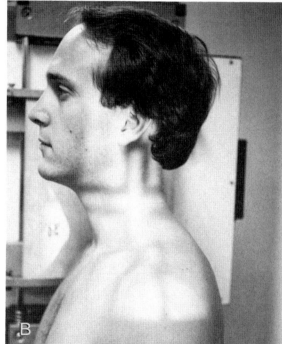

Figure 1.11A. Patient positioning.
Figure 1.11B. Collimation and central ray.

Normal Anatomy (Figure 1.11C–E)

1. Atlas posterior tubercle.
2. Atlas posterior arch.
3. Atlas lateral masses.
4. Atlas anterior arch.
5. Odontoid process.
6. Axis body.
7. C4 body.
8. C4 intervertebral disc.
9. C5 articular pillar and facet.
10. C5 lamina.
11. C5 spinous process.
12. C6 spinolaminar junction.
13. C6 transverse process.
14. Retropharyngeal interspace (RPI).
15. Retrolaryngeal interspace (RLI).
16. Retrotracheal interspace (RTI).
17. Trachea.
18. Thyroid cartilage and larynx.
19. Pharynx.
20. Hyoid bone.
21. Angle of mandible.
22. Sphenoid sinus.
23. Sella turcica.
24. Mastoid air cells.
25. Lambdoidal suture.
26. External occipital protuberance (EOP).

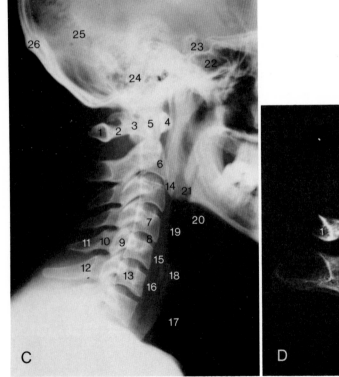
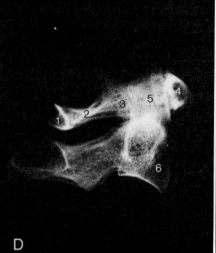
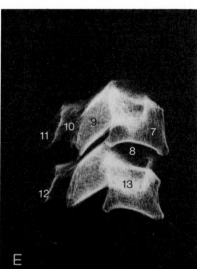

Figure 1.11C. Neutral lateral cervical radiograph.
Figure 1.11D. Specimen radiograph, C1–C2.
Figure 1.11E. Specimen radiograph, C4–C5.

Basic
AP lower cervical
AP open mouth
Lateral
***Obliques**

Cervical Spine
Cervical Obliques
(Figure 1.12A–D)

Optional
Flexion
Extension
Pillars
Moving jaw

Demonstrates: Intervertebral foramina, von Luschka joints, apophyseal joints, pedicles. (1–4,11,12)

Measure: At the C6 level (base of neck).

kVp: 80 (75–85).

Film Size: 8 x 10 inches (18 x 24 cm).

Grid: No. Use nonbucky cassette holder.

TFD: 72 inches (must correct for tube tilt).

Tube Tilt: 15 degrees: 1) Anterior obliques—caudad. 2) Posterior obliques—cephalad.

Patient Position: Upright or recumbent.

Part Position: (1) *Anterior obliques:* Facing the bucky, the body is rotated 45 degrees away. The head is then rotated to be parallel with the plane of the bucky, and the chin is jutted out slightly. (Fig. 1.12A and B) (2) *Posterior obliques:* Facing the tube, the body is rotated 45 degrees away. The head is then rotated to be parallel with the plane of the bucky, and the chin is jutted out slightly. (Fig. 1.12C and D)

CR: C4 level.

Collimation: Top and bottom of the film, with tight lateral collimation.

Side Marker: Under the mandible on posterior obliques; behind spine on anterior obliques when using right or left markers. RPO and LPO or RAO and LAO markers can be placed anywhere outside of the field of interest.

Breathing Instructions: Suspended full expiration.

Special Considerations: In circumstances where these films cannot be performed at 72 inches, they can be done at 60 inches with the bucky, which does compromise detail and increase patient dose. Posterior obliques demonstrate the contralateral foramina (e.g., RPO—left foramina), while anterior obliques demonstrate the homolateral structures (e.g., RAO—right foramina).

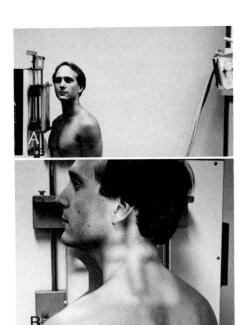

Figure 1.12A. Patient positioning anterior oblique.
Figure 1.12B. Collimation and central ray anterior oblique.

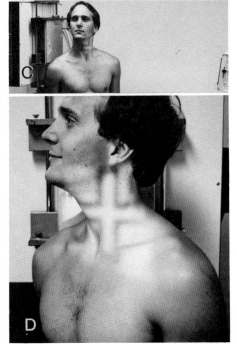

Figure 1.12C. Patient positioning posterior oblique.
Figure 1.12D. Collimation and central ray posterior oblique.

Normal Anatomy (Figure 1.12E)

1. C6 vertebral body.
2. C6 transverse process.
3. C6 pedicle.
4. C5 lamina.
5. C6 articular pillar.
6. C6 spinous process.
7. C6/C7 intervertebral foramen.
8. C5/C6 von Luschka joint.
9. C5 pedicle.
10. C6 transverse process.
11. Mandible.
12. First rib.
13. Trachea.

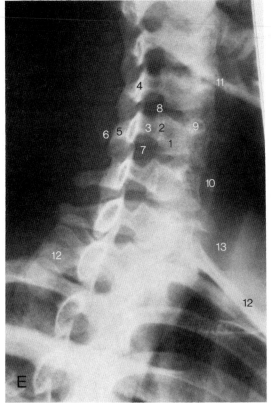

Figure 1.12E. Posterior oblique cervical radiograph.

Basic
AP lower cervical
AP open mouth
Lateral
Obliques

Cervical Spine
Flexion/Extension Lateral Cervical
View Positioning
(Figure 1.13A and B)

Optional
***Flexion**
***Extension**
Pillar
Moving jaw

Demonstrates: As per neutral lateral, but additionally evaluates patterns of intersegmental motion and ligamentous instability. (1–4,13–15)

Measure: At the C4 level.

kVp: 80 (75–85).

Film Size: 8 x 10 inches (18 x 24 cm), 10 x 12 inches (24 x 30 cm).

Grid: No. Use nonbucky cassette holder.

TFD: 72 inches (183 cm).

Tube Tilt: None.

Patient Position: True lateral position aligned to the bucky midline.

Part Position: **(1)** *Flexion.* Tuck chin, then flex the head forward as far as possible; **(2)** *Extension.* Elevate chin, then extend the head backward as far as possible.

CR: At the C4 level.

Collimation: To the film size.

Side Marker: Mark side closest to the film, below the chin.

Breathing Instructions: Suspended expiration.

Special Considerations: These projections must be carefully performed, since the spine is placed into stressful positions. The neutral lateral projection should be evaluated and the patient carefully examined **before** these exposures are taken. (13,14) Special attention to eliminating patient motion is necessary, since the patient is placed in a stressed position. The use of flexion/extension films is often used in cases of trauma and, when part of a seven-view examination (AP open mouth, AP lower cervical, neutral lateral, right and left obliques, and flexion/extension views), has been called a "Davis series." (15)

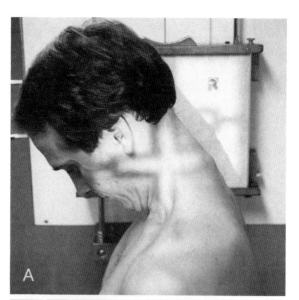

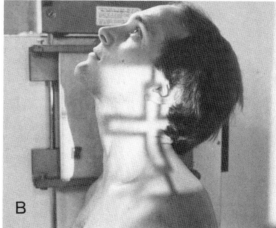

Figure 1.13A. Patient positioning, collimation, and central ray flexion.

Figure 1.13B. Patient positioning, collimation, and central ray extension.

Normal Anatomy (Figure 1.13C and D)

Review the structures seen in the neutral lateral position.

Alignment and Motion Patterns:

1. Posterior vertebral bodies (George's line).
2. Spinolaminar junction lines (posterior cervical line— PCL).
3. Atlantodental interspace (ADI).
4. Interspinous spaces.

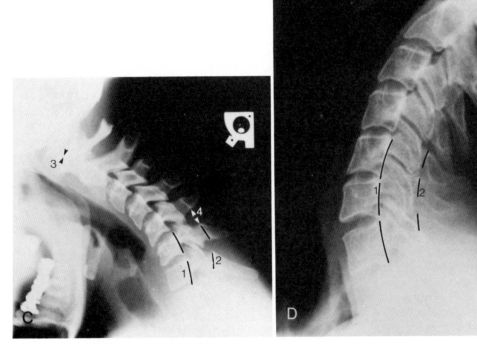

Figure 1.13C. Flexion cervical radiograph.
Figure 1.13D. Extension cervical radiograph.

Cervical Spine

Cervical Articular Pillars Positioning
(Figure 1.14A and B)

Demonstrates: Articular processes and apophyseal joints. Both sides must be done for comparison. (1–4,16,17)

Measure: At C4 level.

kVp: 80 (75–85).

Film Size: 8 x 10 inches (18 x 24 cm).

Grid: Yes.

TFD: 40 inches (must correct for tube tilt).

Tube Tilt: 35 degrees cephalad.

Patient Position: PA.

Part Position: Rotate head 45–50 degrees away from side of interest.

CR: Direct the CR through the C5 vertebra. CR enters neck at superior margin of thyroid cartilage and 1 inch lateral to midline on the side of interest. Center film to CR.

Collimation: Top and bottom of film, side 4 inches wide.

Side Marker: Place appropriate marker, marking side opposite head rotation.

Breathing Instructions: Suspended expiration.

Special Considerations: This view can be taken anteroposterior, with caudad tube tilt. Fractures of the articular pillars are frequently only observed on these special pillar projections. (14)

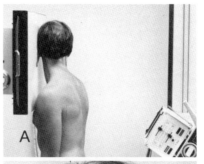
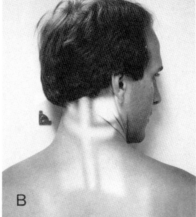

Figure 1.14A. Patient positioning.
Figure 1.14B. Collimation and central ray.

Normal Anatomy (Figure 1.14C)

1. C5 articular pillar.
2. C4-C5 apophyseal joint.
3. C6 lamina.
4. C5 spinous process.
5. First rib.

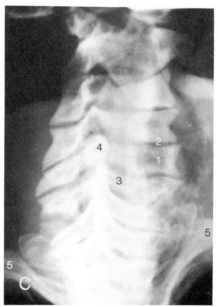

Figure 1.14C. Articular pillar radiograph of the cervical spine.

Basic
***AP**
Lateral

Thoracic Spine

Anteroposterior Thoracic Projection
Positioning
(Figure 1.15A and B)

Optional
Swimmer's lateral
Obliques

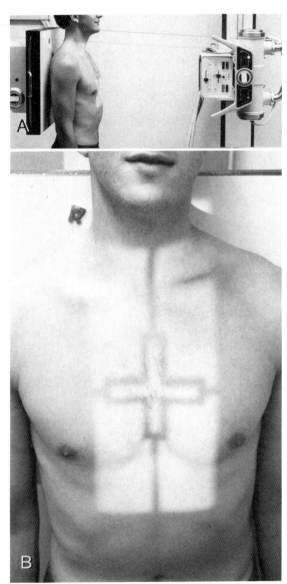

Demonstrates: Thoracic spine, posterior rib heads, lung fields, and mediastinum. (1–3)
Measure: At T6 level.
kVp: 80 (75–85).
Film Size: 7 x 17 inches (18 x 43 cm), or 14 x 17 inches (35 x 43 cm) if significant scoliosis is present.
Grid: Yes.
TFD: 40 inches (102 cm).
Tube Tilt: None.
Patient Position: Upright or supine with hips and knees flexed.
Part Position: Align midsagittal plane of the body to the central ray, with no rotation.
CR: Place the top of the cassette 2 inches above the C7 spinous process. Center CR to film (CR will enter approximately 3 inches inferior to sternal angle).
Collimation: 7 x 17 inches (18 x 43 cm) film—collimate to film size.14 x 17 inches (35 x 43 cm) film—collimate to area of interest.
Side Marker: Place appropriate marker in one of the top corners, preferably above the level of the clavicles.
Breathing Instructions: Suspended inspiration to depress the diaphragm.
Special Considerations: A compensating filter should be used, if available, from the midthoracic to upper thoracic spine.

Figure 1.15A. Patient positioning.
Figure 1.15B. Collimation and central ray.

Normal Anatomy (Figure 1.15C–E)

1. Rib.
2. Transverse process.
3. Costotransverse joint.
4. Costovertebral joint.
5. Pedicle.
6. Spinous process.
7. Inferior end plate.
8. Intervertebral disc space.
9. Clavicle.
10. Diaphragm.
11. Gastric air bubble (magenblasse).
12. Paraspinal line (arrowheads).
13. Aorta (arrows).
14. Pulmonary vessels.

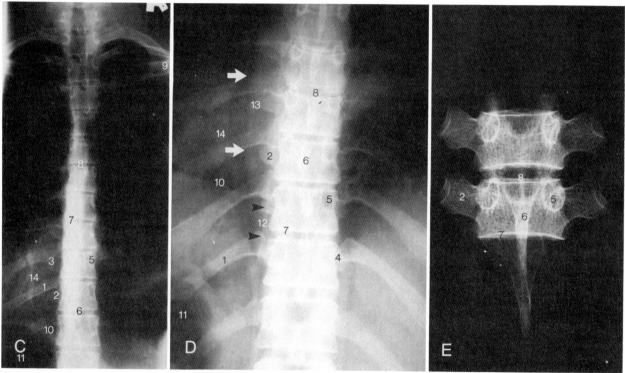

Figure 1.15C. Anteroposterior thoracic radiograph.
Figure 1.15D. Close-up anteroposterior thoracic radiograph.
Figure 1.15E. Specimen radiograph.

Thoracic Spine
Lateral Thoracic Projection
(Figure 1.16A and B)

Demonstrates: Thoracic spine, ribs, lung fields, and heart. (1,2,4)

Measure: At T6 level, under the axilla adjacent to the scapula.

kVp: 90 (85–95).

Film Size: 7 x 17 inches (18 x 43 cm), or 14 x 17 inches (35 x 43 cm) if kyphosis is increased.

Grid: Yes.

TFD: 40 inches (102 cm).

Tube Tilt: None.

Patient Position: Lateral recumbent or upright lateral.

Part Position: Align midaxillary plane to central ray.

CR: Place the top of the cassette 2 inches above the C7 spinous process. Center CR to film (CR will enter approximately 3 inches inferior to sternal angle).

Collimation: 7 x 17 inches (18 x 43 cm) film—collimate to film size. 14 x 17 inches (35 x 43 cm) film—collimate to area of interest.

Side Marker: Place appropriate marker in film corner behind spine.

Breathing Instructions: Suspended inspiration to depress diaphragm.

Special Considerations: The overlying rib structures can be obliterated from the film by allowing shallow respiration during an extended exposure time (approximately 1 second). If this is done, care must be taken to reduce motion of the spinal column by allowing only shallow, quiet respiration and careful patient instruction. A compensating filter should be used, if available, from the midthoracic to lower thoracic spine.

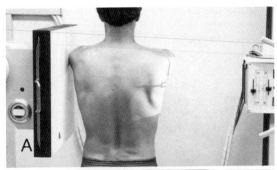

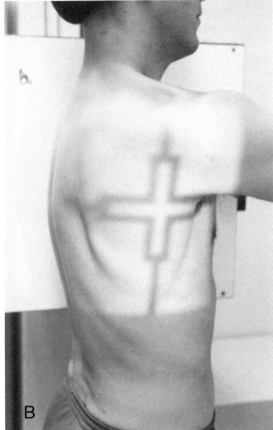

Figure 1.16A. Patient positioning.
Figure 1.16B. Collimation and central ray.

Normal Anatomy (Figure 1.16C–E)

1. Vertebral body.
2. End plate.
3. Intervertebral disc.
4. Pedicle.
5. Intervertebral foramen.
6. Apophyseal joint.
7. Spinous process.
8. Transverse process.
9. Rib head.
10. Posterior rib.
11. Lateral rib.
12. Manubrium.
13. Axillary margin, scapula (arrow).
14. Diaphragm.
15. Posterior costophrenic sulcus.
16. Heart.
17. Lung hilus.
18. Trachea.

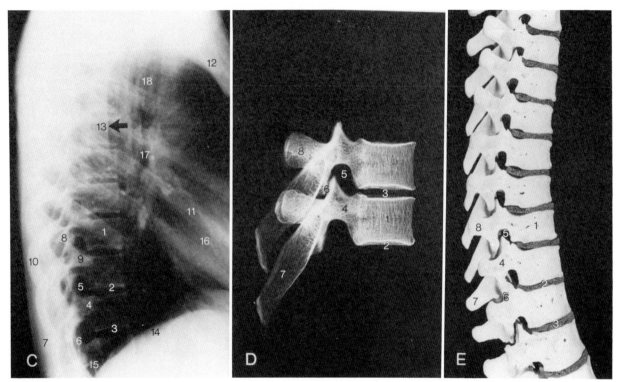

Figure 1.16C. Lateral thoracic spine radiograph.
Figure 1.16D. Specimen radiograph.
Figure 1.16E. Anatomic specimen.

Thoracic Spine
Lateral Cervicothoracic Junction
(Swimmer's Lateral) Positioning
(Figure 1.17A and B)

Demonstrates: Lower cervical and upper thoracic vertebrae, especially the vertebral bodies and intervertebral discs. (5,6)

Measure: As for lateral thoracic, at the T6 level under the axilla adjacent to the scapulae.

kVp: 90 (85–95).

Film Size: 10 x 12 inches (24 x 30 cm).

Grid: Yes.

TFD: 40 inches (102 cm).

Tube Tilt: None.

Patient Position: Upright or recumbent lateral position. Rotate the body 10–20 degrees toward the bucky. The arm closest to the bucky is flexed, with the hand placed on the top of the head. The arm closest to the tube is extended, with the hand placed over the hip.

CR: Passes just anterior to the tube-side shoulder through the sternal notch.

Collimation: To film size.

Side Marker: In top corner of film, posterior to the cervical spinous processes.

Breathing Instructions: Suspended expiration to accentuate shoulder depression.

Special Considerations: This is especially useful following cervicothoracic trauma and in broad-shouldered individuals. (6) A caudal angulation of 5 degrees may assist in separating the overlying shoulders. The lower cervical vertebrae are relatively overexposed, which can be compensated for by appropriate filtration.

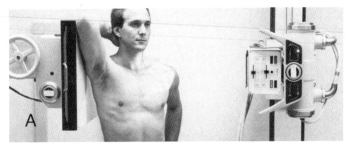

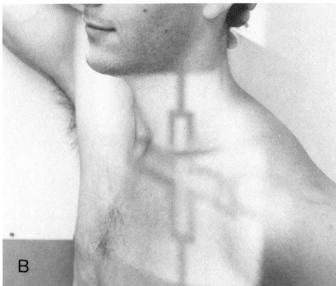

Figure 1.17A. Patient positioning.
Figure 1.17B. Collimation and central ray.

Normal Anatomy (Figure 1.17C)

1. First rib.
2. Medial clavicle.
3. Manubrium.
4. Scapula.
5. Distal clavicle.
6. Posterior ribs.
7. Lateral ribs.
8. Trachea.
9. Retrotracheal space.
10. C6 vertebral body.
11. C6 intervertebral foramen.
12. Spinous process (C7, T5).

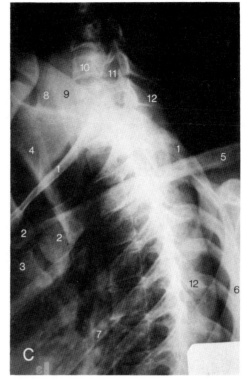

Figure 1.17C. Lateral cervicothoracic "swimmer's" radiograph.

Basic
*AP
Lateral
Obliques
AP spot

Lumbar Spine
Anteroposterior Lumbopelvic
Projection Positioning
(Figure 1.18A and B)

Optional
Lateral lumbosacral spot
Flexion
Extension
Lateral bending

Demonstrates: Lumbar vertebrae, pelvis, hips, proximal femora, and soft tissues of the abdomen. (1–4)

Measure: At L4/L5 level.

kVp: 85 (80–90).

Film Size: 14 x 17 inches (35 x 43 cm).

Grid: Yes.

TFD: 40 inches (102 cm).

Tube Tilt: None.

Patient Position: Upright or supine.

Part Position: Center lumbar spine to the bucky.

CR: 1½ inches below the iliac crest level. Center film to CR.

Collimation: 14 x 17 inch field.

Side Marker: Place appropriate side marker at one of the upper film corners.

Breathing Instructions: Suspended expiration.

Special Considerations: For the AP lumbosacral view without the full pelvis, use 14 x 17 inch (35 x 43 cm) or 7 x 17 inch (18 x 43 cm) film, collimated laterally to include sacroiliac joints, with the CR at the level of the iliac crests. In obese patients a supine view is preferred to compress the abdomen and reduce the time of exposure. Use gonad shielding when appropriate.

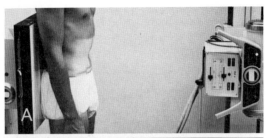

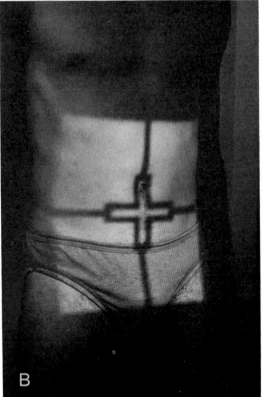

Figure 1.18A. Patient positioning.
Figure 1.18B. Collimation and central ray.

Normal Anatomy (Figure 1.18C and D)

1. Spinous process.
2. Pedicle.
3. Superior articular process.
4. Transverse process.
5. Inferior articular process.
6. Lamina.
7. Pars interarticularis (isthmus).
8. Twelfth rib.
9. Sacral ala.
10. First sacral tubercle.
11. Sacroiliac joint.
12. Transverse colon.

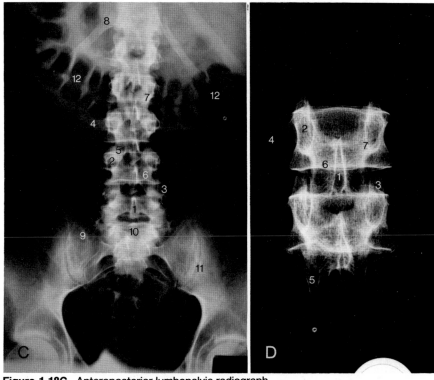

Figure 1.18C. Anteroposterior lumbopelvic radiograph.
Figure 1.18D. Specimen radiograph.

Basic
Anteroposterior
*Lateral
Obliques
Anteroposterior spot

Lumbar Spine

Lateral Lumbosacral Projection
Positioning
(Figure 1.19A and B)

Optional
Lateral lumbosacral spot
Flexion
Extension
Lateral bending

Demonstrates: Lumbar vertebrae, sacrum, coccyx, and soft tissues of the pelvis, abdomen, and lower chest. (1,2,5,6)

Measure: Males—1 inch below the iliac crests. Females—1 inch below the iliac crests and 1 inch above the iliac crests, then average the two.

kVp: 90 (85–95).

Film Size: 7 x 17 inches (18 x 43 cm), or 14 x 17 inches (35 x 43 cm) if lordosis is increased, or with obese patients.

Grid: Yes.

TFD: 40 inches (102 cm).

Tube Tilt: None.

Patient Position: Upright lateral or lateral recumbent.

Part Position: True lateral position, with no rotation or lateral flexion.

CR: 1 inch above iliac crest level, with the vertical central ray passing halfway between the ASIS and PSIS. Center film to CR.

Collimation: Top and bottom of film, side collimation to accommodate the lordosis.

Side Marker: Place appropriate marker in film corner anterior to the spine.

Breathing Instructions: Suspended expiration, to elevate the diaphragm in order to visualize the lower thoracic spine.

Special Considerations: If there is a large discrepancy between the measurements above and below the iliac crests, then a compensating filter should be used. Use gonad shielding when appropriate. If scoliosis is present, it may be helpful to expose and develop the anteroposterior film first, to optimally position the central ray and the patient.

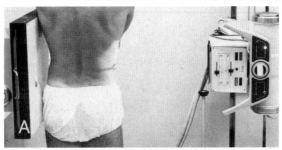

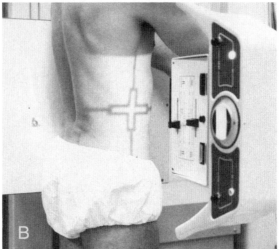

Figure 1.19A. Patient positioning.
Figure 1.19B. Collimation and central ray.

Normal Anatomy (Figure 1.19C and D)

1. Vertebral body.
2. Pedicle.
3. Superior articular process.
4. Spinous process.
5. Inferior articular process.
6. Intervertebral foramen (IVF).
7. Pars interarticularis (isthmus).
8. Intervertebral disc.
9. Vertebral end plate.
10. Sacral promontory.
11. Twelfth rib.
12. Iliac crest.
13. Synovial joint between articular processes.
14. Superior articulating processes, sacrum.

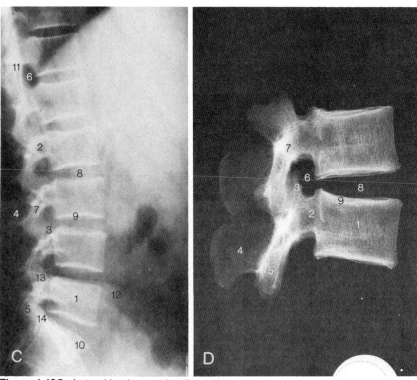

Figure 1.19C. Lateral lumbosacral radiograph.
Figure 1.19D. Specimen radiograph.

Basic
Anteroposterior
Lateral
*Obliques
Anteroposterior spot

Lumbar Spine
Lumbar Oblique Projections
Positioning
(Figure 1.20A and B)

Optional
Lateral lumbosacral spot
Flexion
Extension
Lateral bending

Demonstrates: The "scotty dog"—transverse process, pedicle, articulating processes, facet joints, pars interarticularis, and laminae. Also provides an additional view of the vertebral body and abdominal soft tissues. (1,2,7,8)

Measure: At the central ray at L3.

kVp: 80 (75–85).

Film Size: 10 x 12 inches (24 x 30 cm).

Grid: Yes.

TFD: 40 inches (102 cm).

Tube Tilt: None.

Patient Position: Upright or recumbent.

Part Position: 1) *Anterior oblique.* Semiprone, with the body elevated 45 degrees. On the side elevated, flex the knee and elbow to support the position. Align the spine to the central ray. (Fig. 1.20A) 2) *Posterior oblique.* Semisupine, with the body elevated 45 degrees. Arm along table lays at patient's side. The elevated arm crosses the body to grasp the edge of the table. (Fig. 1.20B)

CR: (1) *Anterior oblique.* 1 inch lateral to L3 spinous process. (2) *Posterior oblique.* 1 inch above the iliac crest and 2 inches medial to the ASIS.

Collimation: Top to bottom, to film size, and 8 inches from side to side.

Side Marker: For anterior obliques, place marker behind the spine; or posterior obliques, place the side marker in front of the spine.

Breathing Instructions: Suspended expiration.

Special Considerations: Anterior obliques show greater structural detail because the lumbar lordosis compliments the diverging x-ray beam. Both right and left obliques must be routinely taken.

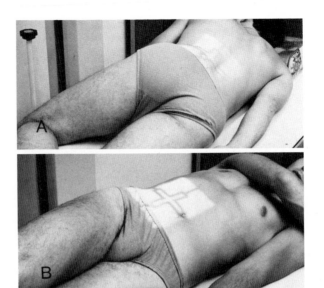

Figure 1.20A. Patient positioning, collimation, and central ray anterior oblique.

Figure 1.20B. Patient positioning, collimation, and central ray posterior oblique.

Normal Anatomy (Figure 1.20C and D)

1. Pedicle.
2. Superior articular process.
3. Pars interarticularis (isthmus).
4. Lamina.
5. Inferior articular process.
6. Transverse process.
7. Spinous process.
8. Intervertebral disc.
9. Interlaminar space.

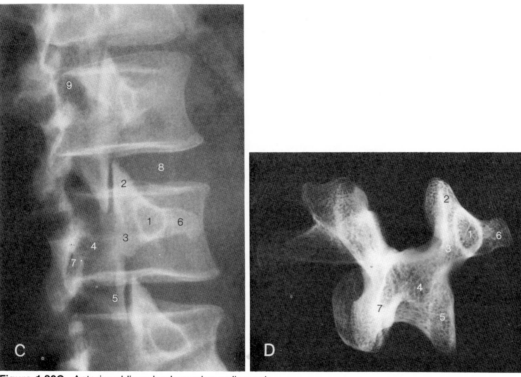

Figure 1.20C. Anterior oblique lumbar spine radiograph.
Figure 1.20D. Specimen radiograph.

Basic
 Anteroposterior
 Lateral
 Obliques
 *****Anteroposterior spot**

Lumbar Spine

Anteroposterior Lumbosacral Spot
Positioning
(Figure 1.21A and B)

Optional
Lateral lumbosacral spot
Flexion
Extension
Lateral bending

Demonstrates: L5 vertebra and disc, upper sacrum and sacroiliac joints. (1,2,9–11)
Measure: Through the central ray.
kVp: 85 (80–90).
Film Size: 8 x 10 inches (18 x 24 cm) anteroposterior, or 10 x 12 inches (24 x 30 cm) posteroanterior.
Grid: Yes.
TFD: 40 inches (must correct for tube tilt).
Tube Tilt: 30 degrees cephalad or to coincide with the plane of the sacral base.
Patient Position: Upright or supine.
Part Position: Supine or erect. Center lumbosacral spine to midline of film.
CR: Enter midline at the level of the inferior aspect of the ASIS level (halfway between the umbilicus and the pubic articulation). Center film to CR.
Collimation: To film size.
Side Marker: Place appropriate marker in the corner of the film.
Breathing Instructions: Suspended expiration.
Special Considerations: For a posteroanterior lumbosacral spot projection done upright or prone, the tube is tilted caudad (20 degrees), with the CR passing through the L5 spinous process. In the evaluation of the sacroiliac joints this is the most optimum view, since oblique views of the sacroiliac joints seldom demonstrate the joint clearly. (12–15) This is due to the great asymmetry of these joints. In order to obtain a film of optimum density, assuming the anteroposterior lumbar spine film is properly exposed, a doubling of the mAs from the anteroposterior lumbar spine and leaving the kVp the same will suffice. Use gonadal shielding when appropriate.

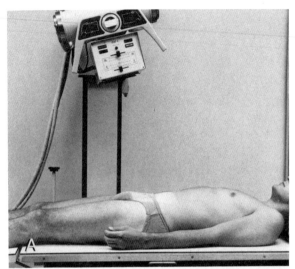

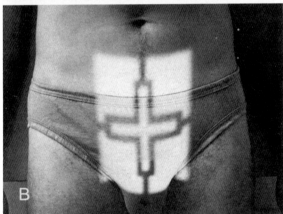

Figure 1.21A. Patient positioning.
Figure 1.21B. Collimation and central ray.

Normal Anatomy (Figure 1.21C)

1. Spinous process of L5.
2. First sacral tubercle.
3. Sacral ala.
4. Posterior surface of the ilium.
5. First sacral foramina.
6. Sacroiliac joint.
7. Posterior superior iliac spine (PSIS).
8. Sacral end plate.
9. Transverse process of L5.

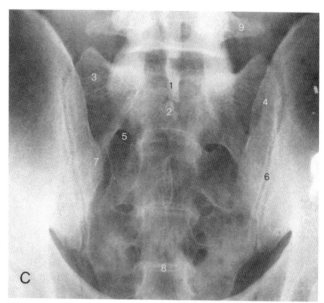

Figure 1.21C. Anteroposterior angulated radiograph of the lumbo-sacral junction.

Lumbar Spine
Lateral Lumbosacral Spot
Positioning
(Figure 1.22A and B)

Demonstrates: L5 vertebra and disc, upper sacrum and adjacent soft tissues. (1,2,16)

Measure: 1 inch below the iliac crests.

kVp: 90 (85–95).

Film Size: 8 x 10 inches (18 x 24 cm).

Grid: Yes.

TFD: 40 inches (102 cm).

Tube Tilt: None.

Patient Position: Upright lateral or lateral recumbent.

Part Position: True lateral position, with CR entering midway between ASIS and PSIS.

CR: 1 inch below the iliac crest level. Center film to CR.

Collimation: 8 x 10 inches (24 x 30 cm)

Side Marker: Place appropriate side marker in film corner.

Breathing Instructions: Suspended expiration.

Special Considerations: This is a supplemental view obtained when the lumbosacral joint is underexposed on the routine lateral film. (17,18)

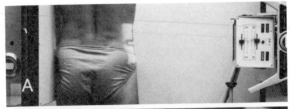

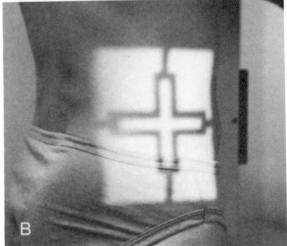

Figure 1.22A. Patient positioning.
Figure 1.22B. Collimation and central ray.

Normal Anatomy (Figure 1.22C)

1. Body.
2. Pedicle.
3. Superior articular process.
4. Pars interarticularis (isthmus)
5. Inferior articular process.
6. Lamina.
7. Intervertebral foramina (IVF).
8. Intervertebral disc.
9. Vertebral end plate.
10. Sacral promontory.
11. Superior articular process of the sacrum.
12. Transverse process.

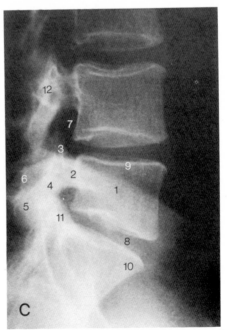

Figure 1.22C. Lateral lumbosacral spot radiograph.

Basic
*Anteroposterior
Lateral

Sacrum
Anteroposterior Sacrum Projection
Positioning
(Figure 1.23A and B)

Demonstrates: Sacrum and sacroiliac joints. (1–5)
Measure: At CR.
kVp: 80 (75–85).
Film Size: 10 x 12 inches (24 x 30 cm).
Grid: Yes.
TFD: 40 inches (must correct for tube tilt).
Tube Tilt: 15 degrees cephalad. Tilt will depend on sacral position. Ultimately, the central ray should be perpendicular to the body of the sacrum.
Patient Position: Supine or upright.
Part Position: Patient is centered to the midline.
CR: Midway between the pubic symphysis and the ASIS. Center film to central ray.
Collimation: 10 x 12-inch field.
Side Marker: Place appropriate marker.
Breathing Instructions: Suspended expiration.
Special Considerations: A preceding enema and voiding of the bladder should be performed to reduce the confusing overlying densities of gas, feces, and urine. (4) It may be helpful to expose and develop the lateral radiograph first, to most accurately determine the necessary tube tilt.

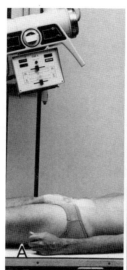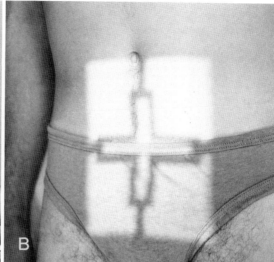

Figure 1.23A. Patient positioning.
Figure 1.23B. Collimation and central ray.

Normal Anatomy (Figure 1.23C and D)

1. First sacral tubercle.
2. Sacral ala.
3. Superior articular process of the sacrum.
4. Second sacral foramen.
5. Sacral/coccygeal junction.
6. Coccyx.
7. Sacroiliac joint.
8. Third sacral tubercle.

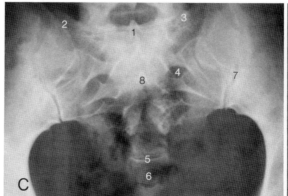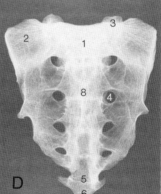

Figure 1.23C. Anteroposterior sacral radiograph.
Figure 1.23D. Specimen radiograph.

Basic
  Anteroposterior
*****Lateral**

Sacrum
Lateral Sacrum Positioning
(Figure 1.24A and B)

Demonstrates: Sacrum and L5/S1 inter-space. (1,2,3,4)
Measure: At CR.
kVp: 80 (75–85).
Film Size: 10 x 12 inches (24 x 30 cm).
Grid: Yes.
TFD: 40 inches (102 cm).
Tube Tilt: None.
Patient Position: Lateral recumbent or upright.
Part Position: Place patient in the lateral position, with the hips and knees flexed for support, if recumbent. Center the sacrum over the midline of the table.
CR: At the ASIS level, 2 inches anterior to the posterior sacral surface. Center the film to central ray.
Collimation: 10 x 12 inch field.
Side Marker: Place appropriate marker in film corner.
Breathing Instructions: Suspended expiration.

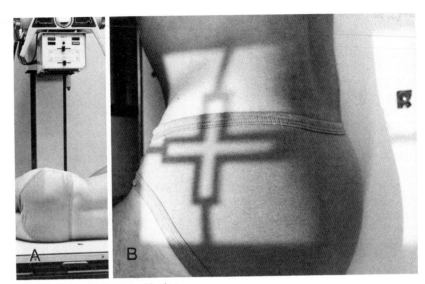

Figure 1.24A. Patient positioning.
Figure 1.24B. Collimation and central ray.

Normal Anatomy (Figure 1.24C and D)

1. Sacral promontory.
2. Second sacral segment.
3. First sacral tubercle.
4. Sacral crest.
5. Sacral canal.
6. Auricular surface.
7. Sacrococcygeal segment.
8. Superior articular process, sacrum.

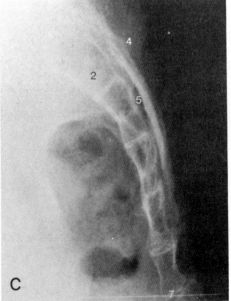
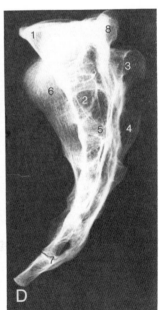
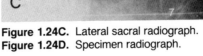

Figure 1.24C. Lateral sacral radiograph.
Figure 1.24D. Specimen radiograph.

Basic
***Anteroposterior**
Lateral

Coccyx
Anteroposterior Coccyx Projection
Positioning
(Figure 1.25A and B)

Demonstrates: Coccyx and lower sacrum. (1–3)

Measure: At the CR.

kVp: 80 (75–85).

Film Size: 8 x 10 inches (18 x 24 cm).

Grid: Yes.

TFD: 40 inches (must correct for tube tilt).

Tube Tilt: 10 degrees caudad. Tilt will depend on coccygeal position. Ultimately, the central ray should be perpendicular to the ventral surface of the coccyx.

Patient Position: Supine or upright.

Part Position: Centered to the bucky.

CR: Enters at a point 2½ inches above the symphysis pubis. Center film to central ray.

Collimation: 5 x 5 inch field.

Side Marker: Place appropriate marker.

Breathing Instructions: Suspended expiration.

Special Considerations: Preliminary patient preparation such as voiding of the bladder and an enema to remove overlying, confusing gas and fecal shadows should be performed. It may be helpful to expose and develop the lateral radiograph first, to most accurately determine the necessary tube tilt for the AP spot projection.

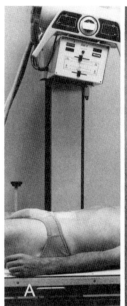
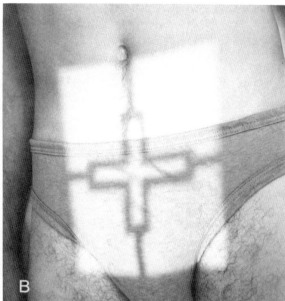

Figure 1.25A. Patient positioning.
Figure 1.25B. Collimation and central ray.

Normal Anatomy (Figure 1.25C and D)

1. First sacral tubercle.
2. Sacral ala.
3. Second sacral foramen.
4. Sacral pedicle.
5. Sacral hiatus.
6. Sacrococcygeal junction.
7. Coccyx.
8. Cornu of the coccyx.

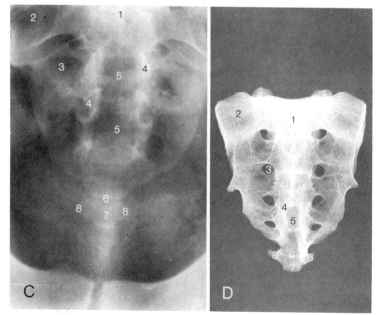

Figure 1.25C. Anteroposterior coccyx radiograph.
Figure 1.25D. Specimen radiograph.

Basic
Anteroposterior
***Lateral**

Coccyx

Lateral Coccyx Projection
Positioning
(Figure 1.25A and B)

Demonstrates: Coccyx and lower sacrum. (1–3)
Measure: At the CR.
kVp: 80 (75–85).
Film Size: 8 x 10 inches (18 x 24 cm).
Grid: Yes.
TFD: 40 inches (102 cm).
Tube Tilt: None.
Patient Position: Lateral recumbent or upright lateral.
Part Position: Lateral position, with the coccyx centered over the midline of the bucky.
CR: Directed through the sacrococcygeal junction, 2 inches anterior to the posterior body surface. Center film to central ray.
Collimation: 8 x 8 inch field.
Side Marker: Place appropriate marker.
Breathing Instructions: Suspended expiration.

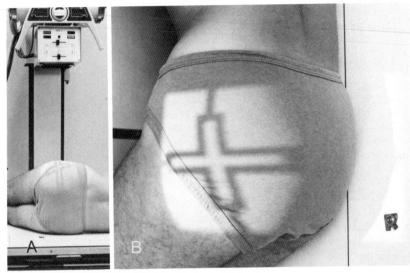

Figure 1.26A. Patient positioning.
Figure 1.26B. Collimation and central ray.

Normal Anatomy (Figure 1.26C and D)

1. Sacrococcygeal joint.
2. First coccygeal segment.
3. Auricular surface.
4. Sacral crest.
5. Sacral canal.
6. Fifth sacral segment.
7. Distal coccygeal segment.
8. Ischial tuberosity.
9. Ischial spine.

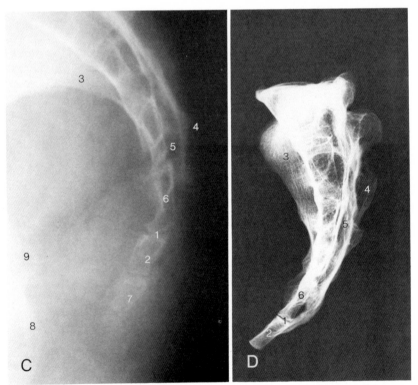

Figure 1.26C. Lateral coccyx radiograph.
Figure 1.26D. Specimen radiograph.

Basic
*Anteroposterior

Pelvis
Anteroposterior Pelvis Projection
Positioning
(Figure 1.27 A and B)

Demonstrates: Both innominates, sacrum, and coccyx, as well as the proximal femora. (1–5)

Measure: At the CR.

kVp: 80 (75–85).

Film Size: 14 x 17 inches (35 x 43 cm) crosswise.

Grid: Yes.

TFD: 40 inches (102 cm).

Tube Tilt: None.

Patient Position: Supine or upright.

Part Position: Center the midsagittal plane of the body to the midline. Internally rotate the feet about 15 degrees (heels apart and big toes together), and use sandbags to stabilize.

CR: Midway between the symphysis pubis and iliac crest. Center film to central ray.

Collimation: 14 x 17 inches.

Side Marker: Place appropriate marker at film corner.

Breathing Instructions: Suspended expiration.

Special Considerations: If the feet are not internally rotated, the femoral necks will appear foreshortened and obscure its anatomical details and relationships. (6)

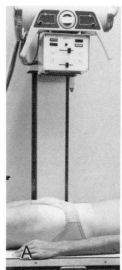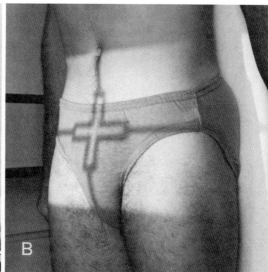

Figure 1.27A. Patient positioning.
Figure 1.27B. Collimation and central ray.

Normal Anatomy (Figure 1.27C)

1. First sacral tubercle.
2. Anterior sacral foramina.
3. Sacroiliac joint.
4. Anterior superior iliac spine (ASIS).
5. Anterior inferior iliac spine (AIIS).
6. Ischial spine.
7. Pelvic brim.
8. Gas in the colon overlying the iliac fossa.
9. Sacral ala.
10. Posterior surface of the ilium.
11. Acetabular rim.
12. Fovea capitus centralis of the femoral head.
13. Superior pubic rami.
14. Inferior pubic rami.
15. Obturator foramen.
16. Inferior edge of the acetabular fossa (Kohler's teardrop).
17. Greater trochanter of the femur.
18. Lesser trochanter of the femur.
19. Pubic symphysis.
20. First coccygeal segment.
21. Iliac fossa.
22. Iliac crest.

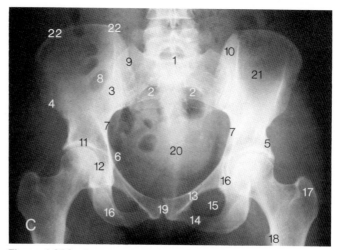

Figure 1.27C. Anteroposterior pelvic radiograph.

Full Spine
Anteroposterior View Positioning
(Figure 1.28A and B)

Demonstrates: Pelvis, lumbar, thoracic, and cervical spine. (1–4)

Measure: Anteroposterior at the lumbosacral joint.

kVp: 90 (85–95).

Film Size: 14 x 36 inches (14 x 91 cm).

Grid: Yes.

TFD: 84 inches (200 cm) optimum; no less than 72 inches (183 cm).

Tube Tilt: None.

Patient Position: Upright.

Part Position: Spine centered to bucky. Film placed 1 inch below inferior gluteal fold.

CR: To the film.

Collimation: To exclude the eyes and include the ischial tuberosities. Laterally to the ASIS bilaterally.

Side Marker: Appropriate marker adjacent to and above the shoulder.

Breathing Instructions: Suspended expiration.

Special Considerations: A compensating filter should be used to prevent overexposure to the upper third of the film. (5–9) Patients with anteroposterior measurements greater than 28 cm should not be subjected to a single anteroposterior full spine projection. (Fig. 1.28B) Use gonad shielding when appropriate.

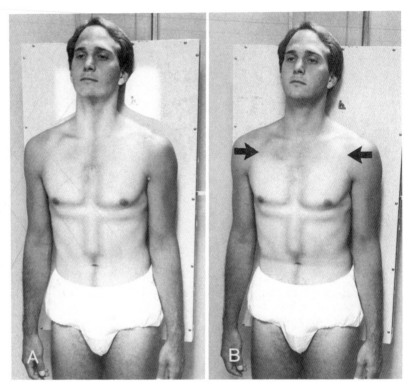

AP FULL SPINE:
WITHOUT FILTRATION

AP FULL SPINE:
WITH FILTRATION

Figure 1.28A. Patient positioning, collimation, and central ray, without compensating filtration.
Figure 1.28B. Patient positioning, collimation, and central ray, with compensating filtration (arrows).

Basic
***Anteroposterior**
Frog-leg

Hip
Anteroposterior Hip Projection
Positioning
(Figure 1.29A and B)

Demonstrates: Acetabulum, adjacent pelvis, joint space, femoral head, neck, trochanters, and proximal diaphysis. (1–4)

Measure: At the CR.

kVp: 80 (75–85).

Film Size: 10 x 12 inches (24 x 30 cm).

Grid: Yes.

TFD: 40 inches (102 cm).

Tube Tilt: None.

Patient Position: Supine or upright.

Part Position: The leg is internally rotated 15 degrees. (4) The femoral neck is centered to the midline.

CR: Make an imaginary line between the ASIS and symphysis pubis and locate its midpoint. From the midpoint, move away from the umbilicus 2 inches to locate the center point.

Collimation: 10 x 12-inch field.

Side Marker: Place appropriate marker in film corner.

Breathing Instructions: Suspended expiration.

Special Considerations: In bilateral hip studies a crosswise film of suitable size can be used and positioned appropriately. Generally, for children under 12 years of age both hips are done for comparison. Use gonadal shielding when appropriate.

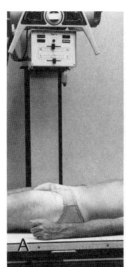
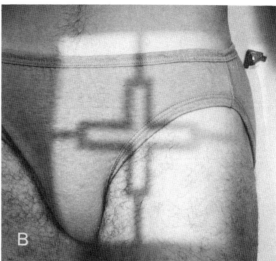

Figure 1.29A. Patient positioning.
Figure 1.29B. Collimation and central ray.

Normal Anatomy (Figure 1.29C and D)

1. Femoral head.
2. Femoral neck.
3. Fovea capitus centralis of the femoral head.
4. Intertrochanteric crest.
5. Greater trochanter.
6. Lesser trochanter.
7. Shaft of the femur.
8. Ischial tuberosity.
9. Superior pubic ramus.
10. Inferior pubic ramus.
11. Obturator foramen.
12. Acetabular rim.
13. Anterior inferior iliac spine (AIIS).
14. Anterior superior iliac spine (ASIS).
15. Iliac fossa.
16. Sacroiliac joint.
17. Sacral ala.
18. Kohler's teardrop.

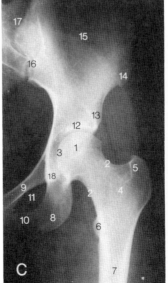
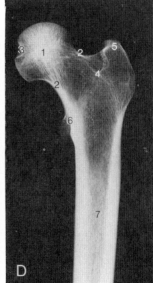

Figure 1.29C. Anteroposterior hip radiograph.
Figure 1.29D. Specimen radiograph.

Basic
Anteroposterior
***Frog-leg**

Hip

Frog-Leg Projection Positioning

(Figure 1.30A and B)

Demonstrates: Acetabulum, adjacent pelvis, joint space, femoral head, neck, trochanters, and proximal diaphysis. (1–3,5,6)
Measure: At the CR.
kVp: 80 (75–85).
Film Size: 10 x 12 inches (24 x 30 cm).
Grid: Yes.
TFD: 40 inches (102 cm).
Tube Tilt: None.
Patient Position: Supine or upright.
Part Position: The femoral neck is centered to the midline of the table. The hip and knee are flexed until the foot reaches the level of the opposite knee. The flexed lower extremity is then abducted as far as possible.
CR: Make an imaginary line between the ASIS and symphysis pubis and locate its midpoint. From this midpoint, move away from the umbilicus 2 inches to locate the center point.
Collimation: 10 x 12-inch field.
Side Marker: Place appropriate marker in film corner.
Breathing Instructions: Suspended expiration.
Special Considerations: In a bilateral frog-leg view a film of suitable size placed cross-wise is used. Generally, for children under 12 years of age both hips are taken for comparison. In a unilateral frog-leg view the cassette may be placed in a diagonal mode to the long axis of the body, thus rendering more available anatomy to be placed on the final radiograph. Use gonadal shielding when appropriate.

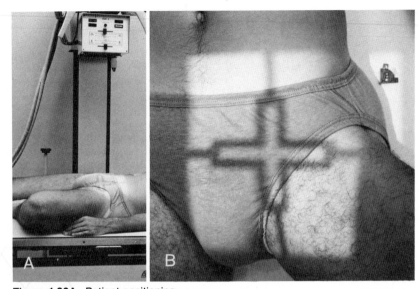

Figure 1.30A. Patient positioning.
Figure 1.30B. Collimation and central ray.

Normal Anatomy (Figure 1.30C and D)

1. Femoral head.
2. Greater trochanter.
3. Lesser trochanter.
4. Intertrochanteric line.
5. Femoral neck.
6. Acetabular rim.
7. Inferior pubic ramus.
8. Superior pubic ramus.
9. Pelvic rim.
10. Sacroiliac joint.
11. Anterior superior iliac spine (ASIS).
12. Anterior inferior iliac spine (AIIS).
13. Obturator foramen.
14. Ischial tuberosity.
15. Inferior acetabular fossa (Kohler's teardrop).

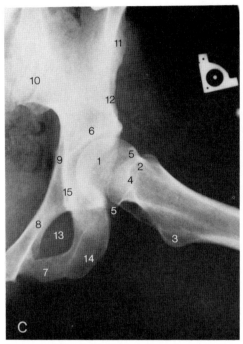

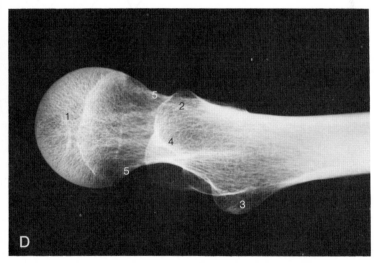

Figure 1.30C. Frog-leg radiograph of the hip.
Figure 1.30D. Specimen radiograph.

Basic
***Anteroposterior**
Lateral
Intercondylar
Tangential

Knee

Anteroposterior View Positioning
(Figure 1.31A and B)

Optional
Obliques

Demonstrates: Distal femur, proximal tibia and fibula, femorotibial joint space, and patella. (1–3)
Measure: At the CR.
kVp: 60 (55–65).
Film Size: 8 x 10 inches (18 x 24 cm).
Grid: Yes, if the knee measures more than 10 cm; below 10 cm, a nongrid technique is used.
TFD: 40 inches (must correct for tube tilt).
Tube Tilt: 5 degrees cephalad.
Patient Position: Supine or upright.
Part Position: Internally rotate the leg slightly so that the knee is in a true anteroposterior position. Sandbag the ankle and foot.
CR: 1 cm inferior to the apex of the patella. Center film to CR.
Collimation: Collimate to area of radiographic interest.
Side Marker: Place appropriate marker at film corner.
Special Considerations: This view can also be performed upright. These erect weightbearing anteroposterior views frequently identify joint space narrowing and/or instability when nonweightbearing views appear normal. (4,5) Tube tilt is utilized to make the central ray coincident with the superior tibial articulating surface.

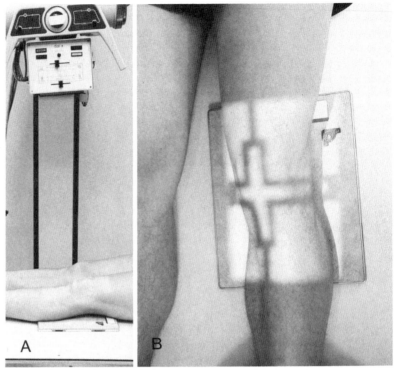

Figure 1.31A. Patient positioning.
Figure 1.31B. Collimation and central ray.

Normal Anatomy (Figure 1.31C and D)

1. Femoral shaft.
2. Medial epicondyle.
3. Lateral epicondyle.
4. Medial condyle.
5. Lateral condyle.
6. Intercondylar notch.
7. Intercondylar eminences (tibial spines)
8. Medial condyle of the tibia.
9. Lateral condyle of the tibia.
10. Head of the fibula.
11. Neck of the fibula.
12. Adductor tubercle.
13. Medial joint space.
14. Lateral joint space.
15. Tibial shaft.
16. Patella.

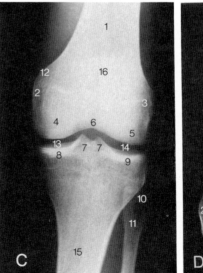

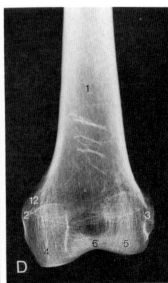

Figure 1.31C. Anteroposterior knee radiograph.
Figure 1.31D. Specimen radiograph.

Basic
Anteroposterior
*Lateral
Intercondylar
Tangential

Knee
Lateral Knee Projection Positioning
(Figure 1.32A and B)

Optional
Oblique

Demonstrates: Distal femur, proximal tibia and fibula, patella, and patellofemoral and tibiofemoral joint spaces. (1–3,6,7)
Measure: At the CR.
kVp: 60 (55–65).
Film Size: 8 x 10 inches (18 x 24 cm).
Grid: Yes. Can be done nonbucky if part measures less than 10 cm.
TFD: 40 inches (102 cm).
Tube Tilt: Optional. 5 degrees cephalad may be used to superimpose the inferior aspects of the medial and lateral femoral condyles.
Patient Position: Lateral recumbent.
Part Position: Place the patient on the table with the side of the leg being examined down. Flex the lower leg about 45 degrees to traction the patella in place. Cross the opposite leg over the leg being examined and support, if necessary, to prevent pelvic rotation. Center the long axis of the femur to the midline of the film. Particular attention should be directed to the posterior surface of the buttocks. When this skin surface is perpendicular to the film, a true lateral view of the distal femur will be assured.
CR: Enters 1 cm distal to the medial epicondyle. Center the film to central ray.
Collimation: By film size.
Side Marker: Place appropriate marker in film corner.
Special Considerations: A crosstable lateral with the knee fully extended will demonstrate fat/fluid levels, if present, in severely traumatized knees.

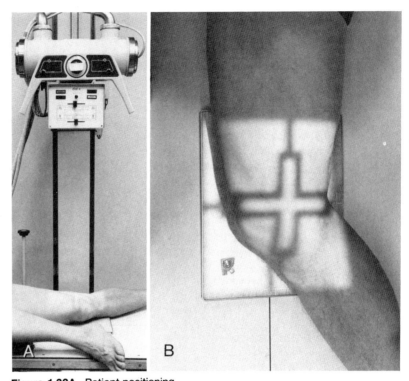

Figure 1.32A. Patient positioning.
Figure 1.32B. Collimation and central ray.

Normal Anatomy (Figure 1.32C and D)

1. Anterior intercondylar area.
2. Posterior intercondylar area.
3. Tibial tuberosity.
4. Tibial shaft.
5. Head of fibula.
6. Fabella (sesamoid bone in the head of the lateral gastrocnemius tendon).
7. Patella.
8. Condyles (medial and lateral).
9. Femoral shaft.
10. Superior pole, patella.
11. Inferior pole, patella.
12. Infrapatellar fat.

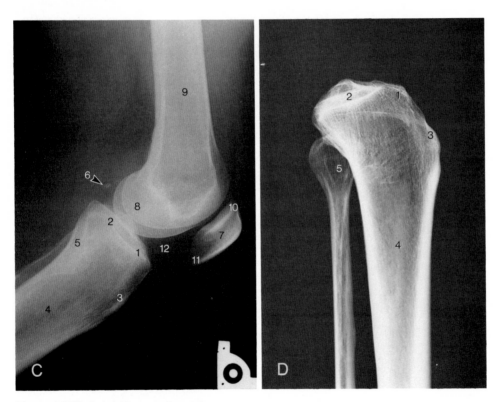

Figure 1.32C. Lateral knee radiograph.
Figure 1.32D. Specimen radiograph.

Basic
Anteroposterior
Lateral
*Intercondylar
Tangential

Knee
Intercondylar (Tunnel) Projection
Positioning
(Figure 1.33A–C)

Optional
Oblique

Demonstrates: Intercondyloid fossa, distal femur, proximal tibia, tibial eminences, proximal fibula, and joint space. (1–3,8,9)
Measure: At the CR.
kVp: 60 (55–65).
Film Size: 8 x 10 inches (18 x 24 cm).
Grid: Yes. Can use nongrid if the knee measures less than 10 cm.
TFD: 40 inches (102 cm) (must correct for tube tilt).
Tube Tilt: 45-degree caudal angulation with the prone position.
Patient Position: Prone or kneeling.
Part Position: (1) *Prone.* The patient is prone on the table. The knee is flexed approximately 45 degrees, with the lower leg and ankle supported. (Fig. 1.33A) (2) *Kneeling.* The patient is on the table in the kneeling position. The patient then leans forward so that the shaft of the femur will form a 25-degree angle with the central ray. (Fig. 1.33B) The unaffected knee is brought forward so that the majority of the weight of the torso is upon this knee.
CR: (1) *Prone.* The central ray is angled 25 degrees caudal and enters the knee joint at the popliteal depression. Center film to the central ray. (2) *Kneeling.* No tube tilt is used, and the central ray passes through the knee joint. Center film to the central ray.
Collimation: Collimate closely.
Side Marker: Place appropriate marker in film corner.
Special Considerations: This is a useful view for depicting the intercondylar notch, which is not demonstrated on the anteroposterior projection. This is a common site for intra-articular loose bodies to collect. The kneeling position is the optimum means of producing this projection. Doubling the mAs value utilized for the anteroposterior view of the knee, with the same kVp, will produce a diagnostic radiograph in this position.

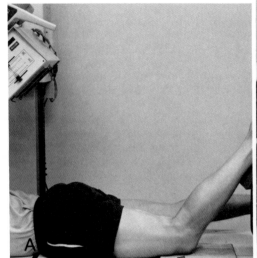
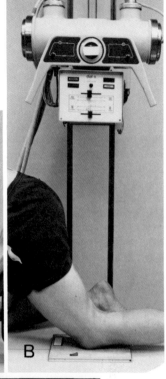
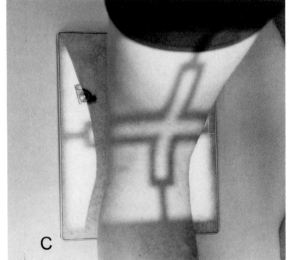

Figure 1.33A. Patient positioning prone.
Figure 1.33B. Patient positioning kneeling.
Figure 1.33C. Collimation and central ray kneeling.

Normal Anatomy (Figure 1.33D and E)

1. Femoral shaft.
2. Adductor tubercle.
3. Medial condyle.
4. Lateral condyle.
5. Medial epicondyle.
6. Lateral epicondyle.
7. Popliteal groove.
8. Intercondylar notch.
9. Intercondylar eminences (tibial spines).
10. Medial condyle, tibia.
11. Lateral condyle, tibia.
12. Styloid process, fibula.
13. Neck of fibula.
14. Tibial shaft.
15. Patella.

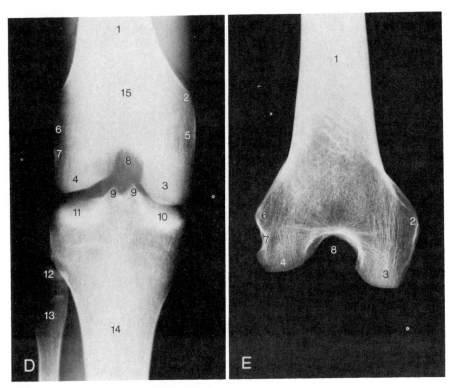

Figure 1.33D. Tunnel radiograph of the knee.
Figure 1.33E. Specimen radiograph.

Basic
Anteroposterior
Lateral
Intercondylar
*Tangential

Knee
**Tangential (Skyline, Sunrise)
Projection Positioning**
(Figure 1.34A and B)

Optional
Oblique

Demonstrates: Patella and patellofemoral joint space. (1–3,10–13)
Measure: At the CR.
kVp: 60 (55–65).
Film Size: 8 x 10 inches (18 x 24 cm).
Grid: Yes. May be done nongrid if part measures less than 10 cm.
TFD: 40 inches (must correct for tube tilt).
Tube Tilt: 10 degrees cephalad.
Patient Position: Prone.
Part Position: The knee is fully flexed. If the patient is unable to fully flex the knee, angle the central ray cephalad so that a 45-degree angle exists between the lower leg and the central ray.
CR: Set the central ray between the patella and the femoral condyles. Center film to central ray.
Collimation: 4 x 4-inch field.
Side Marker: Place appropriate marker in film corner.

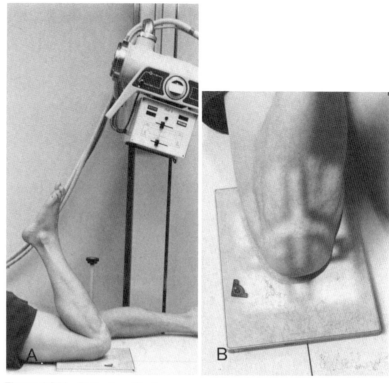

Figure 1.34A. Patient positioning.
Figure 1.34B. Collimation and central ray.

Normal Anatomy (Figure 1.34C and D)

1. Odd facet of the patella.
2. Medial facet of the patella.
3. Lateral facet of the patella.
4. External cortical surface of the patella.
5. Patella.
6. Head of the fibula.
7. Tibiofibular articulation.
8. Patellofemoral articulation.
9. Medial condyle.
10. Lateral condyle.
11. Popliteal groove.
12. Intercondylar notch.
13. Medial epicondyle.
14. Lateral epicondyle.
15. Adductor tubercle.

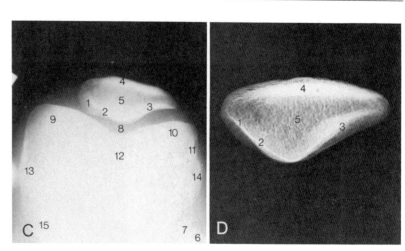

Figure 1.34C. Tangential (skyline) knee radiograph.
Figure 1.34D. Specimen radiograph.

Ankle
Anteroposterior Ankle Projection
Positioning
(Figure 1.35A and B)

Demonstrates: Distal tibia and fibula, talus, and ankle joint. (1–3)

Measure: Anteroposterior at the ankle mortise.

kVp: 55 (50–60).

Film Size: 10 x 12 inches (24 x 30 cm).

Grid: No.

TFD: 40 inches (102 cm).

Tube Tilt: None.

Patient Position: Supine.

Part Position: The ankle is slightly dorsiflexed so that the plantar surface of the foot is perpendicular to the film. Internally rotate the lower leg so that a line through the malleoli is parallel with the film surface.

CR: Center halfway between the medial and lateral malleolus.

Collimation: Collimate to a 6 x 10-inch field.

Side Marker: Place appropriate marker in film corner.

Special Considerations: If the foot is not dorsiflexed, the tibiotalar joint space will not be clearly visualized; (3) however, in subtle fractures of the talar dome plantar flexion will often demonstrate the fracture site. (4)

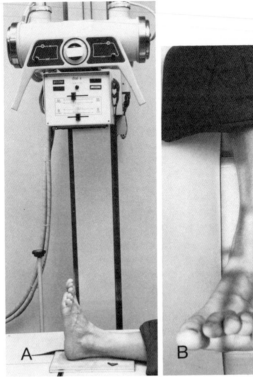
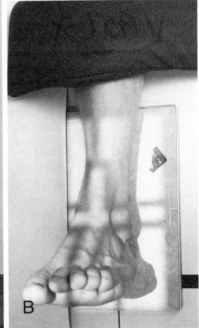

Figure 1.35A. Patient positioning.
Figure 1.35B. Collimation and central ray.

Normal Anatomy (Figure 1.35C and D)

1. Tibia.
2. Fibula.
3. Medial malleolus, tibia.
4. Lateral malleolus, fibula.
5. Plafond of the tibia.
6. Lateral surface of the tibia.
7. Dome of the talus.
8. Neck of the talus.
9. Posterior malleolus.

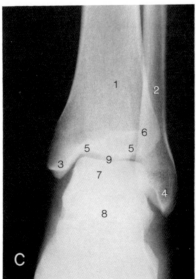
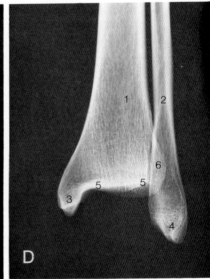

Figure 1.35C. Anteroposterior ankle radiograph.
Figure 1.35D. Specimen radiograph.

Basic
Anteroposterior
*Medial Oblique
Lateral

Optional
Stress views

Ankle
Medial Oblique Ankle Projection
Positioning
(Figure 1.36A)

Demonstrates: Distal tibia and fibula, talus, and ankle joint. (1–3,5)

Measure: Anteroposterior at the ankle mortise.

kVp: 55 (50–60).

Film Size: ½ of a 10 x 12 (24 x 30 cm). Divide in half; the other half is used for the anteroposterior projection.

Grid: No.

TFD: 40 inches (102 cm).

Tube Tilt: None.

Patient Position: Supine.

Part Position: The ankle is slightly dorsiflexed so that the plantar surface of the foot is perpendicular to the film. The lower leg is then internally rotated so that the intermalleolar line forms an angle of 35–45 degrees with the film.

CR: Center halfway between the medial and lateral malleolus. Center film to central ray.

Collimation: Collimate to a 6 x 10-inch field.

Side Marker: Place appropriate marker in film corner.

Special Considerations: This is an important view in the assessment of the posttraumatic ankle for detecting subtle fractures of the distal fibula, posterior tibia, and base of the fifth metatarsal.

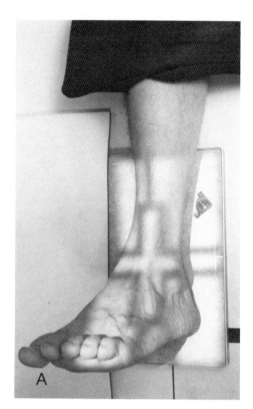

Figure 1.36A. Patient positioning, collimation, and central ray.

Normal Anatomy (Figure 1.36B)

1. Tibia.
2. Fibula.
3. Lateral malleolus, fibula.
4. Medial malleolus, tibia.
5. Plafond of the tibia.
6. Lateral surface of the tibia.
7. Posterior malleolus.
8. Body of the talus.
9. Neck of the talus.
10. Head of the talus.
11. Sinus tarsi (sulcus calcanei).
12. Anterior tubercle, calcaneus.
13. Calcaneus.
14. Navicular.
15. Lateral cuneiform.
16. Cuboid.
17. Fifth metatarsal base.

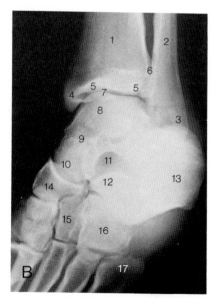

Figure 1.36B. Medial oblique ankle radiograph.

Ankle
Lateral Ankle Projection Positioning
(Figure 1.37A)

Demonstrates: Distal tibia and fibula, ankle joint, talus, and calcaneus. (1–3,6,7)

Measure: Transversely through the malleoli.

kVp: 55 (50–60).

Film Size: 8 x 10 inches (18 x 24 cm).

Grid: No.

TFD: 40 inches (102 cm).

Tube Tilt: None.

Patient Position: Lateral recumbent.

Part Position: The lateral surface of the ankle is in contact with the film, with the foot slightly dorsiflexed. Cross the opposite leg over the leg being examined and support the opposite knee to avoid rotation of the ankle.

CR: Directed to the medial malleolus. Center film to the central ray.

Collimation: 8 x 10-inch field.

Side Marker: Place appropriate marker in film corner.

Special Considerations: The posterior tibial lip is a frequent site of fracture and can be best demonstrated in an off-lateral projection, with slight external rotation of the foot. (7)

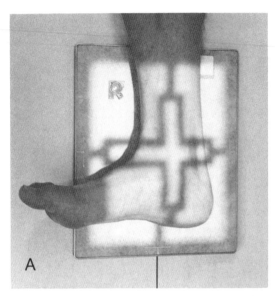

Figure 1.37A. Patient positioning, collimation, and central ray.

Normal Anatomy (Figure 1.37B and C)

1. Tibia.
2. Fibula.
3. Plafond of the tibia.
4. Posterior malleolus, tibia.
5. Lateral malleolus, fibula.
6. Talar dome.
7. Neck of talus.
8. Head of talus.
9. Navicular.
10. Cuboid.
11. Anterior tubercle, calcaneus.
12. Middle tubercle, calcaneus.
13. Posterior tubercle, calcaneus.
14. Posterior surface, calcaneus.

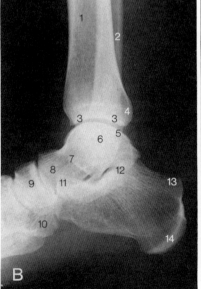
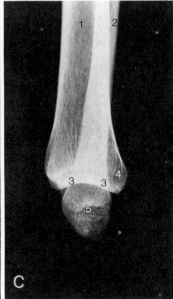

Figure 1.37B. Lateral ankle radiograph.
Figure 1.37C. Specimen radiograph.

Foot
Dorsiplantar Foot Projection
Positioning
(Figure 1.38A and B)

Demonstrates: Phalanges, metatarsals, cuneiforms, cuboid, and navicular. (1–5)

Measure: Through the tarsometatarsal junction at the base of the third metatarsal.

kVp: 55 (50–60).

Film Size: 10 x 12 inches (24 x 30 cm). Divide in half lengthwise; the other half is used for the medial oblique.

Grid: No.

TFD: 40 inches (must correct for tube tilt).

Tube Tilt: 10 degrees cephalad.

Patient Position: Supine, with knee flexed, or standing.

Part Position: The knee is flexed so that the plantar surface of the foot is resting on the film.

CR: Centered to base of third metatarsal. Center film to the central ray.

Collimation: 5 x 12-inch exposure field.

Side Marker: Place appropriate marker in corner of film.

Special Considerations: A compensating filter can be used to prevent overexposure of the metatarsal heads and toes, filtering from the midshaft of the metatarsals distally. Tube tilt utilization will improve visualization of the intertarsal and tarsometatarsal articulations. Weightbearing views of the foot may have some biomechanical value.

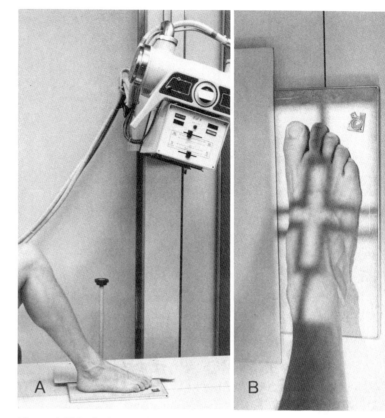

Figure 1.38A. Patient positioning.
Figure 1.38B. Collimation and central ray.

Normal Anatomy (Figure 1.38C and D)

1. Medial malleolus, tibia.
2. Calcaneus.
3. Cuboid.
4. Head of talus.
5. Navicular.
6. First cuneiform (medial).
7. Second cuneiform (intermediate).
8. Third cuneiform (lateral).
9. Base of fifth metatarsal (styloid process).
10. Base of fourth metatarsal.
11. Shaft of third metatarsal.
12. Neck of second metatarsal.
13. Head of first metatarsal.
14. First metatarsal phalangeal articulation.
15. Medial sesamoid in tendon of flexor hallucis brevis.
16. Lateral sesamoid in tendon of flexor hallucis brevis.
17. Proximal phalanx of the fourth toe.
18. Middle phalanx of the third toe.
19. Distal phalanx of the second toe.
20. Distal ungual tuft of the first toe.

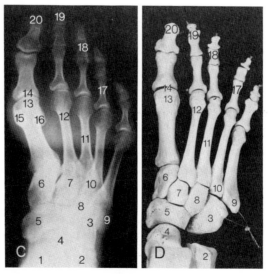

Figure 1.38C. Dorsiplantar foot radiograph.
Figure 1.38D. Anatomic specimen.

Basic
Dorsiplantar
*Medial oblique
Lateral

Foot
Medial Oblique Projection
Positioning
(Figure 1.39A and B)

Demonstrates: Phalanges, metatarsals, cuboid, third cuneiform, navicular, and distal calcaneus. (1–4,6)

Measure: Tarsometatarsal junction at the base of the third metatarsal.

kVp: 55 (50–60).

Film Size: 10 x 12 inches (24 x 30 cm). Divide in half lengthwise.

Grid: No.

TFD: 40 inches (102 cm).

Tube Tilt: None.

Patient Position: Supine, with knee flexed, or standing.

Part Position: The knee is flexed so that the foot is resting flat on the film. The leg is rotated medially so that the plantar surface of the foot forms an angle of approximately 35 degrees, with the plane of the film and the fifth digit being elevated from the film surface.

CR: Center to the base of the third metatarsal. Center film to the central ray.

Collimation: 6 x 12-inch field size.

Side Marker: Place appropriate marker in corner of film.

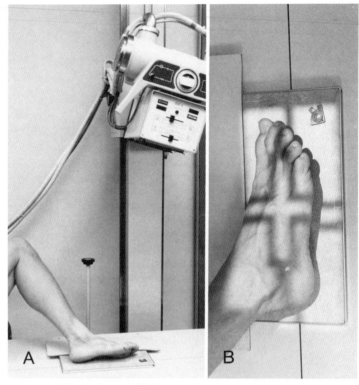

Figure 1.39A. Patient positioning.
Figure 1.39B. Collimation and central ray.

Normal Anatomy (Figure 1.39C and D)

1. Calcaneus.
2. Head of talus.
3. Navicular.
4. First cuneiform (medial).
5. Second cuneiform (intermediate).
6. Third cuneiform (lateral).
7. Cuboid.
8. Calcaneocuboid joint.
9. Base of fifth metatarsal (styloid process).
10. Base of fourth metatarsal.
11. Shaft of third metatarsal.
12. Neck of second metatarsal.
13. Head of first metatarsal.
14. First metatarsal phalangeal articulation.
15. Bipartite medial sesamoid in tendon of flexor hallucis brevis.
16. Lateral sesamoid in tendon of flexor hallucis brevis.
17. Proximal phalanx of the fourth toe.
18. Middle phalanx of the third toe.
19. Distal phalanx of the second toe.
20. Distal ungual tuft of the first toe.

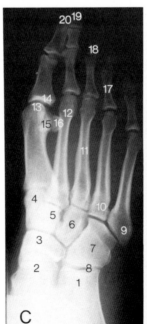
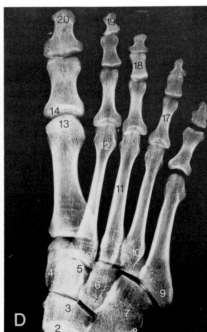

Figure 1.39C. Medial oblique foot radiograph.
Figure 1.39D. Specimen radiograph.

Foot

Basic
Dorsiplantar
Medial oblique
*Lateral

Lateral Foot Projection Positioning
(Figure 1.40A and B)

Demonstrates: Distal tibia and fibula, tarsals, ankle joint, metatarsals, and phalanges. (1–4)
Measure: Navicular to fifth metatarsal.
kVp: 55 (50–60).
Film Size: 8 x 10 inches (18 x 24 cm), or 10 x 12 inches (24 x 30 cm) for large feet.
Grid: No.
TFD: 40 inches (102 cm).
Tube Tilt: None.
Patient Position: Lateral recumbent or standing.
Part Position: Cross the unaffected leg over and forward for patient stability. The affected foot is placed in true lateral projection, with the fifth metatarsal in contact with the film. The plantar surface should be perpendicular to the film.
CR: At the navicular.
Collimation: To the film.
Side Marker: Place appropriate marker in film corner.
Special Considerations: Weightbearing views of the feet may have some biomechanical value.

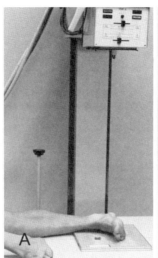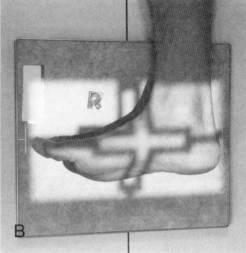

Figure 1.40A. Patient positioning.
Figure 1.40B. Collimation and central ray.

Normal Anatomy (Figure 1.40C)

1. Tibia.
2. Dome of talus.
3. Neck of talus.
4. Head of talus.
5. Navicular.
6. Cuneiforms (superimposed upon each other).
7. Cuboid.
8. Base of fifth metatarsal.
9. Styloid process, fifth metatarsal.
10. Calcaneus.
11. Anterior tubercle, calcaneus.
12. Middle tubercle, calcaneus.
13. Posterior tubercle, calcaneus.
14. Os trigonum

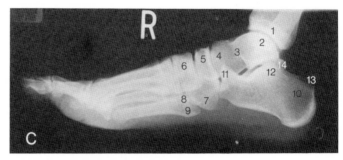

Figure 1.40C. Lateral foot radiograph.

Toes
Dorsiplantar Projection of the Toes
Positioning
(Figure 1.41A)

Demonstrates: Phalanges, distal metatarsals, interphalangeal and metatarsophalangeal joints. (1–3)

Measure: At the proximal interphalangeal joints. For the great toe, at the interphalangeal joint.

kVp: 55 (50–60).

Film Size: 8 x 10 inches (18 x 24 cm) divided into halves; the other half is used for the oblique.

Grid: No.

TFD: 40 inches (102 cm).

Tube Tilt: None.

Patient Position: Supine or sitting on the table top.

Part Position: The knee is flexed so the foot is placed flat on the film.

CR: At the proximal interphalangeal joint.

Collimation: If a general evaluation of the toes is required, all of the toes should be exposed. If a specific toe is being evaluated, then appropriate collimation should be performed.

Side Marker: Appropriate marker in film corner.

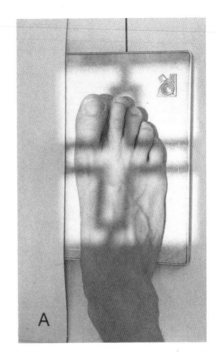

Figure 1.41A. Patient positioning, collimation, and central ray.

Normal Anatomy (Figure 1.41B and C)

1. Medial sesamoid bone in tendon of flexor hallucis brevis.
2. Lateral sesamoid bone in tendon of flexor hallucis brevis.
3. First metatarsal head.
4. Proximal phalanx, fourth toe.
5. Middle phalanx, third toe.
6. Distal phalanx, second toe.
7. Distal ungual tuft, first toe.
8. Metatarsal phalangeal joint, second toe.
9. Interphalangeal joint, second toe.
10. Distal interphalangeal joint, third toe.

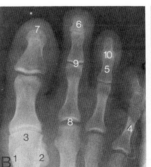 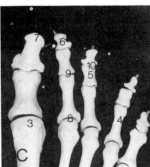

Figure 1.41B. Dorsiplantar toe radiograph.
Figure 1.41C. Anatomic specimen.

Basic
  Dorsiplantar
*Oblique

Toes
Oblique Projection of the Toes
Positioning
(Figure 1.42A–C)

Optional
  Axial (sesamoids)

Demonstrates: Phalanges, distal metatarsals, interphalangeal and metatarsophalangeal joints. (1–3)

Measure: At interphalangeal joints.

kVp: 55 (50–60).

Film Size: 8 x 10 inches (18 x 24 cm) divided into halves; the other half is used for the dorsiplantar view.

Grid: No.

TFD: 40 inches (102 cm).

Tube Tilt: None.

Patient Position: Supine or sitting on the table top.

Part Position: The knee is flexed so the foot is placed flat on the film. (1) *Toes 1, 2, and 3.* Elevate the fifth metatarsal region so the foot forms a 45-degree angle with the film. (Fig. 1.42A) (2) *Toes 4 and 5.* Elevate the great toe region so the foot forms a 45-degree angle with the film. (Fig. 1.42B)

CR: At the proximal interphalangeal joint.

Collimation: If a general evaluation of the toes is required, all of the toes should be exposed. If a specific toe is being evaluated, then appropriate collimation should be performed.

Side Marker: Appropriate marker in film corner.

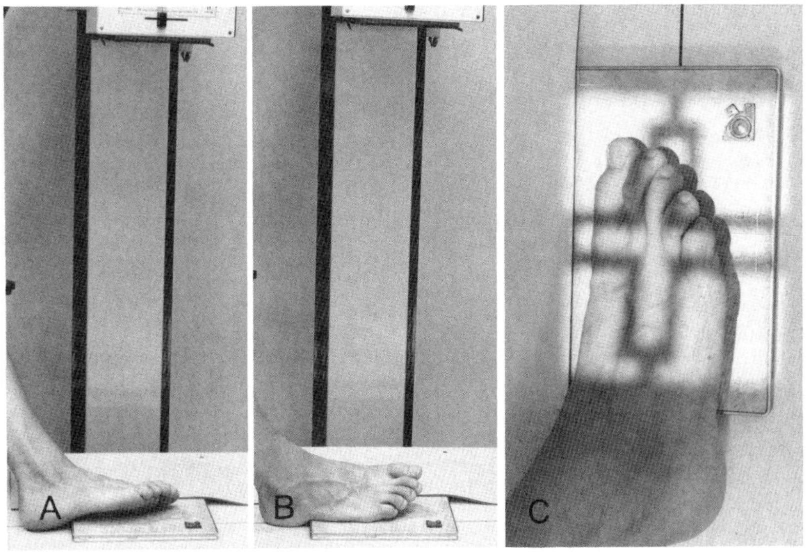

Figure 1.42A. Patient positioning, Toes 1, 2, and 3.
Figure 1.42B. Patient positioning, Toes 4 and 5.
Figure 1.42C. Collimation and central ray.

Normal Anatomy (Figure 1.42D and E)

1. Base of second metatarsal.
2. Shaft of first metatarsal.
3. Neck of second metatarsal.
4. Head of third metatarsal.
5. Proximal phalanx, fifth toe.
6. Middle phalanx, fourth toe.
7. Distal phalanx, third toe.
8. Distal tuft (ungual), second toe.
9. Proximal phalanx, first toe.
10. Interphalangeal joint, first toe.
11. Distal phalanx, first toe.
12. Metatarsal phalangeal articulation, second toe.
13. Proximal interphalangeal joint, fifth toe.
14. Distal interphalangeal joint, second toe.
15. Medial sesamoid bone in the tendon of flexor hallucis brevis.
16. Lateral sesamoid bone in the tendon of flexor hallucis brevis.

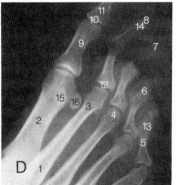
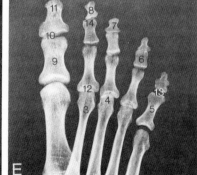

Figure 1.42D. Oblique toe radiograph.
Figure 1.42E. Specimen radiograph.

Basic
*Axial
Lateral

Calcaneus

Axial Projection Positioning
(Figure 1.43A and B)

Demonstrates: Calcaneus. (1,2)
Measure: Through the CR.
kVp: 55 (50–60).
Film Size: 8 x 10 inches (18 x 24 cm) divided in halves; the other half is used for the lateral projection.
Grid: No.
TFD: 40 inches (must correct for tube tilt).
Tube Tilt: 35–40 degrees cephalad.
Patient Position: Supine, with legs extended.
Part Position: Foot is dorsiflexed such that the plantar surface is perpendicular to the film.
CR: 2 inches up from the back of the heel.
Collimation: To the size of the calcaneus (approximately 5 x 5 inches).
Side Marker: Appropriate side marker in film corner.
Special Considerations: A looped strap can be placed around the ball of the foot which the patient can grasp and accentuate the dorsiflexion of the foot.

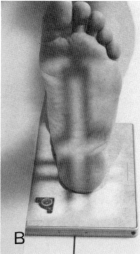
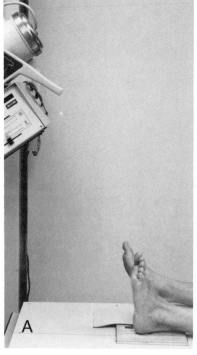

Figure 1.43A. Patient positioning.
Figure 1.43B. Collimation and central ray.

Normal Anatomy (Figure 1.43C and D)

1. Calcaneus.
2. Medial process, calcaneus.
3. Tuberosity, calcaneus.
4. Lateral process, calcaneus.
5. Sustentaculum tali, calcaneus.
6. Trochlear process, calcaneus.

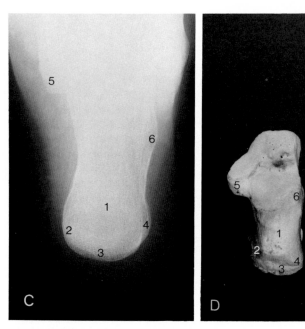

Figure 1.43C. Axial calcaneal radiograph.
Figure 1.43D. Anatomic specimen.

Basic
Axial
*Lateral

Calcaneus
Lateral Projection Positioning
(Figure 1.44A)

Demonstrates: Calcaneus, talus, subtalar joints, and Achilles tendon. (1,2)
Measure: At the CR.
kVp: 55 (50–60).
Film Size: 8 x 10 inches (18 x 24 cm) divided in halves; the other half is used for the axial projection.
Grid: No.
TFD: 40 inches (102 cm).
Tube Tilt: None.
Patient Position: Lateral recumbent.
Part Position: The unaffected leg is crossed over and anterior for patient stability. The lateral side of the foot contacts the film, with the plantar surface perpendicular to the film.
CR: Midcalcaneus (1-½ inches up from the plantar surface of the heel and 2 inches from the posterior surface of the heel).
Collimation: To the calcaneus size (5 x 5 inches).
Side Marker: Appropriate side marker in film corner.

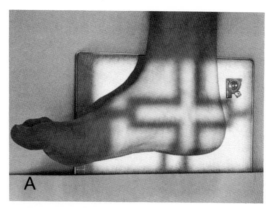

Figure 1.44A. Patient positioning, collimation, and central ray.

Normal Anatomy (Figure 1.44B and C)

1. Tibia.
2. Dome of the talus.
3. Body of the talus.
4. Head of the talus.
5. Navicular.
6. Cuneiforms (superimposed upon each other).
7. Cuboid.
8. Anterior tuberosity of the calcaneus.
9. Subtalar joint.
10. Posterior tuberosity of the calcaneus.
11. Calcaneus.
12. Posterior surface of the calcaneus.
13. Calcaneocuboid joint.

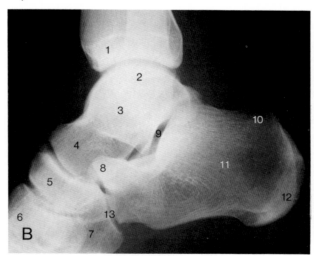
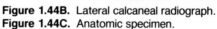
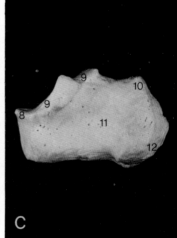

Figure 1.44B. Lateral calcaneal radiograph.
Figure 1.44C. Anatomic specimen.

Basic
***Internal rotation**
External rotation
Abduction (baby arm)

Shoulder

Anteroposterior Internal Rotation Projection
Positioning
(Figure 1.45A)

Optional
Transaxial

Demonstrates: Proximal humerus, scapula, clavicle, ribcage, and lung. (1–6)
Measure: Between the coracoid process and scapula.
kVp: 75 (70–80).
Film Size: 10 x 12 inches (24 x 30 cm) vertical.
Grid: Yes.
TFD: 40 inches (102 cm).
Tube Tilt: None.
Patient Position: Upright or supine.
Part Position: The patient is rotated to be at 30 degrees to the bucky. The coracoid is centered to the bucky and the arm internally rotated until the elbow epicondyles are perpendicular to the film.
CR: Through the coracoid process.
Collimation: To film size.
Side Marker: Appropriate marker placed at film corner above humeral head.
Breathing Instructions: Suspended expiration.
Special Considerations: If the trunk is not rotated, a clear view of the glenohumeral joint will not be obtained. A comfortable positioning alternative for the patient with an acute shoulder is to allow 90 degrees of elbow flexion, then rest the forearm against the abdomen.

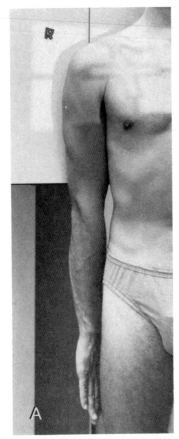

Figure 1.45A. Patient positioning, collimation, and central ray.

Normal Anatomy (Figure 1.45B and C)

1. Coracoid process, scapula.
2. Acromion, scapula.
3. Glenoid fossa.
4. Axillary border, scapula.
5. Subscapular fossa.
6. Lesser tuberosity, humerus.
7. Greater tuberosity, humerus.
8. Humeral head.
9. Pectoralis groove.

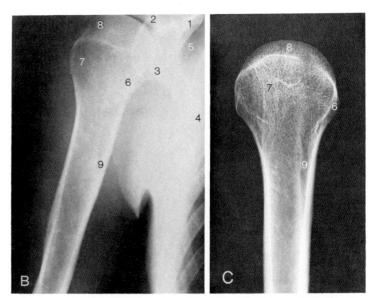

Figure 1.45B. Anteroposterior internal rotation shoulder radiograph.
Figure 1.45C. Specimen radiograph.

Basic
Internal rotation
*****External rotation**
Abduction

Shoulder
Anteroposterior External Rotation Projection
Positioning
(Figure 1.46A)

Optional
Transaxial

Demonstrates: Proximal humerus (especially the greater tuberosity), scapula, clavicle, ribcage, and lung. (1–6)

Measure: Between the coracoid process and scapula.

kVp: 75 (70–80).

Film Size: 10 x 12 (24 x 30 cm) vertical.

Grid: Yes.

TFD: 40 inches (102 cm).

Tube Tilt: None.

Patient Position: Upright or supine.

Part Position: The patient is rotated to be at 30 degrees to the bucky. The coracoid is centered to the bucky and the arm externally rotated until the elbow epicondyles are parallel to the film.

CR: To the coracoid process.

Collimation: To film size.

Side Marker: Appropriate marker placed at film corner above humeral head.

Breathing Instructions: Suspended expiration.

Special Considerations: This is an especially useful view to demonstrate calcific tendinitis and fractures of the greater tuberosity. (7) Greater external rotation may be assured by allowing 90 degrees of elbow flexion, with the patient maximally externally rotating the forearm.

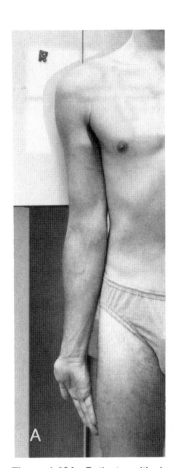

Figure 1.46A. Patient positioning, collimation, and central ray.

Normal Anatomy (Figure 1.46B–D)

1. Coracoid process, scapula.
2. Acromion, scapula.
3. Distal clavicle.
4. Glenoid fossa.
5. Spine of scapula.
6. Superior angle, scapula.
7. Vertebral border, scapula.
8. Axillary border, scapula.
9. Inferior angle, scapula.
10. Posterior rib.
11. Anterior rib.
12. Acromioclavicular joint.
13. Glenohumeral articulation.
14. Humeral head.
15. Greater tuberosity, humerus.
16. Lesser tuberosity, humerus.
17. Intertubercular groove, humerus.
18. Anatomical neck, humerus.
19. Surgical neck, humerus.
20. Shaft of the humerus.

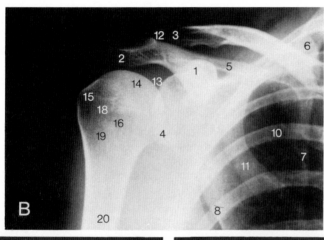

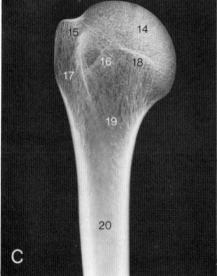

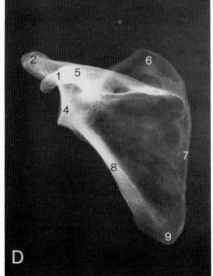

Figure 1.46B. Anteroposterior external rotation shoulder radiograph.
Figure 1.46C. Specimen radiograph humerus.
Figure 1.46D. Specimen radiograph scapula.

Basic
Internal rotation
External rotation
*Abduction (baby arm)

Shoulder
Abduction (Baby Arm) Projection
Positioning
(Figure 1.47A)

Optional
Transaxial

Demonstrates: Proximal humerus, scapula (especially the coracoid and acromion), acromioclavicular joint, upper ribcage, clavicle, and lung apex. (1–5)
Measure: Coracoid process.
kVp: 75 (70–80).
Film Size: 10 x 12 inches (24 x 30 cm) horizontal.
Grid: Yes.
TFD: 40 inches (102 cm).
Tube Tilt: None.
Patient Position: Upright or supine.
Part Position: The patient's back is flat to the bucky. The arm is abducted to 90 degrees, the elbow flexed to 90 degrees, and the palm of the hand faces the x-ray tube.
CR: At the midclavicular line at the level of the coracoid process.
Collimation: To film size.
Side Marker: Appropriate side marker at film corner above humerus.
Breathing Instructions: Suspended expiration.
Special Considerations: An attempt should be made to include the upper thorax to the spine. Attention should be directed to the lung apex to rule out pulmonary pathology and to the C7 vertebra to rule out a cervical rib on the resulting radiograph.

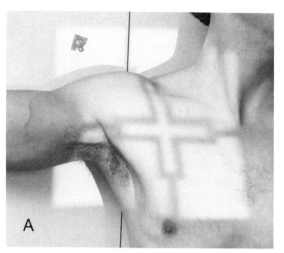

Figure 1.47A. Patient positioning, collimation, and central ray.

Normal Anatomy (Figure 1.47B)

1. Coracoid process, scapula.
2. Acromion, scapula.
3. Distal clavicle.
4. Superior angle, scapula.
5. Spine of scapula.
6. Glenoid fossa.
7. Greater and lesser tuberosities superimposed.
8. Intertubercular groove, humerus.
9. Surgical neck, humerus.
10. Shaft, humerus.
11. Posterior rib.
12. Anterior rib.
13. Axillary border, scapula.
14. Acromioclavicular joint.
15. Conoid tubercle, clavicle.
16. Transverse process, T1.

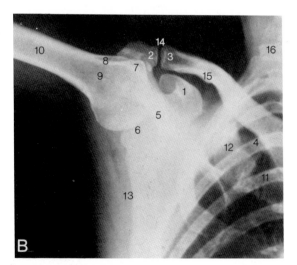

Figure 1.47B. Abduction (baby arm) shoulder radiograph.

Basic
Anteroposterior (cephalad angulation)
***Posteroanterior (caudad angulation)**

Clavicle
Posteroanterior Projection
Positioning
(Figure 1.48A and B)

Demonstrates: Clavicle, upper ribs, scapula, and lung. (1–3)

Measure: At coracoid process.

kVp: 70 (65–75).

Film Size: 10 x 12 inches (24 x 30 cm).

Grid: Yes.

TFD: 40 inches (must correct for tube tilt).

Tube Tilt: (1) Posteroanterior: 10 degrees caudad. (2) Anteroposterior: 10 degrees cephalad.

Patient Position: Upright.

Part Position: (1) Posteroanterior: Facing the bucky, with no body rotation, but the head is turned away from the side being evaluated. Midpoint of the clavicle is centered to the midline of the bucky. (2) Anteroposterior: Facing the tube, with no body rotation. Midpoint of the clavicle is centered to the midline of the bucky.

CR: (1) Posteroanterior: Through the midclavicle and 1 inch above the level of the clavicle at the patient's back. (2) Anteroposterior: Through the midclavicle.

Collimation: Top to bottom, 8 inches; side to side, 12 inches.

Side Marker: Appropriate marker above the humeral head.

Breathing Instructions: Suspended expiration.

Special Considerations: The posteroanterior projection is preferred for anatomic detail and in kyphotic patients.

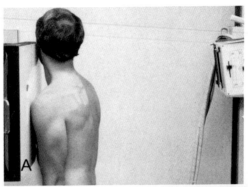

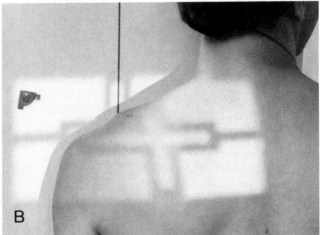

Figure 1.48A. Patient positioning.
Figure 1.48B. Collimation and central ray.

Normal Anatomy (Figure 1.48C and D)

1. Coracoid process, scapula.
2. Acromion, scapula.
3. Distal clavicle.
4. Superior angle, scapula.
5. Superior border, scapula.
6. Axillary border, scapula.
7. Medial clavicle.
8. Sternoclavicular joint.
9. Rhomboid fossa.
10. Midportion, clavicle.
11. Glenoid fossa.
12. Posterior rib.
13. Anterior rib.
14. Humeral head.
15. Shaft of the humerus.

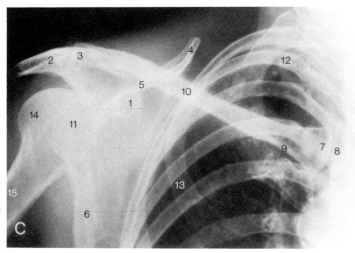
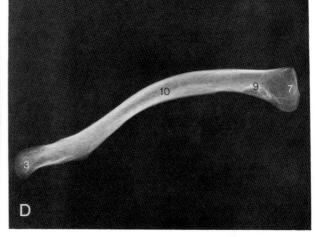

Figure 1.48C. Posteroanterior clavicle radiograph.
Figure 1.48D. Specimen radiograph.

Basic
*Without weights
*With weights

Acromioclavicular Joints
Anteroposterior Projection
Positioning
(Figure 1.49A and B)

Demonstrates: Distal clavicle, acromioclavicular joint. (1–3)

Measure: At the coracoid process; use half the mAs as calculated from the shoulder exposure factors.

kVp: 70 (65–75).

Film Size: 8 x 10 inches (18 x 24 cm) horizontal.

Grid: Yes.

TFD: 40 inches (must correct for tube tilt).

Tube Tilt: 5 degrees cephalad.

Patient Position: Upright.

Part Position: Anteroposterior position, with no body rotation and the acromioclavicular joint centered to the bucky. The same position is done with and without the patient holding 10–15-pound weights. (4)

CR: Through the acromioclavicular joint.

Collimation: To the film.

Side Marker: Appropriate marker placed in upper film corner above the humeral head.

Breathing Instructions: Suspended expiration.

Special Considerations: The purpose of comparing nonweightbearing and weightbearing views is to assess the integrity of the acromioclavicular and costoclavicular ligaments. Bilateral anteroposterior comparison in a single exposure is discouraged, unless appropriate shielding of the thyroid is utilized.

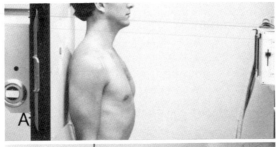

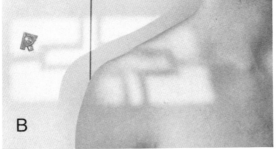

Figure 1.49A. Patient positioning.
Figure 1.49B. Collimation and central ray.

Normal Anatomy (Figure 1.49C)

1. Coracoid process, scapula.
2. Acromion, scapula.
3. Distal clavicle.
4. Superior angle, scapula.
5. Superior border, scapula.
6. Acromioclavicular joint.
7. Humeral head.

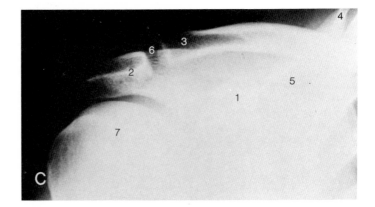

Figure 1.49C. Acromioclavicular joint radiograph.

Basic
*Anteroposterior
  Medial oblique
  Lateral
  Tangential

Elbow
**Anteroposterior Projection
Positioning**
(Figure 1.50A and B)

Optional
Radial head

Demonstrates: Distal humerus, proximal ulna, proximal radius, and elbow joint. (1–3)

Measure: Anteroposterior through the elbow at the epicondyles.

kVp: 55 (50–60).

Film Size: 10 x 12 inches (24 x 30 cm) divided in half; the other half used for the medial oblique projection.

Grid: No.

TFD: 40 inches (102 cm).

Tube Tilt: None.

Patient Position: Seated, with body rotated away from the table.

Part Position: Arm fully extended, and the hand supinated. If the elbow cannot be extended, two AP's are done, one with the forearm on the film and the second with the humerus on the film.

CR: To the elbow, between and 1 inch below the level of the epicondyle.

Collimation: To the arm.

Side Marker: Appropriate marker adjacent to the humerus at the film edge. Lead vinyl must be placed beneath the cassette to reduce primary and secondary radiation to the patient.

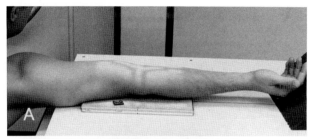

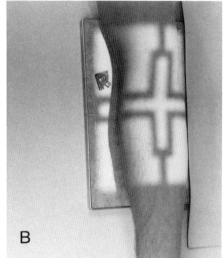

Figure 1.50A. Patient positioning.
Figure 1.50B. Collimation and central ray.

Normal Anatomy (Figure 1.50C and D)

1. Shaft of the humerus.
2. Olecranon fossa, ulna.
3. Medial epicondyle, humerus.
4. Lateral epicondyle, humerus.
5. Capitellum, humerus.
6. Trochlea, humerus.
7. Supracondylar ridge, humerus.
8. Radial head.
9. Neck of the radius.
10. Radial tuberosity.
11. Shaft of the radius.
12. Coronoid process, ulna.
13. Ulna.
14. Olecranon process, ulna.

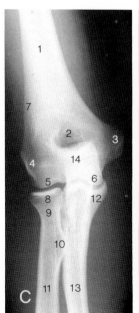
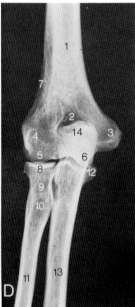

Figure 1.50C. Anteroposterior elbow radiograph.
Figure 1.50D. Specimen radiograph.

Elbow
**Medial Oblique Projection
Positioning**
(Figure 1.51A and B)

Demonstrates: Distal humerus, proximal ulna, proximal radius, and elbow joint. (1–3)

Measure: At the CR.

kVp: 55 (50–60).

Film Size: 10 x 12 inches (24 x 30 cm) divided in half; the other half is used for the anteroposterior projection.

Grid: No.

TFD: 40 inches (102 cm).

Tube Tilt: None.

Patient Position: Seated, with body rotated away from the table.

Part Position: Arm fully extended, and the forearm pronated.

CR: 1 inch below the epicondyles.

Collimation: To the arm.

Side Marker: Appropriate marker adjacent to the humerus at the film edge. Lead vinyl must be placed beneath the cassette to reduce primary and secondary radiation to the patient.

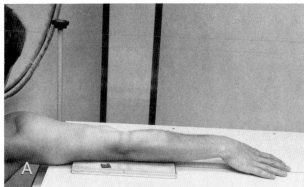

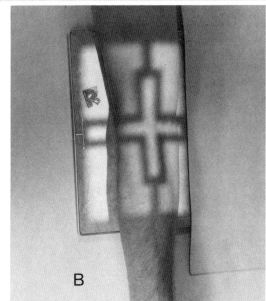

Figure 1.51A. Patient positioning.
Figure 1.51B. Collimation and central ray.

Normal Anatomy (Figure 1.51C)

1. Shaft of the humerus.
2. Olecranon fossa, humerus.
3. Medial epicondyle, humerus.
4. Lateral epicondyle, humerus.
5. Supracondylar ridge, humerus.
6. Olecranon process, ulna.
7. Coronoid process, ulna.
8. Radial head.

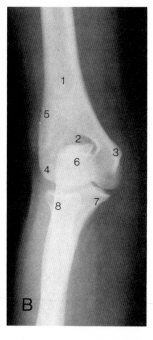

Figure 1.51C. Medial oblique elbow radiograph.

Basic
Anteroposterior
Medial oblique
***Lateral**
Tangential

Elbow
Lateral Projection Positioning
(Figure 1.52A)

Optional
Radial head

Demonstrates: Distal humerus, proximal ulna, proximal radius, and elbow joint. (1–3)

Measure: At the CR.

kVp: 55 (50–60).

Film Size: 10 x 12 inches (24 x 30 cm) divided in half; the other half is used for the tangential projection.

Grid: No.

TFD: 40 inches (102 cm).

Tube Tilt: None.

Patient Position: Seated, with the body rotated away from the table.

Part Position: Elbow flexed to 90 degrees, with the ulnar surface of the forearm flat on the film. The hand is in the true lateral position. The humerus must also be parallel to the film plane.

CR: Mid elbow joint, just anterior to the lateral epicondyle.

Collimation: To the arm, 10 inches along the forearm axis and 6 inches top to bottom.

Side Marker: Appropriate marker placed in the corner of the film adjacent to the olecranon.

Special Considerations: This is a useful view in the evaluation of a post-traumatic elbow in the detection of olecranon process, coronoid process, and radial head fractures. Lead vinyl must be placed beneath the cassette to reduce primary and secondary radiation to the patient.

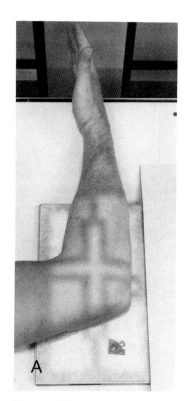

Figure 1.52A. Patient positioning, collimation, and central ray.

Normal Anatomy (Figure 1.52B and C)

1. Shaft of the humerus.
2. Capitellum and trochlea superimposed.
3. Olecranon process, ulna.
4. Coronoid process, ulna.
5. Radial head.
6. Neck of the radius.
7. Radial tuberosity.
8. Coronoid fossa, humerus.
9. Olecranon fossa, humerus.
10. Supinator fat line (arrow).

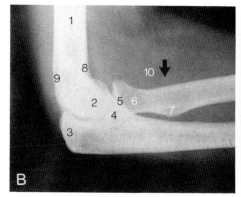
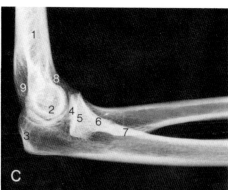
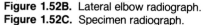

Figure 1.52B. Lateral elbow radiograph.
Figure 1.52C. Specimen radiograph.

Elbow
Tangential (Jones) Projection
Positioning
(Figure 1.53A and B)

Demonstrates: Olecranon, ulnar groove, trochlea, and radial head. (1–4)

Measure: 2 inches above the olecranon tip.

kVp: 55 (50–60).

Film Size: 10 x 12 inches (24 x 30 cm) divided in half; the other half is used for the lateral projection.

Grid: No.

TFD: 40 inches (102 cm).

Tube Tilt: None.

Patient Position: Seated, with the body rotated away from the table.

Part Position: Elbow is fully flexed and the humerus is placed parallel to the film.

CR: 2 inches above the olecranon tip.

Collimation: 6 x 6 inches.

Side Marker: Appropriate marker in film corner adjacent to the olecranon.

Special Considerations: The selective visualization of the olecranon/trochlear joint compartment is useful in the detection of intra-articular loose bodies. Lead vinyl must be placed beneath the cassette to reduce primary and secondary radiation to the patient.

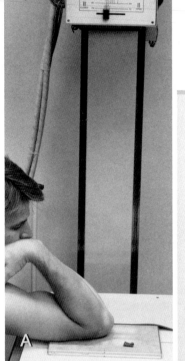
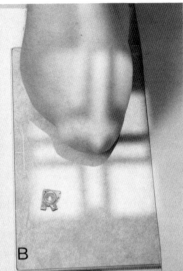

Figure 1.53A. Patient positioning.
Figure 1.53B. Collimation and central ray.

Normal Anatomy (Figure 1.53C)

1. Olecranon process.
2. Trochlea.
3. Head of the radius.
4. Neck of the radius.
5. Tuberosity, radius.
6. Medial epicondyle, humerus.
7. Olecranon fossa.
8. Ulnar groove.

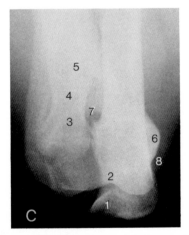

Figure 1.53C. Tangential elbow radiograph.

Basic
*Posteroanterior
Posteroanterior ulnar flexion
Medial oblique
Lateral

Wrist

**Posteroanterior Projection
Positioning**
(Figure 1.54A)

Optional
Carpal tunnel
Scaphoid
Lateral oblique (pisiform)

Demonstrates: Carpal bones and joints, distal radius and ulna. (1–4)

Measure: Posteroanterior at the level of the wrist.

kVp: 55 (50–60).

Film Size: 10 x 12 inches (24 x 30 cm) divided into quarters; the other quarters are used for the other basic projections.

Grid: No.

TFD: 40 inches (102 cm).

Tube Tilt: None.

Patient Position: Seated.

Part Position: Forearm pronated, with a loosely closed fist and the wrist flat on the film.

CR: To the midcarpal region.

Collimation: To the wrist (approximately 6 x 5 inches).

Side Marker: Appropriate marker at film corner.

Special Considerations: The closed fist allows closer wrist/film contact. Lead vinyl must be placed beneath the cassette to reduce primary and secondary radiation to the patient.

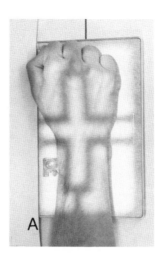

Figure 1.54A. Patient positioning, collimation, and central ray.

Normal Anatomy (Figure 1.54B and C)

1. Styloid process, radius.
2. Metaphysis, distal radius.
3. Metaphysis, distal ulna.
4. Styloid process, ulna.
5. Scaphoid.
6. Lunate.
7. Triquetrum.
8. Pisiform.
9. Trapezium.
10. Trapezoid.
11. Capitate.
12. Hamate.
13. Base, fifth metacarpal.
14. Shaft, fourth metacarpal.
15. Neck, third metacarpal.
16. Hook of the hamate.
17. Radioulnar joint.
18. Radiocarpal joint.
19. Ulnarcarpal joint.
20. Navicular fat stripe.

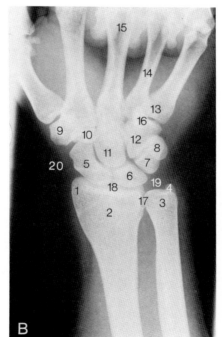

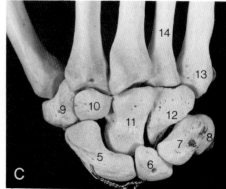

Figure 1.54B. Posteroanterior wrist radiograph.
Figure 1.54C. Anatomic specimen.

Basic
Posteroanterior
*Posteroanterior ulnar flexion
Medial oblique
Lateral

Wrist
**Posteroanterior Ulnar Flexion Projection
Positioning**
(Figure 1.55A)

Optional
Carpal tunnel
Scaphoid
Lateral oblique (pisiform)

Demonstrates: Carpal bones and joints, distal radius and ulna. (1–4) Especially good for assessing the scaphoid. (5,6)
Measure: Posteroanterior at the level of the wrist.
kVp: 55 (50–60).
Film Size: 10 x 12 inches (24 x 30 cm) divided into quarters; the other quarters are used for the other basic projections.
Grid: No.
TFD: 40 inches (102 cm).
Tube Tilt: None.
Patient Position: Seated.
Part Position: Forearm pronated, the wrist moved into ulnar deviation and placed flat on the film.
CR: To the midcarpal region.
Collimation: To the wrist (approximately 6 x 5 inches).
Side Marker: Appropriate marker at film corner.
Special Considerations: This view enhances visualization of scaphoid fractures by distracting the fracture fragments and widening the fracture line. Lead vinyl must be placed beneath the cassette to reduce primary and secondary radiation to the patient.

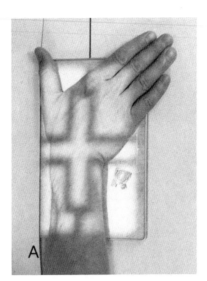

Figure 1.55A. Patient positioning, collimation, and central ray.

Normal Anatomy (Figure 1.55B)

1. Styloid process, radius.
2. Metaphysis, distal radius.
3. Metaphysis, distal ulna.
4. Styloid process, ulna.
5. Scaphoid.
6. Lunate.
7. Triquetrum.
8. Pisiform.
9. Trapezium.
10. Trapezoid.
11. Capitate.
12. Hamate.
13. Base, fifth metacarpal.
14. Shaft, fourth metacarpal.
15. Neck, third metacarpal.
16. Hook of the hamate.
17. Radioulnar joint.
18. Radiocarpal joint.
19. Ulnarcarpal joint.
20. Navicular fat stripe.

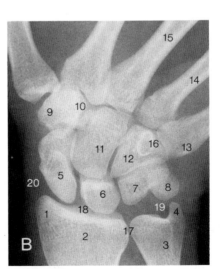

Figure 1.55B. Posteroanterior ulnar flexion wrist radiograph.

Wrist

**Medial Oblique Projection
Positioning**
(Figure 1.56A)

Demonstrates: Carpal bones and joints, distal radius and ulna. (1–4,7)

Measure: Laterally, between radial and ulnar styloid processes.

kVp: 55 (50–60).

Film Size: 10 x 12 inches (24 x 30 cm) divided into quarters; the other quarters are used for the other basic projections.

Grid: No.

TFD: 40 inches (102 cm).

Tube Tilt: None.

Patient Position: Seated.

Part Position: Forearm semipronated so the dorsum of the wrist is 45 degrees to the film (see oblique hand).

CR: To the midcarpal area.

Collimation: To the wrist (approximately 6 x 5 inches).

Side Marker: Appropriate marker at film corner.

Special Considerations: Lead vinyl must be placed beneath the cassette to reduce primary and secondary radiation to the patient.

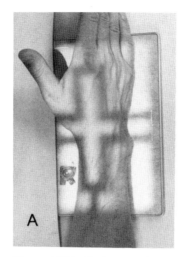

Figure 1.56A. Patient positioning, collimation, and central ray.

Normal Anatomy (Figure 1.56B and C)

1. Styloid process, radius.
2. Metaphysis, distal radius.
3. Metaphysis, distal ulna.
4. Styloid process, ulna.
5. Scaphoid.
6. Lunate.
7. Triquetrum.
8. Pisiform.
9. Trapezium.
10. Trapezoid.
11. Capitate.
12. Hamate.
13. Base, fifth metacarpal.
14. Shaft, fourth metacarpal.
15. Shaft, first metacarpal.
16. Radioulnar joint.
17. Radiocarpal joint.
18. Ulnarcarpal joint.
19. Navicular fat stripe.

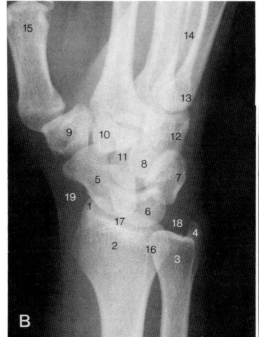

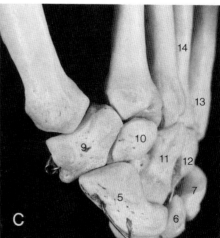

Figure 1.56B. Oblique wrist radiograph.
Figure 1.56C. Anatomic specimen.

Basic
Posteroanterior
Posteroanterior ulnar flexion
Medial oblique
*Lateral

Wrist

**Lateral Projection
Positioning**
(Figure 1.57A)

Optional
Carpal tunnel
Scaphoid
Lateral oblique (pisiform)

Demonstrates: Carpal bones, distal radius and ulna. (1–4)

Measure: Laterally, between the radial and ulnar styloids.

kVp: 55 (50–60).

Film Size: 10 x 12 inches (24 x 30 cm) divided into quarters; the other quarters are used for the other basic projections.

Grid: No.

TFD: 40 inches (102 cm).

Tube Tilt: None.

Patient Position: Seated.

Part Position: Forearm is in true lateral projection.

CR: To the midcarpal area.

Collimation: To the wrist (approximately 6 x 5 inches).

Side Marker: Appropriate marker at film corner.

Special Considerations: This view is especially useful in determining the relationships of the carpal bones (especially the lunate) and distal radius following trauma. Lead vinyl must be placed beneath the cassette to reduce primary and secondary radiation to the patient.

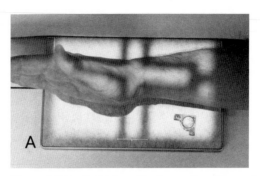

Figure 1.57A. Patient positioning, collimation, and central ray.

Normal Anatomy (Figure 1.57B)

1. Posterior lip, radius.
2. Anterior lip, radius.
3. Styloid process, ulna.
4. Shaft of the ulna.
5. Shaft of the radius.
6. Lunate.
7. Capitate.
8. Scaphoid.
9. Pisiform.
10. Trapezium.
11. Base, first metacarpal.
12. Fatline, pronator quadratus (arrow).

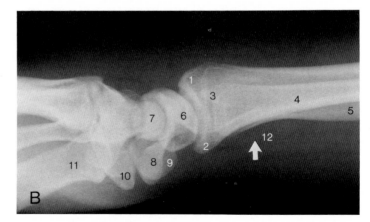

Figure 1.57B. Lateral wrist radiograph.

Hand
Posteroanterior Projection
Positioning
(Figure 1.58A)

Demonstrates: Carpals, metacarpals, phalanges, and joints. (1–3)
Measure: Posteroanterior through metacarpals.
kVp: 55 (50–60).
Film Size: 8 x 10 inches (18 x 24 cm).
Grid: No.
TFD: 40 inches (102 cm).
Tube Tilt: None.
Patient Position: Seated.
Part Position: Hand is placed palm down on the film.
CR: Third metacarpal head.
Collimation: To hand size.
Side Marker: Appropriate marker at film corner adjacent to the little finger.
Special Considerations: Lead vinyl must be placed beneath the cassette to reduce primary and secondary radiation to the patient.

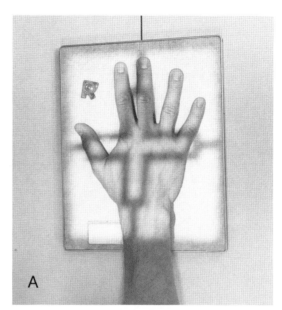

Figure 1.58A. Patient positioning, collimation, and central ray.

Normal Anatomy (Figure 1.58B and C)

1. Styloid process, radius.
2. Metaphysis, radius.
3. Metaphysis, ulna.
4. Styloid process, ulna.
5. Scaphoid.
6. Lunate.
7. Triquetrum.
8. Pisiform.
9. Trapezium.
10. Trapezoid.
11. Capitate.
12. Hamate.
13. Base, second metacarpal.
14. Shaft, third metacarpal.
15. Neck, fourth metacarpal.
16. Head, fifth metacarpal.
17. Metacarpophalangeal joint.
18. Proximal phalanx.
19. Middle phalanx.
20. Distal phalanx.
21. Sesamoid bones (flexor pollicus brevis, adductor pollicus).
22. Distal (ungual) tuft.
23. Vallecula, metacarpal head.
24. Styloid process, third metacarpal.

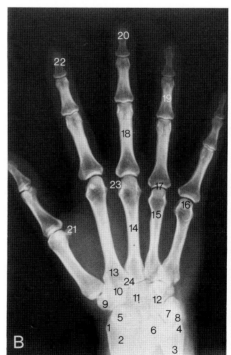
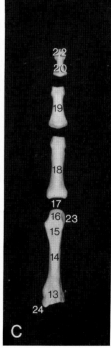

Figure 1.58B. Posteroanterior hand radiograph.
Figure 1.58C. Anatomic specimen.

Hand
**Oblique Projection
Positioning**
(Figure 1.59A)

Demonstrates: Carpals, metacarpals, phalanges, and joints. (1–4)
Measure: Through the CR.
kVp: 55 (50–60).
Film Size: 8 x 10 inches (18 x 24 cm).
Grid: No.
TFD: 40 inches (102 cm).
Tube Tilt: None.
Patient Position: Seated.
Part Position: Hand is semipronated to be 45 degrees to the film. For stability, the fingers are flexed to touch the film and be projected free from each other (see oblique wrist) or may be placed on a foam rubber positioning aid.
CR: Between the second and third metacarpal heads.
Collimation: To hand size.
Side Marker: Appropriate marker at film corner adjacent to the little finger.
Special Considerations: Lead vinyl must be placed beneath the cassette to reduce primary and secondary radiation to the patient.

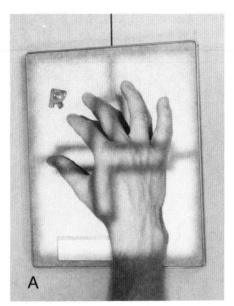

Figure 1.59A. Patient positioning, collimation, and central ray.

Normal Anatomy (Figure 1.59B)

1. Styloid process, radius.
2. Metaphysis, radius.
3. Metaphysis, ulna.
4. Styloid process, ulna.
5. Scaphoid.
6. Lunate.
7. Triquetrum.
8. Pisiform.
9. Trapezium.
10. Trapezoid.
11. Capitate.
12. Hamate.
13. Base, second metacarpal.
14. Shaft, third metacarpal.
15. Neck, fourth metacarpal.
16. Head, fifth metacarpal.
17. Metacarpophalangeal joint.
18. Proximal phalanx.
19. Middle phalanx.
20. Distal phalanx.
21. Sesamoid bones (flexor pollicus brevis, adductor pollicus).

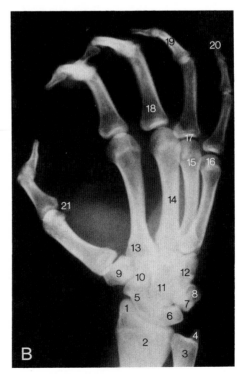

Figure 1.59B. Oblique hand radiograph.

Fingers
Posteroanterior, Oblique, and Lateral Projections
Positioning
(Figure 1.60A–C)

Basic
*Posteroanterior
*Oblique
*Lateral

Demonstrates: Phalanges, metacarpal heads, and interphalangeal joints. (1–4)
Measure: At metacarpal head.
kVp: 55 (50–60).
Film Size: 8 x 10 inches (18 x 24 cm) divided into thirds; the other divisions are used for the other basic views.
Grid: No.
TFD: 40 inches (102 cm).
Tube Tilt: None.
Patient Position: Seated.
Part Position: (1) *Posteroanterior*: Hand prone, with affected finger centered. (Fig. 1.60A) (2) *Oblique*: Hand semiprone to 45 degrees with the film, fingers slightly flexed and spread apart. (3) *Lateral*: Hand in true lateral position, affected finger extended and the remaining fingers flexed. (Fig. 1.60C)
CR: At the proximal interphalangeal joint.
Collimation: To include only the affected digit.
Side Marker: Appropriate marker in film corner adjacent to fingertip.
Special Considerations: In lateral projection the finger should be parallel to the film to adequately show the interphalangeal joints and small chip fractures. Lead vinyl must be placed beneath the cassette to reduce primary and secondary radiation to the patient.

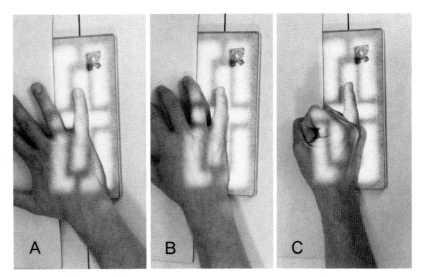

Figure 1.60A. Patient positioning anteroposterior, collimation and central ray.
Figure 1.60B. Patient positioning oblique, collimation and central ray.
Figure 1.60C. Patient positioning lateral, collimation and central ray.

Normal Anatomy (Figure 1.60D–G)

1. Distal (ungual) tuft.
2. Distal phalanx.
3. Distal interphalangeal joint.
4. Middle phalanx.
5. Proximal interphalangeal joint.
6. Proximal phalanx.
7. Metacarpophalangeal joint.
8. Head metacarpal.
9. Vallecula.
10. Neck, metacarpal.
11. Shaft, metacarpal.
12. Base, metacarpal.

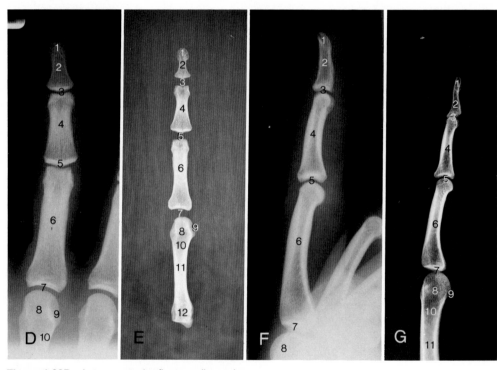

Figure 1.60D. Anteroposterior finger radiograph.
Figure 1.60E. Specimen radiograph anteroposterior.
Figure 1.60F. Lateral finger radiograph.
Figure 1.60G. Specimen radiograph lateral.

Basic
*Anteroposterior
*Lateral

Thumb
Anteroposterior and Lateral Projection Positioning
(Figure 1.61A and B)

Optional
Oblique

54 KV
100 5 @ 40
36"

Demonstrates: Phalanges, first metacarpal, trapezium, scaphoid, and intervening joints. (1–4)
Measure: At the metacarpophalangeal joint.
kVp: 55 (50–60).
Film Size: 8 x 10 inches (18 x 24 cm) divided into halves.
Grid: No.
TFD: 40 inches (102 cm).
Tube Tilt: None.
Patient Position: Seated.
Part Position: (1) *Anteroposterior*: The hand is rotated internally until the posterior surface of the thumb contacts the film. (Fig 1.61A) (2) *Lateral*: The hand is placed prone and the thumb brought to a lateral position. This is assisted by slightly flexing the metacarpophalangeal joints. (Fig. 1.61B)
CR: Through the first metacarpophalangeal joint.
Collimation: To thumb size.
Side Marker: Appropriate marker at film corner adjacent to thumb tip.

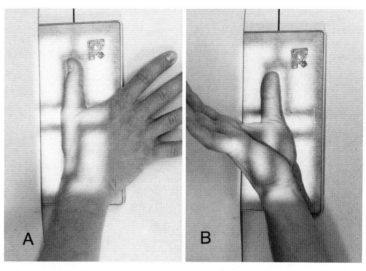

Figure 1.61A. Patient positioning anteroposterior, collimation and central ray.
Figure 1.61B. Patient positioning lateral, collimation and central ray.

Normal Anatomy (Figure 1.61C–E)

1. Distal (ungual) tuft.
2. Distal phalanx.
3. Distal interphalangeal joint.
4. Proximal phalanx.
5. Metacarpophalangeal joint.
6. Metacarpal head.
7. Metacarpal shaft.
8. Metacarpal base.
9. Trapezium.
10. Sesamoid bones (flexor pollicus brevis, adductor pollicus).

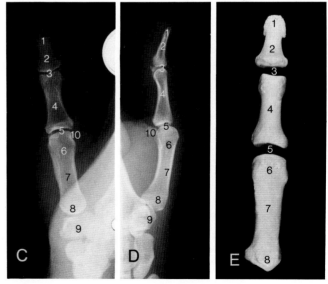

Figure 1.61C. Posteroanterior thumb radiograph.
Figure 1.61D. Lateral thumb radiograph.
Figure 1.61E. Anatomic specimen.

Basic
***Anteroposterior or Posteroanterior
    (above or below diaphragm)**
Anterior oblique (45-degree)
Posterior oblique (45-degree)

Ribs

**Anteroposterior and
Posteroanterior Projections
Positioning**
(Figure 1.62A)

Demonstrates: Ribs, anterior and posterior. (1–5)

Measure: Anteroposterior chest at CR.

kVp: 80 (75–85) (low for ribs above diaphragm; high for ribs below diaphragm).

Film Size: 14 x 17 inches (35 x 43 cm).

Grid: Yes.

TFD: 40 inches (102 cm).

Tube Tilt: None.

Patient Position: Upright or recumbent.

Part Position: (1) *Anteroposterior*: If rib lesion is posterior, centered to bucky. (2) *Posteroanterior*: If rib lesion is anterior, centered to bucky.

CR: To the area of complaint.

Collimation: To the film.

Side Marker: Appropriate marker at film corner.

Breathing Instructions: Above diaphragm rib projection, suspended full inspiration. Below diaphragm rib projection, suspended full expiration.

Special Considerations: Multiple oblique views at varying angles may be necessary to demonstrate rib fractures. If the suspected lesion is located anteriorly, the obliques are taken PA; if posterior, they are taken anteroposterior. Due to normal overlying anatomy the positioning, exposure, and interpretation of rib radiographs is extremely difficult. It is recommended that these patients be referred to a radiology specialist for the production and evaluation of rib radiographs.

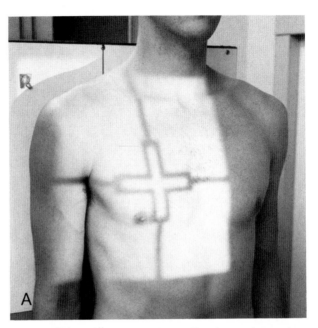

Figure 1.62A. Patient positioning, collimation, and central ray.

Normal Anatomy (Figure 1.62B–D)

1. Anterior rib.
2. Posterior rib.
3. Rib tubercle.
4. Costotransverse joint.
5. Rib head.
6. Transverse process.
7. Superior angle, scapula.
8. Distal clavicle.
9. Transverse aorta.
10. Pulmonary artery.
11. Peripheral pulmonary vessel.
12. Heart.

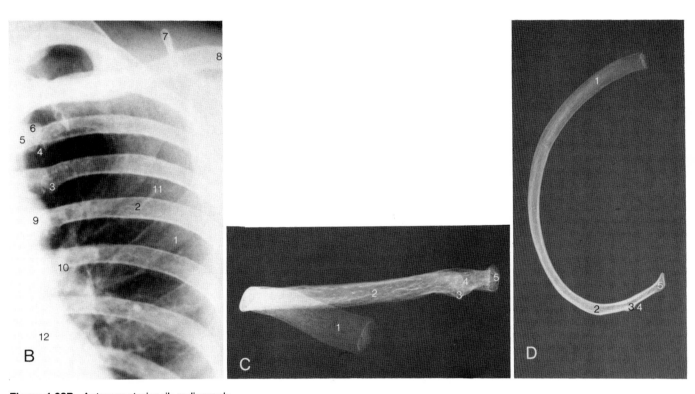

Figure 1.62B. Anteroposterior rib radiograph.
Figure 1.62C. Specimen radiograph.
Figure 1.62D. Specimen radiograph.

Chest
Posteroanterior Projection
Positioning
(Figure 1.63A and B)

Demonstrates: Lung fields, heart, great vessels, ribs, shoulder girdles, thoracic spine, and upper abdomen. (1–4)

Measure: Anteroposterior at greatest diameter in full, deep inspiration.

kVp: 110 (100-120).

Film Size: 14 x 17 inches (35 x 43 cm).

Grid: No.

TFD: 72 inches (183 cm).

Tube Tilt: None.

Patient Position: Upright.

Part Position: Posteroanterior, chin elevated, hands placed over buttocks, and shoulders rolled forward. Thoracic spine centered to the midline of the bucky. Cassette positioned so that its superior border is 2 inches above the shoulders.

CR: To the film.

Collimation: To the film.

Side Marker: Appropriate marker in film corner above shoulder.

Breathing Instructions: Suspended deep inspiration.

Special Considerations: To evaluate if a full inspiratory breath has been achieved, seven anterior ribs or ten posterior ribs should be visible above the diaphragm. Rotational malposition is assessed by the relative positions of the medial clavicles to the thoracic spine. Expiration chest radiography is a useful supplemental view when evaluating for a small, subtle pneumothorax.

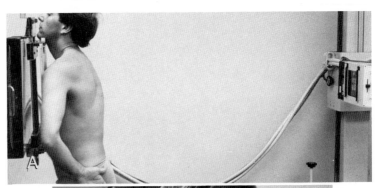

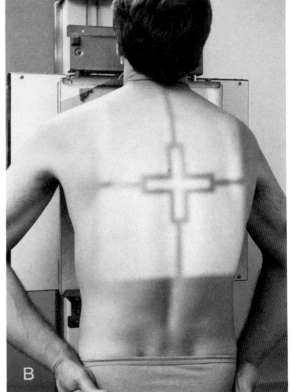

Figure 1.63A. Patient positioning.
Figure 1.63B. Collimation and central ray.

Normal Anatomy (Figure 1.63C)

1. Right atrial border.
2. Left ventricular border.
3. Left atrial border.
4. Pulmonary trunk.
5. Transverse aorta (aortic knob).
6. Ascending aorta.
7. Left pulmonary hilus.
8. Right pulmonary hilus.
9. Right pulmonary vessel.
10. Right cardiophrenic angle.
11. Left cardiophrenic angle.
12. Right costophrenic angle.
13. Left costophrenic angle.
14. Right apex.
15. Breast.
16. Right hemidiaphragm.
17. Left hemidiaphragm.
18. Liver.
19. Gastric air bubble (magenblasse).
20. Humeral head.
21. Axillary border, scapula.
22. Coracoid process, scapula.
23. Acromion, scapula.
24. Superior angle, scapula.
25. Clavicle.
26. Spinous process, T2.
27. Tracheal air shadow.
28. Manubrium.
29. Thoracic spine.

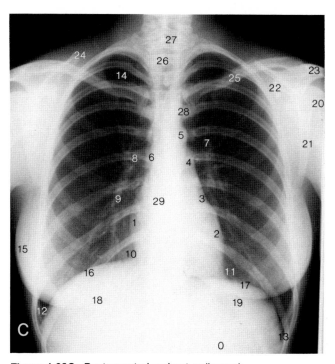

Figure 1.63C. Posteroanterior chest radiograph.

Chest

Lateral Projection
Positioning
(Figure 1.64A)

Demonstrates: Lung fields, heart, great vessels, ribs, sternum, and thoracic spine. (5–7)

Measure: Transversely, under the axilla, at the T6 level.

kVp: 110 (100–120).

Film Size: 14 x 17 inches (35 x 43 cm).

Grid: No.

TFD: 72 inches (183 cm).

Tube Tilt: None.

Patient Position: Upright.

Part Position: Left lateral position, with no rotation. Both arms elevated and crossed on top of the head. Cassette position is 2 inches above the shoulders.

CR: To the film.

Collimation: To patient size.

Side Marker: Left marker placed anterior to the sternum or behind the upper thoracic spine.

Breathing Instructions: Suspended deep inspiration.

Special Considerations: Left laterals are routinely performed to reduce cardiac magnification.

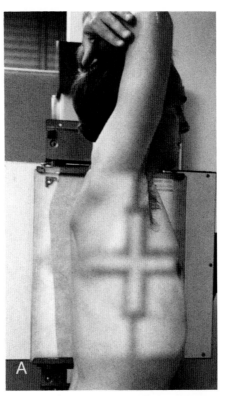

Figure 1.64A. Patient positioning, collimation, and central ray.

Normal Anatomy (Figure 1.64B)

 1. Right ventricular border.
 2. Ascending aorta.
 3. Aortic arch.
 4. Descending aorta.
 5. Left atrial border.
 6. Left ventricular border.
 7. Hilus.
 8. Pulmonary vessels.
 9. Retrosternal space.
10. Retrocardiac space.
11. Body of sternum.
12. Manubriosternal joint.
13. Manubrium.
14. Axillary borders, scapulae.
15. Vertebral body.
16. Intervertebral foramen.
17. Posterior rib.
18. Spinous process.
19. Trachea.
20. Diaphragm.
21. Posterior costophrenic sulcus.
22. Breast shadow.

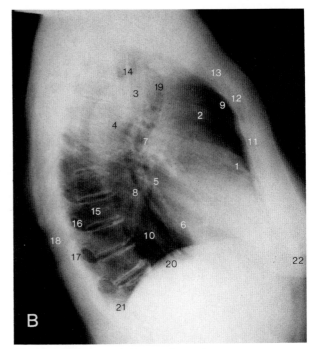

Figure 1.64B. Lateral chest radiograph.

Basic
Posteroanterior
Lateral

Chest

Lordotic Projection Positioning
(Figure 1.65A–C)

Optional
***Lordotic**
Oblique

Demonstrates: Lung apices, right middle lobe and lingular segments. (8–11)
Measure: Through the CR.
kVp: 110 (100–20).
Film Size: 14 x 17 inches (35 x 43 cm).
Grid: No.
TFD: (1) 72 inches (183 cm); no tilt; (2) 72 inches (must correct for tube tilt).
Tube Tilt: (1) No tilt. (2) 30 degrees cephalad.
Patient Position: Upright.
Part Position: (1) *Anteroposterior Patient Tilt*: Patient stands one foot from the bucky and leans back, with shoulders, neck, and back of the head. (Fig. 1.65A) (2) *Anteroposterior Tube Tilt*: Alternatively, the patient stands straight upright and the tube is angled cephalad 30 degrees. The film is placed 2 inches above the shoulders. (Fig. 1.65B and C)
CR: To the film.
Collimation: To the film.
Side Marker: Appropriate marker at film corner above the shoulder.
Breathing Instructions: Suspended full inspiration.
Special Considerations: This is an optional view utilized in the evaluation of lung disease involving the apices, middle lobe, and lingula. (12,13)

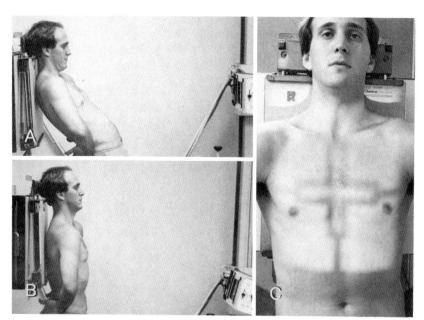

Figure 1.65A. Patient positioning Anteroposterior patient tilt.
Figure 1.65B. Patient positioning Anteroposterior tube tilt.
Figure 1.65C. Collimation and central ray.

Normal Anatomy (Figure 1.65D)

1. Left ventricular border.
2. Left pulmonary vessels.
3. Aortic arch (aortic knob).
4. Superior vena cava.
5. Right pulmonary vessels.
6. Posterior rib.
7. Axillary border, scapula.
8. Coracoid process.
9. Humeral head.
10. Clavicle.
11. C6 vertebral body.

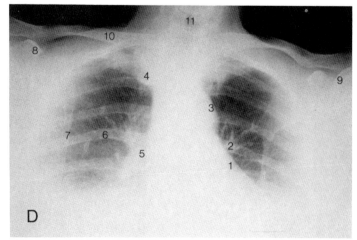

Figure 1.65D. Lordotic chest radiograph.

Abdomen
Anteroposterior (KUB) Projection
Positioning
(Figure 1.66A and B)

Demonstrates: Kidneys, urinary bladder, liver, spleen, large bowel, psoas shadow, pelvis, lumbar spine, and lower ribs. (1–4)

Measure: At the iliac crests.

kVp: (1) 70 (65–75) for calcific densities; (2) 100 (95–105) for soft tissue detail.

Film Size: 14 x 17 inches (35 x 43 cm).

Grid: Yes.

TFD: 40 inches (102 cm).

Tube Tilt: None.

Patient Position: Supine.

Part Position: Spine positioned to the midline.

CR: At the top of the iliac crests.

Collimation: To film size.

Side Marker: Appropriate marker in top corner of film.

Breathing Instructions: Suspended expiration.

Special Considerations: Obese patients should be examined posteroanterior to compress the body tissues and decrease the time of exposure. Exceptionally tall patients may be exposed during a deep inspiration to ensure the abdominal contents from diaphragm to pubic symphysis are included on the radiograph.

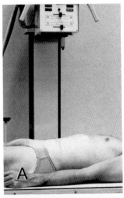

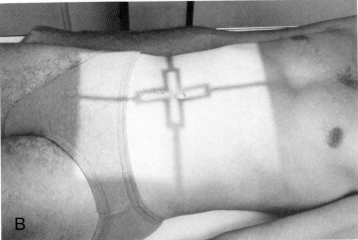

Figure 1.66A. Patient positioning.
Figure 1.66B. Collimation and central ray.

Normal Anatomy (Figure 1.66C)

1. Liver.
2. Right kidney.
3. Gas in splenic flexure.
4. Solid feces in colon.
5. Semifluid feces in colon.
6. Haustra, descending colon.
7. Psoas margin.
8. Flank stripe.
9. T12 vertebral body.
10. Sacral ala.
11. Sacroiliac joint.
12. Iliac fossa.
13. Iliac crest.
14. Anterior superior iliac spine (ASIS).
15. Femoral head.
16. Inferior edge of the acetabular fossa (Kohler's teardrop).
17. Symphysis pubis.
18. Superior pubic ramus.

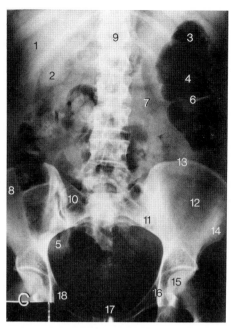

Figure 1.66C. Anteroposterior abdominal radiograph (KUB).

REFERENCES

Introduction

1. Roentgen WC: Üeber eine neue Art von Strahlen. Part I, Sitzungsber, phys-med. Gesellsch, Würzburg, 1895. English translation in *Science*, February, 1896.
2. Grigg ERN: *The Trail of the Invisible Light*, Springfield, Charles C. Thomas, 1965.
3. Eastman TR: History of radiographic technique. *Appl Radiol* 7:97, 1978.
4. Clark KC: *Positioning in Radiography*, ed 9, vol I and II, London, Ilford Limited, William Heinemann Medical Books, 1974.
5. Merrill V: *Atlas of Roentgenographic Positions and Standard Radiologic Procedures*, ed 4, vol I, II, and III, St. Louis, CV Mosby, 1975.
6. Meschan I: *An Atlas of Anatomy Basic to Radiology*, Philadelphia, Lea & Febiger, 1975.
7. Meschan I: *Radiographic Positioning and Related Anatomy*, ed 2, Philadelphia, WB Saunders, 1978.
8. Christensen E, Curry T, Dowdey J: *An Introduction to the Physics of Diagnostic Radiology*, ed 2, Philadelphia, Lea & Febiger, 1978.
9. Eastman TR: Technique charts: The key to radiographic quality. *Radiol Technol* 46:365, 1975.
10. Sherman R, Bauer F: *X-Ray X-Pertise—From A-X*. Ft. Worth, Parker Chiropractic Research Foundation, 1982.
11. Howe JW, Yochum TR: X-ray, pregnancy, and therapeutic abortion: A current perspective. *ACA J Chiro*, April 1985.
12. Gonad shielding in diagnostic radiology. *Bureau of Radiological Health*, Rockville MD, Pub No. (FDA) 75-8024, 1975.
13. Warwick R, Williams PL: *Gray's Anatomy*, ed 35 (British), Philadelphia, WB Saunders, 1973.

Skull

1. Taveras J, Wood E: *Diagnostic Neuroradiology*, ed 2, vol 1, Baltimore, Williams & Wilkins, 1976.
2. Weathers RM, Lee A: Radiologic examination of the skull. *Radiol Clin North Am* 12:215, 1974.
3. Potts DG: A system of skull radiography. *Radiology* 94:25, 1970.
4. Masters SJ: Evaluation of head trauma: Efficacy of skull films. *AJR* 135:539, 1980.
5. Potter GD, Gold RP: Radiographic analaysis of the skull. *Med Radiogr Photogr* 51:2, 1975.

Paranasal Sinuses

1. Macmillan AS Jr: Techniques in paranasal sinus radiography, *Semin Roentgenol* 3:115, 1968.
2. Yanagisawa E, Smith HW: Normal radiographic anatomy of the paranasal sinuses. *Otolaryngol Clin North Am* 6:429, 1973.
3. Waters CA: A modification of the occipitofrontal position in roentgen examination of the accessory nasal sinuses. *Arch Radiol Ther* 20:15, 1915.
4. Spillman R: Early history of roentgenology of the sinuses. *AJR* 54:643, 1945.

Cervical Spine

1. Christenson PC: The radiologic study of the normal spine. Cervical, thoracic, lumbar, and sacral. *Radiol Clin North Am* 15:133, 1977.
2. Bumstead HD: Routine examination of the cervical spine. *Xray Techn* 27:247, 1955.
3. Hadley LA: Roentgenographic studies of the cervical spine. *AJR* 52:173, 1944.
4. DeLuca SA, Rhea JA: Radiographic anatomy of the cervical vertebrae. *Med Radiogr Photogr* 56:18, 1980.
5. Apuzzo, ML, Weiss MH, Heiden JS: Transoral exposure of the atlantoaxial region. *Neurosurg* 3:201, 1978.
6. George AW: Method for more accurate study of injuries to the atlas and axis. *Boston Med Surg J* 181:395, 1919.
7. Ottonello P: New method for roentgenography of the entire cervical spine in ventrodorsal projection. *Rev Radiol Fis Med* 2:291, 1930.
8. Jacobs LG: Roentgenography of the second cervical vertebra by Ottonello's method. *Radiology* 31:412, 1938.
9. Hinck VC, Hopkins CE: Measurement of the atlanto-dental interval in the adult. *AJR* 84:945, 1960.
10. Penning L: Prevertebral hematoma in cervical spine injury. Incidence and etiologic significance. *AJR* 136:553, 1981.
11. Marks JL, Parks SL: A simplified position for demonstrating the cervical intervertebral foramina. *AJR* 63:575, 1950.
12. Boylston BF: Oblique roentgenographic views of the cervical spine in flexion and extension: An aid in the diagnosis of cervical subluxations and obscure dislocations. *J Bone Joint Surg (Am)* 39:1302, 1957.
13. Weir DC: Roentgenographic signs of cervical injury. *Clin Orthop* 109:9, 1975.
14. Miller MD, Gehweiler JA, Martinez S, et al: Significant new observations on cervical spine trauma. *AJR* 130:659, 1978.
15. Davis AG: Injuries of the cervical spine. *JAMA* 127 (3):149, 1945.
16. Hagen DE: Introduction to the pillar projection of the cervical spine. *Radiol Technol* 35:239, 1964.
17. Smith GR, Abel MS: Visualization of the posterolateral elements of the upper cervical vertebrae in the anteroposterior projection. *Radiology* 115:219, 1975.

Thoracic Spine

1. Christenson PC: The radiologic study of the normal spine. Cervical, thoracic, lumbar, and sacral. *Radiol Clin North Am* 15:133, 1977.
2. Fuchs AW: Thoracic vertebrae. *Radiogr Clin Photogr* 17:2, 1941.
3. Scher AT: The diagnostic value of the anteroposterior radiograph for thoracolumbar injuries. *S Afr Med J* 58:415, 1980.
4. Guerreiro, G: Lateral roentgenographic examination of the thoracic spine. *J Bone Joint Surg (Am)* 32:192, 1950.
5. Clarke EK: Visualization of the first and second dorsal and the fifth lumbar vertebrae in lateral or slightly semilateral positions. *X-Ray Techn* 12:5, 1940.
6. Scher A, Vambeck V: An approach to the radiological examination of the cervicodorsal junction following injury. *Clin Radiol* 28:243, 1977.

Lumbar Spine

1. Cornwell WS: Lumbar vertebrae. *Radiogr Clin Photogr* 18:2, 1942.
2. Cornwell WS: Some aspects of radiography of the lumbar vertebrae. *X-Ray Techn* 14:77, 1942.
3. Scavone JG: Latshaw RF, Weidner WA: Anteroposterior and lateral radiographs: An adequate lumbar spine examination. *AJR* 136:715, 1981.
4. Abel MS, Smith GR: Visualization of the posterolateral elements of the lumbar vertebrae in the anteroposterior projection. *Radiology* 122:824, 1977.
5. Hickey PM: Lateral roentgenology of the spine. *AJR* 4:101, 1917.
6. Boyland KG: True lateral positioning of the lumbar spine and pelvis. *Radiography* 13:44, 1947.
7. Etter LE, Carabello NC: Roentgen anatomy of oblique views of the lumbar spine. *AJR* 61:699, 1949.
8. Brown RC, Evans ET: What causes the "eye in the scotty dog" in the oblique projection of the lumbar spine? *AJR* 118:435, 1972.
9. Ferguson AB: The clinical and roentgenographic interpretation of lumbosacral anomalies. *Radiology* 22:548, 1934.
10. Horowitz T, Smith MR: An anatomical, pathological, and roentgenological study of the intervertebral joints of the lumbar spine and of the sacroiliac joints. *AJR* 43:173, 1940.
11. Logroscino D: Das hüftgelenk und das sakroiliakalgelenk in günstiger röntgenographischer projektion. *Röntgenpraxis* 8:433, 1936.
12. Darling BC: The sacroiliac joint: Its diagnosis as determined by x-ray. *Radiology* 3:486, 1924.
13. Kamieth H: What do spot films of the sacroiliac joint accomplish? Pathology of the sacroiliac joint. *Radiol Clin* 26:139, 1957.
14. Johannsen A, Jepsen OL, Winge J: Radiological and scintigraphical examination of the sacroiliac joints in the diagnosis of sacroiliitis. *Dan Med Bull* 21:246, 1974.
15. Resnick D, Niwayama G, Goergen T: Comparison of abnormalities of the sacroiliac joint in degenerative disease and ankylosing spondylitis. *AJR* 128:189, 1977.
16. William PC, Wigby PE: Technique for the roentgen examination of the lumbosacral articulation. *AJR* 33:511, 1935.
17. Curran JT: New approach to positioning for lumbosacral junction in lateral projection. *Radiol Technol* 46:294, 1975.
18. Eisenberg RL, Akin JR, Hedgcock MW: Single, well-centered lateral view of lumbosacral spine: Is coned view necessary? *AJR* 133:711, 1979.

Sacrum

1. Christenson PC: The radiologic study of the normal spine. Cervical, thoracic, lumbar, and sacral. *Radiol Clin North Am* 15:133, 1977.
2. Hoing M: A new technic of coccyxography. *Xray Techn* 7:68, 1935.
3. Zochert RW: The sacrum and coccyx: Location and technic for radiography. *Xray Techn* 4:118, 1933.
4. Turner ML, Mulhern CB, and Dalinka MK: Lesions of the sacrum: Differential diagnosis and radiological evaluation. *JAMA* 245:275, 1981.
5. Amorosa JK, Wintraub S, Amorosa LF, et al: Sacral destruction: Foraminal lines revisited. *AJR* 145:773, 1985.

Coccyx

1. Christenson PC: The radiologic study of the normal spine. Cervical, thoracic, lumbar, and sacral. *Radiol Clin North Am* 15:133, 1977.
2. Hoing M: A new technic of coccyxography. *Xray Techn* 7:68, 1935.
3. Zochert RW: The sacrum and coccyx: Location and technic for radiography. *Xray Techn* 4:118, 1933.

Pelvis

1. Bridgman CF: Radiography of the hip bone. *Med Radiogr Photogr* 28:38, 1952.
2. Liliequist B: Roentgenologic examination of the acetabular part of the os coxae. *Acta Radiol (Diagn)* 4:289, 1966.
3. Armbuster TG, et al: The adult hip: An anatomic study. Part I: The bony landmarks. *Radiology* 128:1, 1978.
4. Katz JF: Precise identification of radiographic acetabular landmarks. *Clin Orthop* 141:166, 1979.
5. Bowerman JW, Sena JM, Chang R: The teardrop shadow of the pelvis: Anatomy and clinical significance. *Radiology* 143:659, 1982.
6. Mitton KL, Auringer EM: Roentgenological study of the femoral neck. *AJR* 66:639, 1951.

Full Spine

1. Farren J: Routine radiographic assessment of the scoliotic spine. *Radiography* 47 (556):92, 1981.
2. Davies WG: Radiography in the treatment of scoliosis and in leg lengthening. Part II—Radiography in scoliosis. *Radiography* 26 (311):349, 1960.
3. Sausser WL: Achievement—Entire body x-ray technic perfected. *ACA J Chiro* 4 (2):17, 1935.
4. Young LW, Oestreich AE, Goldstein LA: Roentgenology in scoliosis: Contribution to evaluation and management. *AJR* 108:778, 1970.
5. Field TJ, Buehler MT: Improvements in chiropractic full spine radiography. *J Manip Physiol Ther* 4:21, 1981.
6. Cartwright PH: The Baulin filtration system: Its effectiveness in patient dose control in chiropractic radiography. Christchurch, NZ: *National Radiation Laboratory, Report NRL 1980/12, 1982.*
7. Merkin JJ, Sportelli L: The effects of two new compensating filters on patient exposure in chiropractic full spine radiography. *J Manip Physiol Ther* 5:25, 1982.

8. Gray JE, Hoffman AD, Peterson NA: Reduction of radiation exposure during radiography for scoliosis. *J Bone Joint Surg (Am)* 65:5, 1983.
9. Bhatnagar JP: X-ray doses to patients undergoing full-spine radiographic examination. *Radiology* 138:231, 1981.

Hip

1. Bridgman CF: Radiography of the hip joint. *Med Radiogr Photogr* 26:2, 1950.
2. Bridgman CF: Radiography of the hip joint. *Med Radiogr Photogr* 27:2, 1951.
3. Bridgman, CF: Radiography of the hip bone. *Med Radiogr Photogr* 28:38, 1952.
4. Hooper AC, Ormond DJ: A radiographic study of hip rotation. *Ir J Med Sci* 144:25, 1975.
5. Armbuster TG, et al: The adult hip: An anatomic study. Part I: The bony landmarks. *Radiology* 128:1, 1978.
6. Mitton KL, Auringer EM: Roentgenological study of the femoral neck. *AJR* 66:639, 1951.

Knee

1. Larsen RM: Radiography of extremities. *Xray Techn* 12:215, 1941.
2. Harris J: Radiography of the lower limb. *Radiography* 31:235, 1965.
3. Funke T: Radiography of the knee joint. *Med Radiogr Photogr* 36:1, 1960.
4. Leach RE, Gregg T, Ferris JS: Weight-bearing radiography in osteoarthritis of the knee. *Radiology* 97:265, 1970.
5. Thomas R, Resnick D, Alazraki N, et al: Compartmental evaluation of osteoarthritis of the knee: A comparative study of available diagnostic modalities. *Radiology* 116:585, 1975.
6. Vaughan FMA: Lateral knees. *Radiography* 16:75, 1950.
7. Alexander OM: Routine lateral radiography of the knee and ankle joints. *Radiography* 17:10, 1951.
8. Camp JD, Coventry MB: Use of special views in roentgenography of the knee joint. *US Naval Med Bull* 42:56, 1944.
9. Holmblad EC: Postero-anterior x-ray view of the knee in flexion. *JAMA* 109:1196, 1937.
10. Settegast: Typische roentgenbilder von normalen menschen. *Lahmanns Med Atlanten* 5:211, 1921.
11. Hughston JC: Subluxation of the patella. *J Bone Joint Surg (Am)* 50:1003, 1968.
12. Laurin CA, Dussault R, Levesque HP: The tangential x-ray investigation of the patello-femoral joint: X-ray technique, diagnostic criteria, and their interpretation. *Clin Orthop* 144:16, 1979.
13. Wiberg G: Roentgenographic and anatomic studies on the femoropatellar joint. *Acta Orthop Scand* 12:319, 1941.

Ankle

1. Larsen RM: Radiography of extremities. *Xray Techn* 12:215, 1941.
2. Harris J: Radiography of the lower limb. *Radiography* 31:235, 1965.
3. Goergen TG, Danzig LA, Resnick D, et al: Roentgenographic evaluation of the tibiotalar joint. *J Bone Joint Surg (Am)* 59:874, 1977.
4. Thompson JP, Loomer RL: Osteochondral lesions of the talus in a sports medicine clinic. A new radiographic technique and surgical approach. *Am J Sports Med* 12 (6):460, 1984.
5. Hutter CG Jr, Scott W: Tibial torsion. *J Bone Joint Surg (Am)* 31:511, 1949.
6. Alexander OM: Routine lateral radiography of the knee and ankle joints. *Radiography* 17:10, 1951.
7. Mandell J: Isolated fracture of the posterior tibial lip at the ankle as demonstrated by an additional projection, the "poor" lateral view. *Radiology* 101:319, 1971.

Foot

1. Larsen RM: Radiography of extremities. *Xray Techr* 12:215, 1941.
2. Harris J: Radiography of the lower limb. *Radiography* 31:235, 1965.
3. Meschan I: Radiology of the normal foot. *Semin Roentgenol* 5:327, 1970.
4. Graham D, Rorrison J: Radiography of the tarsal bones. *Radiography* 28:156, 1962.
5. Santora PJ: Anteroposterior view of the ankle joint and foot. *AJR* 45:127, 1941.
6. Piotrowski Brother D: Oblique view of the ankle joint and foot. *AJR* 45:127, 1938.

Toes

1. Larsen RM: Radiography of extremities. *Xray Techn* 12:215, 1941.
2. Harris J: Radiography of the lower limb. *Radiography* 31:235, 1965.
3. Meschan I: Radiology of the normal foot. *Semin Roentgenol* 5:327, 1970.

Calcaneus

1. Burdick AV: Calcaneus. *Xray Techn* 23:276, 1952.
2. Harris RI, Beath T: Etiology of peroneal spastic flat foot. *J Bone Joint Surg (Br)* 30:624, 1948.

Shoulder

1. Lawrence WS: New position in radiographing the shoulder joint. *AJR* 2:728, 1915.
2. Freedman E: Radiography of the shoulder. *Radiogr Clin Photogr* 10:8, 1934.
3. Jones ML: Radiographic examination of the shoulder. *Xray Techn* 7:104, 1936.
4. Blackett CW, Healy TR: Roentgen studies of the shoulder. *AJR* 37:760, 1937.
5. Knutsson F: An axial projection of the shoulder joint. *Acta Radiol* 30:214, 1948.
6. Stripp WJ: Radiographs of the scapulothoracic region. *Xray Focus* 4:8, 1963.
7. ViGario GD, Keats TE: Localization of calcific deposits in the shoulder. *AJR* 108:806, 1970.

Clavicle

1. Quesada F: Technique for the roentgen diagnosis of fractures of the clavicle.

Surg Gynecol Obstet 42:424, 1926.
2. Stripp WJ: The clavicle and the acromioclavicular joint. *Xray Focus* 4:21, 1963.
3. Zanca P: Shoulder pain: Involvement of the acromioclavicular joint. Analysis of 1000 cases. *AJR* 112:493, 1971.

Acromioclavicular Joints
1. Alexander OM: Radiography of the acromioclavicular joint. *Radiography* 54:139, 1948.
2. Alexander OM: Radiography of the acromioclavicular articulation. *Med Radiogr Photogr* 30:34, 1954.
3. Zanca P: Shoulder pain: Involvement of the acromioclavicular joint. Analysis of 1000 cases. *AJR* 112:493, 1971.
4. Rockwood CA, Green DP: *Fractures*, vol 1, Philadelphia, JB Lippincott, 1975.

Elbow
1. Buxton D: A radiographic survey of normal joints: The elbow joint. *Br J Radiol* 29:395, 1924.
2. Rogers LF: Fractures and dislocations of the elbow. *Semin Roentgenol* 13:97, 1978.
3. Holly EW: Radiography of the radial head. *Med Radiogr Photogr* 32:13, 1956.
4. Jones R: A note on the treatment of injuries about the elbow. *Prov Med J* 14:28, 1895.

Wrist
1. Buxton D: A radiographic survey of normal joints: The wrist joint and hand. *Br J Radiol* 32:199, 1927.
2. Roderick JF: The roentgenographic examination of the carpus. *Xray Techn* 18:8, 1946.
3. Alexander OM: Radiography of the wrist. *Radiology* 4:181, 1938.
4. DeSmet AA, et al: Radiographic projections for the diagnosis of arthritis of the hands and wrists. *Radiology* 139:577, 1981.
5. Bridgman CF: Radiography of the carpal navicular bone. *Med Radiogr Photogr* 25:104, 1949.
6. Fodor J, Malott JC: Radiography of the carpal navicular. *Radiol Technol* 52:175, 1980.
7. Lewis RW: Oblique views in roentgenography of the wrist. *AJR* 50:119, 1943.

Hand
1. Buxton D: A radiographic survey of normal joints: The wrist joint and hand. *Br J Radiol* 32:199, 1927.
2. DeSmet AA, et al: Radiographic projections for the diagnosis of arthritis of the hands and wrists. *Radiology* 139:577, 1981.
3. Yeh HC, Wolf BS: Radiographic anatomical landmarks of the metacarpophalangeal joints. *Radiology* 122:353, 1977.
4. Gramiak R: Oblique radiography of the hands. *Med Radiogr Photogr* 42:28, 1966.

Fingers
1. Buxton D: A radiographic survey of normal joints: The wrist joint and hand. *Br J Radiol* 32:199, 1927.
2. DeSmet AA, et al: Radiographic projections for the diagnosis of arthritis of the hands and wrists. *Radiology* 139:577, 1981.
3. Yeh HC, Wolf BS: Radiographic anatomical landmarks of the metacarpophalangeal joints. *Radiology* 122:353, 1977.
4. Reichmann S, et al: Soft-tissue radiography of finger joints. *Acta Radiol* 15:439, 1974.

Thumb
1. Buxton D: A radiographic survey of normal joints: The wrist joint and hand. *Br J Radiol* 32:199, 1927.
2. DeSmet AA, et al: Radiographic projections for the diagnosis of arthritis of the hands and wrists. *Radiology* 139:577, 1981.
3. Kaye JJ: Fractures and dislocations of the hand and wrist. *Semin Roentgenol* 13:109, 1978.
4. Jones RP, Leach RE: Fracture of the ulnar sesamoid bone of the thumb. *Am J Sports Med* 8:446, 1980.

Ribs
1. Bartsch GW: Radiographic examination of the ribs. *Xray Techn* 14:18, 1942.
2. Rogers NJS: A technique of x-ray examination of the ribs. *Radiography* 9:7, 1943.
3. Bridgeman CF, Holly EW, Zariquiey MO: Radiography of the ribs and costovertebral joints. *Med Radiogr Photogr* 32:38, 1956.
4. Hohmann D, Gasteiger W: Roentgen diagnosis of the costovertebral joints. *Fortschr Roentgenstr* 112:783, 1970.
5. Morris L, Bailey J: A simple method to demonstrate the ribs and sternum. *Clin Radiol* 21:320, 1970.

Chest
1. Pesauera GS: The evolution of chest roentgenographic technique. *AJR* 40:405, 1938.
2. Kattan KR, Wiot JF: How was this roentgenogram taken, AP or PA? *AJR* 117:843, 1973.
3. Bauer RG: High kilovoltage chest radiography with an air gap. *Radiol Techn* 42:10, 1970.
4. Kattan K: High kilovoltage oblique roentgenography of the chest; its advantage in differential diagnosis in diseases of the lung and pleura. *Dis Chest* 50:605, 1966.
5. Proto AV, Speckman JM: The left lateral radiograph of the chest. *Med Radiogr Photogr* 55:30, 1979.
6. Riggs W Jr, Parvey L: Differences between right and left lateral chest radiographs. *AJR* 127:997, 1976.
7. Bachman DM, Ellis K, Austin JH: The effects of minor degrees of obliquity on the lateral chest radiograph. *Radiol Clin North Am* 16:465, 1978.
8. Bray HA: A suggestion for improving the visibility of the apical field on the chest radiogram. *AJR* 8:602, 1921.
9. Lavner G, Copelman B: The anteroposterior lordotic projection in the roentgenographic examination of the lungs. *Radiology* 43:135, 1944.
10. Zinn B, Monroe J: The lordotic position in fluoroscopy and roentgenography of the chest. *AJR* 75:682, 1956.
11. Jacobson G, Sargent EN: Apical roentgenographic views of the chest. *AJR* 104:822, 1968.
12. Baum F, Black LT: The importance of the apical roentgenogram in pulmonary tuberculosis. *Am Rev Tuber* 12:228, 1925.
13. Flaxman AJ: Apical tuberculosis with roentgen technique. *Am Rev Tuber* 54:1, 1946.

Abdomen
1. Williams FH: X-ray examinations of the abdomen. *Boston Med Surg J* 23:1900.
2. Kelly JF, Dowell DH: The value of the preliminary film without opaque media in the diagnosis of abdominal conditions. *Radiology* 29:104, 1937.
3. Levitin J: Scout film of the abdomen. *Radiology* 47:10, 1946.
4. Miller RE: The technical approach to the acute abdomen. *Semin Roentgenol* 8:267, 1973.

Congenital Anomalies and Normal Skeletal Variants

GARY M. GUEBERT
TERRY R. YOCHUM
LINDSAY J. ROWE

Introduction

Congenital anomalies and normal skeletal variants are a common occurrence in clinical practice. In this chapter a large number of skeletal anomalies of the spine and pelvis are reviewed. Some of the more common skeletal anomalies of the extremities are also presented. Pertinent comments relating to the clinical significance of various anomalies are included.

The second section of this chapter deals with normal skeletal variants. Some of these variants may simulate certain disease processes. In some instances there are no clear-cut distinctions between skeletal variants and anomalies; therefore, there may be some overlap of material. The congenital anomalies are presented initially with accompanying text, photos, and references, beginning with the skull and proceeding caudally through the spine to then include the pelvis and extremities. The normal skeletal variants section is presented in an anatomical atlas format without text or references. A full and thorough understanding of these congenital anomalies and skeletal variants will assist the reader in being better prepared to approach the pathological interpretation of skeletal radiographs.

Anomalies of the Craniovertebral Region

OCCIPITALIZATION OF THE ATLAS

Description

Also known as assimilation of C1, Macalister (1) was the first to describe fusion of the atlas to the base of the occiput. This maldevelopment of the craniovertebral junction represents the most cephalic "blocked vertebra" encountered in the spine. Embryologically, there is a lack of segmentation and separation of the most caudal occipital sclerotome during the first few weeks of fetal life which results in this deformity of the atlanto-occipital junction.

Generally, young patients will be asymptomatic, and the condition is of radiographic interest only. Older children or young adults may develop degenerative joint changes at the subadjacent freely articulated segments or possible laxity of the transverse ligament with attendant cord compression syndrome. (2) Occipitalization of C1 may occur as an isolated anomaly but has been seen in association with Sturge-Weber syndrome and Klippel Feil syndrome.

Radiological Features

The lateral film demonstrates a decreased or nonexistent space between the posterior arch of C1 and the base of the occiput. (Fig. 2.1) On the frontal view, even with the head in optimal position, visualization of the atlanto-occipital joints usually is not possible because of the relative basilar impression that is present, so that the teeth of the maxilla overlie the atlas and axis. Flexion and extension views will demonstrate an absence of motion between the posterior arch of C1 and the lower margin of the occiput. Tomograms in the frontal plane demonstrate fusion of one or both atlanto-occipital joints.

OCCIPITAL VERTEBRAE

Developmental anomalies of the spine occur with the greatest frequency at transitional areas such as the atlanto-occipital junction or lumbosacral junction. They may occur as isolated defects or in association with other spinal or soft tissue malformations. Development of the occiput begins when the first four somites of the embryo unite to

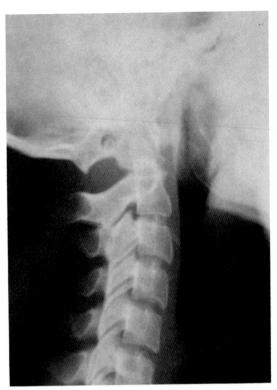

Figure 2.1. OCCIPITALIZATION OF THE ATLAS. Observe the fusion of the posterior arch of C1 to the base of the occiput.

form the basiocciput. The caudal aspect of the fourth somite then fuses with the cranial half of the C1 somite. The disc anlage at this level becomes the apical and alar ligaments.

Failure of normal fusion of the terminal segments of the basiocciput may result in what are called "occipital vertebrae." If the defective fusion is anterior, the result is called a "third condyle." Laterally placed anomalies are termed "paracondyloid," "paramastoid, or "epitransverse" processes, depending upon their exact anatomical relationships relative to the occiput and atlas. Manifestations of occipital vertebrae also include various other accessory ossicles around the foramen magnum.

Third Condyle

Description. The first mention of a third condyle in the radiological literature is by Hadley in 1948. (1) It results from a failure of fusion of the most caudal occipitoblast, near the midline, resulting in a small bony ossicle near the anteroinferior margin of the foramen magnum. Lombardi considers the third condyle to be the most frequent manifestation of occipital vertebrae. (2) Generally, this accessory bone is of no clinical significance; however, if large enough, it may restrict head movement.

Radiological Features. Small third condyles may be impossible to visualize on lateral plain film radiographs due to the superimposed mastoid processes and the petrous portion of the temporal bone. Larger third condyles may be seen on true lateral radiographs of the upper cervical spine as oval or round bone densities equal in size or smaller than the anterior arch of the atlas. Some are sufficiently large and caudally placed, forming an articulation with the superior aspect of the anterior arch of C1. A third condyle will not be evident on open mouth radiographs, but conventional tomography or CT evaluation is ideally suited for imaging this anomaly.

Epitransverse and Paracondylar Processes

Description.   An epitransverse process may be unilateral or bilateral. It may originate from the transverse process of the atlas and will either articulate with the skull near the jugular process or form a solid bony union with the skull base. If, however, the bony process begins at the jugular process of the occiput and projects toward the transverse process of C1, the appropriate name would be a paracondylar process or paramastoid process. (3) The significance of this finding is that a decreased range of motion, particularly lateral flexion, may be perceived at the atlanto-occipital junction. Manipulation of the occiput/C1 articulation would be impossible, as the occiput and atlas are effectively fused and move as a unit.

Radiological Features.   The diagnosis of this anomaly may require the use of sophisticated tomography, as the teeth of the maxilla often obstruct the view of this area on well positioned open mouth radiographs. (Fig. 2.2A and B) A slightly rotated open mouth view will shift the

molars on the side opposite the direction of head rotation away from the area of interest so that the bony connection between the occiput and transverse process may be clearly seen. An accessory joint may be present between the anomalous process and the superior aspect of the C1 transverse process, or a solid bony union may be present. (Fig. 2.3A–C) Occasionally, this process will act like a shim and cause a lateral tilt of the head.

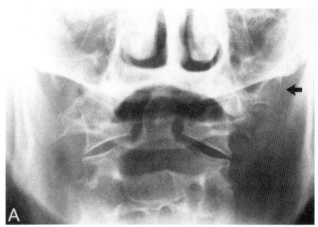

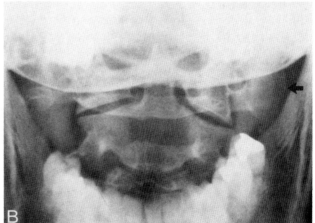

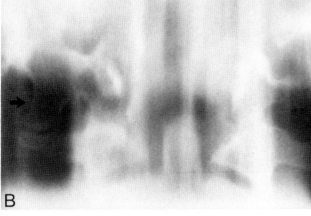

Figure 2.2. PARACONDYLAR PROCESS. A. AP Open Mouth. Observe the bony protuberance projecting from the paracondylar area directed towards the transverse process of the atlas (arrow). This should not be confused with the slender styloid process of the temporal bone (arrowhead). **B. AP Tomogram.** Tomography clearly shows the paracondylar process (arrow), forming an accessory articulation with the transverse process of C1.

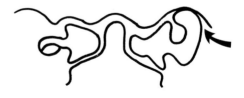

C

Figure 2.3. EPITRANSVERSE AND PARACONDYLAR PROCESS. A. AP Open Mouth. An epitransverse process (arrow), along with an accessory articulation, is present at the atlas. The clarity of the open mouth radiograph is the result of two factors: the patient is edentulous, and the patient's jaw was moving intentionally during the exposure. **B. AP Open Mouth.** An osseous bar is noted between the paracondylar area and the transverse process of the atlas, to which it is fully fused (arrow). **C. Schematic Diagram: Epitransverse Process.**

Accessory Ossicles

Description.   A variety of small bone fragments may develop in the ligaments around the foramen magnum. The embryological evolution of these pieces of bone have been theorized to be expressions of occipital vertebrae, (4) while others consider them to be examples of secondary ossification within the ligaments around the foramen magnum. (5)

Radiological Features.   These accessory bones are usually seen above the anterior arch of the atlas as small round or oval sesamoid-like bones.

PLATYBASIA

Description

Platybasia literally means "broad base" and is the result of congenital maldevelopment of the sphenoid and/or occipital bones. This flattening of the skull base is determined from mensuration performed on lateral skull radiographs. The method of measuring the skull base angle (Martin's basilar angle) has been described in Chapter 3. If this angle is greater than 152 degrees, platybasia exists. Platybasia alone is clinically insignificant, but it is often found in association with occipitalization of C1 and Klippel Feil syndrome.

Platybasia must be differentiated from basilar impression, although Chamberlain incorrectly used the terms interchangeably. (1) The terms "basilar impression" or "basilar invagination" may be used synonymously. There are two types of basilar impression—primary and secondary.

Primary Basilar Impression.   Primary basilar impression is congenital in origin and is often associated with a variety of vertebral defects such as occipitalization of the atlas, spina bifida occulta of the atlas, odontoid anomalies, agenesis or hypoplasia of the atlas, Klippel Feil syndrome, and Arnold Chiari malformation. (2)

Secondary Basilar Impression.   Secondary basilar impression is usually an acquired condition which results from softening of the occipital bone. The weight of the skull causes the occiput to settle around the upper cervical spine so that the distance between the occiput and atlas is reduced, the odontoid process encroaches upon the foramen magnum, and there is elevation in the floor of the posterior fossa.

Three bone softening disorders which are commonly associated with basilar impression are Paget's disease, osteomalacia, and fibrous dysplasia. (2)

Radiological Features

On a lateral x-ray of the skull, platybasia may be diagnosed when Martin's basilar angle, formed by the plane of the clivus and the plane of the floor of the anterior fossa, is unusually flat (i.e., greater than 152 degrees). (3) There is no evidence of a bone softening pathology.

Basilar impression will show evidence of elevation of the floor of the posterior fossa and upward convexity of the posterior aspect of the foramen magnum. The apex of the odontoid process may extend above the plane of the foramen magnum, giving a positive finding to Chamberlain's or McGregor's lines. (See Chapter 3) (Fig. 2.4A

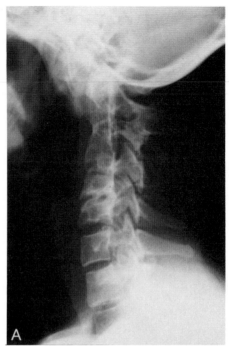

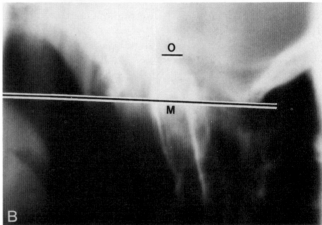

Figure 2.4. BASILAR IMPRESSION.   A. Lateral Cervical. The important plain film finding is the lack of interosseous spacing between the occiput and the posterior arch of the atlas. Note, additionally, the congenital malformations affecting the C2–C5 vertebral bodies and neural arches.   **B. Lateral Tomogram: Upper Cervical.** The odontoid process (O) has projected well above McGregor's line (M), proving basilar impression. Patients with this degree of basilar impression often exhibit profound neurological symptoms.

and B) Additional signs of the associated bone-softening pathology (i.e., Paget's disease, osteomalacia, fibrous dysplasia) will also be observed. (See Chapters 11 and 14)

Anomalies of the Cervical Spine

ANOMALIES OF THE ATLAS

Agenesis of the Posterior Arch

Embryology.   Ossification of the first cervical vertebra begins about the seventh fetal week at the lateral masses and proceeds perichondrally, in a dorsal direction, creating the posterior arch of the atlas. In the second year of life a secondary growth center for the posterior tubercle develops between these neural arches. Complete fusion of the posterior arch should be noted between the third and fifth years. (1)

Description.   The basic defect in agenesis of the posterior arch of the atlas is the lack of a cartilage template for the ossification process to build upon. Complete or partial agenesis of the posterior arch is rare, and posterior arch defects, by themselves, should not be the cause of neurological or biomechanical findings unless found in association with other anomalies such as Klippel Feil syndrome.

Radiological Features.   Radiographically, an absent posterior arch can be easily visualized on standard lateral cervical radiographs by the lack of a bony posterior neural arch. (Fig. 2.5A–C) A commonly associated finding is enlargement of the superior aspect of the second cervical spinous process, which has been referred to as a "megaspinous" process, representing fusion of the rudimentary posterior arch and posterior tubercle of the atlas. (2) (Fig. 2.6) One may also observe increased size of the anterior arch of C1, which is thought to be stress related. This is a helpful radiographic sign and suggests a longstanding and probable congenital origin to the defect. The integrity of the transverse ligament may also be compromised in the maldevelopment process; therefore, a cervical flexion radiograph should be performed to evaluate the atlanto-dental interspace.

Spina Bifida Occulta

See discussion under "Anomalies of the Thoracic and Lumbar Spine." (Fig. 2.7A and B)

Posterior Ponticle

Description.   A posterior ponticle of the atlas is present when there is a calcification which bridges the posterior aspect of the lateral mass and the posterior arch. A foramen is then formed which transmits the vertebral artery and/or the first cervical nerve as they pass over the posterior arch of C1 and is called the "arcuate foramen." It has been given the eponym "Kimmerly anomaly" (1) or "posticus ponticus."

The clinical significance to practitioners of spinal manipulative therapy relates to possible basilar insufficiency during rotary manipulations of the cervical spine. (2,3) It would appear that the ponticle may compress or restrict the vertebral artery, which may temporarily diminish blood flow to the base of the brain. This does not occur in all patients with a posterior ponticle. Proper testing for vertebrobasilar insufficiency must be performed prior to forceful manipulations of the cervical spine when a posterior ponticle is found on x-ray to avoid the potentially catastrophic effects of vertebrobasilar insufficiency.

Radiological Features.   It is best seen radiographically on the lateral view of the cervical spine, forming a partial or complete foramen at the ventral and superior aspect of the posterior arch. (Fig. 2.8A and B) This calcification may be unilateral or bilateral and is found in approximately 15 percent of white patients. (1) It must be differentiated from an overlying pneumatized mastoid air cell.

Agenesis of the Anterior Arch

Description.   Congenital absence of the anterior arch of the atlas is a rare condition. The initial literature account of this condition was in 1886, (1) but further reports are scarce, except for one case in 1972. (2) A case of absent anterior arch of C1 and the odontoid process was published, but the patient had extensive rheumatoid arthritis and it is unclear if the missing bones were congenitally absent or were destroyed by the rheumatoid pannus formation. (3)

Radiological Features.   Lateral radiographs demonstrate absence of the "D" shaped, corticated anterior arch of the first cervical vertebra. Tomograms or computed tomography (CT) better defines the extent of osseous agenesis. Flexion and extension views may be in order to

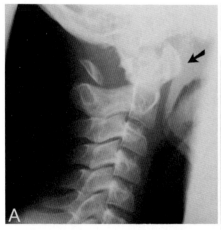
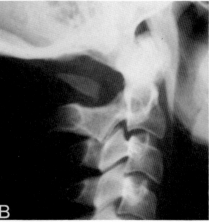
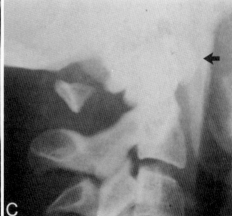

Figure 2.5. PARTIAL AGENESIS OF THE POSTERIOR ARCH OF THE ATLAS.   A. Lateral Cervical. Observe the agenesis of the posterior arch of the atlas, with the posterior tubercle being present. Stress hypertrophy of the anterior tubercle of the atlas is present (arrow).   **B. Lateral Cervical.** Failure of development of the midportion of the posterior arch of the atlas is noted along with stress enlargement of the anterior tubercle of the atlas.   **C. Lateral Cervical.** A focal agenesis of the midportion of the posterior arch of the atlas is noted. Observe the stress hypertrophy of the anterior tubercle of the atlas (arrow).

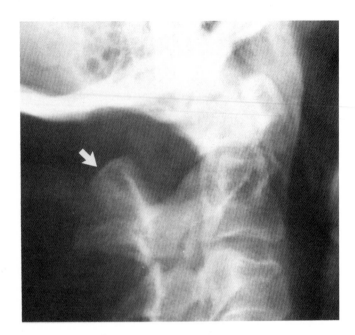

Figure 2.6. COMPLETE AGENESIS OF THE POSTERIOR ARCH OF THE ATLAS: MEGASPINOUS PROCESS OF C2. There is complete agenesis of the posterior arch of the atlas. Observe the "megaspinous" process at C2, representing fusion of the rudimentary posterior arch and posterior tubercle of the atlas (arrow).

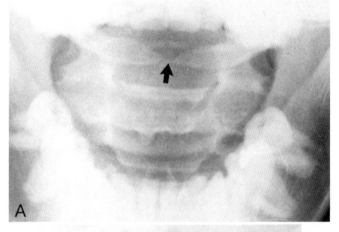

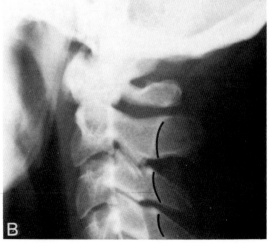

Figure 2.7. SPINA BIFIDA OCCULTA: ATLAS. A. AP Open Mouth. Observe the radiolucent cleft in the posterior arch of the atlas (arrow). **B. Lateral Cervical.** Note the artist enhanced lines at C2, C3, and C4, representing the posterior cervical line and the lack of this line at the atlas. Lack of the spinolaminar junction line (posterior cervical line) on the lateral film may be the only radiographic sign of spina bifida occulta of the atlas on the lateral projection.

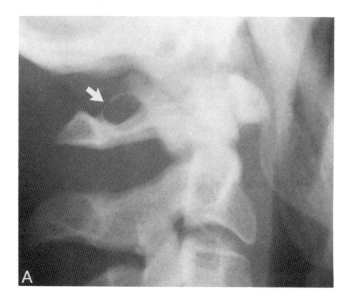

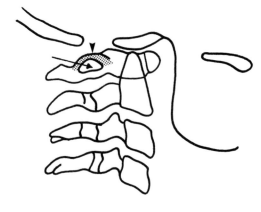

B

Figure 2.8. POSTERIOR PONTICLE OF THE ATLAS. A. Lateral Cervical. A posterior ponticle of the atlas is noted (arrow). **B. Schematic Diagram.** A posterior ponticle of the atlas is present (arrowhead), which creates an arcuate foramen (arrow).

determine if hypermobility exists between C1 and C2. Apparently, retrosubluxation of C1 on C2 may be possible.

Down's Syndrome (Mongolism)

Description. Down's syndrome is the most common autosomal syndrome, occurring once in every 600 births. (1) It is the result of trisomy of the 21st chromosome. Patients affected with Down's syndrome are recognizable at birth, with a decreased anteroposterior diameter of the skull, a small nose with a flat bridge, slanting eyes, and a protruding tongue. Mental retardation is a constant feature. Leukemia is significantly more common in patients with Down's syndrome than in an otherwise normal individual.

Radiological Features. The most clinically significant radiographic finding concerns the integrity of the transverse ligament of the atlas. Up to 20 percent of these patients are born without a transverse ligament; (2,3) therefore, before cervical spinal manipulative therapy is undertaken a flexion radiograph must be seen to ensure

the stability of the atlantoaxial motion segment. (See Chapter 3) (Fig. 2.9)

Other radiographic findings include a decreased iliac index (see Chapter 3); hypoplasia of the middle phalanx of the fifth finger, with clinodactyly; multiple ossification

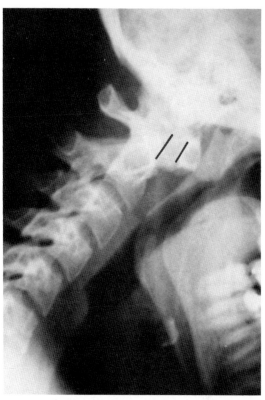

Figure 2.9. DOWN'S SYNDROME: UPPER CERVICAL INVOLVEMENT. There is a significant increase in the atlantodental interspace (ADI represented by distance between artist enhanced lines) as a result of agenesis of the transverse ligament of the atlas. *Comment:* Up to 20 percent of patients with Down's syndrome are born without a transverse ligament of the atlas. Upper cervical spinal manipulative therapy is contraindicated until a flexion radiograph of the upper cervical spine has been performed and the atlantodental interspace is proven normal.

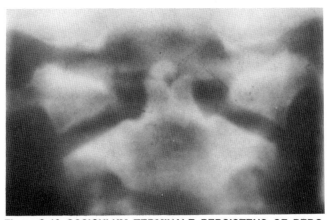

Figure 2.10. OSSICULUM TERMINALE PERSISTENS OF BERGMAN. Observe the failure of union of the cephalic ossification center for the odontoid process tip. A symmetrical "V" shaped lucent cleft helps differentiate this finding from fracture.

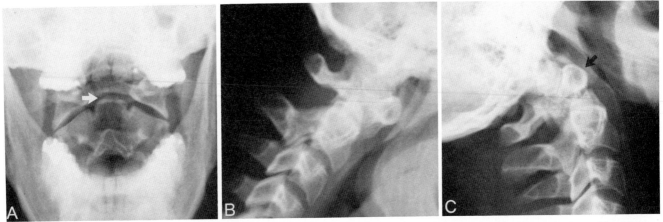

Figure 2.11. OS ODONTOIDEUM WITH INSTABILITY. A. AP Open Mouth. Note the incomplete odontoid process with a wide radiolucent band (arrow) just above its base. **B. Lateral Cervical Flexion. C. Lateral Cervical Extension.** Note the forward excursion of the atlas in flexion and the posterior movement in extension, signifying instability. There is a stress enlargement of the anterior tubercle of the atlas (arrow) as a result of this underlying instability. **Comment:** The presence of a horizontal radiolucent band at the base of the odontoid process may represent mach lines, an odontoid fracture, or the cleft of an os odontoideum and must be differentiated.

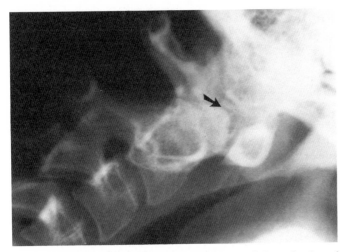

Figure 2.12. OS ODONTOIDEUM. Observe the failure of union of the odontoid process to the base of the body of the axis, as demonstrated by a radiolucent band (arrow). Cortical thickening of the anterior tubercle of the atlas, as well as an angular deformity of the posterior surface of the anterior tubercle, suggests a congenital etiology. (Courtesy of Robert J. Longenecker, DC, DACBR, Irving, Texas)

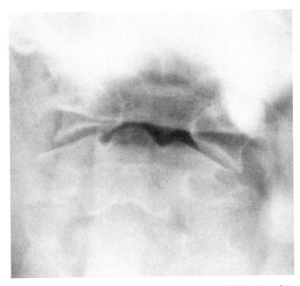

Figure 2.13. AGENESIS OF THE ODONTOID PROCESS. Observe the abbreviated peg of the odontoid process, with the remainder of its substance lacking. The lateral shift of C1 upon C2 indicates instability. (Courtesy of Klaus W. Weber, MD, Hechingen, West Germany)

centers for the manubrium; underpneumatization of the paranasal sinuses; decreased anteroposterior diameter of the lumbar vertebral bodies; and either 11 or 13 pairs of ribs. (4)

Spina Bifida Occulta

See discussion under "Anomalies of the Thoracic and Lumbar Spine."

ANOMALIES OF THE AXIS

Ossiculum Terminale Persistens of Bergman

Description. The cephalic portion of the odontoid process develops from a secondary growth center which appears about the second year and usually unites at 10–12 years of age. (1) Occasionally, this secondary growth center does not unite with the subadjacent process and remains as a separate ossicle.

Radiological Features. The x-ray finding of a discrete, round, oval, or diamond-shaped piece of bone at the most cephalic portion of the dens in a patient over the age of 12 years is considered an ossiculum terminale and is a normal variant of development which is of no clinical significance. (Fig. 2.10) It must be differentiated from other anomalies of development of the odontoid process such as an os odontoideum and fracture.

Odontoid Anomalies

Differentiation of the odontoid anomalies (os odontoideum, hypoplasia of the odontoid or agenesis of the odontoid) is possible by x-ray examination. Most patients

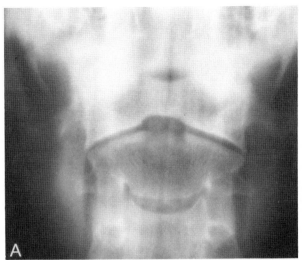

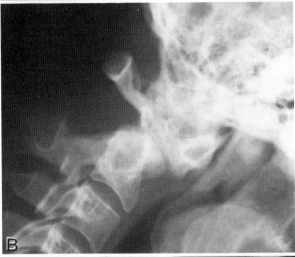

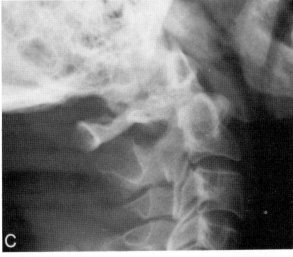

Figure 2.14. AGENESIS OF THE ODONTOID PROCESS WITH IN-STABILITY. A. AP Tomogram. Observe the complete lack of an osseous shadow of the odontoid. **B. Flexion, Lateral Cervical. C. Extension, Lateral Cervical.** There is no odontoid process, allowing significant movement of the atlas in flexion and extension. **Comment:** Patients with this degree of instability are destined for surgical arthrodesis. (Courtesy of Bryan Hartley, MD, Melbourne, Australia)

with these conditions proceed to develop atlantoaxial instability. High-velocity spinal manipulative techniques are contraindicated in patients with these conditions. Surgical consultation must be considered for a patient with progressive instability or neurological symptoms.

Os Odontoideum

Description. Anomalies of the odontoid process are considered uncommon (1) and are usually discovered by the principle of "traumatic determinism." This means that the underlying condition predated the injury and is not caused by the current trauma. These anomalies may be associated with Down's syndrome, Klippel Feil syndrome, Morquio's syndrome, and spondyloepiphyseal dysplasia.

An understanding of the developmental anatomy is necessary due to the potential for significant neurological damage (e.g., paralysis or death) that may result from a trivial trauma or even spinal manipulative therapy. In os odontoideum the cephalic portion of the odontoid process develops normally from its two lateral ossification centers but remains ununited with the body of the second cervical vertebra, above the level of the neurocentral synchondrosis. (2) Since the osseous defect is not found at the site of the growth plate (neurocentral synchondrosis), it has been hypothesized that os odontoideum is actually a longstanding and unrecognized fracture of the base of the odontoid process. (3) It must be noted that many authors still consider this entity to constitute an event of congenital nonunion. The transverse ligament is usually intact and, occasionally, in association with this fact, the posterior arch of the atlas may be hypoplastic or absent.

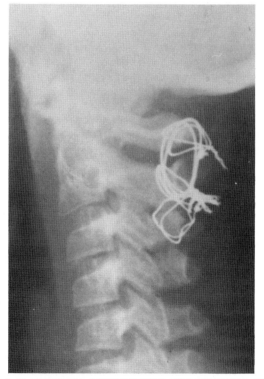

Figure 2.15. SURGICAL ARTHRODESIS FOR AGENESIS OF THE ODONTOID PROCESS. Posterior interspinous wiring of C1, C2, and C3 as treatment for agenesis of the odontoid process.

Any symptoms the patient may manifest are usually the result of atlantoaxial instability, with resultant cord compression (Fig. 2.11A–C); however, if there is compression of the vertebral artery due to stretching during subluxation, then the symptoms may be considerably greater. Increased deep-tendon reflexes, proprioceptive loss, or sphincter incompetence may be encountered.

Radiological Features. The x-ray diagnosis of os odontoideum in a child below the age of 5 years can be made if there is demonstration of hypermobility of the odontoid process on the body of C2 during flexion and extension. In the adult an x-ray diagnosis is certain if a smooth, wide, lucent defect is seen to separate the odontoid process from the C2 body at the level of the superior articular processes and there is an associated stress hypertrophy of the anterior tubercle of the atlas. (4) (Fig. 2.12) This finding will not be present in the child, as the biomechanical stresses on the anterior arch of the atlas will not have been present for a long enough period of

time to allow the hypertrophy to develop. Os odontoideum must be differentiated from a fracture of the odontoid process. (See Chapter 9) A helpful radiographic sign which may be present and confirms a developmental defect of the odontoid process is a "molding" of the anterior arch of C1 into the ventral aspect of the odontoid process. (Fig. 2.12)

Hypoplastic and Agenetic Odontoid Process

Radiological Features. A patient with hypoplasia of the odontoid process will show an abbreviated peg or stump of bone projecting slightly above the C1/C2 articulations on an open-mouth radiograph (Fig. 2.13). Complete agenesis of the odontoid process appears to be extremely rare, although the true incidence is unknown. (1) This anomaly can be diagnosed at birth, on radiographs through the open mouth, as the ossification center for the odontoid process should be present at that time. Flexion and extension radiographs should be performed to rule out hypermobility between C1 and C2. (Fig.

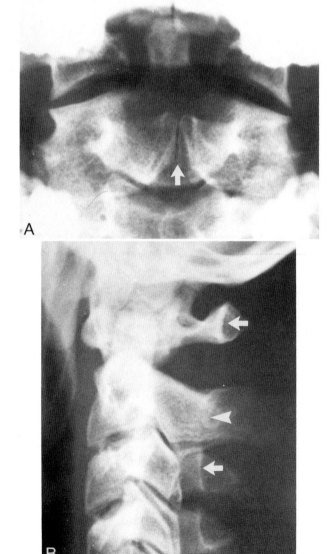

Figure 2.16. SPINA BIFIDA OCCULTA OF THE AXIS.   A. AP Open Mouth. Observe the midline radiolucent cleft of the spinous process of C2 (arrow).   **B. Lateral Cervical.** The cortical white line created by the junction of the lamina and spinous process is clearly noted at C1 and C3 (arrows). The white line represents the spinolaminar junction line or the posterior cervical line (PCL) and is a line drawn to connect the spinolaminar lines of the cervical vertebrae. The lack of a spinolaminar junction line at C2 (arrowhead) signifies spina bifida occulta. (Courtesy of Kenneth E. Yochum, DC, St. Louis, Missouri)

2.14A–C) If present, spinal manipulation is contraindicated, and referral for a surgical opinion concerning arthrodesis is recommended. (Fig. 2.15)

Spina Bifida Occulta

See description in "Anomalies of the Thoracic and Lumbar Spine." (Fig. 2.16A and B)

ANOMALIES OF C3 THROUGH C7

Block Vertebra

Description. When two adjacent vertebrae are osseously fused from birth, this joined unit is called a "congenital block vertebra." Embryologically, this is the result of failure of the normal segmentation process of the somites during the period of differentiation, at 3–8 fetal weeks. (1)

The block vertebra, by itself, is clinically insignificant. As there is no motion allowed at the fused level, there is no potential for degenerative disease of the disc or neurocentral or posterior apophyseal joints. The foramina at the blocked level may be smaller than normal, normally sized, or enlarged, but have not been shown to cause nerve compression. However, due to the lack of a motion segment the free articulations above and below the block segment are stressed and usually result in premature degenerative discogenic spondylosis and arthrosis at the fully articulated levels, especially below the fusion site.

(Fig. 2.17A and B) Fusions which are partial (i.e., do not completely involve the anterior and posterior spinal units) may result in abnormal spinal curvature, usually scoliosis, due to a unilateral bar. Block vertebra are most commonly found at C5/C6, C2/C3, T12/L1, and L4/L5, in decreasing order of incidence. (1,2)

A recent report suggests that longstanding congenital or acquired fusion of upper cervical vertebrae may lead to stretching and laxity of the ligaments between the occiput and the atlas, resulting in excessive motion and brainstem or cord compression. (2)

Radiological Features. A typical congenital block vertebra will demonstrate the following roentgen signs: 1) a diminished AP diameter of the vertebral body; 2) a hypoplastic or rudimentary disc space which may show faint calcification; 3) possible fusion of the apophyseal joints (50% of cases); and 4) possible malformation or fusion of the spinous processes. (Fig. 2.18A and B)

If one traces the anterior margin of the vertebral bodies at the involved level, due to the decreased AP diameter a concavity will be observed. In order to remember that this is a congenital malformation, visualize the concavity as having a "C" shape. This narrowing at the disc level has been called the "wasp waist" appearance. (3) (Fig. 2.19A and B) Osseous fusion of the neural arches is almost never associated with infectious or traumatic processes and is another helpful sign of this congenital anomaly. (4)

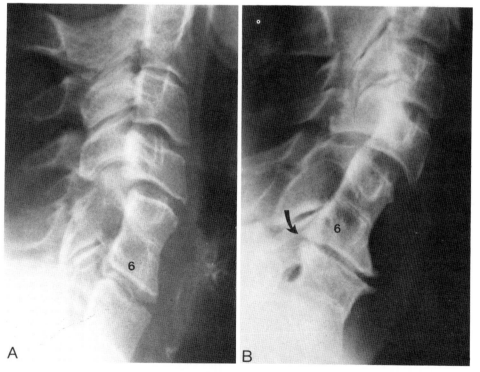

Figure 2.17. CERVICAL BLOCK VERTEBRAE. **A. Lateral Cervical: Single Block Vertebra.** Observe the block vertebra present at the C5/C6 level. The arrested growth of the vertebral bodies results in an anterior concavity which has been referred to as the "wasp-waist" appearance. Facet structures at C5/C6 are also fused. **B. Lateral Cervical: Multiple Block Vertebrae.** There are block vertebrae present at C5/C6 and C7/T1. Facet joint fusion is noted at the C5/C6 level. Premature degenerative discopathy with spondylosis is present at the C6 disc level. Posterior osteophyte formation affecting the C6/C7 vertebrae (arrow) may result in spinal stenosis. **Comment:** Fifty percent of patients with block vertebra have associated apophyseal joint fusion, as is present in both of these cases.

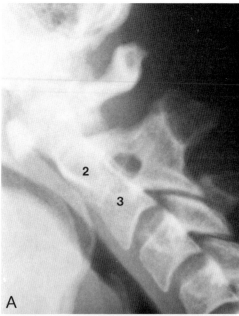

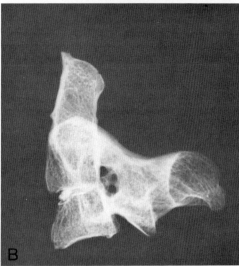

Figure 2.18. CERVICAL BLOCK VERTEBRAE. A. Lateral Cervical Flexion. Observe the block vertebra present between C2/C3, with posterior fusion of the apophyseal joints. **B. Specimen Radiograph.** Observe the rudimentary calcified disc at C2 in this blocked specimen. **Comment:** Block vertebrae are most commonly found at C5/C6, C2/C3, T12/L1, and L4/L5, in decreasing order of incidence.

Klippel Feil Syndrome

Description. In 1912 Klippel and Feil (1) described a 46-year-old man with congestion of the lungs and nephritis. They described his physical appearance as follows: The head seemed to be resting directly on the trunk, and the spine was compressed without apparent pain. This original description is typical of the patient affected with Klippel Feil syndrome (i.e., a patient with a short, webbed neck (pterygium colli), low hairline, and a decreased range of cervical motion) and has become known as the classic triad of this abnormality. This triad is completely expressed in only 52 percent of patients with the disease. (2) Men and women are equally affected.

Facial asymmetry, torticollis, or webbing of the neck, may be seen in 20 percent of patients. (3) The thoracic cage may also be deformed due to scoliosis or Sprengel's deformity. (Fig. 2.20A and B, 2.21A and B)

Other organ systems may be involved beyond the spine. These include the genitourinary, nervous, and cardiopulmonary systems. An alternative name for this condition, which can be found in the literature, is "brevicollis." An embryological basis for this problem has been offered which explains the association of genitourinary anomalies, a fact not completely appreciated in the Klippel and Feil case. The original patient died of complications of renal disease and uremia. (1) Duncan states: "Existing embryologic data suggest that the blastema of the cervical vertebrae, scapulae, and the genitourinary system have an intimate spatial relationship at the end of the fourth or beginning of the fifth week of fetal life. An alteration in this region can affect the cervical vertebrae and scapulae directly, and the genitourologic changes are mediated indirectly through the inductive capacity of the pronephric duct." (4)

Radiological Features: X-ray examination of the spine will reveal multiple block vertebrae (two or more) of the cervical and upper thoracic spine. Anomalies of rib development may also be evident. (Fig. 2.20 A and B) These block vertebrae are responsible for scoliosis, which is the most commonly associated condition with Klippel Feil syndrome. (2) Platybasia of the skull may be noted on the lateral cervical film. Congenital elevation of the scapula, Sprengel's deformity, is found in 25 percent of Klippel Feil patients. (3) (Fig. 2.21 A and B).

Sprengel's Deformity

Description. Although congenital elevation of the scapula appears to have been first described in 1863 by Eulenberg, (1) this defomity currently bears Sprengel's name. In Sprengel's original description he relates his observations on four children with similar deformities of the scapula. (2) All four of these patients had elevation of the left scapula. In spite of his postulates on etiology, the reason for this deformity remains a mystery. At the third fetal week the scapula develops in the neck, at the C4/C5 level. Under ordinary conditions, the scapula migrates to its normal position by the 50th day of gestation. It would appear, therefore, that a failure to descend, rather than elevation of the scapula, is a more accurate description of the pathology. It is felt that the problem then must develop prior to the third month of skeletal development. A 2:1 female predominance has been noted. (3) The deformity can be detected at birth and is usually unilateral but may be seen bilaterally. (3)

Examination of a patient with Sprengel's deformity will show elevation of the scapula, with reduction of abduction of the arm. Torticollis, with or without muscle spasm, may be noted. It is recommended that a determination of the degree of fixation, as well as the quantity of malrotation and maldevelopment, be made. (3)

Sprengel's deformity may occur alone, but it is also associated in 20–25 percent of the cases of Klippel Feil syndrome. Another association is the presence of the omovertebral bone in 30–40 percent of cases of Sprengel's

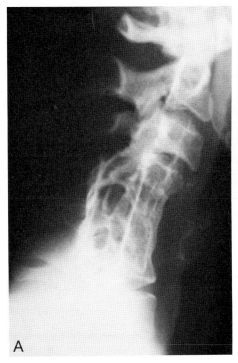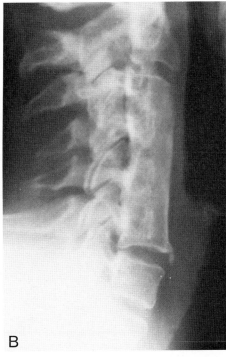

Figure 2.19. CONGENITAL VERSUS SURGICAL BLOCK VERTEBRAE. A. Lateral Cervical: Congenital. Observe the congenital block vertebra at C4 through C7, with the characteristic anterior "C" shaped ("wasp-waist") deformity signifying the congenital origin of this fusion. **B. Lateral Cervical: Surgical.** There is surgical fusion of C3 through C6. The lack of anterior concavity, rudimentary discs, and fusion of the apophyseal joints are radiographic signs suggesting surgical intervention rather than a fusion of congenital origin.

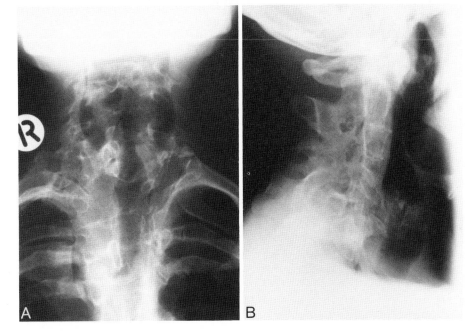

Figure 2.20. KLIPPEL FEIL SYNDROME. A. AP Lower Cervical. There are multiple block vertebrae noted throughout the lower cervical and upper thoracic spine, as evidenced by the lack of disc spacing. Anomalous rib development is also noted. **B. Lateral Cervical.** There are multiple block vertebrae throughout the cervical spine. The zygapophyseal joints are additionally fused. Of incidental notation is spina bifida occulta of the atlas.

deformity. (4) (Fig. 2.22) It is not always bone; it may be cartilage or fibrous tissue. The omovertebral bone usually runs between the C5 or C6 spinous process, lamina, or transverse process to the superior angle of the scapula. The earliest description of the omovertebral bone is attributed to Willett and Walsham in 1880. (5)

Concerning Sprengel's deformity, Lovell and Winter state: "The treatment of choice is surgery. The deformity does not progress, but it does not spontaneously improve without surgery. Conservative treatment does not result in any improvement. Physical therapy also is not helpful." Surgery is best considered between the ages of 4 and 7 years. (3)

Radiological Features. The scapula is hypoplastic, shortened vertically, and is broad on x-ray examination. It is rotated so that the glenoid process is directed inferiorly. The inferior angle rests above the normal T7 level. The amount of elevation may be from 2 to 10 cm. Two thirds of patients presenting with these features demonstrate associated scoliosis, hemivertebrae, block vertebrae, spina bifida occulta, or cervical ribs. (6)

Cervical Spondylolisthesis

Description. The original reference to this rare anomaly is credited to Perlman and Hawes in 1951. (1) There is absence of the pedicles bilaterally, with dysplasia of the

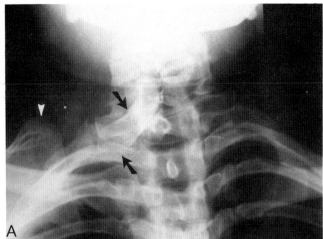

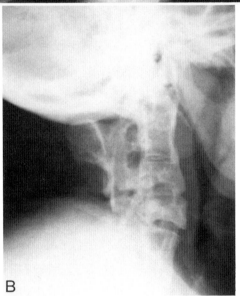

Figure 2.21. KLIPPEL FEIL SYNDROME WITH OMOVERTEBRAL BONE. A. AP Lower Cervical. Observe the omovertebral bone projecting from the lamina of C7 toward the superior angle of the scapula (arrows). There is associated congenital failure of descent of the scapula (Sprengel's deformity) (arrowhead). **B. Lateral Cervical.** There are multiple congenital block vertebrae. (Courtesy of James R. Brandt DC, FACO, Coon Rapids, Minnesota) *Comment:* Sprengel's deformity is found in 25 percent of patients with Klippel Feil syndrome.

Figure 2.22. SPRENGEL'S DEFORMITY WITH OMOVERTEBRAL BONE. Observe the congenital failure of descent of the scapula (arrow), denoting a Sprengel's deformity. There is a large, bony bar projecting from the lamina and spinous process of C7 to the vertebral border of the scapula, representing an omovertebral bone (arrowhead). *Comment:* Thirty to 40 percent of the cases of Sprengel's deformity will have an associated omovertebral bone.

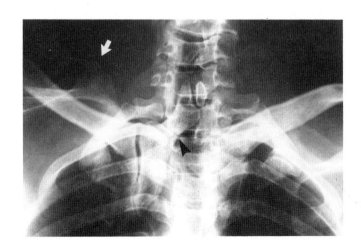

articular processes, and spina bifida occulta is a constant feature. The sixth cervical vertebra is most commonly involved, but other cervical levels have been described. (2) Males are more commonly affected. The patient may have no complaints or may report symptoms which include nuchal rigidity, dysphagia, and radicular arm pain. (2)

Radiological Features.   Abnormalities will be seen on anteroposterior, lateral, and oblique radiographs of the cervical spine. The lateral film will show dysplasia of the neural arch, and there may be slight anterolisthesis of the involved level. (Fig. 2.23A and B) The anteroposterior radiograph will reveal a spina bifida occulta. (Fig. 2.24A and B) Spina bifida occulta at C6 is a rare, isolated anomaly and is a highly suggestive sign of cervical spondylolisthesis. Enlarged foramina will be present bilaterally due to the absent pedicles. Flexion and extension radiographs may demonstrate intersegmental instability. (See Chapter 5)

Absent Pedicle of the Cervical Spine

Description.   In 1946 Hadley (1) is credited with the first report of congenital absence of a cervical pedicle. As of 1982 the literature had reported 17 cases. The cartilage anlage of the cervical vertebra develops from six centers—one for each side of the vertebral body, one in each costal process, and one for each neural arch—which then becomes the pedicle, articular process, transverse process, and lamina. It is a failure of development of the latter which results in this vertebral anomaly. The most common levels in the cervical spine to be affected are C6 (44 percent), C5 (31 percent), C4 (12.5 percent), and C7 (12.5 percent). (2) The left side is affected more often than the right. (2)

Clinically, this finding is insignificant, in itself. Dissection has demonstrated one common dural pouch with two nerve roots inside and a fibrous band at the site of the missing pedicle. The importance of recognizing this entity is so as not to confuse it with the tumor destruction of the pedicle which is seen in neurofibromatosis or metastasis.

Radiological Features.   An absence of the pedicle at the affected level creates an enlarged intervertebral foramen on oblique films. The superior aspect of the articular process at this same level may be dysplastic, as will a portion of the transverse process. The articular dysplasia is seen on lateral views but is best visualized on pillar projections. (Fig. 2.25A–C) Hypertrophy of the contralateral pedicle may also be present and should be considered a hallmark of this congenital dysplasia. This radiographic sign of a sclerotic contralateral pedicle is far more commonly seen with agenesis of a lumbar pedicle as a result of greater weightbearing in this area. The vertebral body is unaffected, in distinction to the posterior scalloping of the body which is seen with neurofibromas (dumbbell tumors) at the intervertebral foramen.

Cervical Rib

Description.   A cervical rib is a separate piece of bone that articulates with the transverse process of a cervical vertebra or vertebrae. It is most common at the C7, C6, and C5 levels, in descending order of occurrence. These ribs may be differentiated from elongation of a cervical transverse process, which would demonstrate no joint at the transverse process, as well as a rudimentary first thoracic rib, which may require the counting of all thoracic ribs.

Cervical ribs are present in 0.5 percent of the popula-

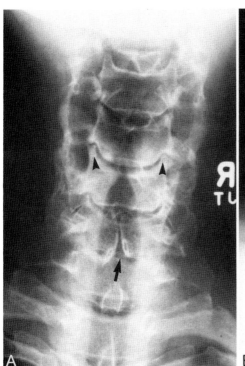
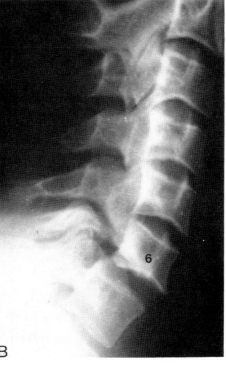

Figure 2.23. CERVICAL SPONDYLO-LISTHESIS: C6.   A. AP Lower Cervical. There is a spina bifida occulta present at C6 (arrow). Considerable joint of von Luschka arthrosis is present bilaterally at the C4/C5 levels (arrowheads).   **B. Lateral Cervical.** Note the marked dysplasia of the pedicles and articular pillars of C6. There is anterior translation of the vertebral body of C6 upon C7.

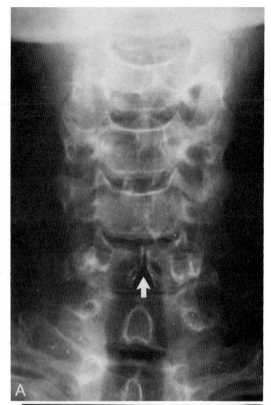

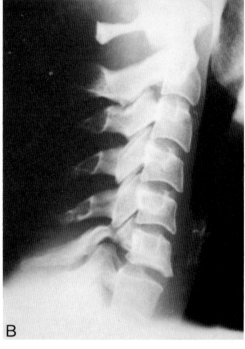

Figure 2.24. CERVICAL SPONDYLOLISTHESIS: C6. A. AP Lower Cervical. Observe the spina bifida occulta present at C6 (arrow). **B. Lateral Cervical.** Congenital malformation of the articular pillar and pedicles is present. *Comment:* Spina bifida occulta at C6 is a rare, isolated anomaly and is seen in association with cervical spondylolisthesis in 50 percent of cases.

tion and are twice as common in females. (1) They are bilateral in 66 percent of cases. (1) If these ribs cause symptoms, it is usually after middle age, when the shoulders begin to droop, resulting in neurovascular compression.

Radiological Features. The radiographic diagnosis is made when the anomalous rib is seen to form a joint with a transverse process which is oriented in a caudal direction

(thoracic transverse processes normally point cephalically, while cervical transverse processes are directed caudally). The length of the cervical rib is quite variable, from a rudimentary stump to a fully developed rib which may also articulate with the sternoclavicular junction. (Fig. 2.26A and B) Sutton considers cervical ribs to be a common anomaly. (2) Cervical ribs may be differentiated from elongation or enlargement of the transverse process. An

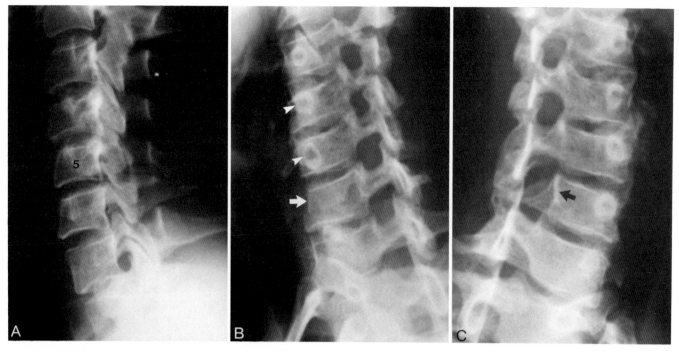

Figure 2.25. ABSENT PEDICLE OF THE CERVICAL SPINE.   A. Lateral Cervical. Observe the altered appearance of the articular pillar of C6.   **B. Oblique Cervical.** There is no pedicle shadow present on C6 (arrow). Observe the normal pedicle shadow on C4, 5 (arrowheads).   **C. Oblique Cervical.** The failure of pedicle development has resulted in an abnormally large intervertebral foramen (arrow). (Courtesy of Gary M. Guebert, DC, DACBR, St. Louis, Missouri)

Figure 2.26. CERVICAL RIBS.   A. AP Lower Cervical. There is a complete cervical rib present at C7 on the right side. An attenuated cervical rib is present at C7 on the left side.   **B. AP Lower Cervical.** There is a cervical rib with an accessory articulation (arrow). A small cervical rib is also noted on the opposite side. (Courtesy of Donald E. Freuden, DC, FACO, Denver, Colorado)

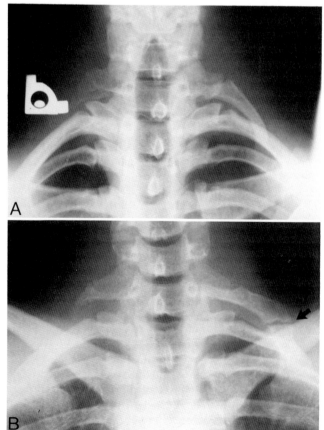

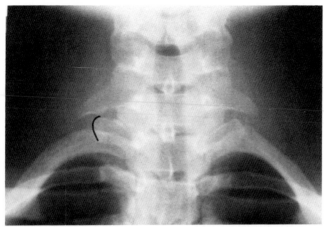

Figure 2.27. ELONGATED TRANSVERSE PROCESSES: C7. Observe the bilateral elongation of the transverse processes of C7. The transverse process of T1 is outlined as a reference point, with the elongated transverse process of C7 beyond the distal tip of the first thoracic transverse process.

enlarged transverse process extends laterally beyond the transverse of the first thoracic vertebra and does not reveal a joint. (Fig. 2.27)

"Cervical ribs vary greatly in size and shape, and clinical symptoms bear little relation to the radiographic abnormality." (2) One should be aware that a fibrous band may extend from the end of a small cervical rib and be the actual source of neural or vascular compression. Unfortunately, this band is unappreciated on plain film radiographs. Contrast radiographic examination demonstrating vascular occlusion would be necessary to make a preoperative diagnosis of a fibrous band creating a thoracic outlet syndrome.

Anomalies of the Thoracic and Lumbar Spine

VERTEBRAL BODY ANOMALIES

Block Vertebra

See description in the section "Anomalies of the Cervical Spine." (Fig. 2.28A–C, 2.29A and B, 2.30A and B).

Butterfly Vertebra

Description.   The embryological explanation for this radiologically distinctive entity has been variously described as failure of regression of the chorda dorsalis, persistence of the ventrodorsal extension of the perichordal sheath, or failure of the lateral ossification centers to unite. (1,2) Tanaka and Uhthoff, (3) regarding coronal cleft vertebrae, show conclusive histopathological correlation of lack of involvement of the notochord in development of this anomaly and attribute the defect to the placement of the intraosseous blood vessels. This opinion directly disputes the theories of Schmorl and Junghans (1) and is corroborated by the work of Emery. (4) The initial description of butterfly vertebra is attributed to von Rokitansky, (5) in 1844, where the two halves of the

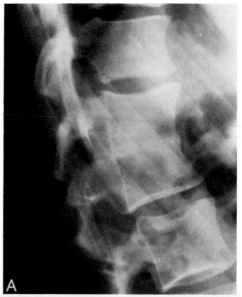

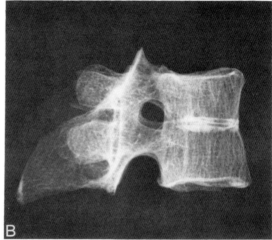

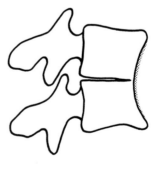

C

Figure 2.28. LUMBAR BLOCK VERTEBRA.   A. Lateral Lumbar. There is a block vertebra present at the T12/L1 vertebral bodies. Observe the "C" shaped deformity present at the anterior surface of the blocked vertebra ("wasp-waist" appearance). (Reprinted with permission: Yochum TR et al: A radiographic anthology of vertebral names. *J Manip Physiol Ther* 8:87, June 1985). **B. Specimen Radiograph.   C. Schematic Diagram.** Observe the "wasp-waist" appearance, signifying the congenital nature of the vertebral fusion.

fly. It is created by indentation of the end plate cortices toward the central body, creating an hourglass central lucency which anatomically represents continuous disc material from the adjacent disc spaces above and below. The pedicles may appear slightly enlarged, and the interpediculate distance may be minimally increased. (6) (Fig. 2.31)

The most common areas to be affected are the thoracic and lumbar spine. (6) It is usually clinically insignificant if occurring as an isolated anomaly. The development of the ununited lateral body halves is generally symmetrical; therefore, scoliosis or kyphoscoliosis are not associated. (Fig. 2.32A and B) Dysraphic spinal conditions such as meningocele, myelomeningocele, or diastematomyelia may have multiple butterfly vertebrae present. (6)

Hemivertebrae

Description. The vertebral body normally develops from two lateral ossification centers. When one of these centers fails to grow, the resultant triangular deformity of the body is called a "lateral hemivertebra." Lateral hemivertebra is the most common type of presentation. As a rule, a hemivertebra does not exist singularly, and there are usually other coexistent vertebral anomalies. (1) Rarely, a dorsal hemivertebra occurs which is characterized by absence of the anterior portion of the vertebral body. (1) Even more rare is a ventral hemivertebra, where the posterior portion of the body is absent. (Fig. 2.33) The most commonly affected areas of the spine are the upper lumbar and lower thoracic regions. (1)

An isolated hemivertebra will cause a structural scoliosis with an angular lateral curvature, the hemivertebra occurring at the apex of the scoliosis. There is no hope of reducing this type of scoliosis without surgical intervention; however, if two hemivertebrae are balanced by their wedges being based on opposite sides, they produce little or no visible deformity. (2) The interposed discs at the affected level are normally developed. (3)

Hemivertebrae constitute approximately 6 percent of anomalies associated with congenital spinal deformities. (4) Lateral hemivertebrae have been shown to occur with other vertebral anomalies such as block vertebrae, diastematomyelia, Klippel Feil syndrome, meningocele, multiple enchondromatosis (Ollier's disease), and spondylothoracic dysplasia. (1,3) Dorsal hemivertebrae may be seen with achondroplasia, cretinism, chondrodystrophy, Morquio's disease, and gargoylism. (3)

Radiological Features. The x-ray appearance of hemivertebrae is quite characteristic and may be diagnosed from anteroposterior plain film radiographs. The body of the involved vertebra has a triangular shape, as the end plates taper to a point, creating a laterally wedged vertebra. (Fig. 2.34) Disc spacing above and below the site of involvement is of normal vertical height, but the end plates of the adjacent vertebrae are slightly deformed, resulting in a trapezoid shape to those vertebrae. If the anomaly is isolated, there will be an angular scoliosis (Fig. 2.35); but there are more likely to be multiple congenital anomalies besides the hemivertebra. The presence of multiple hemivertebrae with block vertebrae distorts the appearance of the spine and has been referred to as the

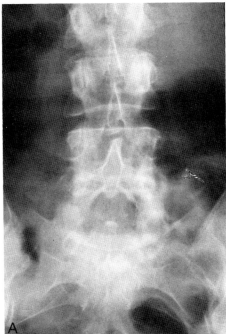
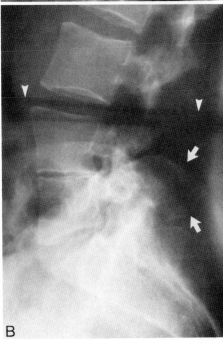

Figure 2.29. LUMBAR BLOCK VERTEBRA. A. AP Lumbar Spine. Observe the single, large, common spinous process at the L4/L5 level. **B. Lateral Lumbar.** There is a remnant disc present between the L4/L5 block vertebra. Underdevelopment of the anterior surface of the vertebral bodies of L4/L5 has created the "wasp-waist" appearance. A single common spinous process for L4/L5 is noted (arrows). A radiolucent band (arrowheads) represents a fat fold artifact. (Courtesy of Douglas B. Hart, DC, Carina, Queensland, Australia)

vertebra assume the appearance of a butterfly's wings when viewing the vertebral body from the front.

Radiological Features. The x-ray appearance on an AP radiograph has been likened to the wings of a butter-

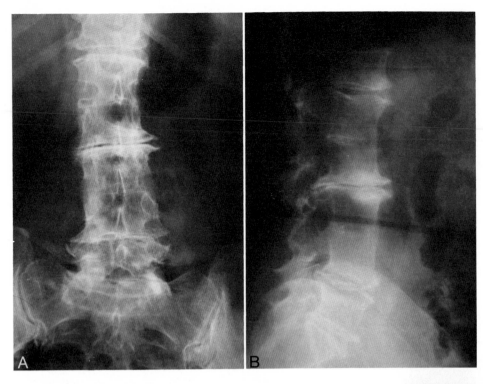

Figure 2.30. MULTIPLE LUMBAR BLOCK VERTEBRAE. A. AP Lumbar Spine. B. Lateral Lumbar Spine. There are multiple block vertebrae throughout the lumbar spine. There is significant degenerative change noted at the freely articulated, unfused levels. (Courtesy of James F. Winterstein, DC, DACBR, Chicago, Illinois)

"scrambled spine." (5,6) A dorsal hemivertebra is pointed toward the anterior and results in a gibbus formation, but it is best visualized on lateral radiographs. (Fig. 2.36)

Schmorl's Nodes

Description. Schmorl's nodes occur when the nucleus pulposus herniates through the vertebral end plate. (Fig. 2.37A and B) These defects have also been called cartilaginous nodes and intraspongy nuclear herniations. There may be an inherent developmental weakness of the end plate, such as occurs with regression of the chorda dorsalis or penetrating blood vessels, (1) allowing for disc protrusion or a pathological weakening of the bone, as is seen in osteoporosis or osteomalacia, which permits the cartilaginous end plate and softened subchondral bone to yield to the pressure of the fluid and noncompressible nucleus pulposus. The incidence of cartilaginous nodes varies from 2 percent to 76 percent, depending on the method of assessment. (2,3)

Other causes for or associations with Schmorl's nodes include idiopathic, post-traumatic, Scheuermann's disease, Paget's disease, degenerative joint disease, sickle cell anemia, and malignant tumors.

Radiological Features. The radiographic appearance of a Schmorl's node looks as though the eraser end of a pencil has been pushed through the end plate, resulting in a squared-off or sharp, rectangular rim of sclerosis protruding above the end plate. (Fig. 2.38A and B) The lesion may appear to be central or peripherally located. (Fig. 2.39) Giant Schmorl's nodes have been noted to occur as anteriorly placed end plate defects and have erroneously been called Scheuermann's disease. (4) (Fig. 2.40) An occasional associated finding with large anteriorly-placed Schmorl's nodes is a slightly increased anteroposterior diameter of the vertebral body. These nodes are most common in the lumbar and thoracic spine and

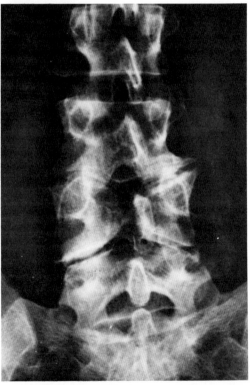

Figure 2.31. BUTTERFLY VERTEBRA. There is a butterfly vertebra present at L4. Note the widened interpediculate distance. (Reprinted with permission: Yochum TR et al: A radiographic anthology of vertebral names. *J Manip Physiol Ther* 8:87, June 1985) (Courtesy of Robert J. Hooke, BAppSc(Chiro), Cootamundra, New South Wales, Australia)

are usually best seen on lateral radiographs. Occasionally, a narrowing of the adjacent disc space may be noted, particularly if the herniation is large, with a significant loss of nuclear material. (5) (Fig. 2.40)

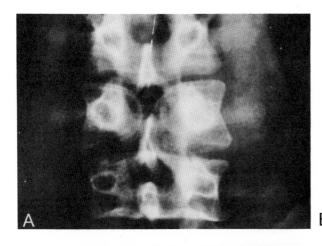

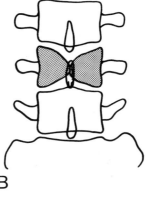

Figure 2.32. BUTTERFLY VERTE-BRA. A. AP Lumbar Spine. There is a symmetrically formed butterfly vertebra present at L3. **B. Schematic Diagram: Butterfly Vertebra.**

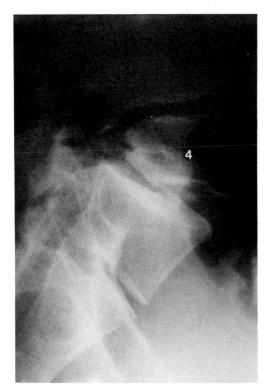

Figure 2.33. VENTRAL HEMIVERTEBRA: LUMBAR SPINE. Observe the anterior hemivertebra present at the L4 lumbar level. (Courtesy of Frank S. Grayson, DC, Rochester, New York)

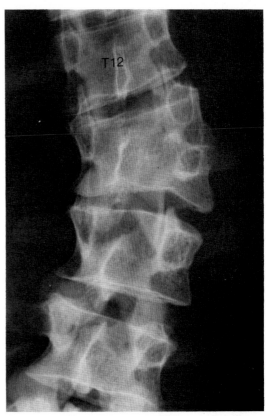

Figure 2.34. LATERAL HEMIVERTEBRA: LUMBAR SPINE. Observe the duplicated pedicles and transverse processes on the L1 vertebra. There is a lateral wedging of the vertebral body consistent with a lateral hemivertebra.

Schmorl's nodes must be differentiated from nuclear impressions (notochordal persistence). These variants of development also cause irregularity of the end plates, but there is a smooth, undulating cortical surface which involves almost the entire end plate. (Fig. 2.41A–C) On a lateral radiograph of nuclear impression there is an indentation of the inferior end plate, while on an anteroposterior radiograph a "double hump" will be noted and has been referred to as the "Cupid's bow contour." (6) (Fig. 2.42A–E) A named appearance has been described due to the characteristic computed tomographic presentation of this anomaly. The "owl's eyes" appearance is present when paired, well-corticated radiolucencies are noted in the vertebral end plate, and the central area has the CT value of disc material. This finding has been

described in the typical inferior end plate location and also in superior vertebral end plates. (7) (Fig. 2.42E)

VATER Syndrome

Description.   The VATER syndrome (vertebral anomalies, anal atresia, tracheo-esophageal fistula with esophageal atresia, and renal and radial dysplasia) was first proposed by Quan and Smith, (1) where they described seven patients with the association of vertebral maldevelopment and multiple visceral anomalies. The reason proposed for this constellation of defects is a nonrandom

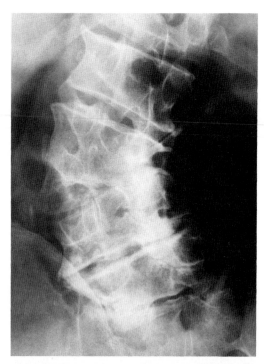

Figure 2.35. LATERAL HEMIVERTEBRA: LUMBAR SPINE. An isolated hemivertebra at L2/L3 is present. This congenital deformity has created a significant structural scoliosis throughout the lumbar spine. Observe the resultant advanced degenerative spondylophyte formation and substantial disc space narrowing present on the concave margins of this scoliotic spine. (Courtesy of Donald E. Freuden, DC, FACO, Denver, Colorado)

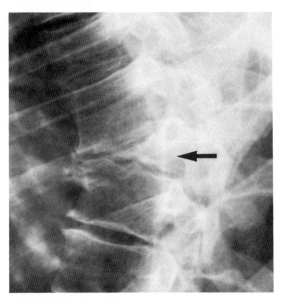

Figure 2.36. DORSAL HEMIVERTEBRA: THORACIC SPINE. Observe the dorsal hemivertebra present in the midthoracic spine (arrow). This congenital abnormality has created an increase in the thoracic kyphosis.

association of congenital anomalies of mesodermal structures that must occur before the seventh fetal week of development, which is a tendency of concurrence and not an absolute interrelationship. The vertebral anomalies are

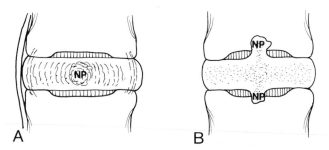

Figure 2.37. DEVELOPMENT OF SCHMORL'S NODES. A. Schematic Diagram: Normal Disc. Observe the normal location of the nucleus pulposus (NP). **Schematic Diagram: Schmorl's Node.** Observe the herniated nucleus pulposus (NP) through the cartilaginous end plate.

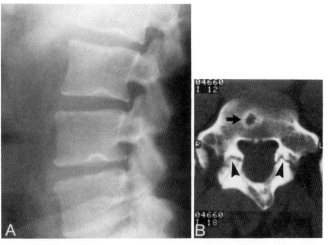

Figure 2.38. SCHMORL'S NODES: LUMBAR SPINE. A. Lateral Lumbar Spine. The short, sharply defined defects involving the vertebral end plates on multiple lumbar levels represent Schmorl's nodes. **B. Computed Tomographic Appearance of a Schmorl's Node.** (Not the same patient as Fig. A) Observe the clearly defined defect present within the vertebral body, representing a Schmorl's node (arrow). This patient has, additionally, bilateral pars defects (arrowheads).

usually hypoplastic or aplastic. (2) Ventricular septal defect and single umbilical artery have occurred frequently; therefore, the "V" may also be considered to stand for vascular. (3) Karyotyping with advanced banding techniques is recommended in the diagnosis of this disorder to determine if any chromosome deletion abnormalities coexist. (4)

The reason for including this rather rare entity is to demonstrate that all anomalies of the spine do not occur as isolated incidents and may be associated with other, multiple defects which may have great clinical significance in the management of the patient. A generalization to keep in mind: If you see one anomaly, search for and rule out others, as they may occur in groups.

POSTERIOR ARCH ANOMALIES

Agenesis of a Lumbar Pedicle

See discussion under "Absent Pedicle of the Cervical Spine." (Fig. 2.43A–C, 2.44)

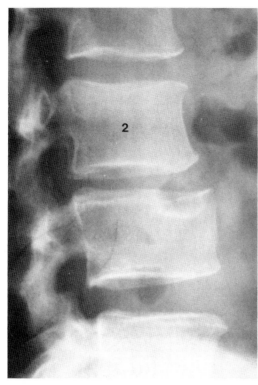

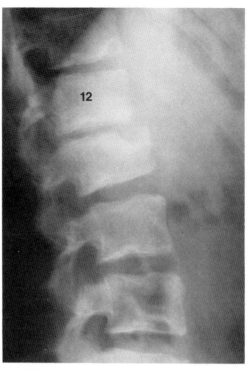

Figure 2.39. A UNIQUE MANIFESTATION OF A SCHMORL'S NODE. There is a giant Schmorl's node present on the anterosuperior corner of the third lumbar vertebra. Associated disc space narrowing is present at the L2/L3 level. Observe the increase in the anteroposterior diameter of the L3 vertebral body. This constellation of changes appears to be a unique manifestation of anteriorly placed giant Schmorl's nodes.

Figure 2.40. GIANT SCHMORL'S NODE. There is a large, anteriorly placed, giant Schmorl's node present on the superior end plate of L1. Significant disc space narrowing is present at the T12/L1 level, associated with the giant Schmorl's node formation. Smaller Schmorl's node formations are present at the anteroinferior corner of T11 and at the vertebral end plates of L3 and L4. **Comment:** Multiple giant Schmorl's nodes have been previously misdiagnosed as representing Scheuermann's disease.

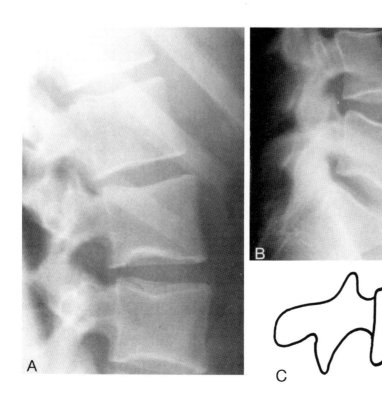

Figure 2.41. NUCLEAR IMPRESSIONS: LUMBAR SPINE. A. Lateral Lumbar Spine. There are multiple nuclear impressions affecting the inferior vertebral end plates of the midlumbar spine. **B. Lateral Lumbosacral Spine.** Observe the broad-based nuclear impression affecting the inferior end plate of the L5 vertebra. **C. Schematic Diagram: Nuclear Impression.** Observe the smooth and long depression of the inferior end plate found associated with nuclear impression.

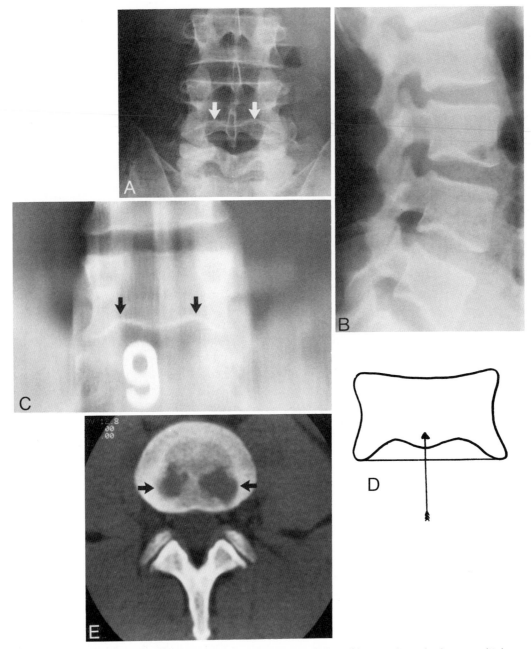

Figure 2.42. "CUPID'S BOW" CONTOUR: LUMBAR SPINE. A. AP Lumbar Spine. Observe the paired parasagittal concavities affecting the inferior end plate of the L4 vertebra (arrows). **B. Lateral Lumbar Spine.** Note the multiple nuclear impressions affecting the inferior end plates of L2 through L5. **C. AP Tomogram: L5 Vertebra.** Observe the "cupid's bow" contour affecting the inferior end plate of the L5 vertebra (arrows). **D. Schematic Diagram: "Cupid's Bow" Contour. E. Computed Tomogram: "Owl's Eyes" Appearance.** The computed tomographic features of nuclear impressions with the "Cupid's bow" contour is that of paired, well-corticated, round areas of intervertebral disc density within the vertebral bodies ("Owl's eyes" appearance) (arrows). ***Comment:*** The "Cupid's bow" contour is associated with nuclear impression deformities usually of the inferior vertebral end plates. They commonly affect the L4 and L5 vertebrae. The bilateral smooth indentations help differentiate this from a vertebral end plate fracture.

Spina Bifida Occulta and Vera

Spina Bifida Occulta. There is a small defect in closure of the laminae in order to form the spinous process which results in a cleft spinous. This defect may be mild, with a small void of osseous development, and is known as "spina bifida occulta (SBO)," and is of no clinical significance since it is not a cause of back pain. (1) Spina bifida occulta does not predispose to low back pain, nor

does it influence the chronicity of low back pain. (2) Spina bifida occulta occurs more commonly in males at the L5 and S1 levels in a 1:9 ratio. (2) Magora and Schwartz convincingly state, "All pre-employment surveys of candidates for any type of work should disregard this [SBO] finding." (2)

Spina Bifida Vera. The defect may be quite large, with no protection of the spinal cord by a bony shield, and is known as "spina bifida vera" or "spina bifida

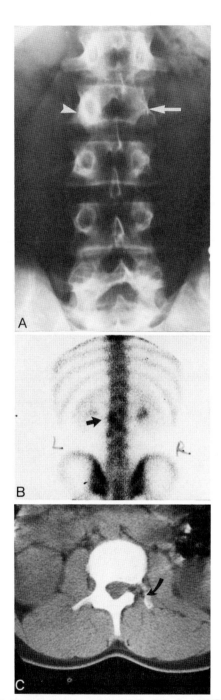

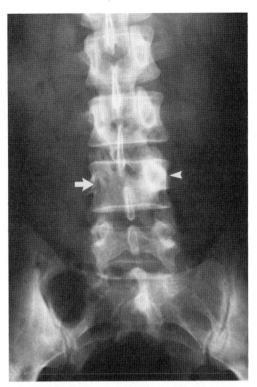

Figure 2.44. CONGENITAL ABSENCE OF A LUMBAR PEDI-CLE. There is congenital agenesis of the pedicle of L4 (arrow), with contralateral reactive sclerosis and hypertrophy of the opposite pedicle (arrowhead). **Comment:** The absence of a vertebral pedicle should be considered the result of metastatic carcinoma unless the contralateral pedicle demonstrates hypertrophy and reactive sclerosis, indicating a longstanding congenital lesion with stress response.

Figure 2.43. CONGENITAL AGENESIS OF A LUMBAR PEDI-CLE. A. AP Lumbar Spine. Agenesis of the L2 pedicle (arrow) has created instability in the neural arch, allowing for stress to be placed upon the opposite pedicle and neural arch, producing significant reactive sclerosis (arrowhead). **B. Bone Scan: Lumbar Spine.** There is an area of increased radionuclide uptake present in the area of stress hypertrophy opposite the agenetic pedicle (arrow). **C. Computed Tomogram.** Computed tomography clearly demonstrates the agenesis of the pedicle (arrow). (Reprinted with permission: Albers VL: Congenital absence of the lumbar pedicle, with sclerosis and hypertrophy of the contralateral pedicle. *ACA J Chiro, Radiology Case Report*, April 1984)

manifesta," allowing protrusion of the spinal cord. There is no simple genetic explanation, but it appears that inheritance is polygenic and that 60 percent are genetic in origin. (3)

Spina bifida vera may be diagnosed in utero through analysis of the amniotic fluid, looking for an elevated level of alpha fetoprotein. The postpartum diagnosis of spina bifida manifesta can be suspected when, on physical examination, there is discovered the cutaneous signature in the form of a hair patch, lipoma, or dimple. The clinical effects of spina bifida manifesta are related to the extent of local cord and nerve root deficit, plus the delayed effects of hydrocephalus and infection of the cord.

Radiological Features.

Spina Bifida Occulta. This defect is well seen on anteroposterior radiographs of the spine. A lucent cleft is noted between the laminae, and the spinous process at that level is diminutive or absent. (Fig. 2.45A–D) A lateral view of the cervical spine may suggest the presence of a spina bifida occulta by absence of the posterior cervical line (spinolaminar junction line) and is found most commonly at C1. (Fig. 2.7B)

Spina Bifida Vera. This defect will be seen on anteroposterior and lateral views of the spine due to the wide defect in the posterior neural arch structures at multiple levels. A soft tissue mass posterior to the spine may also be present, representing the meningocele or myelomeningocele. (Fig. 2.46)

Meningocele/Myelomeningocele

Description. If a defect of the neural arch of a vertebra or vertebrae allows protrusion of the protective

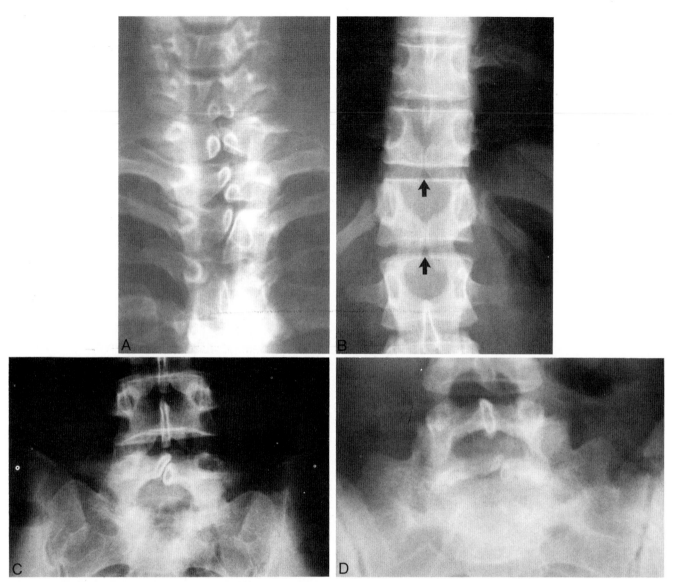

Figure 2.45. SPINA BIFIDA OCCULTA: MULTIPLE LOCATIONS.   A. AP Thoracic. There are multiple spina bifidae affecting C6, C7, T1, and T2.   **B. Lower Thoracic Spine.** Failure of formation of the spinous processes of the 11th and 12th thoracic vertebrae has left a clearly defined midline radiolucent cleft (arrows).   **C. AP Lumbosacral Junction.** Spina bifida occulta is present at the fifth lumbar vertebra.   **D. AP Lumbosacral Junction.** Spina bifida occulta is present at the first sacral tubercle.

coverings of the spinal cord (the leptomeninges) or also allows herniation of the spinal cord itself into the meningeal diverticulum, then there exists a meningocele or myelomeningocele, respectively. (1,2) Failure of fusion of the neural arch halves, resulting in a spina bifida vera, must take place during the 21st to the 29th fetal day in order for a posterior myelomeningocele to result. (2)

There are related problems seen with myelomeningocele, but differentiation based on clinical findings may not be possible. These problems include skin manifestations such as a hairy or pigmented patch, malformed fibrous tissue and blood vessels, and fatty tumors (lipomas). In patients with severe manifestations the protruding sac will be evident at birth, along with bilateral clubbed feet and paralysis, depending on the level of involvement. With mild expression, the child may not begin to show motor disturbances in gait until the age of

5 or 6. The prenatal diagnosis of spinal canal closure defects can be performed by assay of alpha fetoprotein from maternal serum or from amniotic fluid aspirate about the 18th fetal week. (3) All meningoceles do not protrude to the posterior. Commonly, in the upper thoracic spine a lateral herniation of the meninges through the intervertebral foramen may be seen as a water density mass on thoracic or chest radiographs in association with neurofibromatosis. (4) Meningoceles have also been reported to occur anteriorly through the sacrum, creating a curvilinear defect on the anterior aspect of the sacral canal, when viewed laterally. This has been called the "scimitar sacrum," since the lytic defect appears like a curved Turkish sword. (5,6)

Radiological Features.   The roentgenographic findings demonstrate spina bifida vera at one or more vertebral levels. The interpediculate distance will usually be

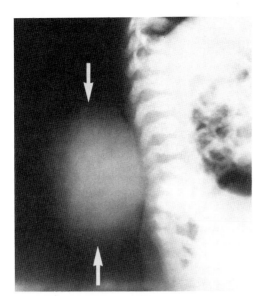

Figure 2.46. SPINA BIFIDA VERA: MYELOMENINGOCELE. There is a large myelomeningocele posterior to the lower lumbar spine and upper sacral area in this infant (arrows).

increased at the site of involvement. Rarely, there is erosion of the vertebral body. The presence of a water density mass may be seen, representing the sac filled with cerebrospinal fluid. Myelography or ultrasonography is necessary to determine if the sac contains spinal cord elements. Water-soluble contrast media is preferred over oil-based contrast, as the communication of subarachnoid space and meningocele may be quite small. (7)

Diastematomyelia

Description. The term "diastematomyelia" was first coined by Ollivier in 1837. (1) It represents a congenital anomaly wherein an osseous, cartilaginous, or fibrous bar divides the spinal cord or cauda equina and fixes it in the midline, effectively tethering the cord. The thoracolumbar area is most commonly affected.

Radiological Features. If an osseous bar is present, it may be demonstrable on plain film radiographs; a fibrous septum will not be seen. There is usually widening of the interpediculate distance at the level of the abnormality. Vertebral body deformities such as spina bifida occulta, hemivertebrae, and congenital bar and scoliosis are present in 50 percent of cases. (2) (Fig. 2.47A and B)

Transitional Vertebrae

Introduction. Transitional vertebrae occur at those regions of the spine where the morphological characteristics of the vertebrae normally markedly change from one area to the next, i.e., cervicothoracic, thoracolumbar, lumbosacral regions. When a transitional segment occurs, it has some features of both adjacent spinal segments. The result may be a fifth "lumbar" vertebra that has some or all of the anatomic characteristics of the first sacral segment. The lumbosacral junction is the most common area of the spine for transitional vertebrae to occur.

Description. Much time and effort has been spent determining the appropriate name for these affected segments, such as "sacralization of the fifth lumbar vertebra,"

where the segment has more characteristics of the sacrum, or "lumbarization of the first sacral segment," which has more characteristics of a lumbar vertebra. "Transitional segment" is less descriptive but encompasses both lumbarization and sacralization. The name is considerably less important than the biomechanical or clinical significance.

If the transitional segment is partially or completely fused to the adjacent segment, then a motion segment is lost. The clinical significance of transitional vertebrae, especially at the lumbosacral junction, is still being debated and researched. The exhaustive study of Tini, Wieser, and Zinn (1) examined the radiographs of 4,000

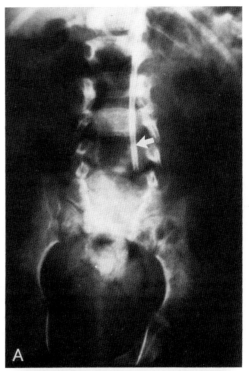

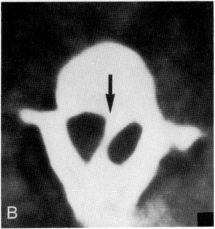

Figure 2.47. DIASTEMATOMYELIA: LUMBAR SPINE. A. AP Lumbar Spine. Observe the widened interpediculate spaces present throughout the lumbar spine. Observe an osseous bar dividing the spinal canal (arrow). **B. Computed Tomogram.** Note the osseous bar dividing the spinal canal (arrow).

Swiss workers and concluded that "... carriers of a lumbosacral transitional vertebra do not have more backache than controls." These findings corroborate the work of Nachemson; (2) however, Castellvi and coworkers (3) found that there is a significant incidence of herniation of the nucleus pulposus at the next disc level above some lumbosacral transitional vertebra. They feel this may be due to abnormal mechanical forces placed on the superior disc which may lead to premature degeneration of the disc. The disc between transitional segments is usually rudimentary in nature, but it has been shown that there is a potential for nuclear herniation with certain classifications of transitional vertebrae. (3) It is known that the accessory joints that develop between the enlarged lumbar transverse processes and the sacral alae may eventually degenerate, due to the asymmetrical forces of movement, and, therefore, may also be a source of low back pain. (4) The combination of transitional vertebrae that cause scoliosis and sciatica is known as Bertolotti's syndrome. (5)

Radiological Features.   The radiographic appearance of transitional lumbosacral vertebra may vary greatly. An increase in the vertical dimension of one or both of the L5 transverse processes greater than 19 mm is considered the least anatomic change necessary to be considered transitional. (Fig. 2.48A–D) Complete fusion of the L5 transverse process to the remaining sacrum, either unilaterally or bilaterally, may be seen, or the enlarged transverse process may form an accessory joint with the sacrum. (Fig. 2.49A and B) When the development of the transitional segment is asymmetrical and longstanding, it is not uncommon to see signs of degenerative joint disease at this accessory articulation in the form of subchondral sclerosis and marginal osteophytes. The body of L5 is usually normal in size and shape, but the interposed disc is generally vestigial.

Facet Tropism

Description.   The joint formed between articulating processes in the lumbar spine is not planar but curved.

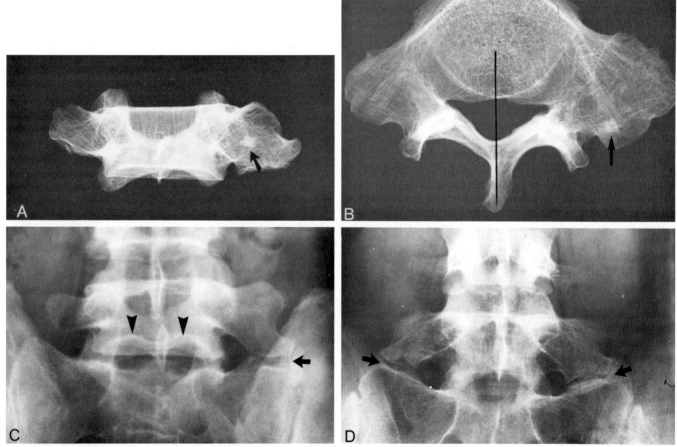

Figure 2.48. TRANSITIONAL SEGMENT: LUMBOSACRAL JUNCTION.   A. Specimen Radiograph. The large, spatulated transverse process of the fifth lumbar vertebra is noted in this transitional anatomical specimen. Of incidental notation is a benign bone island within the spatulated transverse process of L5 (arrow).   **B. Specimen Radiograph.** An axial projection of the specimen demonstrates the large, spatulated transverse process of the transitional segment. A benign bone island is noted (arrow).   **C. AP Lumbosacral Junction.** A unilateral transitional segment is noted, with an accessory articulation (arrow). Of incidental notation is a "Cupid's bow" contour on the inferior end plate of L5 (arrowheads), resulting from nuclear impression.   **D. AP Lumbosacral Junction.** Observe the bilateral transitional segment present at the lumbosacral junction, with bilateral accessory joints (arrows).

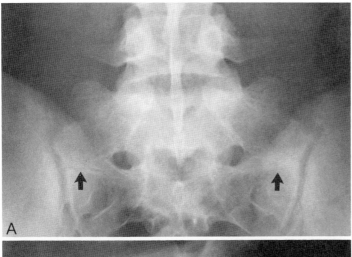

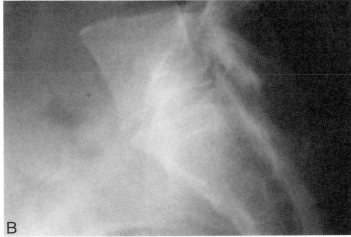

Figure 2.49. TRANSITIONAL SEGMENT: LUMBOSAC-RAL JUNCTION. A. AP Lumbosacral Junction. There is a bilateral, nearly completely fused transitional segment (arrows) present at the lumbosacral junction. **B. Lateral Lumbosacral View.** Observe the hypoplastic disc between the transitional segment and the sacral base.

Biomechanically, bilaterally symmetrical sagittal joints at each level should allow equal ranges of motion, but these circumstances also limit flexion and rotation of the lumbar spine. (1)

In some individuals the planes of articulations at a single level are asymmetrical. When this condition exists, the term "tropism" (literally meaning, "turning") is applied. The significance of this anomaly has not been clearly delineated and remains an area of clinical controversy. (2, 3)

Radiological Features. Facet tropism may be seen on the anteroposterior projection of the lumbar spine. In the normal lumbar spine the facet joints are visible as linear radiolucent regions between each superior and inferior articular process. Tropism at any level will manifest as an absence of the joint space on one side, while being clearly delineated on the opposite side. (Fig. 2.50A and B) This is most frequently encountered at the lumbosacral joint but may be seen at any lumbar level. In the presence of scoliosis or intersegmental rotation the appearance of tropism may be simulated, as the facet joints are displaced, to be no longer oriented tangential to the x-ray beam.

Knife Clasp Syndrome

Description. This syndrome is named for the painful effect created upon extension of the lumbar spine in a patient who has a spina bifida of the first sacral segment and an associated caudal enlargement of the fifth lumbar spinous process. The enlargement of the spinous process may be the result of inclusion of the first sacral tubercle with the ossification center for the spinous process of the fifth lumbar. DeAnguin (1) reported 15 patients with this defect and surmised that, due to the absence of the sacral tubercle, the L5 vertebra demonstrated an increased range of motion and, further, that low back pain may be due to pressure on the laminar stumps at S1 or by pressure on a membrane that covers the sacral defect.

Radiological Features. AP roentgenograms will reveal a spina bifida occulta of the S1 level and an increased vertical dimension of the L5 spinous process. (Fig. 2.51A and B, 2.52) A lateral film will clearly demonstrate the distal enlargement of the L5 spinous process. Myelography, with the patient in extension, may demonstrate a complete block to the flow of subarachnoid contrast. (2)

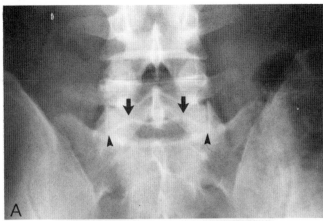

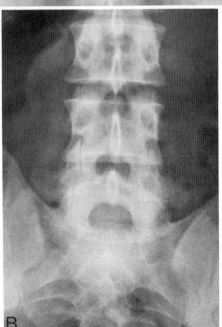

Figure 2.50. ABNORMALITIES OF FACET ORIENTATION: LUMBOSACRAL JUNCTION. A. AP Lumbosacral View. There are bilateral sagittal facet facings (arrowheads) present at the lumbosacral junction. Asymmetrical facet facings (tropism) are noted at the L4/L5 level. A "Cupid's bow" deformity is present, affecting the inferior end plate of L5 (arrows). **B. AP Lumbosacral View.** There is facet asymmetry present at the lumbosacral junction (tropism). **Comment:** Computed tomography has clearly demonstrated that patients with plain film radiographic demonstration of bilateral sagittal facet facings at the lumbosacral junction in fact may have "cupped" facet facings rather than purely sagittal joints in many instances.

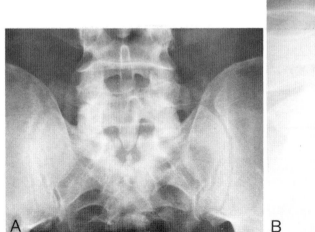

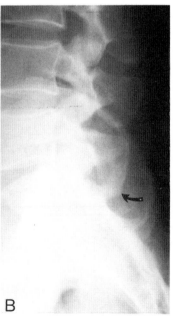

Figure 2.51. "KNIFE CLASP" DEFORMITY. A. AP Lumbosacral View. Observe the large spinous process of L5, which projects into a spina bifida affecting the first sacral segment. **B. Lateral Lumbosacral View.** The elongated spinous process of L5 (arrow) projects caudally into the first sacral cleft. (Courtesy of James R. Brandt, DC, FACO, Coon Rapids, Minnesota)

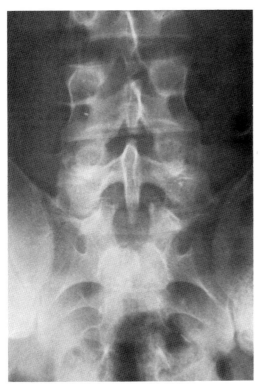

Figure 2.52. "KNIFE CLASP" DEFORMITY. Observe the large spina bifida present in the first sacral segment, which allows the elongated spinous process of L5 to enter this defect.

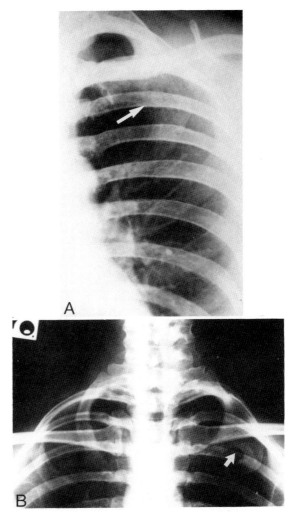

Figure 2.53. SRB'S ANOMALY. **A. PA Ribs.** Observe the partial congenital synostosis of the first and second ribs (arrow). **B. PA Ribs.** There is nearly complete congenital fusion of the first and second ribs on the right side (arrow).

Anomalies of the Thorax

RIB ANOMALIES

Srb's Anomaly

Description. Involution of one or both first ribs as a result of diminished length and incomplete fusion of the first and second ribs to form a solid bony plate is known as Srb's anomaly. (1)

Radiological Features. Views taken for the chest or ribs will demonstrate this anomaly. The normal rib interspace between the first and second ribs is absent. (Fig. 2.53A and B) A pseudarthrosis may be seen in the midportion of the fused rib.

Luschka's Bifurcated Rib

Occasionally, the anterior aspect of an upper thoracic rib may be split or bifurcated. It is clinically insignificant but must not be mistaken for a cavity within the lung. (1) (Fig. 2.54A–C)

Rib Foramen

Anomalous foraminal development in a rib may rarely be noted and is of no clinical significance. (Fig. 2.55)

Intrathoracic Rib

Occasionally, an anomalous rib is present which protrudes through instead of around the thoracic cavity. (Fig. 2.56)

CHEST ANOMALIES

Pectus Excavatum/Carinatum

Pectus Excavatum. This is the commonest deformity of the chest wall. It is also known as funnel chest, due to the midline depression of the sternum which is seen on physical examination. A lateral radiograph of the chest will confirm the physical examination finding of posterior displacement of the sternum. (Fig. 2.57A and B)

Pectus Carinatum. This deformity is produced by an anterior displacement of the sternum. An alternate name for this condition is "pigeon breast." It has been found associated with Morquio's syndrome. A lateral chest film will demonstrate a prominent sternum, with an increased retrosternal clear space.

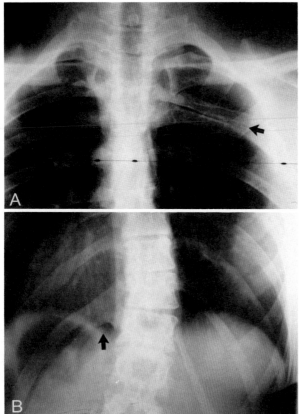

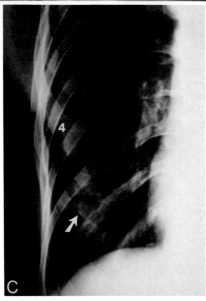

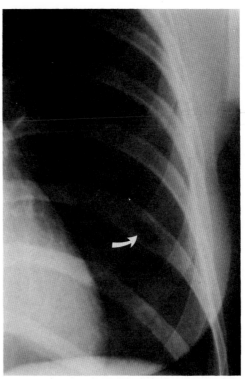

Figure 2.55. RIB FORAMEN. Observe the radiolucent foramen present within the posterolateral aspect of the eighth left rib (arrow). (Courtesy of Kenneth E. Yochum, DC, St. Louis, Missouri)

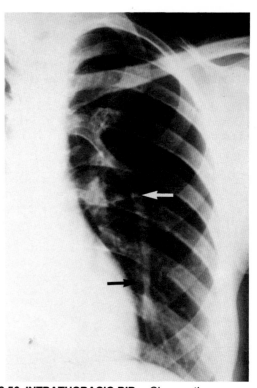

Figure 2.54. LUSCHKA'S BIFURCATED RIB. A. AP Ribs. Observe the congenital fusion of the posterolateral surface of the third and fourth rib on the right side (arrow). The black transverse line through the lower half of the radiograph represents the perforated crease of a folding film. **B. AP Ribs.** There is congenital synostosis of the posterior surface of the 11th and 12th ribs on the left side (arrow). **C. AP Ribs.** A focal bifurcation of the anterior surface of the right fourth rib is present. The circular radiopaque density present over the right lower lung field represents a nipple shadow (arrow). **Comment:** Luschka's bifurcated rib is clinically insignificant but must not be mistaken for a cavity within the lung.

Figure 2.56. INTRATHORACIC RIB. Observe the accessory intrathoracic rib (arrows). This is a rare congenital anomaly. (Courtesy of Bryan Hartley, MD, Melbourne, Australia)

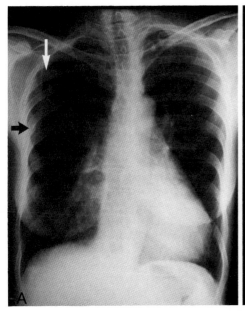
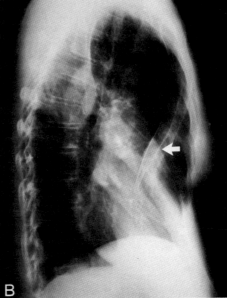

Figure 2.57. PECTUS EXCAVATUM. A. PA Chest. As a result of posterior protrusion of the sternum, the right atrial heart border cannot be visualized on this PA radiograph. There is excessive caudal angulation of the ribs anteriorly. Of incidental notation are old healed fractures present on the right at ribs 4, 5, 6, and 7 (arrows). **B. Lateral Chest.** Observe the posterior protrusion of the sternum (arrow), which has displaced the cardiac shadow, thereby overlapping the lower thoracic spine.

Anomalies of the Hip and Pelvis

CONGENITAL HIP DYSPLASIA

Description

Congenital hip dysplasia includes deformities of the acetabulum as well as dislocation of the femur from a malformed acetabulum. The diagnosis of congenital hip dislocation may be suspected at birth if there is an index of suspicion and the appropriate orthopedic tests are performed (Ortolani's and Barlow's tests). The main reason for the dislocation is inversion of the fibrocartilaginous limbus and capsular contraction, which makes reduction of the dislocation difficult or impossible. (1)

Radiological Features. The description of congenital hip dislocation by Putti in 1929 remains accurate today. The combination of an absent or small proximal femoral epiphysis, lateral displacement of the femur, and increased inclination of the acetabular roof is known as Putti's triad. (2) (Fig. 2.58) With longstanding dislocations and attempted weightbearing the proximally and posteriorly luxated femoral head may create a shallow pseudoacetabulum superior to the deformed primary acetabulum. (Fig. 2.59A–C)

SACRAL DYSPLASIA

Sacral Agenesis

Description. Congenital absence of the distal portion of the spinal column, also known as caudal regression, was first reported by Hohl in 1850. (1) Lack of development of the caudal spine has been reported as high as the 10th thoracic level. (2) An extensive study of 853 British infants (3) demonstrated that the incidence of all congenital malformations occurs at a rate three times higher than normal when it is shown that the mother had diabetes and the association of maternal diabetes with sacral agenesis has been well documented. (4)

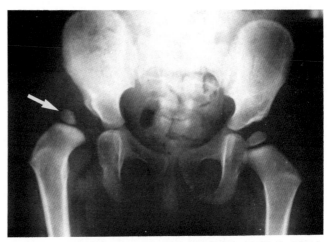

Figure 2.58. CONGENITAL HIP DISLOCATION: PUTTI'S TRIAD. There is lateral displacement of the affected proximal femur, with underdevelopment of the femoral capital epiphysis (arrow). Additionally, a shallow acetabulum is associated.

The diagnosis is usually apparent at birth. The child has a flat or depressed sacral area with deficient musculature of the lower extremities. Associated problems include spinopelvic instability, scoliosis (most common), myelomeningocele, hip dislocation or contracture, knee contracture, and foot deformity. Renshaw has described four types, based on the variable sacral/vertebral development seen radiographically. (4)

There is evidence that this condition is teratogenically induced or is a spontaneous genetic mutation. This evidence includes 1) the association with maternal diabetes; 2) the relationship of insulin-dependent diabetes mellitus with the major histocompatibility system; and 3) demonstration of a defect at a locus or loci on the sixth chromosome. This site codes for the major histocompatibility system of cell surface antigens. (4)

Radiological Features. Radiographs will demon-

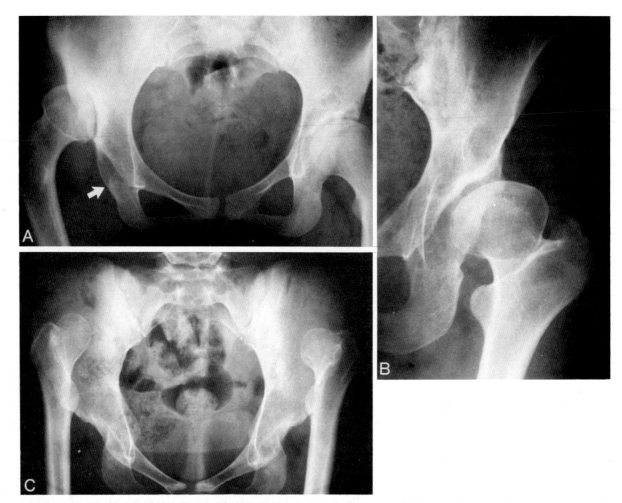

Figure 2.59. EXAMPLES OF LONGSTANDING CONGENITAL HIP DYSPLASIA.   A. AP Pelvis. Observe the shallowness of the original acetabulum (arrow), as compared to the accessory acetabulum, which has formed on the lateral edge of the ilium.   **B. AP Hip.** There is deformity and flattening of the femoral head. The acetabulum is shallow.   **C. AP Pelvis.** There is complete bilateral dislocation of the femoral heads from the acetabuli, both of which are shallow. (Courtesy of Lynton G. F. Giles, MSc, DC, Perth, Australia).

strate absence of the sacrum and possibly some of the caudal lumbar segments. If the patient ever assumes a weightbearing posture, abnormal biomechanics will cause typical degenerative joint changes to occur where the two ilia articulate. (Fig. 2.60)

COXA VARA/VALGA

Description

The noun "coxa" loosely refers to the hip, while the terms "varus" and "valgus" are adjectives which describe angulation of a part toward or away from the midline, respectively. The normal angle of incidence of the proximal femur is 120–130 degrees (Mikulicz's angle). If this angle measures less than 120 degrees, coxa vara exists. An angle greater than 130 degrees indicates coxa valga.

Coxa Vara.   This femoral deformity is the result of eccentric cessation of growth of the medial aspect of the growth plate between the proximal femoral epiphysis and the femoral neck. It may occur in isolation or accompany proximal femoral focal deficiency, osteogenesis imperfecta, rickets, fibrous dysplasia, (2) and cleidocranial dysplasia. (3) The sex incidence is equal, and it is unilateral

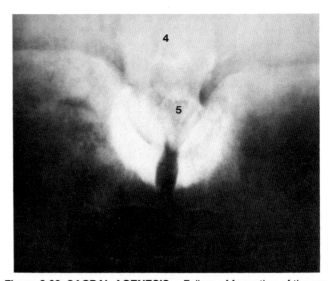

Figure 2.60. SACRAL AGENESIS.   Failure of formation of the sacrum creates close proximity of the posterior iliac surfaces. Degenerative reactive sclerosis is present on the approximated iliac surfaces. (Courtesy of Appa L. Anderson, DC, DACBR, Portland, Oregon).

in 75 percent of cases. Acquired coxa vara may also complicate proximal femoral fractures.

Coxa Valga. This deformity appears to be the result of muscular imbalance of the abductor mechanism of the hip. (1) This imbalance, in turn, reduces the traction effect on the physis at the base of the greater trochanter. Histological studies show that this growth plate is continuous (along the lateral aspect of the femoral neck) with the growth plate of the proximal femoral epiphysis. Therefore, this region of growth has great influence on the developing angulation of the femoral neck/shaft.

Radiological Features

Coxa Vara. Patients with coxa vara will have a decreased femoral angle, an inverted radiolucent "V" in the proximal metaphysis of the femur, an enlarged greater trochanter, and, depending on the length of existence, some deformity of the acetabulum may be present. (Fig.

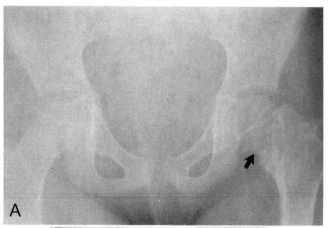
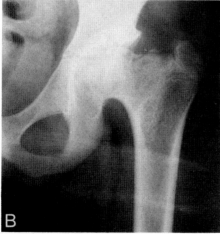

Figure 2.61. COXA VARA. A. AP Pelvis. There is a decreased femoral angle, with an inverted radiolucent "V" in the proximal metaphysis of the femur (arrow). This is a characteristic appearance for infantile coxa vara. An associated widening of the metaphysis is related to the deformity. There is no evidence of degenerative joint changes at this time. (Courtesy of C. H. Quay, MD, Melbourne, Australia). **B. AP Hip.** There is significant reduction of the femoral angle, with broadening of the metaphysis. A characteristic enlargement of the greater trochanter is noted. Associated deformity and osteophyte formation is present, affecting the lateral edge of the acetabulum.

2.61A and B) Degenerative joint changes may be superimposed findings in longstanding cases.

Coxa Valga. Patients with coxa valga will demonstrate an increased femoral angle (greater than 130 degrees). Partial lateral dislocation of the femoral head out of the acetabular cavity is frequently found. Coxa valga is common with lesions which predispose to atrophy or disease of the structures contiguous to the hip such as chronic injuries to the lower extremities.

Anomalies of the Extremities

PATELLAR ANOMALIES

Bipartite, Tripartite, and Multipartite Patellae

Description. The patella is a sesamoid bone which usually develops from a single ossification center about the fifth or sixth year of life. Occasionally, this ossification center may be fragmented and fail to osseously unite (although there is usually a fibrous bridge), resulting in a mature patella that is made up of two or more separate pieces of bone. A *bipartite patella* is the most common presentation of this anomaly (two separate pieces of bone) and is commonly bilateral (80%). (1) If there are three pieces to the patella, it is termed a *tripartite patella*. More than three pieces is called *multipartite* or *segmented* patella. These patellar anomalies affect 2–3 percent of the population, with an equal sex incidence. (1) These anomalies are usually clinically insignificant but must be differentiated from fracture.

It should be noted, there have been recent reports of pain associated with bipartite patella. (1–3) The pain appears to be the result of traumatic loosening of the fibrous connection and is localized to the area of the osseous defect, is exacerbated with activity, and does not abate with conservative treatment. Surgical excision of the accessory portion of the patella appears to have the best results.

Radiological Features. Anteroposterior, lateral, and axial views of the knee are most helpful in the diagnosis of congenital maldevelopments of the patella and differentiating them from a fractured patella. The ununited segment is usually in the superolateral aspect of the patella, although bone fragments have been demonstrated in various quadrants. (4) (Fig. 2.62, 2.63) Particular attention should be directed to the margins of the separated bone. The bone edges should be smooth, rounded, and corticated. Soft tissue swelling is unrelated to bipartite patellae.

Fong's Syndrome

Description. Also known as iliac horn syndrome and may be associated with the nail-patella syndrome, hereditary osteo-oncho dysplasia, this hereditary syndrome is transmitted as an autosomal dominant. The patient demonstrates abnormalities of the nails of the hand and feet, renal dysplasia, and bone deformities. (1,2)

Radiological Features. The patellae are hypoplastic and laterally placed. Exostoses from the posterior aspect of the ilia are noted (iliac horns). The articulations of the

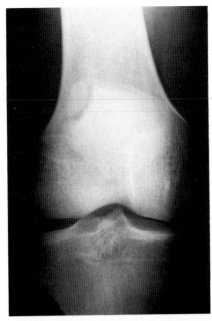

Figure 2.62. OSSIFICATION ABNORMALITIES OF THE PATELLA: BIPARTITE PATELLA. *Comment:* Bipartite and tripartite patellae almost always occur on the superolateral margin of the patella. They should not be confused with patellar fracture, since fractures usually occur through the waist of the patella. (Courtesy of Kenneth E. Yochum, DC, St. Louis, Missouri)

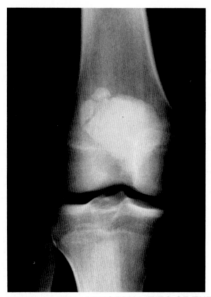

Figure 2.63. OSSIFICATION ABNORMALITIES OF THE PATELLA: TRIPARTITE PATELLA. (Courtesy of Kenneth E. Yochum, DC, St. Louis, Missouri)

elbow are malformed. (For further discussion, see Chapter 8.)

TARSAL AND FOOT ANOMALIES

Tarsal Coalition (Tarsal Bars)

Description. Tarsal coalition is due to a congenital fibrous union or a bony bar between two or more tarsal bones. Some coalitions are acquired post-traumatically or

are the sequellae of inflammatory arthritic conditions. The majority of tarsal coalitions seen in clinical practice are present from birth. (1,2) Symptoms appear after the first decade. The majority of symptoms are secondary to biomechanically induced osteoarthritis. It affects 1–2 percent of the population. (3)

The patient may complain of pain, which may be severe, in the tarsal area. Limited subtalar or midtarsal joint motion, a rigid or semirigid flatfoot deformity, and prominence of the peroneal tendons may be noted. (4) Coalitions with peroneal spasm may present, or peroneal prominence without spasm. (5) Tarsal coalition can be a cause of chronic inversion injuries to the ankle. It should be looked for in patients with such histories, since it may be corrected surgically, re-establishing normal subtalar joint weightbearing.

Tarsal coalitions are known to be present in phocomelia, hemimelia, and other gross limb anomalies. (6) An extensive and authoritative account of tarsal coalition by Jacobs et al should be consulted. (3)

Radiological Features. The diagnosis of tarsal coalition can usually be made on plain film radiographs by performing dorsoplantar, lateral, and medial oblique

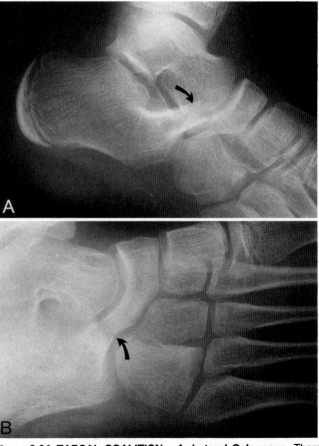

Figure 2.64. TARSAL COALITION. **A. Lateral Calcaneus.** There is a large bony bar projecting from the anterior process of the calcaneus (arrow). **B. Oblique Foot.** An accessory articulation (arrow) has formed between the anterior calcaneal bar and the tarsal navicular. This coalition is fibrous in nature. **Comment:** Tarsal coalition often goes unrecognized and may be the underlying etiology in patients with chronic inversion injuries of the ankle.

views of the foot and an axial view of the calcaneus to visualize the subtalar joints. When an expected normal joint is obliterated by a bony bar which is continuous with the normally articulated adjacent bones, the diagnosis is certain. (Fig. 2.64A and B) The two most common sites for tarsal coalition are the talocalcaneal and calcaneonavicular articulations. (3) Fusion of bones by syndesmoses, synchondroses, or synostoses may require tomography or CT evaluation.

Vertical Talus

Description. Congenital vertical talus is a developmental anomaly where a primary dislocation of the talonavicular joint is present and the talus assumes a more upright position. This appears to be the result of a short Achille's tendon. (1) The characteristic foot deformity is known as "rocker bottom" foot because of the rounded prominence on the medial plantar surface. It is often associated with spina bifida manifesta, myelomeningocele, and Down's syndrome. The sex ratio is equal, and it is bilateral in 50 percent of patients. (2)

Radiological Features. On the dorsoplantar film a calcaneus valgus is present, along with metatarsus adduc-

tus. The lateral film will show plantar flexion of the calcaneus and an increased plantar inclination of the talus. (Fig. 2.65A and B) The navicular then articulates with the dorsal aspect of the talus. The altered plane of articulations for the talus predisposes these patients to development of degenerative joint disease later in life.

Morton's Syndrome

Description. Morton's syndrome, named after Dudley Morton, (1) occurs in the presence of an abnormally short first metatarsal, and the second metatarsal is unusually broad at its base. The patient complains of pain upon activity at the plantar surface of the foot, in the vicinity of the second cuneiform-metatarsal joint. On observation a significant callus may be present under the second and third metatarsal heads. This condition is also known as Morton's foot or first ray insufficiency syndrome, while Morton suggested the term "metatarsus atavicus." (1)

Radiological Features. A dorsoplantar view of the affected foot will reveal the first metatarsal bone to be significantly shorter than the second metatarsal. There is a varus deformity of the first metatarsal. Due to the increased biomechanical forces placed upon the second metatarsal bone, its shaft and base will be increased in transverse diameter through periosteal bone deposition. The tibial and fibular sesamoids are proximally displaced. Stress fractures of the second and third metatarsals may complicate this condition. (2)

Polydactyly

See discussion under "Finger Anomalies." (Fig. 2.66)

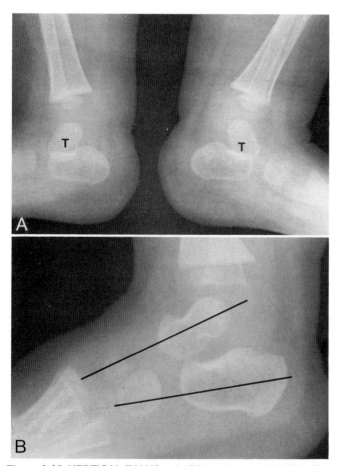

Figure 2.65. VERTICAL TALUS. A. Bilateral Lateral Ankles. The talus (T) has assumed a vertical position bilaterally. (Courtesy of David M. Walker, DPM, Melbourne, Australia). **B. Lateral Foot: Normal Axial Relationships.** The enhanced lines demonstrate the normal axial relationships of the talus with the remainder of the forefoot, and the calcaneus with the talus.

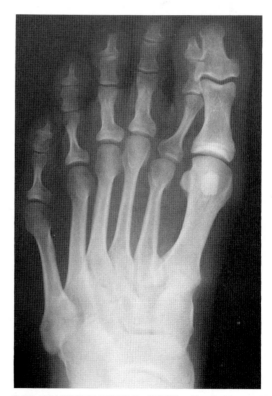

Figure 2.66. POLYSYNDACTYLY: FOOT. Duplication and hypoplasia of the second ray with soft tissue fusion to the great toe is noted. (Courtesy of Bryan Hartley, MD, Melbourne, Australia)

ELBOW ANOMALIES

Supracondylar Process of the Humerus

Description. A rudimentary exostosis of bone seen in man and lower animals may be present on the anteromedial aspect of the distal humeral metaphysis and is known as a supracondylar process. It can be differentiated from an osteochondroma by the fact that the supracondylar process grows toward the adjacent joint, whereas, osteochondroma grows away from the joint. It may occur in approximately 3 percent of the population and is slightly more common in Europe. (1) It has been variously called "supracondyloid," "supraepitrochlear," or "epicondylic process." (2)

The presence of a supracondylar process may have clinical significance in two instances: Firstly, it is bone and is therefore subject to fracture; secondly, it may compress the median nerve and the brachial, radial, or median arteries, if they happen to travel in the course of the median nerve. (2) Rarely, compression of the median nerve may create a median nerve neuralgia; however, most remain asymptomatic. (2,3) Anatomically, a fibrous or fibro-osseous ligament may extend from the end of the process to the medial epicondyle of the humerus and is known as Struther's ligament. (4)

Radiological Features. Radiographically, a supracondylar process is composed of cortical and trabeculated bone, forming a beak-like bony spur at the anterior and medial portions of the distal humeral metaphysis. This excrescence of bone is angled toward the elbow joint and is usually not larger than 2 cm in length. (Fig. 2.67) It is not well seen on frontal radiographs but is clearly defined in lateral or oblique projections.

Radioulnar Synostosis

Description. When there is a failure of longitudinal segmentation of the proximal radius and ulna, a bone fusion results. This defect is transmitted as an autosomal dominant, with an equal sex incidence. It may be seen unilaterally, but 80 percent of the time it is bilateral. (1) The length of the fusion may extend from 3–6 cm and may be osseous or fibrous. From a clinical standpoint, pronation and supination may be limited to nonexistent, depending on the degree and type of fusion. The defect may be diagnosed at birth, but diagnosis is delayed in most instances until childhood. Surgery may result in a more normal position for hand function. (2) Associated conditions include congenital dislocated hip, club foot, Madelung's deformity, and syndactyly or polydactyly. (3)

Radiological Features. This diagnosis can be made on anteroposterior and lateral views of the elbow. These will demonstrate bone in the area between the proximal radius and ulna, usually occupied by the interosseous membrane for a distance of up to 6 cm. (Fig. 2.68)

WRIST ANOMALIES

Madelung's Deformity

Introduction. This entity was first defined in 1878 by a German surgeon, Madelung, (1) who described a young woman with a deformity of her wrist. He also reported that this deformity had been described as early

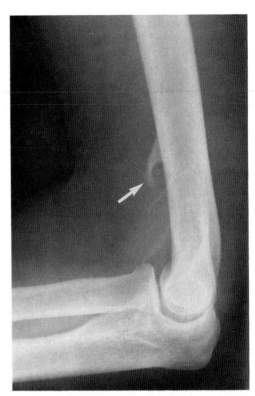

Figure 2.67. SUPRACONDYLAR PROCESS: DISTAL HUMERUS. A slender bony spur projects from the anterior distal diaphyseal surface of the humerus (arrow). The supracondylar process projects towards the joint, a helpful differential point from an osteochondroma, which projects away from the joint. ***Comment:*** The supracondylar process is usually asymptomatic; however, it may be complicated with fracture or, if large, may compress the median nerve, creating a median nerve palsy.

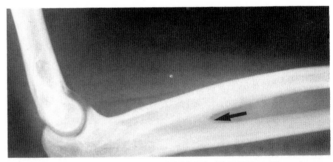

Figure 2.68. RADIOULNAR SYNOSTOSIS: ELBOW. There is congenital fusion of the proximal interosseous space between the radius and ulna (arrow). This usually occurs as an isolated congenital anomaly.

as 1834, but it is his name that has persisted as the eponym of this congenital anomaly. It now seems that Madelung's deformity of the wrist may exist alone or as part of a more generalized condition known as dyschondrosteosis.

Description. The problem is passed on as an autosomal dominant trait and is usually more manifest in females. The deformity is twice as common in bilateral form. The diagnosis is usually made in early adolescence, during periods of rapid growth, when associated wrist pain develops. This pain will usually subside after the growth period; therefore, observation of the patient is recommended until closure of the growth plate before any operation is considered. (2,3)

The fundamental abnormality is retarded growth of the medial portion of the distal radial epiphysis, resulting in asymmetrical growth. This results in ulnar deviation of the hand and a dorsal prominence of the ulnar styloid process due to posterior subluxation of the distal ulna. Manual reduction of the subluxation may be attempted but is only a temporary measure. The physical appearance of the resulting wrist deformity has been called the "bayonette" appearance. (4)

Radiological Features.   On a posterior to anterior film of the wrist the x-ray appearance shows a triangular shape to the distal radial epiphysis, with retarded growth of its medial aspect, resulting in an ulnar slant to the distal articulating surface. The radius is shortened, and a lucent defect is noted along its medial metaphysis. The distal radioulnar joint is widened. The carpal angle is decreased (less than 117 degrees). A lateral film usually shows a volar tilt of the distal radial articular surface greater than the normal 5 degrees and dorsal subluxation of the ulna. The carpal alignment is altered to accommodate the radial changes, with the lunate being at the proximal apex of the carpal deformity. (Fig. 2.69A and B)

Carpal Coalition

Description.   Carpal coalition is the fusion of two or more carpal bones. It may occur as an isolated anomaly or as part of a more widespread anomalous development. The cause for congenital fusion of the carpal bones is lack of segmentation and cavitation in the cartilage template for the affected bones. Carpal coalition is twice as com-

mon in females and slightly more common in blacks. (1) Bridging between the lunate and triquetral bones is the most common fusion in the wrist. (2) Some of the associated conditions include Madelung's deformity, Holt-Oram syndrome, Turner's syndrome, Ellis-van Creveld syndrome. (1,2) Generally, isolated fusions affect the bones in one row of the wrist, (1) whereas fusions that cross from one row to the other tend to be associated with congenital syndromes. (2) The greatest clinical risk associated with carpal coalition is fracture.

Radiological Features.   Due to the incomplete fusion in some examples, plain film demonstration of the osseous bridge may be difficult and require multiple views of the affected wrist. The diagnosis can be made when continuity of cortical and trabecular bone between adjacent carpal bones is demonstrated. (Fig. 2.70) Diagnosis will be delayed until ossification is radiographically evident. Fusions secondary to acquired disease, such as psoriatic arthritis, rheumatoid arthritis, or septic arthritis, may be differentiated through historical data.

FINGER ANOMALIES

Polydactyly

Description.   Polydactyly is an increased number of fingers or toes. There is a predominance for this condition in black patients. The significance of polydactyly depends on whether the extra digit is on the radial (pre-axial) or ulnar (post-axial) side of the hand. Pre-axial polydactyly is seen in Apert's syndrome, Fanconi's syndrome, and Holt-Oram syndrome. Post-axial polydactyly is associated with Ellis-van Creveld syndrome and Laurence-Moon-Biedl syndrome. (1)

Radiological Features.   The diagnosis of polydactyly

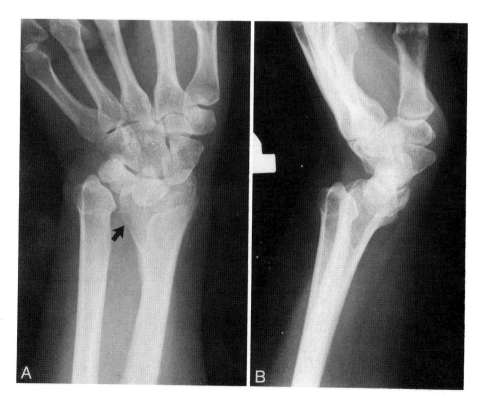

Figure 2.69. MADELUNG'S DEFORMITY: WRIST. A. PA Wrist. Premature closure of the medial portion of the distal radial physis (growth plate) has created an ulnar slant to the distal articulating surface of the radius. A characteristic "V" shaped deformity is present on the ulnar side of the distal radius (arrow). There is a widening of the radioulnar articulation and disorientation of the radiocarpal articulation. This has created a decreased carpal angle. **B. Lateral Wrist.** There is characteristic posterior subluxation in the ulna, which has been referred to in Madelung's deformity as the "bayonette" appearance.

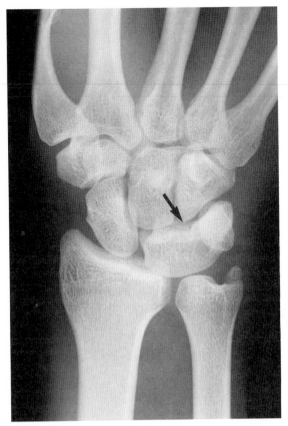

Figure 2.70. CARPAL COALITION: WRIST. There is congenital synostosis affecting the lunate and triquetrum. The arrow indicates where the normal articulation should have occurred. Of incidental notation is nonunion of the ulnar styloid tip.

is evident clinically. The role of x-ray is to determine the nature of osseous development within the extra finger, as well as any additional bony maldevelopment associated with coexisting syndromes.

Syndactyly

Description. Syndactyly is the most common developmental anomaly of the hand, but it may also affect the foot and is manifest in the form of fusion of the skin between the digits (syndactyly) or fusion of the osseous phalanges of adjacent digits (synostosis). The incidence is thought to be one in 2,500 births, (1) with a distinct male predominance, (2) and is more common in whites than blacks in a 10:1 ratio. (3) It may be considered partial when the fusion involves the proximal segments, or complete if the fusion extends to the distal aspect. If the fusion is distal, with the proximal segments free, the appropriate name is acrosyndactyly. It is not a bone or cartilage disease but a defect of mesenchymal organization during the 5th fetal week, resulting in failure of an interphalangeal joint to develop. (4)

Five types of syndactyly have been described: 1) zygodactyly (most common type), involving the third and fourth fingers and/or the second and third toes; 2) synpolydactyly of the third and fourth fingers, with partial or complete reduplication of fingers three and four in the web (or may be toes four and five); 3) ring and little finger syndactyly, where the middle phalanx of the fifth finger

is rudimentary or absent; 4) complete syndactyly, involving all fingers; and 5) syndactyly associated with metacarpal and/or metatarsal synostosis. (5) It more commonly affects the medial side of the hand. (6)

Syndactyly may be associated with other syndromes, including Poland, Apert, Saethre, and Pfeiffer syndromes. (5)

Radiological Features. X-ray examination of the affected extremity will show soft tissue fusion between the fingers or toes and any osseous anomalies of development. In some instances fusion of the phalanges of the same finger or toe may be present; in other cases, fusion of the phalanges between adjacent digits may be noted.

Kirner's Deformity

Description. Kirner's deformity, a type of curvature of the fifth finger, is also known as dystelephalangy. (1) It occurs sporadically or is transmitted as an autosomal dominant trait. This abnormality usually affects the fifth fingers bilaterally. (2) Physical examination will show a palmar curvature of the distal phalanx in a patient beyond 5 years of age. Before this age, the deformity is usually unnoticeable. Soft tissue swelling may precede the bone deformity. (3)

Radiological Features. Radiographically, there is volar curvature of the fifth digits, with separation (widening) of the growth plate and deformity of the epiphysis. There is no apparent clinical significance of this deformity.

An Atlas of Normal Skeletal Variants

Introduction

In order to properly interpret skeletal radiographs, a thorough understanding of normal radiographic anatomy and its skeletal variations is essential. Often, the skeletal variations from normal may simulate various disease processes. The authors therefore offer the following pictorial atlas of "skeletal variants" in order to familiarize the reader with the more common variations from normal.

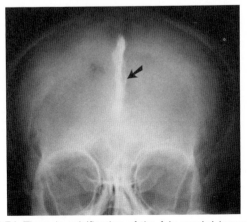

Figure 2.71. There is calcification of the falx cerebri (arrow), which is of no clinical significance.

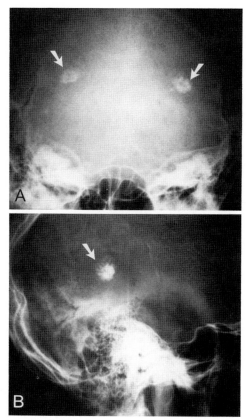

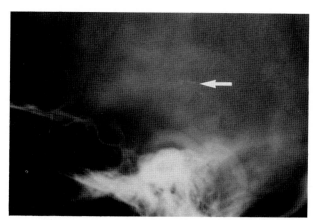

Figure 2.72. A and B. There are calcifications noted in the choroid plexuses (arrows), which are of no clinical significance.

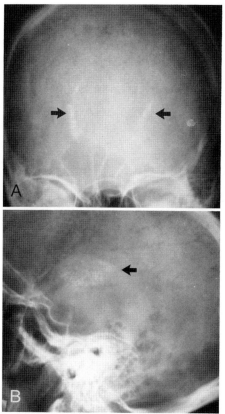

Figure 2.74. A and B. There is calcification noted within the basal ganglia (arrows). *Comment:* Calcification of the basal ganglia may occur as a normal variant or can be associated with pseudohypoparathyroidism and pseudopseudohypoparathyroidism.

Figure 2.73. There is calcification present within the pineal gland (arrow), which is of no clinical significance. (Courtesy of Kenneth E. Yochum, DC, St. Louis, Missouri).

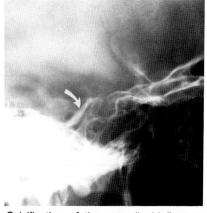

Figure 2.75. Calcification of the petroclinoid ligament is present (arrow), which is a normal variant.

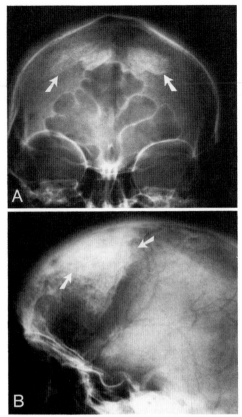

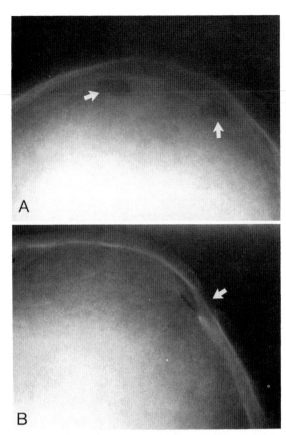

Figure 2.76. A and B. Hyperostosis Frontalis Interna (arrows). *Comment:* Hyperostosis in this area must be differentiated from meningioma.

Figure 2.78. A and B. Observe the parietal foramina which serve as a conduit for the emissary veins of Santorini (arrows).

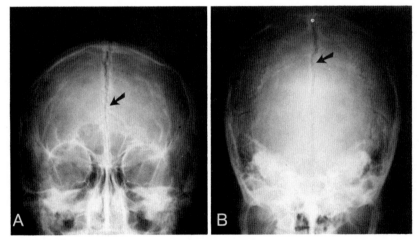

Figure 2.77. A and B. There is persistence of the metopic suture (arrows). *Comment:* This suture may persist throughout life and be mistaken for a fracture. It is also found associated with cleidocranial dysplasia.

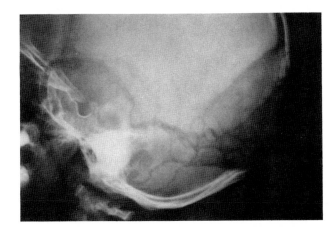

Figure 2.79. There are multiple Wormian bones present at the lambdoidal suture.   ***Comment:*** Wormian bones represent isolated intrasutural bones occurring along the course of the cranial sutures. They may be seen as a normal variant or can occur with cleidocranial dysplasia, osteogenesis imperfecta, and other congenital anomalies. (Courtesy of C. H. Quay, MD, Melbourne, Australia)

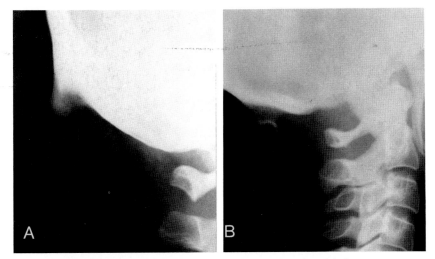

Figure 2.80. A and B. There is a prominent external occipital protuberance, which is considered a variation of normal.

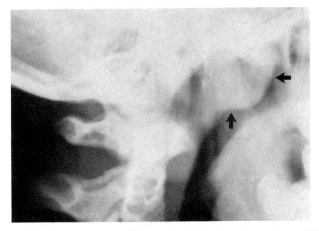

Figure 2.81. There is an indentation on the posterior surface of the nasopharyngeal air space from slight enlargement of adenoidal tissue (arrows).

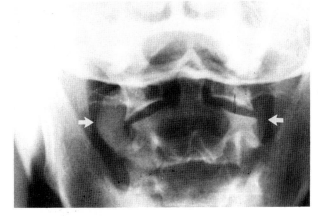

Figure 2.82. The radiopaque density seen adjacent to the lateral mass and articular pillars of C2 (arrows) represents the water density of the tongue and not an ossific or calcific abnormality.

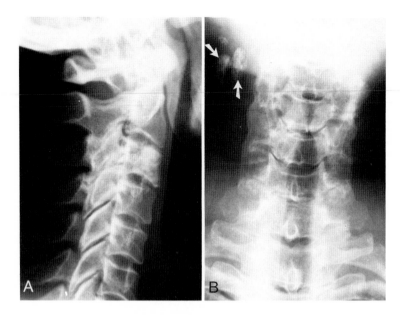

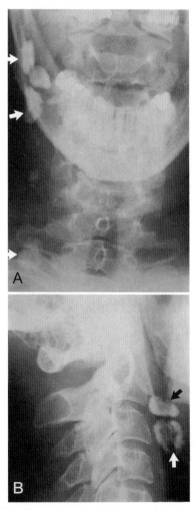

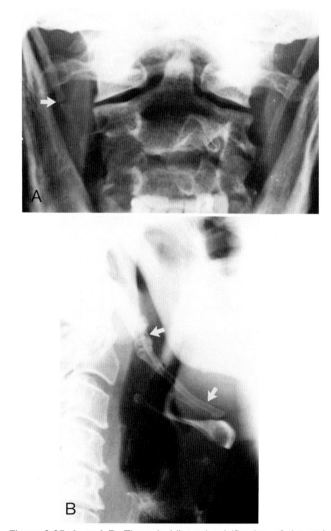

Figure 2.83. A and B. Calcification of the cervical lymph nodes (arrows) are noted lateral to the cervical spine. ***Comment:*** The superimposition of the calcified cervical lymph nodes over the cervical vertebrae on the lateral projection may mimic the appearance of an ivory vertebra. This emphasizes the point of having two views at 90 degrees to each other as a minimum radiological investigation. (Courtesy of Allan J. Warrener, DC, Melbourne, Australia)

Figure 2.84. There is unilateral calcification of the cervical chain of lymph nodes (arrows). ***Comment:*** Calcifications of this degree frequently follow prior inflammatory disease of the lymph nodes but are otherwise of no clinical significance.

Figure 2.85. A and B. There is bilateral calcification of the stylo-hyoideus ligament (arrows).

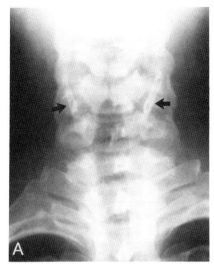

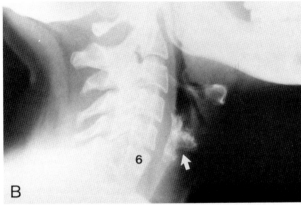

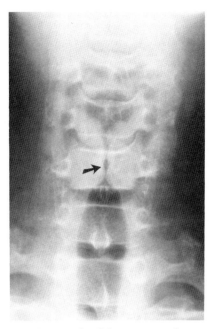

Figure 2.88. The thin area of radiolucency superimposed on the C6 vertebral body represents the contracted larynx (arrow). This should not be confused with a spina bifida occulta or a vertical fracture line.

Figure 2.86. A and B. Calcification of the wings of the thyroid cartilage simulates vertebral artery calcification (arrows). Note the oblique orientation is wrong for vertebral artery calcification. There is a congenital block vertebra present between C6 and C7.

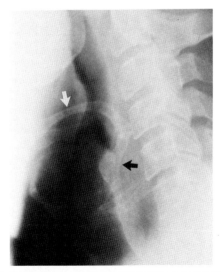

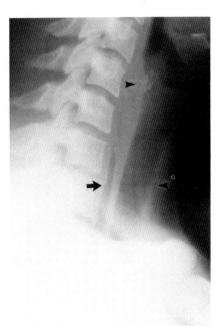

Figure 2.87. Calcification of the superior cornua of the thyroid cartilage is noted (arrows).

Figure 2.89. Observe the air present in the esophagus (arrow). The normal air density of the pharynx and trachea are identified (arrowheads).

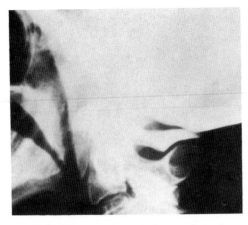

Figure 2.90. Observe the peculiar knife-like configuration to the posterior arch and tubercle of the atlas.

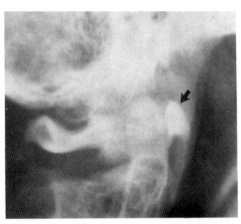

Figure 2.91. The area of increased density in the anterior tubercle of the atlas is considered a variation of normal (arrow). ***Comment:*** If the anterior tubercle of the atlas appears radiopaque and enlarged it signifies compensatory stress hypertrophy. The lack of enlargement signifies a variation of normal.

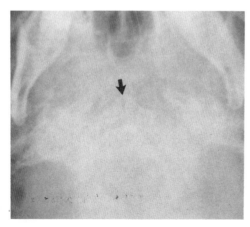

Figure 2.92. There is a cleft in the anterior arch of the atlas (arrow).

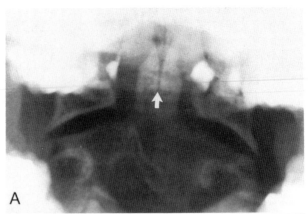

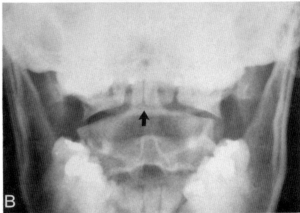

Figure 2.93. A and B. Observe the vertical radiolucent line which appears to split the odontoid process (arrows). This represents the space between the central incisors. ***Comment:*** This may appear to simulate a vertical fracture of the odontoid process; however, these have not been reported.

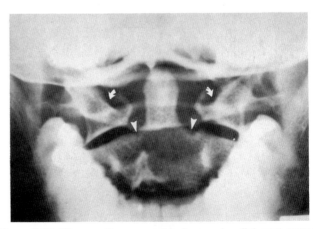

Figure 2.94. Observe the symmetrical normal radiolucent appearance of the concave medial surfaces of the lateral masses of the atlas (arrows). Observe, also, the normal paraodontoid notches (arrowheads) near the base of the odontoid process.

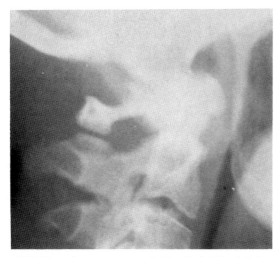

Figure 2.95. There is an accessory joint noted at the inferior aspect of the posterior tubercle of the atlas and the superior surface of the lamina of the axis.

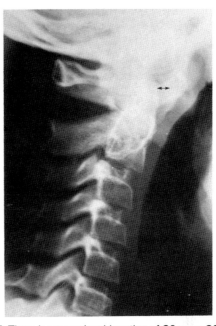

Figure 2.97. There is a pseudosubluxation of C2 upon C3 as a result of hypermobility in this area in children, which is frequently misinterpreted as a pathological instability. Note the trapezoid appearance of the cervical vertebral bodies, which is normal in a child of this age (10 years old). Observe the normal appearance of the atlantodental interspace (ADI) (double-headed arrow). This measured 5 mm, representing the upper limit of normal in a pediatric patient.

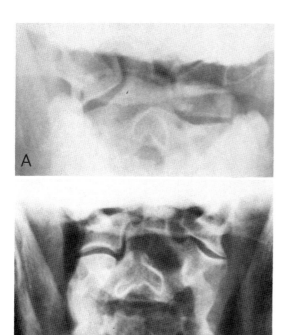

Figure 2.96. A and B. These are two examples of anomalous development of the base of the odontoid process and a right angle formation of the lateral mass of C1 and the superior facet of the axis on one side. (Courtesy of Donald E. Freuden, DC, FACO, Denver, Colorado)

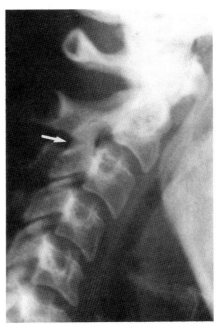

Figure 2.98. There is an apparent ankylosis of the C2/C3 zygapophyseal joints demonstrated on this flexion lateral radiograph (arrow). This is a pseudofusion, since the zygapophyseal joint spaces at C2/C3 are seldom seen clearly on the neutral lateral cervical spine because of their oblique anatomic orientation.

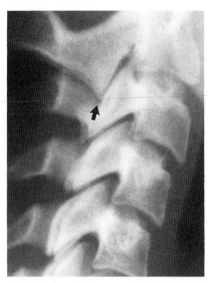

Figure 2.99. Observe the normal notching of the apophyseal joint surface of the C3 vertebra (arrow). This should not be mistaken for erosion or fracture.

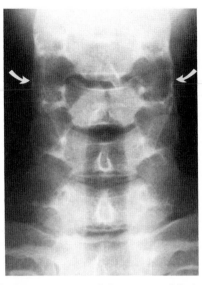

Figure 2.101. Observe the two radiolucent pseudolesions (arrows) present in the lower cervical spine. These radiolucent areas may simulate destructive osteolytic lesions; however, they actually represent projectional distortion in the area of the normal articular pillars.

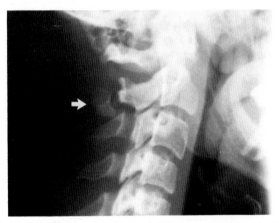

Figure 2.100. There is nonunion of the spinous process (arrow) to the lamina of C2. The sclerotic margins help differentiate this lesion from recent fracture.

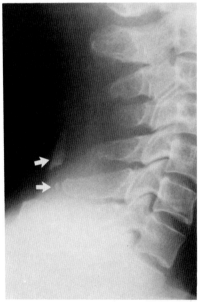

Figure 2.102. Note the calcification in the ligamentum nuchae, creating "nuchal bones" (arrows).

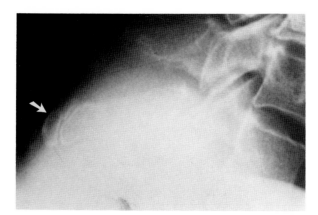

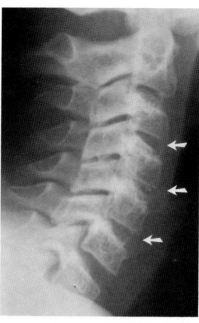

Figure 2.103. Nonunion of the secondary growth center for the spinous process is present at C7 (arrow). **Comment:** This must be differentiated from a "clay shoveler's" avulsion fracture. This is accomplished by the demonstration of the sclerotic margins between the bony segments and the lack of caudal displacement of the distal portion of the spinous process, which is usually present in avulsion fractures.

Figure 2.104. Observe the bony densities superimposed on the intervertebral discs, representing elongated transverse processes of the midcervical spine (arrows).

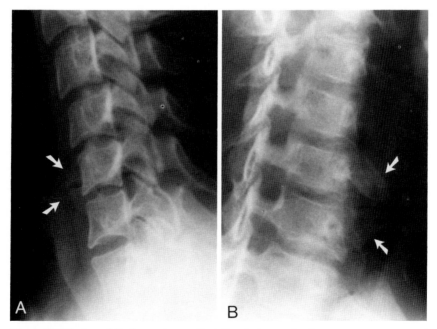

Figure 2.105. A and B. Anomalous articulation between the transverse processes of C5 and C6 has occurred due to elongation of the anterior tubercles (arrows). (Courtesy of Gary M. Guebert, DC, DACBR, St. Louis, Missouri)

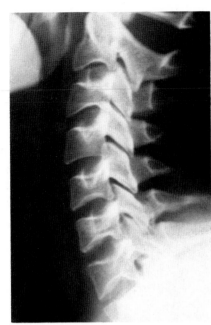

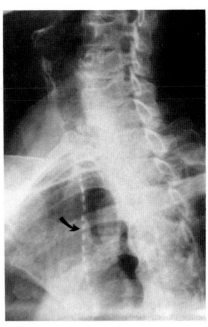

Figure 2.106. There are multiple, long, broad-based, smooth indentations affecting the superior and inferior vertebral end plates throughout the cervical spine. These represent nuclear impressions (notochordal persistency) and are a variation of normal.

Figure 2.107. Clinically insignificant calcification of the tracheal cartilages is present (arrow). (Courtesy of Kenneth E. Yochum, DC, St. Louis, Missouri)

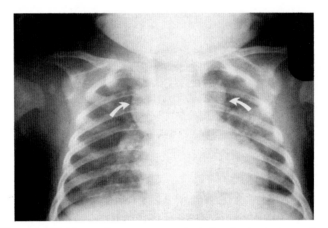

Figure 2.108. The radiopaque paraspinal density just above the heart (arrows) represents the normal infant thymus gland.

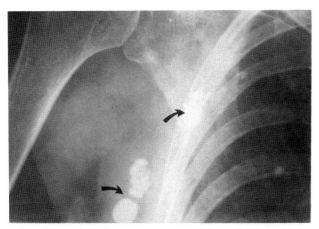

Figure 2.109. There is calcification in multiple axillary lymph nodes (arrows). These should not be confused with blastic bone lesions or pulmonary nodules when they overlie these anatomic structures. It is unusual for the axillary lymph nodes to calcify. (Courtesy of Kenneth E. Yochum, DC, St. Louis, Missouri)

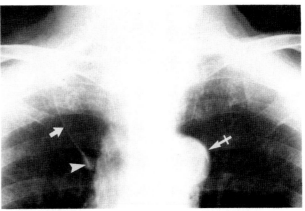

Figure 2.110. Observe the fine radiopaque line present in the right upper lung apex, representing the azygos fissure (arrow). The radiopaque density at the base of this fissure represents the azygos vein (arrowhead). Extensive atherosclerotic plaquing is present within the aortic knob, demonstrating a "thumbnail" sign (crossed arrow). ***Comment:*** The azygos fissure creates an accessory lobe, referred to as the azygos lobe. This is of no clinical significance to the patient.

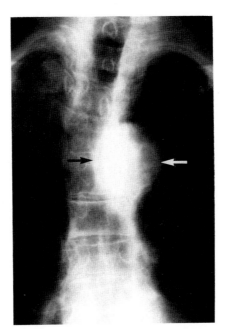

Figure 2.111. The large radiopaque density represents the aortic arch (knob) (arrows). ***Comment:*** Patients with systemic hypertension often will have significant prominence of the aortic arch.

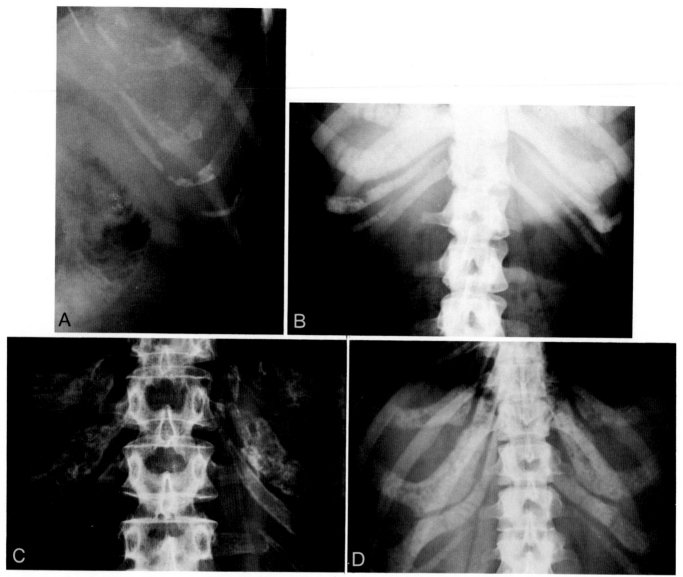

Figure 2.112. A–D. Observe the extensive costochondral calcification involving the lower ribs bilaterally. These may appear very dense, symmetrical, and homogeneous; however, they have no pathologic significance. Costochondral calcification may occur in children, as well as in adults, and is a variation of normal.

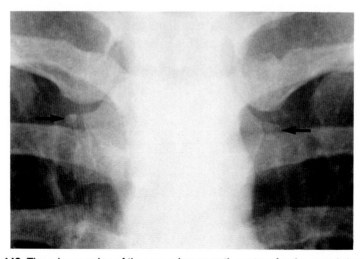

Figure 2.113. There is nonunion of the secondary growth centers for the manubrium (arrows).

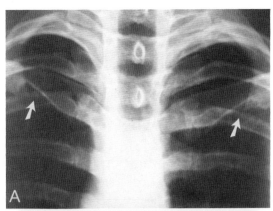

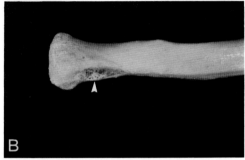

Figure 2.114. A and B. There are bilateral rhomboid fossae present on the inferior surface of the medial aspect of the clavicles (arrows). A photograph of an anatomical specimen clearly defines the indentation of the rhomboid fossae (arrowhead). **Comment:** The rhomboid fossa represents a developmental variation at the insertion of the rhomboid ligament, which is of no clinical significance.

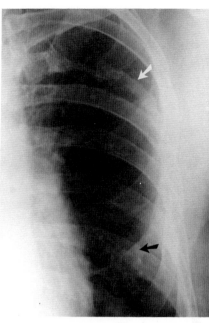

Figure 2.116. Reformation and growth of a previously resected rib is present (arrows). This is a common occurrence following rib resection if residual periosteum is left behind. **Comment:** The patient's history of previous surgery is very helpful, since the radiographic appearance may simulate a destructive rib lesion.

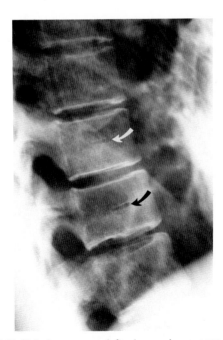

Figure 2.115. Hahn's venous clefts (arrows) are seen throughout the central portion of the thoracic vertebral bodies. **Comment:** These venous grooves are most frequently seen in the lower thoracic spine and should not be confused with any pathologic process.

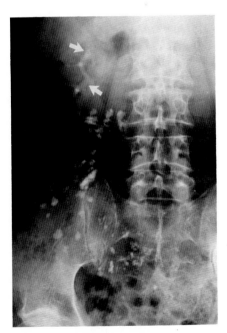

Figure 2.117. There are multiple, scattered, irregular areas of calcification present in the right lower abdomen, representing mesenteric lymph nodes. Contrast media is noted within the collecting system of the kidney (arrows). (Courtesy of Kenneth E. Yochum, DC, St. Louis, Missouri)

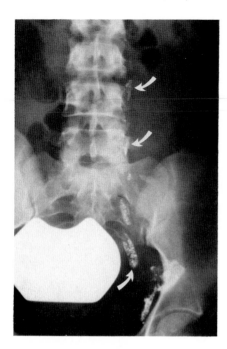

Figure 2.118. The radiopaque material present adjacent to the lumbar spine and extending into the pelvic basin (arrows) represents residual contrast media from a previous lymphangiogram. Note the ovarian shield superimposed upon the pelvic inlet.

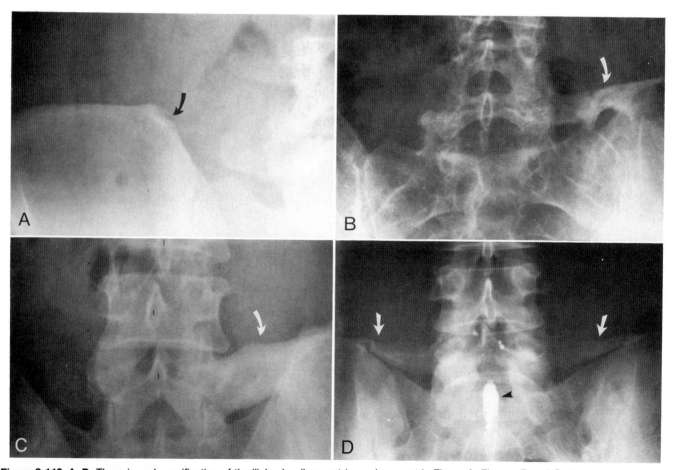

Figure 2.119. A–D. There is early ossification of the iliolumbar ligament (arrow) present in Figure A. Figures B and C demonstrate unilateral ossification of the iliolumbar ligaments (arrows). Figure D demonstrates bilateral ossification of the iliolumbar ligaments (arrows) and contrast media present within the subarachnoid space above the first sacral level (arrowhead) as a result of previous myelographic investigation. (Fig. B courtesy of William E. Litterer, DC, DACBR, Elizabeth, New Jersey; Fig. C courtesy of David J. Byrnes, DC, Coffs Harbor, New South Wales, Australia)

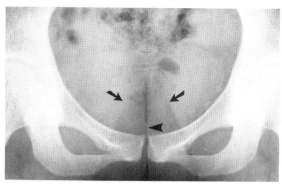

Figure 2.120. The radiolucent shadows above the pubic rami (arrows) represent the fascial planes within the gluteus maximus muscles. The clear, sharply demarcated radiolucent linear line (arrowhead) represents the fold between the buttocks.

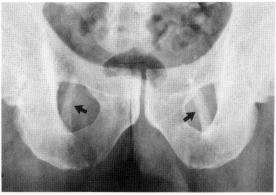

Figure 2.121. Calcification of the sacrotuberous ligaments is noted (arrows). **Comment:** Calcification of the sacrotuberous ligaments is more commonly found in diffuse idiopathic skeletal hyperostosis (DISH) and fluorosis. It may, however, occur as an isolated variant, as was the case in this patient.

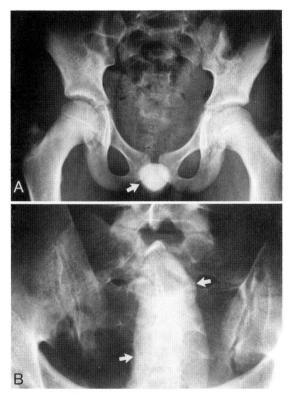

Figure 2.122. A and B. The radiopaque circular density present in the area of the pubic articulation in Figure A represents the penis seen *en face* (arrow). The elongated radiopacity seen superimposed on the sacrum (arrows) in Figure B represents the water density of the penis.

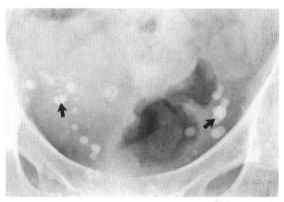

Figure 2.123. The multiple radiopacities above the superior pubic rami represent phleboliths. The radiolucent center (arrows) is typical of phleboliths, which are located within the pelvic veins. **Comment:** Phleboliths in this location are of no clinical significance to the patient.

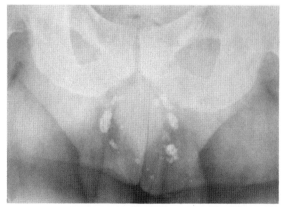

Figure 2.124. The irregular calcifications seen below the pubic rami bilaterally represent calcified scrotal lymph nodes. **Comment:** Calcification of the scrotal lymph nodes are of no clinical significance.

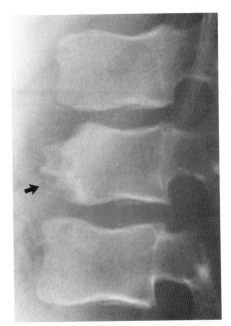

Figure 2.125. Observe the normal "step" defect (arrow) present on the anterior surface of this juvenile lumbar vertebra. This is a developmental variation of normal and will disappear with ossification of the ring apophysis.

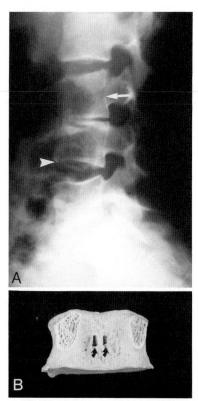

Figure 2.127. A and B. There is a partial congenital block vertebra present at L3/L4. A posterior venous cleft is present at the L3 vertebra (arrow). Observe the persistent secondary growth center at the anteroinferior aspect of L4 (arrowhead). The posterior venous cleft is clearly demonstrated in the photograph of the anatomical specimen (arrows) and represents a growth variant. The neural arch has been removed at the pedicles.

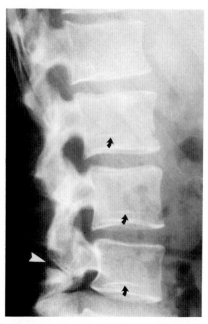

Figure 2.126. There are Harris' growth arrest lines which parallel the end plates of the lumbar vertebrae (arrows). A defect in the pars interarticularis is noted at a single lumbar vertebra (arrowhead). No evidence of spondylolisthesis is present. **Comment:** Harris' growth arrest lines are seldom seen within the spine and should not be interpreted as lead lines or associated with any other metabolic abnormality or bone-sclerosing dysplasia.

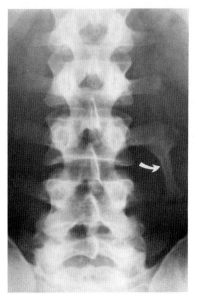

Figure 2.128. A rare lumbar rib is present, projecting from the inferior aspect of the third lumbar transverse process (arrow). (Courtesy of Gary M. Guebert, DC, DACBR, St. Louis, Missouri)

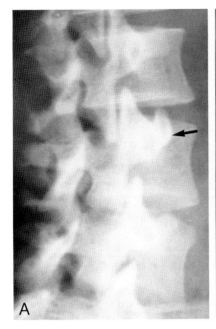

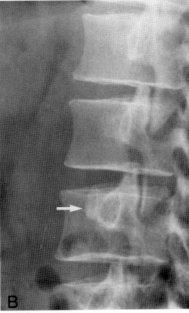

Figure 2.129. A and B. An anomalous malformation of the transverse process (arrows) of a lumbar vertebra creates the "pig snout" appearance of the scotty dog. (Fig. A, Reprinted with permission: Keats, TE: *Atlas of Normal Roentgen Variants That May Simulate Disease*, ed. 3. Chicago Year Book Medical Publishers, 1984. Courtesy of William E. Litterer, DC, DACBR, Elizabeth, New Jersey)

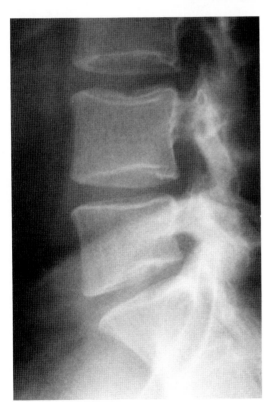

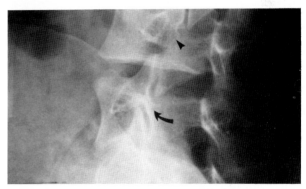

Figure 2.131. The pars interarticularis of the L5 vertebra are congenitally thin (arrow) in comparison to the normal width present at the L4 vertebra (arrowhead). ***Comment:*** Patients born with a thin pars interarticularis may be predisposed to spondylolysis.

Figure 2.130. Observe the trapezoidal shape of the L5 vertebral body. This is a developmental variation of normal and should not be confused with a compression fracture.

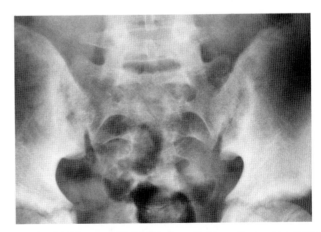

Figure 2.132. The sacroiliac joints in pediatric patients may appear ill defined, with the joints being somewhat wide. This is a normal appearance in younger patients.

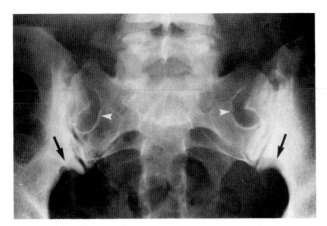

Figure 2.133. There are bilateral accessory sacral foramina noted (arrowheads). Bilateral paraglenoid sulci are present (arrows).

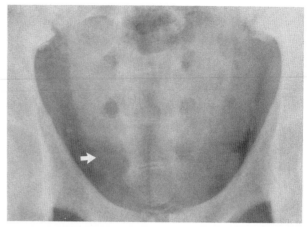

Figure 2.135. Observe the failure of ossification of the lateral margin of the distal sacral foramina (arrow). This is a growth variant which is of no clinical significance and should not be interpreted as a destructive lesion.

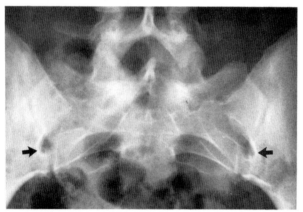

Figure 2.134. There are bilateral fossae present within the ilium (arrows), creating the appearance of a sacroiliac defect. This is a variation of normal.

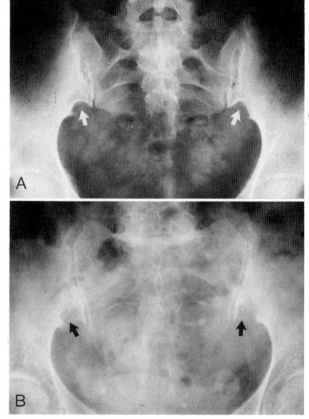

Figure 2.136. A and B. Observe the deep paraglenoid sulci (arrows) affecting the iliac portion of the lower aspect of the area of the sacroiliac joint. ***Comment:*** This sulcus transmits the superior branch of the gluteal artery and supplies insertion for a portion of the sacroiliac ligament. It is a characteristic of the female pelvis, since it is rarely found in the male pelvis. It is occasionally unilateral but is most often found bilaterally, although asymmetrical in its presentation. It has also been referred to as the "preauricular" sulcus.

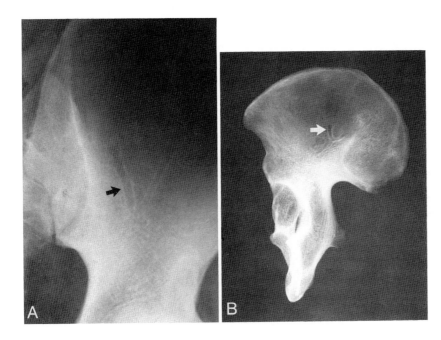

Figure 2.137. A and B. The "V" and "Y" shaped grooves (arrows) represent the passageway for the nutrient arteries of the ilium.

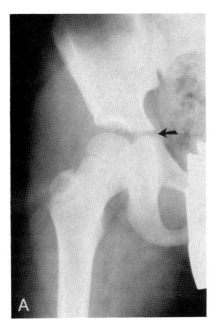

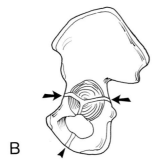

Figure 2.138. TRIRADIATE CARTILAGE. A. AP Hip. The radiolucent defect present on the medial surface of the acetabulum represents the normal triradiate cartilage (arrow).   **B. Schematic Diagram.** This represents a lateral perspective of the ilium, demonstrating the triradiate cartilage (arrows) and the ischiopubic synchondrosis (arrowhead).

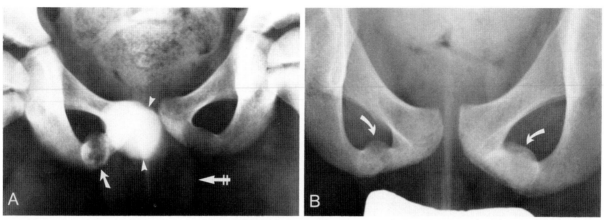

Figure 2.139. ISCHIOPUBIC SYNCHONDROSIS GROWTH VARIANT.   A. The area of radiolucency and bulbous deformity of the ischiopubic synchondrosis (arrow) denotes a developmental growth variant. The adjacent radiopacity (arrowheads) represents the penis. The linear radiopaque margin (crossed arrow) represents the lateral edge of the scrotum.   **B.** There are bilateral areas of bony expansion at the junction of the ischiopubic synchondrosis (arrows). These represent a growth abnormality.   ***Comment:*** The growth irregularity occurring at the ischiopubic synchondrosis often creates a expansile abnormality at the junction of the growth center or the previous site of same. This should not be referred to as an area of ischemic necrosis, as had been described by van Neck.

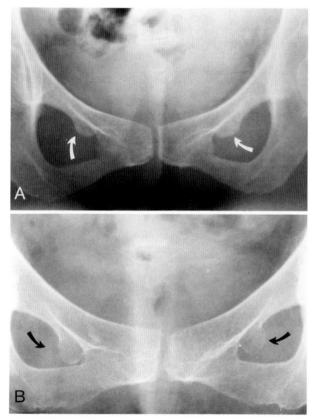

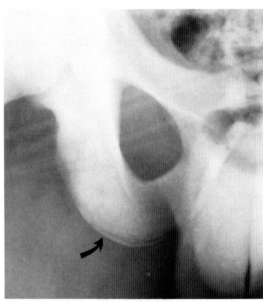

Figure 2.141. Observe the fine linear area of radiopacity below the ischial tuberosity, representing the ischial apophysis (arrow).

Figure 2.140. A and B. There are congenital protuberances noted projecting towards the obturator foramen (arrows), representing a variation of normal referred to as "pubic ears."

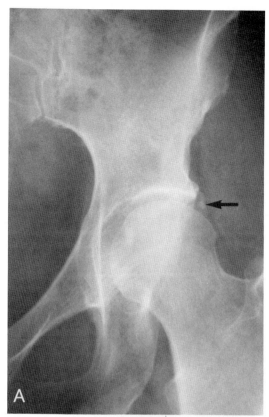

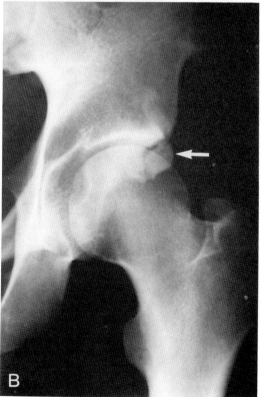

Figure 2.142. A and B. These are two examples of os acetabulae (arrows), accessory bones. (Courtesy of Kenneth E. Yochum, DC, St. Louis, Missouri)

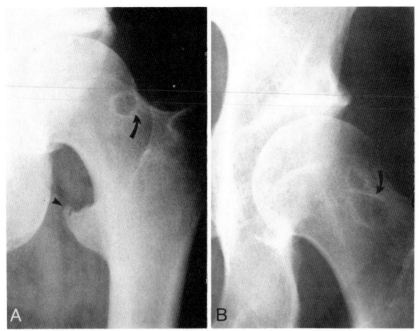

Figure 2.143. A and B. The well-corticated, geographic areas of radiolucency present within the femoral neck (arrows) represent herniation pits (also Pitt's pits), a bone reaction to an irregular capsular surface. They should not be confused with smaller linear defects on the superior and lateral border of the femoral neck caused by penetrating blood vessels known as perforation grooves. Previously, herniation pits have erroneously been called benign fibrocystic conversion defects. Note the small osteophyte formation on the lesser trochanter at the insertion of the psoas muscle (arrowhead). (Fig. A).

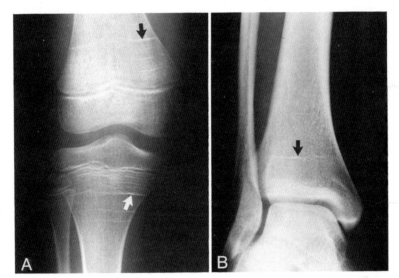

Figure 2.144. A and B. There are Harris' growth arrest lines present in the distal metaphysis of the femur, proximal metaphysis of the tibia, and distal metaphysis of the tibia (arrows). *Comment:* These radiopaque transverse bands should not be confused with heavy metal intoxication, bone-sclerosing dysplasia, or any metabolic underlying abnormalities.

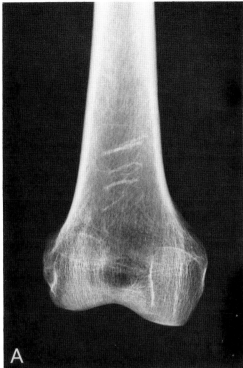

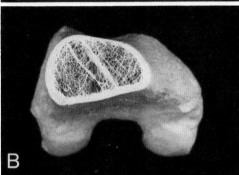

Figure 2.145. A and B. The radiopaque densities present through the metaphysis of the distal femur represent confluent trabeculae known as "bone bars." This appearance on the radiograph is a variation of normal.

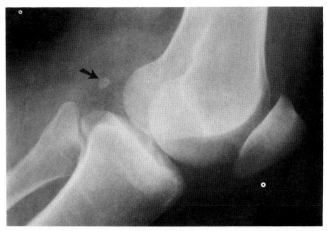

Figure 2.146. The small spherical radiopacity present in the popliteal fossa (arrow) represents a fabella. ***Comment:*** A fabella represents a normal sesamoid bone present within the lateral gastrocnemius tendon. This should not be confused with an osteochondral fragment within the joint capsule, as found in patients with osteochondritis dissecans.

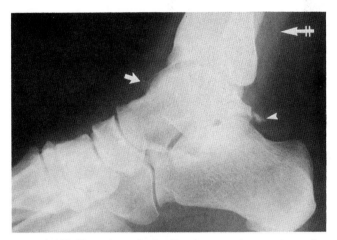

Figure 2.147. There is a talar beak present on the anterior surface of the talus (arrow). An os trigonum is present in the area of the posterior aspect of the talus (arrowhead). There is calcification in the posterior tibial artery of the Mönkeberg medial sclerosis variety in this diabetic patient (crossed arrow). ***Comment:*** The talar beak is a developmental variant that should not be confused with hypertrophic spurring seen adjacent to the talonavicular joint. The os trigonum is a variation of normal and should not be mistaken for a fracture of the posterior process of the talus.

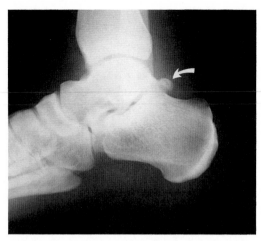

Figure 2.148. An os trigonum is noted posterior to the talus (arrow). *Comment:* The os trigonum represents an accessory ossicle and should not be mistaken for a fracture of the posterior process of the talus.

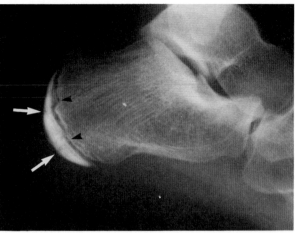

Figure 2.149. The increase in density in the secondary ossification center for the calcaneal apophysis (arrows) is a normal manifestation of the growing pediatric calcaneus. The multiserrated margins to the parent calcaneus (arrowheads) additionally represent a normal manifestation of growth before complete closure of the calcaneal growth center occurs. *Comment:* Young patients with pain in the calcaneus should always have the opposite calcaneus radiographed for comparison. The normal increased radiopacity of the calcaneal apophysis has often been erroneously referred to as "avascular necrosis" (Sever's disease).

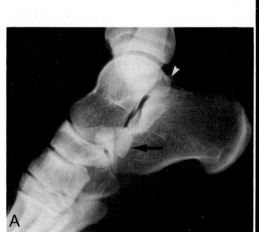
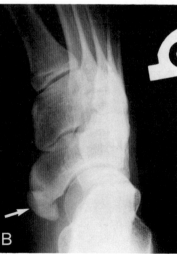

Figure 2.150. A and B. An accessory ossicle is noted medial to the tarsal navicular bone (arrows), representing an os tibiale externum. An os trigonum is also noted (arrowhead).

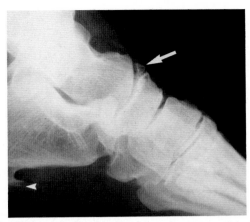

Figure 2.151. An os supranaviculare, an accessory ossicle, is noted (arrow). A large plantar calcaneal exostosis is also seen (arrowhead). *Comment:* The os supranaviculare should not be mistaken for an avulsion fracture. The os supranaviculare has been referred to as "Pirie's bone."

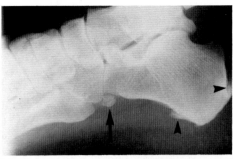

Figure 2.152. There is an accessory ossicle present near the cuboid (arrow). This is referred to as an "os peroneum." There are large calcaneal spurs projecting from the Achilles and plantar surfaces of the calcaneus (arrowheads).

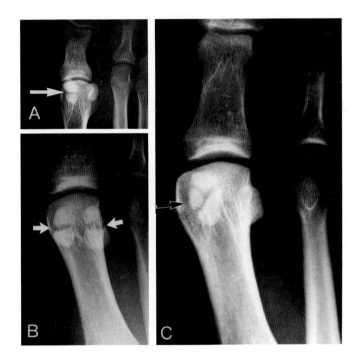

Figure 2.153. A. Bipartite Single Sesamoid (arrow). B. Bipartite Double Sesamoid (arrows). C. Tripartite Single Sesamoid (arrow). *Comment:* The sesamoids outlined here are found in the flexor hallucis brevis tendons. These sesamoid bones lie below the first metatarsophalangeal articulation and are occasionally subjected to stress fracture.

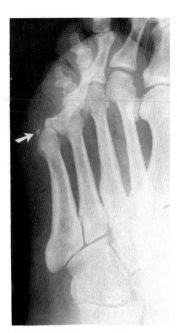

Figure 2.154. There is a small sesamoid bone noted adjacent to the fifth metatarsophalangeal articulation (arrow).

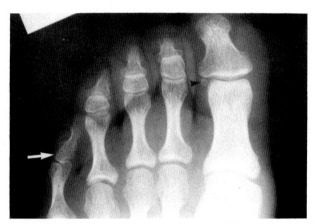

Figure 2.155. There is congenital synostosis of the mid and distal phalanges of the fifth toe (arrow). This is a frequent congenital variation of normal and should not be confused with any underlying pathology. A small accessory ossicle is noted adjacent to the distal interphalangeal articulation of the great toe (arrowhead).

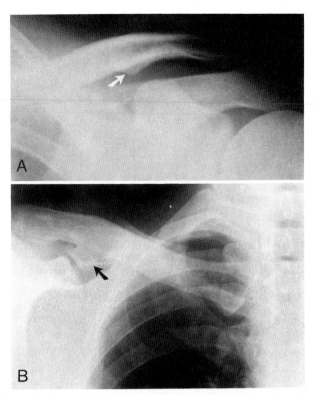

Figure 2.156. A. A small bony process projecting from the inferior surface of the clavicle (arrow) represents the conoid tubercle and should not be confused with any underlying pathology. **B.** There is an enlarged conoid tubercle projecting as an exostosis and forming an accessory articulation with the coracoid process of the scapula (arrow).

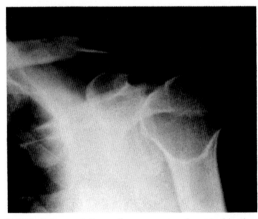

Figure 2.157. A "pseudotumor" appearance is noted in the humeral head. This is created with internal rotation and represents the ball-shaped articular surface of the humeral head, along with superimposition of the tuberosities. This appearance is frequently seen on PA chest radiographs and should be regarded as a variation of normal.

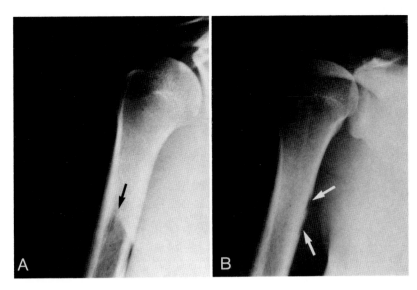

Figure 2.158. A and B. The radiolucencies noted in the humeral cortex (arrows) are produced by the insertion of the pectoralis major muscle.

Figure 2.159. A and B. The radiolucent defect in the area of the humeral cortex represents the area of insertion of the pectoralis major muscle (arrows). The slight cortical bump on the lateral surface of the humerus represents the normal deltoid tuberosity (arrowheads).

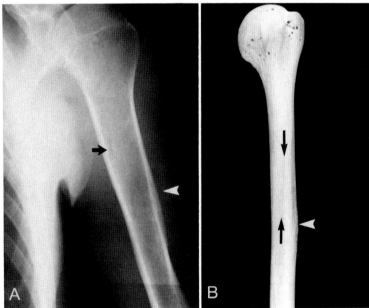

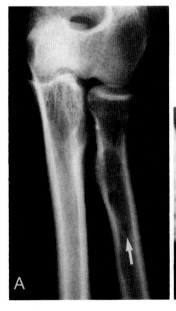

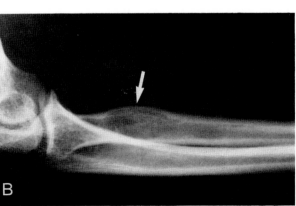

Figure 2.160. A and B. There is a "pseudotumor" appearance noted in the proximal metaphysis of the radius (arrows). This is created by an unusually large radial tuberosity. (Courtesy of Gary M. Guebert, DC, DACBR, St. Louis, Missouri)

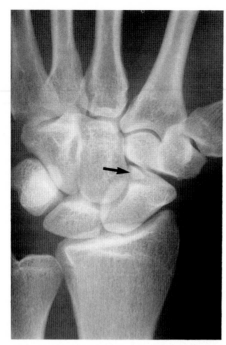

Figure 2.161. An os centrale is present on the dorsum of the carpus (arrow), lying among the scaphoid, trapezoid, and capitate.

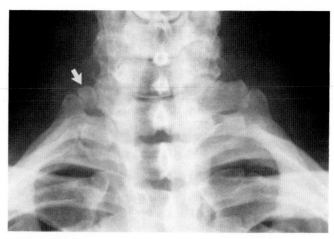

Figure 2.163. Nonunion of the secondary growth center for the transverse process (arrow) is present. ***Comment:*** This must be differentiated from fracture, done by noting its smooth margins and sclerotic borders. Fractures of the transverse processes of the lower cervical and upper thoracic spine are rare and, when present, are found associated with severe trauma and other fractures.

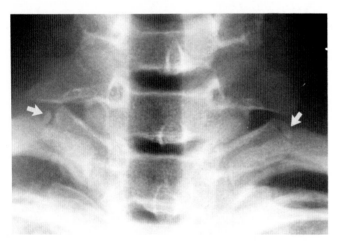

Figure 2.162. Normal ossification centers at the distal ends of the transverse processes of T1 in an adolescent (arrows). ***Comment:*** The smooth margins and sclerotic rims differentiate these secondary growth centers from fractures. Isolated fracture in this area is exceedingly rare, and its bilateral presentation is an additional sign that this is not a fracture.

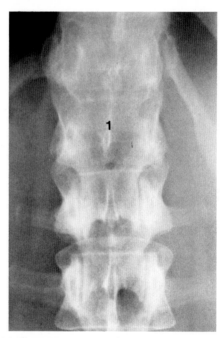

Figure 2.164. There is agenesis of the transverse processes of L1 bilaterally. This is a rare anomaly. (Courtesy of Kenneth E. Yochum, DC, St. Louis, Missouri)

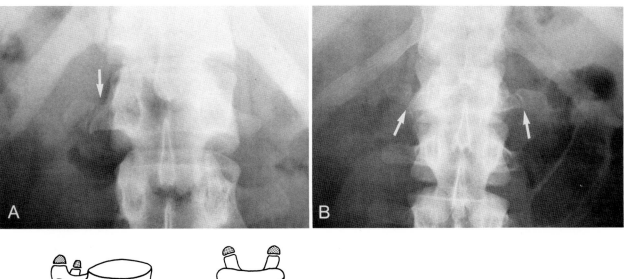

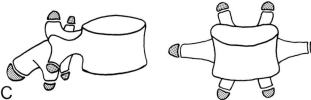

Figure 2.165. SECONDARY OSSIFICATION CENTERS OF THE SPINE. **A.** Unilateral nonunion of the ossification center for the transverse process (arrow). **B.** Bilateral nonunion (arrows). **C.** This schematic diagram demonstrates the normal secondary growth centers for the spine.

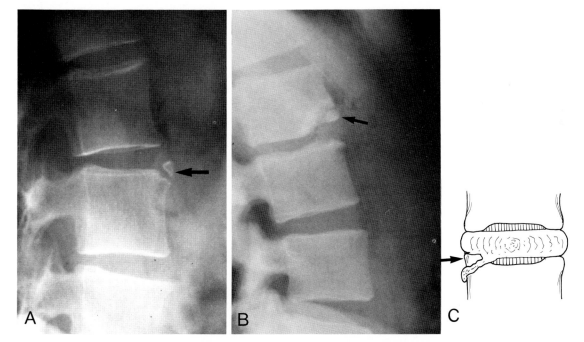

Figure 2.166. LIMBUS BONE. **A and B.** The small ossicles present at the anterior corners of the vertebral bodies (arrows) represent limbus bones. **C.** This schematic diagram demonstrates herniation of nuclear material as the basis for the production of the limbus bone (arrow). *Comment:* The limbus bone is produced as a result of migration and herniation of nuclear material through the secondary growth center for the corner of the vertebral body. This nuclear migration results in nonunion of the secondary growth center.

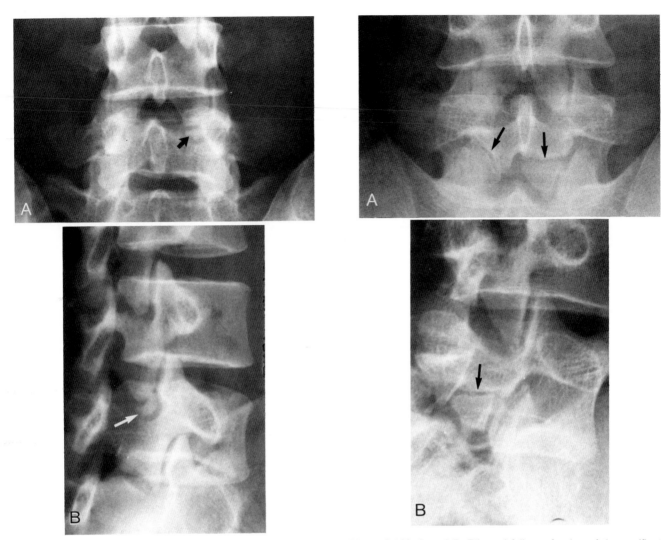

Figure 2.167. A. Frontal View.   B. Oblique View. There is nonunion of the secondary ossification center for the end of the inferior articulating process of L4 (arrows), which may be mistaken for a fracture.

Figure 2.168. A and B. Bilateral failure of union of the ossification centers for the inferior articulating processes of L5 is identified (arrows).

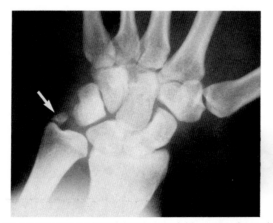

Figure 2.169. Observe the nonunion of the ulnar styloid process (arrow).   ***Comment:*** This should not be mistaken for a fracture and is differentiated from same by its smooth sclerotic margins and lack of displacement.

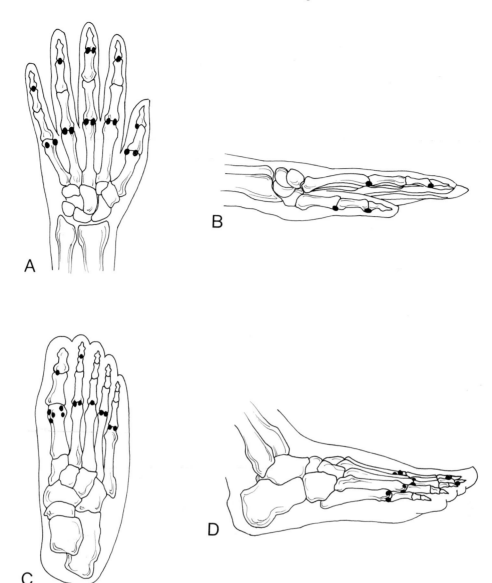

Figure 2.170. NORMALLY OCCURRING SESAMOID BONES: HAND AND FOOT. A. PA Hand. B. Lateral Hand. C. Dorsoplantar Foot. D. Lateral Foot.

REFERENCES

Anomalies of the Craniovertebral Region

Occipitalization of the Atlas

1. Macalister A: Notes on the development and variations at the atlas. *J Anat Phys* 27:519, 1893.
2. Dunsker SB, Brown O, Thompson N: Craniovertebral anomalies. *Clin Neurosurg* 27:430, 1980.

Occipital Vertebrae

1. Hadley LA: Atlanto-occipital fusion, ossiculum terminale and occipital vertebra as related to basilar impression with neurological symptoms. *Am J Roentgenol Rad Therapy* 59:511, 1948.
2. Lombardi G: The occipital vertebra. *AJR* 86:260, 1961.
3. Tulsi RS: Some specific anatomical features of the atlas and axis: Dens, epitransverse process and articular facets. *Aust NZ J Surg* 48:570, 1978.
4. Schumacher S: Ein Beitrag zur Manifestation des Okcipitalwirbels. *Anat Anz* 31:145, 1907.
5. Fischer E: Akzessorische freie Knochenelemente in der umgebung des Foramen Occipitale magnum. *Fortschr Geb Roentgenstrahlen Nuklearmedizin* 91:638, 1959.

Platybasia

1. Chamberlain WE: Basilar impression (platybasia). *Yale J Biol Med* 11:487, 1939.
2. Rothman RH, Simeone FA: *The Spine*, ed 2, Philadelphia, WB Saunders, 1982.

3. Keats TE, Lusted LB: *Atlas of Roentgenographic Measurement*, ed 5, Chicago, Year Book Medical Publishers, 1985.

Anomalies of the Cervical Spine

Agenesis of the Posterior Arch of the Atlas

1. Gehweiler JA, Daffner RH, Roberts L: Malformations of the atlas simulating the Jefferson fracture. *AJR* 140:1083, 1983.
2. Page GT and Yock DH: Total aplasia of the posterior arch of the atlas. *Minn Med* 64:666, 1981.

Posterior Ponticle of the Atlas

1. Kimmerly: Roentgenpraxis 2:479, 1930. Cited by Dugdale LM: The ponticulus posterior of the atlas. *Australas Radiol* 25:237, 1981.
2. Buna M, Coghlan W, deGruchy M, et al: Ponticles of the atlas: A review and clinical perspective. *J Manip Physiol Ther* 7:261, 1984.
3. Gatterman MI: Contraindications and complications of spinal manipulative technique. *ACA J Chiro* 15:75, 1981.

Agenesis of the Anterior Arch of the Atlas

1. Dwight T: Account of two spines with cervical ribs, one of which had a vertebra suppressed, and absence of the anterior arch of the atlas. *J Anat Physiol* 21:539, 1886.
2. Carella A: Slight anomalies of the atlas: Their pathogenetic meaning. *Neuroradiol* 3:224, 1972.
3. Verjaal A, Harder NC: Backward luxation of the atlas: Report of a case. *Acta Radiol* 3:173, 1965.

Down's Syndrome

1. Greenfield GB: *Radiology of Bone Diseases*, ed 3, Philadelphia, JB Lippincott, 1980.
2. Martel W, Tishler JM: Observation on the spine in mongoloidism. *AJR* 97:630, 1966.
3. Ozonoff MB: *Pediatric Orthopedic Radiology*, Philadelphia, WB Saunders, 1979.
4. Yochum TR: Mongolism. *Euro J Chiro* 30:158, 1982.

Ossiculum Terminale Persistens of Bergman

1. Rothman RH, Simeone FA: *The Spine*, ed 2, Philadelphia, WB Saunders, 1982.

Os Odontoideum

1. Minderhound JM, Braakman R, Penning L: Os odontoideum: Clinical, radiological, and therapeutic aspects. *J Neurol Sci* 8:521, 1969.
2. Rothman RH, Simeone FA: *The Spine*, ed 2, Philadelphia, WB Saunders, 1982.
3. Fielding JW, Hensiger RN, Hawkins RJ: Os odontoideum. *J Bone Joint Surg (Am)* 62:376, 1980.
4. Epstein BS: *The Spine—A Radiological Text and Atlas*, ed 4, Philadelphia, Lea & Febiger, 1976.

Hypoplastic and Agenetic Odontoid Process

1. McRae DL: The significance of abnormalities of the cervical spine. *AJR* 84:3, 1960.

Block Vertebra

1. Lovell WW, Winter RB: *Pediatric Orthopedics*, Philadelphia, JB Lippincott, 1978.
2. Wiesel SW, Rothman RH: Occipitoatlantal hypermobility. *Spine* 4:187, 1979.
3. Meschan I: *Analysis of Roentgen Signs*, Philadelphia, WB Saunders, 1973.
4. Sutton D: *A Textbook of Radiology and Imaging*, ed 3, New York, Churchill Livingstone, 1980.

Klippel Feil Syndrome

1. Klippel M, Feil A: Un cas d'absence des vertebres cervicales. Avec cage thoracique remontant jusqu'a la base du crane (cage thoracique cervicale). *Nouv Iconog Salpetriere* 25:223, 1912.
2. Hensinger RN, Lang JE, MacEwen GD: Klippel Feil syndrome. A constellation of associated anomalies. *J Bone Joint Surg (Am)* 56:1246, 1974.
3. Lovell WW, Winter RB: *Pediatric Orthopedics*, Philadelphia, JB Lippincott, 1978.
4. Duncan PA: Embryologic pathogenesis of renal agenesis associated with cervical vertebral anomalies (Klippel Feil phenotype). *Birth Defects* 13:91, 1977.
5. Morrison SG, Perry LW, Scott LP: Congenital brevicollis (Klippel Feil syndrome) and cardiovascular anomalies. *Am J Dis Child* 115:614, 1968.

Sprengel's Deformity

1. Eulenberg M: Casuistis Mittheilungen aus dem Gebiete der Orthopadie. *Arch Klin Chir* 4:301, 1863.
2. Sprengel OGK: Die angeborene Verschiebung des Schulterblattes nach oben. *Arch Clin Chir* 42:545, 1891.
3. Lovell WW, Winter RB: *Pediatric Orthopedics*, Philadelphia, JB Lippincott, 1978.
4. Ogden JA, Conlogue AB, Phillips SB, et al: Sprengel's deformity. Radiology of the pathologic deformation. *Skel Radiol* 4:204, 1979.
5. Willett A, Walsham WJ: An account of the dissection of the parts removed after death from the body of a woman the subject of congenital malformation of the spinal column, bony thorax, and left scapular arch. With remarks on the probable nature of the defects in development producing the deformities. *Med Chir Trans* 63:257, 1880.
6. Jenkinson SG: Undescended scapula associated with omovertebral bone: Sprengel's deformity. *J La State Med Soc* 129:13, 1977.

Cervical Spondylolisthesis

1. Perlman R, Hawes LE: Cervical spondylolisthesis. *J Bone Joint Surg (Am)* 33:1012, 1951.
2. Niemeyer T, Penning L: Functional roentgenographic examination in a case of cervical spondylolisthesis. *J Bone Joint Surg (Am)* 45:1671, 1963.

Absent Pedicle of the Cervical Spine

1. Hadley LA: Congenital absence of pedicle from cervical vertebra. *Am J Roent Rad Ther Nucl Med* 55:193, 1946.
2. Tiyaworabun S, Beeko D, Bock WJ: Congenital absence of a pedicle in the cervical spine. *Acta Neurochir* 61:303, 1982.

Cervical Rib

1. DuToit J, DeMuelenaere P: Isolated fracture of a cervical rib. *S Afr Med J* 18:62, 1982.
2. Sutton D: *A Textbook of Radiology and Imaging*, ed 3, New York, Churchill Livingstone, 1980.

Anomalies of the Thoracic and Lumbar Spine

Butterfly Vertebra

1. Schmorl G, Junghans H: *The Human Spine in Health and Disease*, ed 2, New York, Grune & Stratton, 1971.
2. Murray RO, Jacobson HG: *The Radiology of Skeletal Disorders*, New York, Churchill Livingstone, 1977.
3. Tanaka T, Uhthoff HK: Coronal cleft vertebrae, a variant of normal enchondral ossification. *Acta Orthop Scand* 54:389, 1983.
4. Emery JL: Deformities of the vertebral bodies. *Dev Med Child Neurol* 24:692, 1982.

5. von Rokitansky C: *Handbuch der Pathologischen Anatomie*, Wein, Braumüller und Seidel, 1844.
6. Epstein BS: *The Spine—A Radiological Text and Atlas*, ed 4, Philadelphia, Lea & Febiger, 1976.

Hemivertebrae

1. Epstein BS: *The Spine—A Radiological Text and Atlas*, ed 4, Philadelphia, Lea & Febiger, 1976.
2. Murray RO, Jacobson HG: *The Radiology of Skeletal Disorders*, New York, Churchill Livingstone, 1977.
3. Gjorup PA: Dorsal hemivertebrae. *Acta Orthop Scand* 35:117, 1964.
4. Blummel J: An analysis of the charts and roentgenograms of 264 patients. *Am Surg* 28:501, 1962.
5. Wilkinson RH, Strand RD: Congenital anomalies and normal variants. *Semin Roentgenol* 1:7, 1979.
6. Yochum TR, Hartley B, Thomas DP, et al: A radiographic anthology of vertebral names. *J Manip Physiol Ther* 8:87, 1985.

Schmorl's Node

1. Coventry MB, Ghormley RK, Kernohan JW: Intervertebral disc; its microscopic anatomy and pathology: Changes in the intervertebral disc concomitant with age. *J Bone Joint Surg (Am)* 27:233, 1945.
2. Coventry MB, Ghormley RK, Kernohan JW: Intervertebral disc; its microscopic anatomy and pathology: Pathologic changes in the intervertebral disc. *J Bone Joint Surg (Am)* 27:460, 1945.
3. Hilton RC, Ball J, Benn RT: Vertebral end-plate lesions (Schmorl's nodes) in the dorsolumbar spine. *Ann Rheum Dis* 35:127, 1976.
4. Resnick D, Niwayama G: *Diagnosis of Bone and Joint Disorders*, Philadelphia, WB Saunders, 1981.
5. Rothman RH, Simeone FA: *The Spine*, ed 2, Philadelphia, WB Saunders, 1982.
6. Dietz GW, Christensen EE: Normal "Cupid's bow" contour of the lower lumbar vertebrae. *Radiology* 121:577, 1976.
7. Ramirez H, Navarro JE, Bennett WF: "Cupid's bow" contour of the lumbar vertebral endplates detected by computed tomography. *J Comput Assist Tomogr* 8:121, 1984.

VATER Syndrome

1. Quan L, Smith DW: The VATER association: Vertebral defects, anal atresia, tracheo-esophageal fistula with esophageal atresia, radial and renal dysplasia: A spectrum of associated defects. *J Pediatr* 82:104, 1973.
2. Barne JC, Smith WL: The VATER association. *Radiology* 126:445, 1978.
3. Temtamy SA, Miller JD: Extending the scope of the VATER association: Definition of the VATER syndrome. *J Pediatr* 85:345, 1974.
4. McNeal RM, Skoglund RR, Francke U: Congenital anomalies including the VATER association in a patient with a del (6) q deletion. *J Pediatr* 91:957, 1977.

Spina Bifida Occulta and Vera

1. Nachemson A: The lumbar spine—An orthopedic challenge. *Spine* 1:59, 1976.
2. Magora A, Schwartz A: Relation between the low back pain syndrome and x-ray findings. 3. Spina bifida occulta. *Scand J Rehabil Med* 12:9, 1980.
3. Carter CO: Genetics of spina bifida. In *Proceedings of Symposium on Spina Bifida*, London, Christofer Foss, 1965.

Meningocele/Myelomeningocele

1. Epstein BS: *The Spine—A Radiological Text and Atlas*, ed 4, Philadelphia, Lea & Febiger, 1976.
2. Turek SL: *Orthopedic Principles and Their Application*, ed 4, Philadelphia, JB Lippincott, 1984.
3. Adams MJ, Windham GC, James LM, et al: Clinical interpretation of maternal alpha fetoprotein concentrations. *Am J Ob Gyn* 148:241, 1984.
4. Greenfield GB: *Radiology of Bone Diseases*, ed 3, Philadelphia, JB Lippincott, 1980.
5. Epstein BS: *The Vertebral Column: An Atlas of Tumor Radiology*, Chicago, Year Book Medical Publishers, 1974.
6. Yochum TR, Hartley B, Thomas DP, et al: A radiographic anthology of vertebral names. *J Manip Physiol Ther* 8:87, 1985.
7. Resnick D, Niwayama G: *Diagnosis of Bone and Joint Disorders*, Philadelphia, WB Saunders, 1981.

Diastematomyelia

1. Ollivier CP: *Traites des Maladies de la Moelle Epiniere*, ed 3, Paris, Mequignon-Marvis, 1837.
2. Hilal S, Marton D, Pollack E: Diastematomyelia in children. *Radiology* 112:609, 1974.

Transitional Vertebrae

1. Tini PG, Wieser C, Zinn WM: The transitional vertebra of the lumbosacral spine: Its radiological classification, incidence, prevalence, and clinical significance. *Rheumatol Rehabil* 16:180, 1977.
2. Nachemson A: Towards a better understanding of low-back pain. *Rheumatol Rehabil* 14:129, 1975.
3. Castellvi AE, Goldstein LA, Chan DPK: Lumbosacral transitional vertebrae and their relationship with lumbar extradural defects. *Spine* 9:493, 1984.
4. Hadley LA: *Anatomico-Roentgenographic Studies of the Spine*, ed 2, Springfield, IL, Charles C. Thomas, 1973.
5. Bertolotti M: Contributo alla conoscenza dei vizi di differenziazione regionale del rachide con speciale riquardo all assimilazione sacrale della V lombare. *Radiol Med* 4:113, 1917.

Facet Tropism
1. Rothman, RH, Simeone FA: *The Spine*, ed 2, Philadelphia, WB Saunders, 1982.
2. Nachemson A: The lumbar spine—An orthopaedic challenge. *Spine* 1:59, 1976.
3. Farfan HF, Sullivan JD: The relationship of facet orientation to intervertebral disc failure. *Can J Surg* 10:179, 1967.

Knife Clasp Deformity
1. DeAnguin CE: Spina bifida occulta with engagement of the fifth lumbar spinous process. *J Bone Joint Surg (Br)* 41:486, 1959.
2. Starr WA: Spina bifida occulta and engagement of the fifth lumbar spinous process. *Clin Orthop* 81:71, 1971.

Anomalies of the Thorax

Srb's Anomaly/Luschka's Rib
1. Srb: Med Jb kk Ges Artze, Vienna, 1862. Cited in Kohler A, Zimmer EA: *Borderlands of the Normal and Early Pathologic in Skeletal Radiology*, ed 3, New York, Grune & Stratton, 1968.

Anomalies of the Hip and Pelvis

Congenital Hip Dysplasia
1. Resnick D, Niwayama G: *Diagnosis of Bone and Joint Disorders*, Philadelphia, WB Saunders, 1981.
2. Putti V: Early treatment of congenital dislocation of the hip. *J Bone Joint Surg (Am)* 11:798, 1929.

Sacral Dysplasia
1. Hohl AF: *Die Geburten Missgestalteter, Kranker und Todter Kinder*, Verlag der Buchhandlung des Waisenhauses, 1850.
2. Friedel G: Defekt der Wirbelsäule vom 10. Brust an abwärts bei einem Neugeborenen. *Arch Klin Chir* 93:944, 1910.
3. Pedersen LM, Tygstrup I, Pedersen J: Congenital malformations in new born infants of diabetic women. *Lancet* 1:1124, 1964.
4. Renshaw TS: Sacral agenesis: A classification and review of 23 cases. *J Bone Joint Surg (Am)* 60:373, 1978.

Coxa Vara/Coxa Valga
1. Katz JF, Siffert SS: *Management of Hip Disorders in Children*, Philadelphia, JB Lippincott, 1983.
2. Calhoun JD, Pierret G: Infantile coxa vara. *AJR* 115:561, 1972.
3. Sutton D: *A Textbook of Radiology and Imaging*, ed 3, Edinburgh, Churchill Livingstone, 1980.

Anomalies of the Extremities

Bipartite, Tripartite, and Multipartite Patellae
1. Weaver JK: Bipartite patellae as a cause of disability in the athlete. *Am J Sports Med* 5:137, 1977.
2. Green WT: Painful Bipartite Patellae. *Clin Orthop* 110:197, 1975.
3. Halpern AA, Hewitt O: Painful medial bipartite patellae. *Clin Orthop* 134:180, 1978.
4. Keats TE: *An Atlas of Normal Roentgen Variants that May Simulate Disease*, ed 3, Chicago, Year Book Medical Publishers, 1984.

Fong's Syndrome
1. Fong EE: Iliac horns (symmetrical bilateral central posterior iliac processes): Case report. *Radiology* 47:517, 1946.
2. Murray RO, Jacobson HG: *Radiology of Skeletal Disorders*, Edinburgh, Churchill Livingstone, 1977.

Tarsal Coalition
1. Harris BA: Anomalous structures in the developing human foot. *Anat Rec* 121:1339, 1955.
2. Leonard MA: The inheritance of tarsal coalitions and its relationship to spastic flatfoot. *J Bone Joint Surg (Br)* 56:520, 1974.
3. Jacobs AM, Sollecito V, Oloff L, et al: Tarsal coalitions: An instructional review. *J Foot Surg* 20:214, 1981.
4. Outland T, Murphy ID: Relation of tarsal anomalies in spastic rigid flatfeet. *Clin Orthop* 1:217, 1953.

5. Kaplan EG, Kaplan GS, Vaccari OA: Tarsal coalition: Review and preliminary conclusions. *J Foot Surg* 16:136, 1977.
6. O'Rahilly R: A survey of carpal and tarsal anomalies. *J Bone Joint Surg (Am)* 35:626, 1953.

Vertical Talus
1. Patterson WR, Fitz DA, Smith WS: The pathologic anatomy of congenital convex pes valgus. *J Bone Joint Surg (Am)* 50:458, 1968.
2. Jacobsen ST, Crawford AH: Congenital vertical talus. *J Pediatr Orthop* 3:306, 1983.

Morton's Syndrome
1. Morton D: *The Human Foot*, New York, Columbia University Press, 1948.
2. Jahss MH: *Disorders of the Foot*, Philadelphia, WB Saunders, 1982.

Supracondylar Process of the Humerus
1. Terry RJ: A study of the supracondyloid process in the living. *Am J Phys Anthropol* 4:129, 1921.
2. Laha RK, Dujovny M, DeCastro SC: Entrapment of median nerve by supracondylar process of the humerus. *J Neurosurg* 46:252, 1977.
3. Barnard LB, McCoy SM: The supracondyloid process of the humerus. *J Bone Joint Surg (Am)* 28:845, 1946.
4. Struthers J: On a peculiarity of the humerus and humeral anatomy. *Month J Med Sci* 9:264, 1849.

Radioulnar Synostosis
1. Hansen OH, Anderson NO: Congenital radio-ulnar synostosis. Report of 37 cases. *Acta Orthop Scand* 41:225, 1970.
2. Turek SL: *Orthopedic Principles and Their Application*, ed 4, Philadelphia, JB Lippincott, 1984.
3. Freyer B: Ungewöhnliche Beobachtung doppelseitiger kongenitaler Synostosen zwischen Radius und Ulna. *Radiologie* 6:253, 1966.

Madelung's Deformity
1. Madelung OW: Die spontane Subluxation der Hand nach vorne. *Verh Dtsch Ges Chir* 7:259, 1878.
2. Lichenstein JR, Sundaran M, Burdge R: Sex influenced expression of Madelung's deformity in a family with dyschondrosteosis. *J Med Genet* 17:41, 1980.
3. Nielsen JB: Madelung's deformity. A followup study of 26 cases and a review of the literature. *Acta Orthop Scand* 48:379, 1977.
4. Kaitila II, Leisti JT, Rimoin DL: Mesomelic skeletal dysplasias. *Clin Orthop* 114:94, 1976.

Carpal Coalition
1. Cope JR: Carpal coalition. *Clin Radiol* 25:261, 1974.
2. Poznanski AK, Holt JF: The carpals in congenital malformation syndromes. *AJR* 112:443, 1971.

Polydactyly
1. Poznanski AK: *The Hand in Radiologic Diagnosis*, ed 2, WB Saunders, 1984.

Syndactyly
1. MacCollum DW: Webbed fingers. *Surg Gynecol Obstet* 71:782, 1940.
2. Nylen B: Repair of congenital finger syndactyly. *Acta Chir Scand* 113:310, 1957.
3. Kelikian H: *Congenital Deformities of the Hand and Forearm*, Philadelphia, WB Saunders, 1974.
4. Castilla EE, Paz JE, Orioli-Parreiras IM: Syndactyly: Frequency of specific types. *Am J Med Genet* 5:357, 1980.
5. Temtamy SA, McKusick VA: The genetics of hand malformations. *Birth Defects* 14:1, 1978.
6. Poznanski AK: *The Hand in Radiologic Diagnosis*, ed 2, Philadelphia, WB Saunders, 1974.

Kirner's Deformity
1. Kirner J: Doppelseitige Verkrümmungen des Kleinfingerendgliedes als selbständiges Krankheitsbild. *Fortschr Geb Roentgenstrahlen* 36:804, 1927.
2. Poznanski AK: *The Hand in Radiologic Diagnosis*, ed 2, WB Saunders, 1984.
3. Steinback H, Gold R, Preger L: *Roentgen Appearance of the Hand in Diffuse Disease*, Chicago, Year Book Medical Publishers, 1975.

Measurements in Skeletal Radiology

LINDSAY J. ROWE
TERRY R. YOCHUM

Introduction

Since the time of the first roentgen image measurements have been used to evaluate normal and abnormal skeletal relationships. Many measurements have been determined by astute observation and appropriate statistical evaluation.

In all analytical assessments of these spatial relationships the outcome is dependent on the quality of the radiographic data collected and its correct interpretation. Any attempt to measure and quantify the human frame has inherent, uncontrolled error. The major errors arising in the mensuration process include 1) image unsharpness, 2) projectional geometric distortion, 3) patient positioning, 4) anatomic variation, 5) locating standard reference points, and 6) observer error.

The clinical interpretation and application of these lines has also been a source of confusion. This would seem particularly applicable in the spine and pelvis, where small measurements derived from various systems of analysis have often exerted a strong influence on treatment regimes. Between the various systems of analysis there appears to be little correlation in the results obtained. (1–3) Many measurements have been used to evaluate spinal segmental motion abnormalities from static radiographs which inadequately reflect motion biomechanics.

In general, any measurement is meaningless unless performed accurately and correlated clinically. To rely on a radiographic measurement as the sole criteria for a particular treatment method represents a frail approach to patient care.

In this chapter each measurement is described according to *synonyms, optimum projections, normal values, special considerations, and significance*. Whenever numerical data are given, these have been rounded for simplicity. Unless otherwise stated the measurements are film image sizes and not corrected for true anatomic dimensions. References are included so the reader may seek further information.

Correction of Geometric Distortion

Numerous methods can be used to determine the anatomic dimensions demonstrated on a given radiograph. These include nomograms and algebraic formulations. (1,2) The roentgen image is always larger than the true anatomic size due to the effect of the diverging rays on a structure not in close contact with the film.

To algebraically arrive at the correct object size (O), three values must be known: (Fig. 3.1)

(1) Film image dimension (cm) (I)
(2) Target film distance (cm) (D)
(3) Object film distance (cm) (d)

Initially, a correction factor (CF) is calculated:

$$CF = \frac{D - d}{D}$$

The film image dimension (I) is then multiplied by this correction factor:

$$O = I \times CF$$

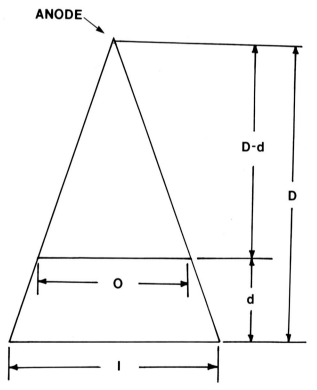

Figure 3.1. Geometric Distortion in Image Production.

Skull

Vastine-Kinney Method of Pineal Gland Localization

Synonyms: None.
Technique.
  Projection: Lateral skull.
  Landmarks: The pineal gland must be visible as a result of calcium deposition before four measurements are made: (1) (Fig. 3.2)
    A. The greatest distance from the pineal gland to the inner table of the frontal bone.
    B. The greatest distance from the pineal gland to the inner aspect of the occipital bone.
    C. The greatest distance from the pineal gland to the inner table of the skull vertex.
    D. The greatest distance from the pineal gland to the posterior margin of the foramen magnum.
  Normal Measurements: A and B are used to assess anterior or posterior pineal displacement while C and D for superior or inferior displacement.
    1. Anteroposterior position. Measurement A is plotted against the sum of A and B and should fall within the specified range.
    2. Superoinferior position. Measurement C is plotted against the sum of C + D and also should fall within a specified range. (2)
  Special Considerations: An alternative and more accurate method for pineal gland localization is the Pawl-Walter method. (3)
Significance. A pineal shift may be due to a space occupying mass such as a tumor, hemorrhage, or localized atrophic cerebral disease.

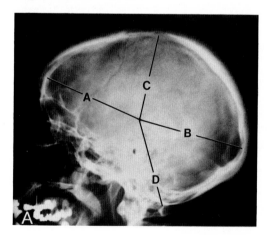

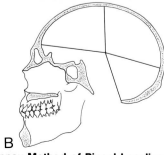

Figure 3.2. A and B. Vastine-Kinney Method of Pineal Localization (see text).

Sella Turcica Size

Synonyms. Pituitary fossa size.
Technique.
Projection: Lateral skull.
Landmarks: Two measurements are made—the greatest anteroposterior diameter and greatest vertical diameter. The anteroposterior value is the widest distance between the anterior and posterior surfaces of the pituitary fossa. The vertical dimension is between the fossa floor and the plane between the opposing surfaces of the anterior and posterior clinoid processes. (4,5) (Fig. 3.3)
Normal Measurements: The anteroposterior dimension averages about 11 mm with a normal range of 5–16 mm. The vertical measurement averages about 8 mm with a normal range of 4–12 mm. (4–6) (Table 3.1) In children these values will be progressively smaller with decreasing age.

Table 3.1.
Normal Values of Sella Turcica Size

	Average (mm)	Minimum (mm)	Maximum (mm)
Anteroposterior	11	5	16
Vertical	8	4	12

Special Considerations: All lateral flexion and rotation of the skull should be eliminated for these measurements to be accurate.
Significance. The finding of a small sella is of debatable significance. (7) However, an enlarged sella may be associated with a pituitary neoplasm, empty sella syndrome, extrapituitary mass (neoplasm, aneurysm) or may even be a normal variant.

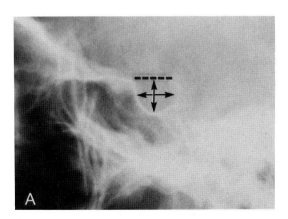

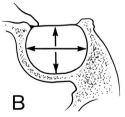

Figure 3.3. A and B. Lateral Measurements of the Sella Turcica (see text).

Basilar Angle

Synonyms. Welker's basilar angle, Martin's basilar angle.
Technique.
Projection: Lateral skull.
Landmarks: Three points are located, joined together by two lines, and the subsequent angle is measured. The three points are the nasion (frontal-nasal junction), center of the sella turcica (midpoint between the clinoid processes) and the basion (anterior margin of the foramen magnum). (Fig. 3.4)
Normal Measurements: The average normal angle subtended by these two lines is 137 degrees with a normal variation of 123–152 degrees. (8) (Table 3.2)

Table 3.2.
Normal Values of the Basilar Angle

Average (deg)	Minimum (deg)	Maximum (deg)
137	123	152

Significance. The measurement is an index of the relationship between the anterior skull and its base. The angle will increase beyond 152 degrees in platybasia where the base is elevated in relation to the rest of the skull. This may or may not be associated with basilar impression.

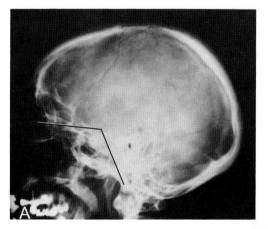

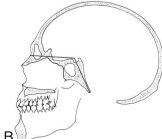

Figure 3.4. A and B. Basilar Angle (see text).

McGregor's Line

Synonyms.   Basal line.
Technique
  Projection: Lateral skull, lateral cervical.
  Landmarks: A line is drawn from the posterosuperior margin of the hard palate to the most inferior surface of the occipital bone. (9) The relationship of the odontoid apex to this line is then examined. (Fig. 3.5)
  Normal Measurements: In 90 percent of individuals the odontoid apex should not lie above this line more than 8 mm in males and 10 mm in females. (9) Under the age of 18 these maximum values diminish with decreasing chronologic age.
  Special Considerations: Of all methods used to evaluate for basilar impression on the lateral projection McGregor's line appears to be the most accurate and reproducible. (10)
Significance.   An abnormal superior position of the odontoid is indicative of basilar impression. Common precipitating causes include platybasia, atlas occipitalization, and bone-softening diseases of the skull base such as Paget's disease and osteomalacia. Occasionally rheumatoid arthritis may also precipitate this deformity.

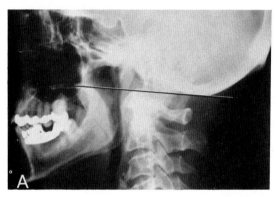

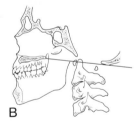

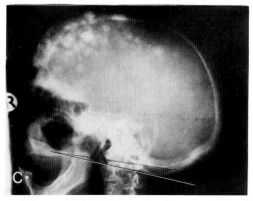

Figure 3.5. A and B. McGregor's Line (see text). **C. Abnormal McGregor's Line.** Note the tip of the odontoid (retouched) is well above the line due to basilar invagination from Paget's disease.

Chamberlain's Line

Synonyms.   Palato-occipital line.
Technique.
  Projection: Lateral skull, lateral cervical.
  Landmarks: A line is constructed from the posterior margin of the hard palate to the posterior aspect of the foramen magnum. The relationship of this line to the tip of the odontoid process is then assessed. (11) (Fig. 3.6)
  Normal Measurements: In the majority of patients the tip of the odontoid process should not project above this line; however, a normal variation of 3 mm above this line may occur. (8) A measurement of 7 mm or more is definitely abnormal.
  Special Considerations: This relationship can also be evaluated on lateral cervical views but is best done on lateral skull films preferably with tomography. To locate the posterior aspect of the foramen magnum, identify the inner table of the occipital bone and follow it anteriorly and observe for an oblique cortical white line crossing the diploe to merge with the outer table. This should be found slightly posterior to the plane of the atlas spinolaminar junction.
Significance.   An abnormal superior position of the odontoid is indicative of basilar impression. Common precipitating causes include platybasia, atlas occipitalization, and bone softening of the skull base such as Paget's disease and osteomalacia. Occasionally rheumatoid arthritis may also precipitate this deformity.

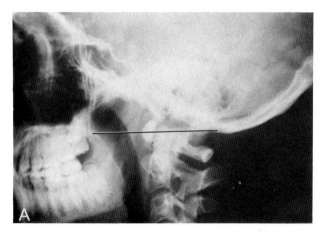

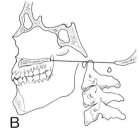

Figure 3.6. A and B. Chamberlain's Line (see text).

MacRae's Line

Synonyms.   Foramen magnum line.
Technique.
   Projection: Lateral skull.
   Landmarks: A line is drawn between the anterior (basion) and posterior (opisthion) margin of the foramen magnum. Two assessments are then made in relation to this line: (1) the occipital bone, and (2) the odontoid process. (Fig. 3.7)
   Normal Measurements: The inferior margin of the occipital bone should lie at or below this line. Additionally a perpendicular line drawn through the odontoid apex should intersect this line in its anterior quarter. (10,12)
   Special Considerations: A true lateral view with no lateral flexion distortion should be obtained for this positional line to be applied.
Significance.   If the inferior margin of the occipital bone is convex in a superior direction and/or lies above this line, then basilar impression is present. Predisposing causes include platybasia, occipitalization, rheumatoid arthritis, and bone-softening diseases such as Paget's disease and osteomalacia. If the odontoid apex does not lie in the ventral quarter of this line a dislocation of the atlanto-occipital joint, a fracture or dysplasia of the dens may be present.

Digastric Line

Synonyms.   Biventor line.
Technique.
   Projection: Anteroposterior open mouth.
   Landmarks: The digastric groove medial to the base of the mastoid process is located on each side and a line is drawn between them. The vertical distance to the odontoid apex and atlanto-occipital joints is then measured. (Fig. 3.8)
   Normal Measurements: The digastric line-odontoid apex average measurement is 11 mm but may range between 1 mm and 21 mm. The odontoid should not project above this line. The digastric line/atlanto-occipital joint average measurement is 12 mm with a normal range between 4 mm and 20 mm. (10,13) (Table 3.3)

Table 3.3.
Normal Digastric Line Values

	Average (mm)	Minimum (mm)	Maximum (mm)
Digastric-Odontoid	11	1	21
Digastric-Cl-OCC Joint	12	4	20

   Special Considerations: Tomographic evaluation is the most accurate method in obtaining clear visualization of the necessary anatomical landmarks.
Significance.   Both measurements will decrease in basilar impression due to platybasia, occipitalization, and bone-softening diseases such as Paget's disease and osteomalacia.

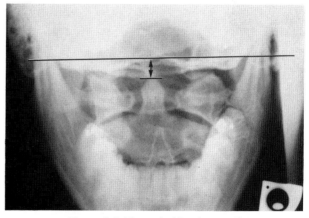

Figure 3.8. Digastric Line (see text).

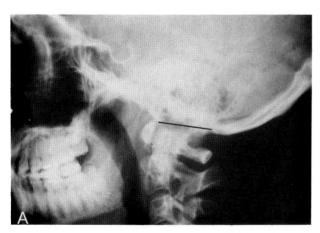

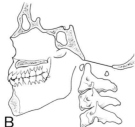

Figure 3.7. A and B. MacRae's Line (see text).

Height Index of Klaus

Synonyms.   None.
Technique.
   Projection: Lateral skull, lateral cervical spine.
   Landmarks: A line is drawn from the tuberculum sellae to the internal occipital protuberance. The vertical distance between this line and the apex of the odontoid is measured. (14) (Fig. 3.9)
   Normal Measurements: (Table 3.4)

Table 3.4.
Normal Values for the Height Index of Klaus

Average (mm)	Minimum (mm)
40–41	30

Significance.   A measurement less than 30 mm indicates basilar impression. Values between 30–36 mm reflect a tendency toward basilar impression. (10,14) The wide range of normal variation casts doubt upon the merit of this measurement. (12)

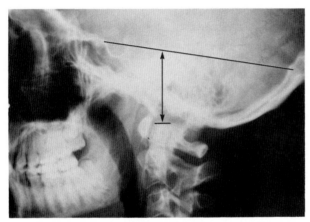

Figure 3.9. Height Index of Klaus (see text).

Boogard's Line and Angle

Synonyms.   None.
Technique.
   Projection: Lateral skull, lateral cervical spine.
   Landmarks:
      Boogard's line: A line is drawn connecting the nasion to the opisthion. (15) (Fig. 3.10A)
      Boogard's angle: A line is drawn between the basion and opisthion (MacRae's line). A second line is drawn from the dorsum sellae to the basion along the plane of the clivus. The angle between these two lines is measured. (15) (Fig. 3.10B)
   Normal Measurements:
      Boogard's line: The basion should lie below this line.
      Boogard's angle: (Table 3.5)

Table 3.5.
Normal Values for Boogard's Angle

Average (deg)	Minimum (deg)	Maximum (deg)
122	119	135

Significance.   Both measurements will be altered in basilar impression—the basion will be above Boogard's line and the angle is greater than 135 degrees.

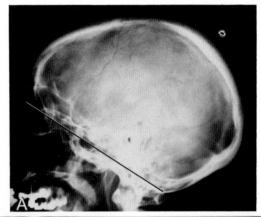

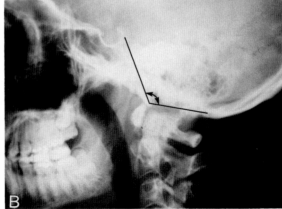

Figure 3.10. A. Boogard's Line. B. Boogard's Angle (see text).

Anterior Atlanto-Occipital Dislocation Measurement

Synonyms. None.

Technique.

Projection: Lateral cervical spine, lateral skull.

Landmarks: Four osseous landmarks are located—the basion, opisthion, as well as the anterior and posterior arches of the atlas. Two measurements are then made:

1. The distance between the basion and posterior arch at the spinolaminar junction (B-P).
2. The distance between the opisthion and posterior margin of the anterior arch (O-A).

The ratio of these two measurements (B-P:O-A) is then calculated. (16) (Fig. 3.11)

Normal Measurements: In the normal individual the ratio is always less than one.

Special Considerations: This relationship can only be assessed when there are not associated fractures or dislocations of the atlas and odontoid process.

Significance. When the ratio is equal or greater than one, then an anterior atlanto-occipital dislocation probably exists.

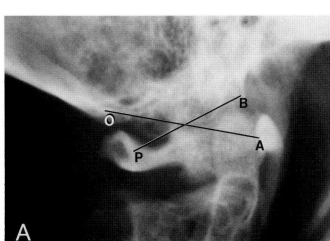

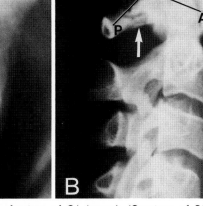

Figure 3.11. A. Normal Atlanto-Occipital Relationship. B. Anterior Atlanto-Occipital Dislocation (see text). Observe the posterior arch fracture of C1 (arrow). (Courtesy of Steven B. Wasserman, DC, Long Beach, California).

Cervical Spine

Atlantodental Interspace (ADI)

Synonyms. Atlas-odontoid space, predental interspace, atlas-dens interval.

Technique.

Projection: Lateral, flexion, extension cervical spine.

Landmarks: The distance measured is between the posterior margin of the anterior tubercle and the anterior surface of the odontoid. (Fig. 3.12)

Normal Measurements: A small but insignificant difference exists between males and females. The measurement is slightly increased in normal children. (1,2) (Table 3.6) The shape of the interspace will alter in flexion to be a "V" configuration while in extension an inverted "V" pattern will be visible.

Special Considerations: Flexion is the most optimum view to assess the interspace since in this position the most stress is placed on the transverse ligament of the atlas.

Table 3.6.
Normal Values of the Atlantodental Interspace

	Minimum (mm)	Maximum (mm)
Adults	1	3
Children	1	5

Significance. There are numerous disorders which may alter the interspace. A decreased space is to be expected with advancing age due to degenerative joint disease of the atlantodental joint. A more significant change is an abnormally widened space. The most frequent causes include trauma, occipitalization, Down's syndrome, pharyngeal infections (Grisel's disease), and inflammatory arthropathies such as ankylosing spondylitis, rheumatoid arthritis, psoriatic arthritis, and Reiter's syndrome. (3)

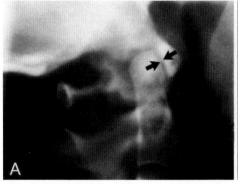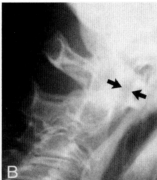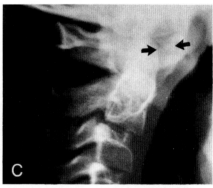

Figure 3.12. A. Adult atlantodental interspace (less than 3 mm) (arrows). **B.** Abnormal atlantodental interspace in a patient with rheumatoid arthritis (5 mm) (arrows) (see text). **C.** Childhood atlantodental interspace (less than 5 mm) (arrows).

Method of Bull

Synonyms.   None.
Technique.
Projection: Lateral skull, lateral cervical.
Landmarks: Two lines are drawn and the resultant angle measured. The first line is drawn between the posterior aspect of the hard palate to the posterior margin of the foramen magnum (Chamberlain's line). The second line is drawn through the midpoints of the anterior and posterior tubercles of the atlas (atlas plane line). The angle formed posteriorly is then measured. (4) (Fig. 3.13)
Normal Measurements: The posterior angle formed by these two lines should be 13 degrees. If this angle is greater than 13 degrees this is abnormal. (2)
Special Considerations: The accuracy of this measurement is readily affected in individuals with acute neck pain due to muscular spasm.
Significance.   The angle will decrease if the odontoid is tilted posteriorly due to congenital malformation or fracture displacement. In some individuals the atlas may be altered in position to change this angle even in the absence of odontoid abnormality.

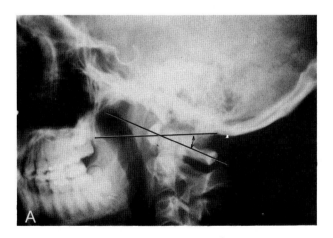

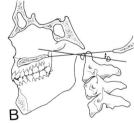

Figure 3.13. A and B. Method of Bull (see text).

George's Line

Synonyms.   Posterior vertebral alignment line, posterior body line.
Technique.
Projection: Lateral cervical.
Landmarks: The posterior vertebral body surfaces are connected with a continuous line which traverses across the intervertebral disc. A straight line cannot be drawn due to the normal concavity of the posterior surface. The key landmarks are the alignment of the superior and inferior posterior body corners. (Fig. 3.14)
Normal Measurements: Normally there is a smooth vertical alignment of each posterior body corner.
Special Considerations: Flexion and extension films are especially useful in determining disruptions in George's line. Care should be taken to eliminate positional rotation since this will create a projectional disruption of the line at consecutive levels ("stair stepping"). This line can be applied throughout the entire spine.
Significance.   Attention to this normal relationship was made by George in 1919 as he commented on detecting post-traumatic cervical injuries. (5,6) Proper alignment of the posterior vertebral bodies signified no fracture, dislocation or ligamentous laxity. If an anterolisthesis or retrolisthesis is present then this may be a radiologic sign of instability due to fracture, dislocation, ligamentous laxity or degenerative joint disease.

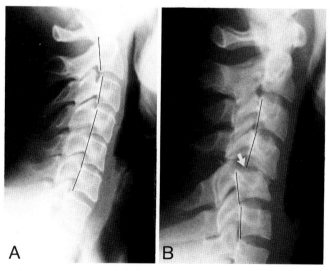

Figure 3.14. A. **George's Line** (see text). **B. Abnormal George's Line**. Due to traumatic bilateral facet dislocation (arrow).

Posterior Cervical Line

Synonyms.   Spinolaminar junction line.
Technique.

Projection: Lateral cervical, (neutral, flexion, extension).

Landmarks: The cortical white line of the spinolaminar junction is first identified at each level C1 to C7. Each spinolaminar junction will be curved anteriorly slightly from superior to inferior. For consistency the most anterior part of the convexity will be compared between levels. (Fig. 3.15)

Normal Measurements: When each spinolaminar

junction point is joined, a smooth arc-like curve results. At the C2 level the spinolaminar junction line in children should not be more than 2 mm anterior to this line.

Significance.   If the drawn curve is discontinuous at any level, then an anterior or posterior displacement may be present. This line is especially useful in the detection of subtle odontoid fractures and atlantoaxial subluxation (anterior) which otherwise may be easily overlooked. (7) A disruption in the mid to lower cervical spine may also be a sign of anterolisthesis, retrolisthesis, or frank dislocation.

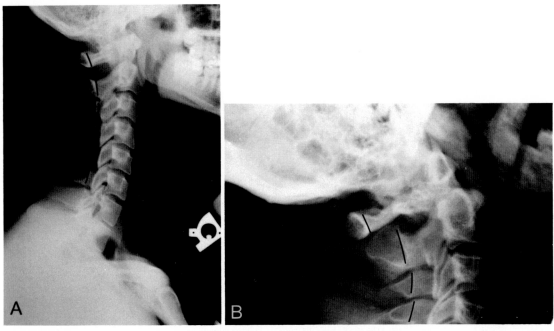

Figure 3.15. A. Posterior Cervical Line (see text). **B. Abnormal Posterior Cervical Line.** Due to posterior displacement of the atlas secondary to os odontoideum.

Sagittal Dimension of the Cervical Spinal Canal

Synonyms.   None.
Technique.
   Projection: Lateral cervical (neutral, flexion, extension).
   Landmarks: The sagittal diameter is measured from the posterior surface of the midvertebral body to the nearest surface of the same segmental spinolaminar junction line. (8) (Fig. 3.16)

Table 3.7.
Normal Sagittal Diameter of the Cervical Spine Canal

Level	Average (mm)	Minimum (mm)	Maximum (mm)
C1	22	16	31
C2	20	14	27
C3	18	13	23
C4	17	12	22
C5	17	12	22
C6	17	12	22
C7	17	12	22

Normal Measurements: These will vary according to the cervical level. (9) (Table 3.7) These values will alter in children (8,10).
Significance.   Narrowing of the canal (stenosis) may be present when the measurement is less than 12 mm. If degenerative posterior osteophytes are present the measurement can be made from its tip to examine the magnitude of the stenotic effect. The degree of stenosis from these spurs is best measured on extension films. (9) An abnormally widened canal may be associated with a spinal cord neoplasm or syringomyelia.

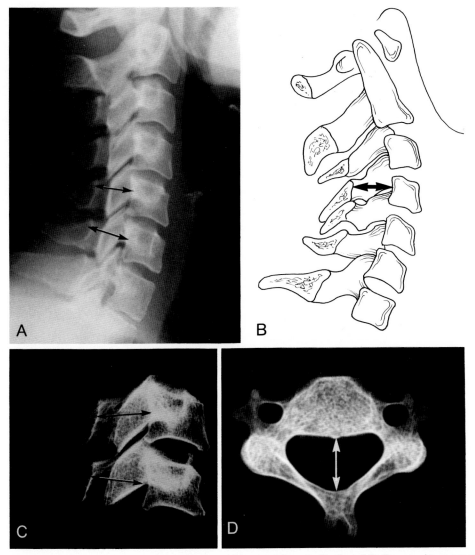

Figure 3.16. A and B. Sagittal dimensions of the cervical spinal canal (arrows) (see text). **C and D.** Dry specimen correlation demonstrating the distance being evaluated (arrows).

Atlantoaxial Alignment

Synonyms.   None.
Technique.
   Projection: Anteroposterior open mouth, cervical spine.
   Landmarks: The lateral margins of the atlas lateral masses are compared to the opposing lateral corner of the axis articular surface. (Fig. 3.17)
   Normal Measurements: These two landmarks should be in vertical alignment.
Significance. If the lateral margin of the atlas lateral mass lies lateral to the lateral axis margin, this may be a radiologic sign of Jefferson's fracture, odontoid fracture, alar ligament instability or rotatory atlantoaxial subluxation. (11)

Cervical Gravity Line

Synonyms.   None.
Technique.
   Projection: Lateral cervical spine (neutral).
   Landmarks: A vertical line is drawn through the apex of the odontoid process. (12) (Fig. 3.18)
   Normal Measurements: This line should pass through the seventh cervical body.
Significance. The line allows a gross assessment of where the gravitational stresses are acting at the cervicothoracic junction.

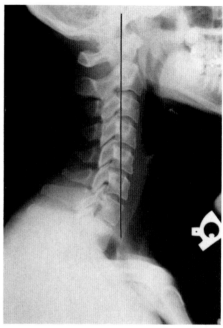

Figure 3.18. Cervical Gravity Line (see text).

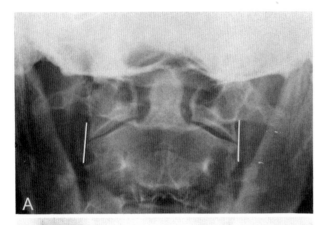

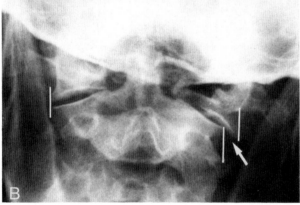

Figure 3.17. A. Normal Atlantoaxial Alignment. B. Abnormal Atlantoaxial Alignment. Due to Jefferson's fracture of the atlas (arrow).

Cervical Lordosis

Synonyms. Angle of the cervical curve, cervical angle.
Technique.
  Projection: Cervical spine, neutral.
  Landmarks: Numerous methods have been proposed, four of which are described:
    Depth of cervical curve. (13) A line is drawn from the superior posterior aspect of the odontoid to the posterior inferior corner of the seventh cervical vertebra. The greatest transverse distance between this line and the posterior vertebral bodies is measured. (Fig. 3.19A)
    Method of Jochumsen. (14) A line is drawn from the anterior border of the atlas anterior tubercle to the anterosuperior corner of the seventh cervical body. The distance from this line to the anterior border of the fifth cervical body is then measured. (Fig. 3.19B)
    Angle of cervical curve. (15) Two lines are drawn, one through and parallel to the inferior end plate of the seventh cervical body, the other through the midpoints of the anterior and posterior tubercles of the atlas (atlas plane line). Perpendiculars are then constructed to the point of intersection and the resultant angle measured. (Fig. 3.19C)

Method of Drexler. (16) This is a laborious but accurate method. Each individual segment is assessed by drawing lines along the body end plates and measuring the resultant angle. The lordosis value is the cumulative total of each intersegmental measurement.
Normal Measurements: (Table 3.8)
Special Considerations: The position of the head is a critical factor in determining the lordosis. If the chin is lowered, tucked downward or retracted, the effect is to straighten the lordosis. (17,18)

Table 3.8.
Normal Values of the Cervical Lordosis

Method	Average	Minimum	Maximum
Depth (mm)	12	7	17
Jochumsen (mm)	3–8	1	9
Angle (deg)	40	35	45
Drexler (deg)	40	16	60

Significance. Many authors have stressed the lack of correlation in relation to altered cervical curvature and clinical symptomatology; however, a reduced or reversed curve may be observed following trauma, muscle spasm, and degenerative spondylosis. (13,17–19)

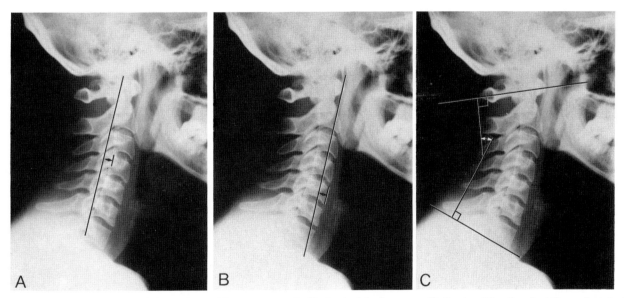

Figure 3.19. CERVICAL LORDOSIS. A. Depth Measurement. B. Method of Jochumsen. C. Angle of the Cervical Curve (see text).

Stress Lines of the Cervical Spine

Synonyms. Ruth Jackson's lines.
Technique.
  Projection: Lateral cervical spine (flexion, extension).
  Landmarks: On each film two lines are constructed. The first line is drawn along the posterior surface of the axis. The second line is drawn along the posterior surface of the seventh cervical body until it intersects the axis line. (19) (Fig. 3.20)

Normal Measurements:
  1. Flexion. These lines normally should intersect at the level of the C5/C6 disc or facet joints.
  2. Extension. These lines normally should intersect at the level of the C4/C5 disc or facet joints.
Significance.   The intersection point represents the focus of stress when the cervical spine is placed in the respective position. Muscle spasm, joint fixation, and disc degeneration may alter the stress point.

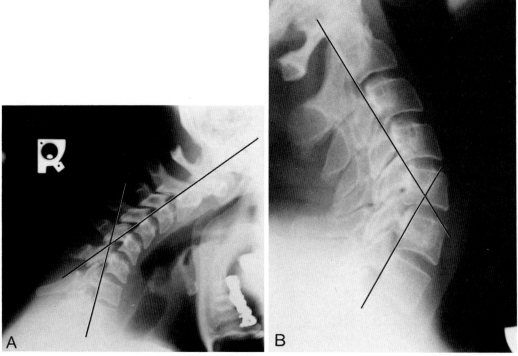

Figure 3.20. CERVICAL STRESS LINES. A. Flexion. B. Extension (see text).

Prevertebral Soft Tissues

Synonyms.   Retropharyngeal interspace (RPI), retrolaryngeal interspace (RLI), retrotracheal space (RTI).

Technique.

Projection: Lateral cervical (neutral, flexion, extension).

Landmarks: The soft tissue in front of the vertebral bodies and behind the air shadow of the pharynx, larynx, and trachea is measured. The bony landmarks are the anterior arch of the atlas, inferior corner of the axis and C3, superior corner of C4, and inferior corner of C5, C6, and C7. (20) At C2/C3 this is called the retropharyngeal interspace, behind the larynx the retrolaryngeal interspace (C4/C5), and behind the trachea (C5–C7) the retrotracheal interspace. (Fig. 3.21)

Normal Measurements: These will vary according to the level being measured and patient position at the time of the exposure. (Table 3.9)

Special Considerations: The values at the C4 and C5 levels may alter dependent on the position of the larynx which may change with swallowing. If anterior spurs are present measure from the body, not the spur.

Table 3.9.
Normal Cervical Prevertebral Soft Tissue Values

Level	Flexion (mm)	Neutral (mm)	Extension (mm)
C1	11	10	8
C2	6	5	6
C3	7	7	6
C4	7	7	8
C5	22	20	20
C6	20	20	19
C7	20	20	21

Significance.   Any soft tissue mass may increase these measurements. These include post-traumatic hematoma, retropharyngeal abscess, or neoplasm from the adjacent bone and soft tissue structures.

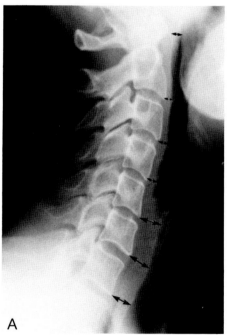

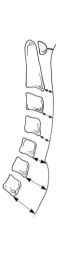

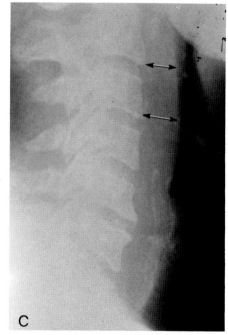

A   **B**   **C**

Figure 3.21. A and B. Prevertebral Soft Tissues (arrows) (see text). **C. Abnormal Retropharyngeal Soft Tissue Measurement.** This is due to hematoma formation following cervical trauma (arrows). (Courtesy of Norman W. Kettner, DC, DACBR, St. Louis, Missouri)

Thoracic Spine

Cobb Method of Scoliosis Evaluation

Synonyms.   Cobb-Lippman method.
Technique.
   Projection: Anteroposterior spine.
   Landmarks:
      End vertebrae.   There are two, one each located at the superior and inferior extremes of the scoliosis. They are defined as the last segment which contributes to the spinal curvature. They appear as being the last segment at the extreme ends of the scoliosis, where the end plates tilt to the side of curvature concavity.
      End plate lines.   On the superior end vertebra a line is drawn through and parallel to the superior end plate. On the inferior end vertebra a line is constructed in a similar manner through and parallel to the inferior end plate.
      Perpendicular lines.   At right angles to both end plate lines another line is drawn until they intersect and the angle measured. (Fig. 3.22)
   Special Considerations: This is the preferred method in scoliosis assessment. In those with double scoliotic curves each component should be measured. Care should be taken to assure common landmarks are utilized in progressive evaluations.
Significance.   This procedure was introduced by Lippman in 1935 and popularized later by Cobb. (1) Essentially, curvatures under 20 degrees require no bracing or surgical intervention; however, if present in a patient between 10–15 years of age, careful monitoring should be implemented to assess for progression of 5 degrees or more in any 3-month period. (2) Curves between 20 and 40 degrees should be braced to prevent progression in the growth period. Surgical intervention may be contemplated for cosmetic reasons, underlying anomaly, curvature progression in an immature spine or curvature in excess of 40 degrees (see Chapter 4).

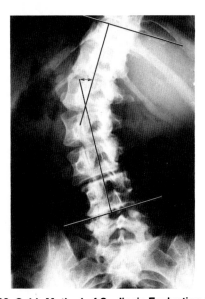

Figure 3.22. Cobb Method of Scoliosis Evaluation (see text).

Risser-Ferguson Method of Scoliosis Evaluation

Synonyms.   None.
Technique.
   Projection: Anteroposterior spine.
   Landmarks:
      1. *End vertebrae.* As per Cobb method.
      2. *Apical vertebra.* The vertebral segment which is the most laterally placed in the curve and usually is the most rotated.
      3. *Vertebral body center.* For each end vertebra and apical segment diagonals are drawn from opposing corners of the body to locate the body center.
      4. *Connecting line.* Two lines are constructed connecting the body centers of the apical segment with each end vertebra and the resultant angle measured. (Fig. 3.23)
   Special Considerations: This method gives values approximately 25 percent below the Cobb method (10 degrees) and some investigators have advocated its use in larger curves, but this practice is to be discouraged. (3) (See Chapter 4)
Significance.   Ferguson first introduced this methodology in the early 1920's and later published his findings in the 1930's and 1940's. (4,5) Like the Cobb method, this assesses the degree of scoliosis and provides data used in the therapeutic decision process.

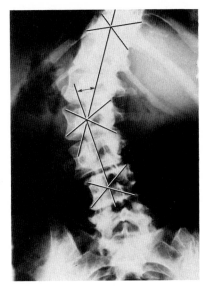

Figure 3.23. Risser-Ferguson Method of Scoliosis Evaluation (see text).

Thoracic Kyphosis

Synonyms. None.
Technique.
Projection: Lateral thoracic spine.
Landmarks: A line is drawn parallel and through the superior end plate of the first thoracic vertebral body. A similar line is drawn through the inferior end plate of the twelfth thoracic vertebral body. Perpendicular lines to these end plate lines are then constructed and the resultant angle is measured at their intersection. (Fig. 3.24)
Normal Measurements: These will vary according to age and sex. (6) (Tables 3.10, 3.11)
Special Considerations: Frequently the vertebral bodies at the ends of the thoracic spine will not be clearly visible. In these circumstances the first visible segment will suffice but may alter the angular value.

Table 3.10.
Degree of Normal Kyphosis in Females by Age

| Age (yr) | Kyphosis (deg) | | | |
	Mean	SD	Minimum	Maximum
2–9	24	7	8	36
10–19	26	7	11	41
20–29	27	8	7	40
30–39	28	9	10	42
40–49	33	7	21	50
50–59	41	10	22	53
60–69	45	8	34	54
70–79	42	9	30	56

Table 3.11.
Degree of Normal Kyphosis in Males by Age

| Age (yr) | Kyphosis (deg) | | | |
	Mean	SD	Minimum	Maximum
2–9	21	8	5	40
10–19	25	8	8	39
20–29	26	8	13	48
30–39	29	8	13	49
40–49	30	7	17	44
50–59	33	6	25	45
60–69	35	5	25	62
70–79	41	8	32	66

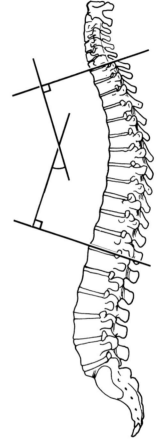

Figure 3.24. Thoracic Kyphosis Measurement (see text).

Significance. The kyphosis may be altered in many disorders. An increased kyphosis may be seen in old age, osteoporosis, Scheuermann's disease, congenital anomalies, muscular paralysis, and even cystic fibrosis. (6) The degree of kyphosis increases with age, and the rate of increase is greater in females than in males.

A reduction in the kyphosis (straight back syndrome) may alter the dynamics of intracardiac blood flow and manifest as apparent cardiac murmurs. (7,8)

Thoracic Cage Dimension

Synonyms. Straight back syndrome evaluation.
Technique.
  Projection: Lateral chest.
  Landmarks: The distance between the posterior sternum and anterior surface of the eighth thoracic vertebral body is measured. (Fig. 3.25)
  Normal Measurements: The sagittal dimension will normally vary slightly. (8) (Table 3.12)

Table 3.12.
Normal Sagittal Dimensions of the Thoracic Cage

	Average (cm)	Minimum (cm)	Maximum (cm)
Male	14	11	18
Female	12	9	15

Significance. A measured sagittal dimension below 13 cm in males and 11 cm in females may indicate the presence of the straight back syndrome. (Table 3.13) If an abnormal measurement is found the chest should be auscultated for a cardiac murmer. If detected an organic cause should be searched for although one may not be found. The decreased anteroposterior diameter may create such a murmer by creating cardiac compression and altered intracardiac hemodynamics. (7,8)

Table 3.13.
Sagittal Dimensions in the Straight Back Syndrome

	Average (cm)	Minimum (cm)	Maximum (cm)
Male	11	9	13
Female	10	8	11

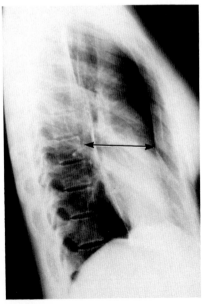

Figure 3.25. Sagittal Thoracic Cage Dimension in Straight Back Syndrome (arrows) (see text).

Lumbar Spine

Intervertebral Disc Height

Synonyms. None.
Technique.
  Projection. Lateral, lumbar spine.
  Landmarks: A number of methodologies have been described, but only two are presented. (1)
    Hurxthal method. (2) The distance between the opposing end plates at the midpoint between the anterior and posterior vertebral body margins is measured. (Fig. 3.26A)
    Farfan's method. (3) The anterior and posterior disc heights are measured and expressed as a ratio to disc diameter. These two ratios are then reduced to a ratio of each other. (Fig. 3.26B)

$$\text{Anterior Height Ratio (AHR)} = \frac{\text{Anterior Height (A)}}{\text{Diameter (D)}}$$

$$\text{Posterior Height Ratio (PHR)} = \frac{\text{Posterior height (P)}}{\text{Diameter (D)}}$$

$$\text{Disc Height (DH)} = \frac{\text{AHR}}{\text{PHR}}$$

  Normal Measurements: Considerable variation exists in disc height according to the lumbar interspace being assessed.
  Special Considerations: Where segmental rotation exceeds 40 degrees or lateral flexion is greater than 20 degrees these methods become unreliable.
Significance. Disc spaces can be altered in many conditions. The most common causes for a decreased disc height include disc degeneration, postsurgery, postchemonucleolysis, infection, and congenital hypoplasia.

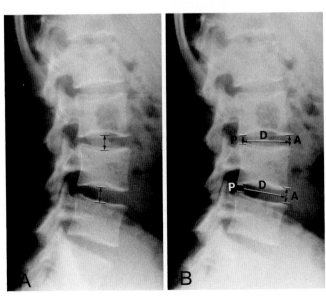

Figure 3.26. INTERVERTEBRAL DISC HEIGHT MEASUREMENT.
A. Hurxthal Method (arrows) (see text). **B. Farfan Method** (arrows) (see text).

Lumbar Intervertebral Disc Angles

Synonyms. None.
Technique.
  Projection: Lateral lumbar spine.
  Landmarks: Lines are drawn through and parallel to each lumbar body end plate, the lines being extended posteriorly until they intersect. The angles formed at each interspace are then measured. (Fig. 3.27)
  Normal Measurements: These vary according to the lumbar level. (4) (Table 3.14)
  Special Considerations: An alternative method of measurement is to include the vertebral bodies in the calculation. (5)

Table 3.14.
Normal Lumbar Intervertebral Disc Angles

Disc Level	Average Angle (deg)
L1	8
L2	10
L3	12
L4	14
L5	14

Significance. The mean angular values will be altered in conditions of antalgia, muscular imbalance, and posture. These measurements may be of assistance in distinguishing the origins of low back pain. In facet syndrome the angles may be increased while in acute discal injuries a reduction in the angle may be seen. (5)

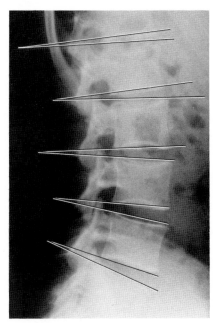

Figure 3.27. Lumbar Intervertebral Disc Angles (see text).

Lumbar Lordosis

Synonyms. Lumbar curve, lumbar spinal angle, lumbar angle.
Technique.
  Projection: Lateral lumbar spine.
  Landmarks: A line is drawn through and parallel to the superior end plate of the first lumbar segment. A second line is drawn through the superior end plate of the first sacral segment. Perpendiculars are then erected and the angle at their intersection measured. (Fig. 3.28)
  Normal Measurements: A wide variation exists within normal individuals. However, an average appears to be approximately 50–60 degrees. (4,5)
  Special Considerations: Some investigators prefer to use the inferior end plate of the fifth lumbar body to eliminate the effects of an altered sacral position. (6)
Significance. The significance of an altered lumbar curve has not been delineated. A wide spectrum of opinions have been expressed, from being of no importance (7) to a prime consideration as it relates to low back pain. (5,8–10)

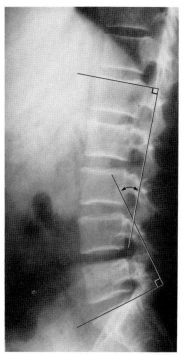

Figure 3.28. Lumbar Lordosis Measurement (see text).

Lumbosacral Lordosis Angle

Synonyms. None.
Technique.
Projection: Lateral lumbar spine.
Landmarks: Two lines are drawn and the angle formed is measured.
  1. The centers of the third and fifth lumbar bodies are located by intersecting diagonal lines from opposing corners for each of the two vertebra. A line is then constructed joining these two body midpoints.
  2. The midpoint of the first sacral segment is located in a similar manner, and a second line is then drawn between the fifth lumbar and first sacral midpoints.
  3. The angle formed posteriorly is then measured. (Fig. 3.29)
Normal Measurements: A wide normal variation in this angle exists. (11) (Table 3.15)
Special Considerations: There appears to be small changes in this angle between the recumbent and upright positions.

Table 3.15.
Normal Values of the Lumbosacral Lordosis

Average (deg)	Minimum (deg)	Maximum (deg)
146	124	162

Significance. The role of an excessive or diminished lumbosacral lordosis angle has not been adequately assessed; however, this is a measurement which can be applied when the upper lumbar segments are not included in the field of study.

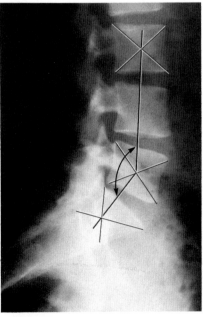

Figure 3.29. Lumbosacral Lordosis Angle (see text).

Sacral Inclination

Synonyms. Sacral tilt angle.
Technique.
Projection: Lateral sacrum, lumbar spine.
Landmarks: Two lines are drawn:
  1. A tangential line parallel and through the posterior margin of the first sacral segment and,
  2. A vertical line intersecting the tangential sacral line. The angle formed is then measured. (Fig. 3.30)
Normal Measurements: A wide variation occurs. (11) (Table 3.16)

Table 3.16.
Normal Sacral Inclination

Average (deg)	Minimum (deg)	Maximum (deg)
46	30	72

Significance. This measurement can be used in the assessment of sacral position and provides additional data on the static mechanics of the low lumbar spine.

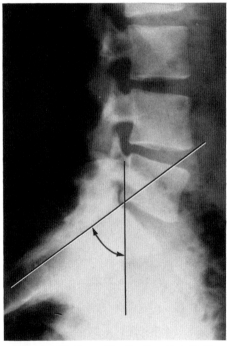

Figure 3.30. Sacral Inclination (see text).

Lumbosacral Angle

Synonyms.   Sacral base angle, Ferguson's angle.
Technique.
  Projection: Lateral lumbar, lumbosacral.
  Landmarks: Two lines are drawn and the resultant angle measured.
   1. A horizontal line is made parallel to the bottom edge of the film
   2. An oblique line is drawn through and parallel to the sacral base. (12–14) (Fig. 3.31)
  Normal Measurements: A wide normal variation is encountered. (15) (Table 3.17) The value will also increase from the recumbent to upright positions by 8–12 degrees.

Table 3.17.
Normal Lumbosacral Angle Values

	Average (degrees)	One Standard Deviation	Minimum (degrees)	Maximum (degrees)
Upright	41	±7	26	57

Significance.   There is no consensus of opinion on the exact role and significance of either a decreased or increased lumbosacral angle. (16–18) An increased angle has been implicated as a mechanical factor in producing low back pain by increasing shearing and compressive forces on the lumbosacral posterior joints. (12,19,20)

Lumbosacral Disc Angle

Synonyms.   Sacrovertebral disc angle.
Technique.
  Projection: Lateral lumbar, lumbosacral spine.
  Landmarks: A line is drawn parallel and through the inferior end plate of the fifth lumbar and superior endplate of the first sacral segment. The angle formed by these lines is then measured. (12) (Fig. 3.32)
  Normal Measurements: The normal range appears to be between 10–15 degrees. (5,21)
Significance.   An increase in the lumbosacral disc angle more than 15 degrees has been linked with the presence of low back pain due to facet impaction. (21) Also there may be a decrease in the value in the presence of acute disc herniation at the fifth lumbar disc. (5)

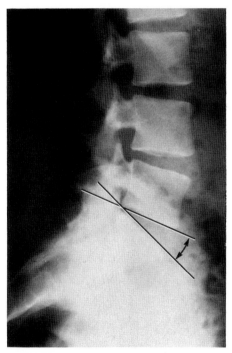

Figure 3.32. Lumbosacral Disc Angle (see text).

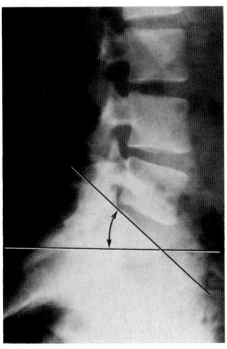

Figure 3.31. Lumbosacral Angle (see text).

Static Vertebral Malpositions

Synonyms. Static intersegmental subluxations.
Technique.

Projection: Anteroposterior and lateral spine.
Landmarks: Numerous terms are applied to describe static vertebral malpositions: (22) (Fig. 3.33)

1. Flexion. The end plates of the opposed segments diverge posteriorly in the lateral view.
2. Extension. (Fig. 3.33A) The end plates of the opposed segments converge more than normal posteriorly in the lateral view.
3. Lateral flexion. (Fig. 3.33B) The end plates of the opposed segments diverge laterally on one side and converge on the other side in the anteroposterior view.
4. Rotation. (Fig. 3.33C) The pedicles will be asymmetrical in shape, and the spinous may be deviated in the anteroposterior view.
5. Anterolisthesis. (Fig. 3.33D) An anterior displacement of one vertebral body in relation to the vertebra below.
6. Retrolisthesis. (Fig. 3.33D) A posterior displacement of one vertebral body in relation to the vertebra below.
7. Laterolisthesis. (Fig. 3.33C) A sideways displacement of one vertebral body in relation to the vertebra below.

Special Considerations: This classification system and terminology can be used for the entire vertebral column. The position of the superior vertebra is always described relative to the subadjacent vertebra, i.e., there is a retrolisthesis of C4 upon C5.

Significance. These various interbody disrelationships may be related to degenerative processes, antalgia, or abnormal mechanics; however, the recognition of these displacements does not necessarily confirm a clinically significant finding.

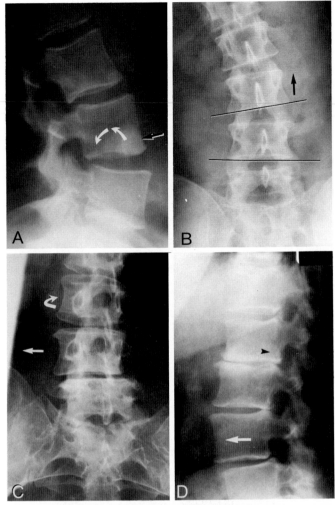

Figure 3.33. STATIC VERTEBRAL MALPOSITIONS. A. Extension (curved arrows). Of incidental notation, observe the domed sclerosis at the anteroinferior aspect of the L3 vertebral body (arrow). This has been called hemispherical spondylosclerosis. **B. Lateral Flexion** (arrow). **C. Laterolisthesis** (arrow), **Rotation** (curved arrows). **D. Anterolisthesis** (arrow), **Retrolisthesis** (arrowhead).

Lumbar Gravity Line

Synonyms. Ferguson's weightbearing line, Ferguson's gravitational line.

Technique.

Projection: Lateral lumbar.

Landmarks: The center of the third lumbar body is located by intersecting diagonals from opposing body corners. A vertical line is then constructed through this point and the relationship to the upper sacrum is assessed. (12,13) (Fig. 3.34)

Normal Measurements: According to Ferguson the center of gravity of the trunk passes through the center of the third lumbar body and continues vertically to intersect the sacral base. (12,13)

Special Considerations: This original description was performed on recumbent lateral lumbar projections; however, some studies suggest that the patient position whether upright or recumbent is irrelevant. (5)

Significance. If this line passes anterior to the sacrum by more than 10 mm (one-half inch) an increase in shearing stresses in an anterior direction between the lumbosacral apophyseal joints may be occurring. (12) Conversely it has been suggested that a posterior shift in this gravity line may be an indicator of increased weightbearing forces on these same lumbosacral joints which may also be active in the production of low back pain. (8,9,19) Increased stress on the pars interarticularis may also be incurred from this posterior shift in weightbearing, although a direct relationship to the formation of spondylolysis has not been demonstrated, only inferred. (20)

Macnab's Line

Synonyms. None.

Technique.

Projection: Lateral lumbar.

Landmarks: A line is drawn through and parallel to the inferior end plate at the level to be evaluated. The relationship of the adjacent tip of the superior articular process of the vertebra below is then assessed. (Fig. 3.35)

Normal Measurements: The line should lie above the tip of the adjacent superior articular process. (23)

Significance. If the line intersects the superior articulating process facet imbrication (subluxation) may be present. The effect of these facets overriding each other is to mechanically infringe on the size of the intervertebral foramen and lateral recess. The reliability of this line, however, has not been documented. (5) It should be noted that the original description of this line was with respect to recumbent radiographs, and their application to weightbearing films is uncertain.

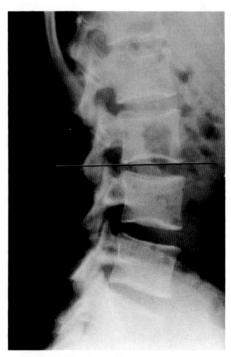

Figure 3.35. Macnab's Line (see text).

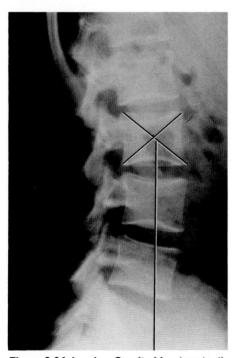

Figure 3.34. Lumbar Gravity Line (see text).

Hadley's "S" Curve

Synonyms.   None.
Technique.
  Projection: Oblique, anteroposterior lumbar spine.
  Landmarks: A curvilinear line is constructed along the inferior margin of the transverse process and down along the inferior articular process to the apophyseal joint space. The line is then continued across the articulation to connect with the outer edge of the opposing superior articular process. (24,25) (Fig. 3.36)
  Normal Measurements: The resultant configuration of this line will be that simulating the letter "S." The key region of the "S" to observe is the normally smooth transition across the joint space.
Significance.   An abrupt interruption in the smooth contour of this line signifies facet imbrication (subluxation).

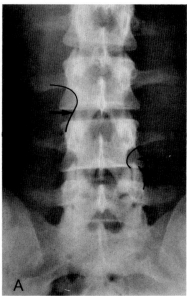

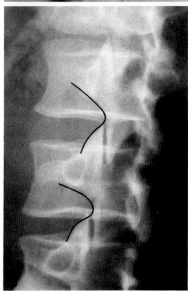

Figure 3.36. Hadley's "S" Curve. A. Anteroposterior Normal (arrow), **Anteroposterior Abnormal** (arrowhead). **B. Oblique Normal** (see text).

Van Akkerveeken's Measurement of Lumbar Instability

Synonyms.   None.
Technique.
  Projection: Lateral lumbar spine (neutral, flexion, extension).
  Landmarks: Two lines are drawn through and parallel to opposing segmental endplates until they intersect posteriorly. The distance from the posterior body margins to the point of intersection is then measured. Alternatively the displacement can be assessed by measuring the offset in the opposing body corners. (Fig. 3.37)
  Normal Measurements: There should be less than 1.5 mm displacement as determined by either measurement method. (26)
  Special Considerations: This evaluation is best performed on the extension film when the most stress is applied to the lower lumbar discs.
Significance.   If there is greater than 1.5 mm difference in measurement then it is likely that nuclear, annular, and posterior ligament damage at the displaced segment is present. Other investigators have cited 3 mm displacement to be of clinical significance. (27)

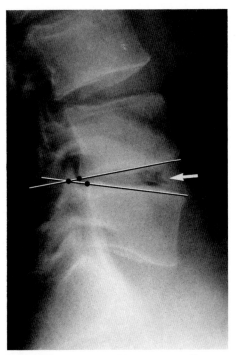

Figure 3.37. Van Akkerveeken's Measurement Demonstrating Intersegmental Instability (see text). Observe the vacuum phenomenon within the L4 disc (arrow).

Degenerative Lumbar Spinal Instability—Flexion/Extension

Synonyms.   Horizontal displacement measurement.
Technique.
   Projection: Lateral lumbar, with flexion and extension.
   Landmarks: The landmarks apply on both flexion and extension. Two methods of assessment can be made—gross and accurate mensuration. (28)
   1. Gross assessment. The alignment of the posterior lumbar bodies is examined by visually observing the relationship of the opposing posterior body corners (George's line).
   2. Accurate measurement—horizontal displacement. The posterior body corners of each body are located. At each segment the superior corners are joined by a line. At the segment which is normal, draw a line parallel to the posterior corner line through the posterior corner of the displaced segment above. The interspace between these two lines is then measured which represents the displaced distance (DD). To remove the effects of radiographic magnification, measure the width of the unstable vertebral body (W) and express the horizontal disrelationship measurement as a percentage (HD%).

$$HD\% = (DD/W) \times 100$$

   3. Accurate measurement—angular displacement. A line is drawn perpendicular to the posterior corner line at opposing body surfaces and the subtended angle measured.
   Normal Measurements: During flexion and extension there should be no detectable anterior or posterior translation of the vertebral bodies in relation to each other. This is assessed by noting the alignment of the posterior body corners in both flexion and extension. (Fig. 3.38) Additionally only one posterior corner of each vertebra should be seen.
Significance.   If anterior or posterior displacement is seen on flexion or extension then this is indicative of degenerative or traumatically induced instability. More specifically if anterior displacement is seen during flexion this denotes laxity of the posterior ligamentous complex (interspinous, supraspinous, capsular, flaval ligaments, and annular disc fibers). Conversely a posterior displacement during extension implies an anterior ligamentous complex failure (anterior longitudinal ligament and annular disc fibers). These may frequently occur together as a manifestation of total segmental ligamentous failure.

Another sign of instability during flexion/extension is the recognition of intersegmental rotation. This can be identified by the observation of two posterior body corners at one segment and implies posterior joint ligamentous instability.

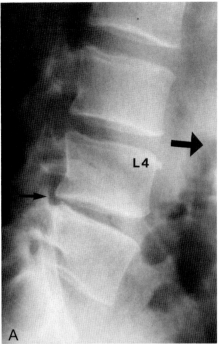

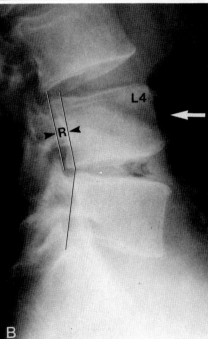

Figure 3.38. FLEXION/EXTENSION INTERSEGMENTAL INSTABILITY EVALUATION. A. Flexion. Note the alignment at the fourth lumbar level (arrow). **B. Extension.** Note the degree of retrolisthesis (R) indicative of extension instability (arrow).

Degenerative Lumbar Instability—Lateral Bending

Synonyms.   None.
Technique.
Projection: Lateral bending, lumbar spine.
Landmarks: Three structures are evaluated—the vertebral body margins, pedicles, and spinous process (28) (Fig. 3.39)
Normal Measurements: On normal lateral bending the following should be noted:

1. Vertebral body alignment. No lateral segmental displacement (shear) should be seen, and the disc space should be less on the concave side.
2. Pedicle position. Each segment should show progressive rotation as evidenced by the altered shape of the pedicle contour along the concave side of the induced curve.
3. Spinous position. Similarly, the normal rotational segmental coupling will be shown by gradual spinous deviation of each successive segment into the concavity of the curve.

Significance.   If there is lateral segmental displacement (shear) this usually indicates laxity of the discal ligaments and is a sign of degenerative lumbar instability.

Abnormalities in normal posterior joint coupling movements where there is a lack of or even complete reversal of rotatory motion (paradoxical motion) indicate ligamentous laxity of the posterior joints or altered joint mechanics.

Lateral Bending Sign

Synonyms.   None.
Technique.
Projection: Right and left lateral bending, lumbar spine.
Landmarks: Transverse lines are drawn on each segment through either of two locations: 1) the tips of the superior articulating process or 2) the superior border of the pedicles. (Fig. 3.40)
Normal Measurements: On each lateral bending study the constructed lines will converge toward the bending side in a gradually increasing manner from the lumbosacral junction up. (28)
Significance.   In the presence of appropriate clinical symptoms a localized segmental failure to laterally flex may indicate the presence of a posterolateral (axillary) disc herniation. (29) However, altered biomechanical function of the posterior joints may produce an identical radiographic appearance. (28)

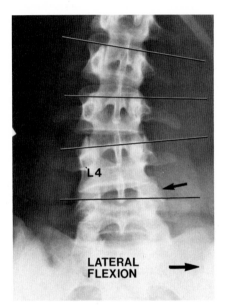

Figure 3.40. LATERAL BENDING SIGN. Observe the failure of intersegmental lateral flexion at the fourth lumbar segment due to a posterolateral disc herniation (arrows).

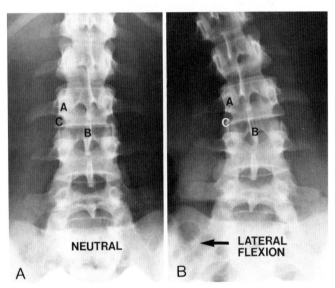

Figure 3.39. LATERAL FLEXION INSTABILITY EVALUATION. A. Neutral Position. Three structures are observed: (A) pedicle position and configuration; (B) spinous position; and (C) adjacent vertebral margin alignment. **B. Lateral Flexion**. The changes in these structures from the neutral to lateral flexion position are assessed.

Meyerding's Grading Method in Spondylolisthesis

Synonyms.   None.
Technique.
   Projection: Lateral lumbar, lumbosacral.
   Landmarks: The superior surface of the first sacral segment is divided into four equal divisions. The relative position of the posterior-inferior corner of the fifth lumbar body to these segments is then made. (30) (Fig. 3.41)
   Normal Measurement: The posterior-inferior corner of the fifth lumbar body should be aligned with the posterior-superior corner of the first sacral segment.
   Special Considerations: The same assessment can be applied to other spinal levels by dividing the superior end plate of the segment below the spondylolisthesis into four.
Significance.   The degree of anterolisthesis of the affected vertebral body can be categorized according into which division the posterior-inferior corner of the body lies. These are designated into "grades":
   Grade 1.   The posterior-inferior corner is aligned within the first division.
   Grade 2.   The posterior-inferior corner is aligned within the second division.
   Grade 3.   The posterior-inferior corner is aligned within the third division.
   Grade 4.   The posterior-inferior corner is aligned within the fourth division. If the vertebral body has completely slipped beyond the sacral promontory then this is called "spondyloptosis."

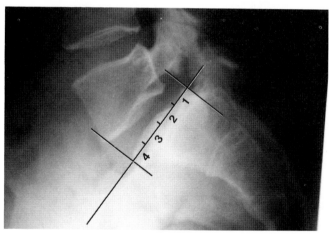

Figure 3.41. Meyerding Classification of Spondylolisthesis.

Ullmann's Line

Synonyms.   Garland-Thomas line, right angle test line.
Technique.
   Projection: Lateral lumbar, lumbosacral.
   Landmarks: Two lines are drawn: (1) parallel and through the sacral base, and (2) a perpendicular line through the anterior margin of the sacral base. The relationship of the fifth lumbar body to this perpendicular line is then assessed. (31–33) (Fig. 3.42)
   Normal Measurements: The fifth lumbar body should lie posterior or just contact this perpendicular line.
Significance.   If the anterior margin of the fifth lumbar body crosses the perpendicular line then anterolisthesis may be present. This is a useful line when there is poor visualization of the pars region in detecting the presence of spondylolisthesis. Application of this line must be interpreted in light of lumbar biomechanics; i.e., if there is a significant loss of the lumbar lordosis, a false positive finding may be present.

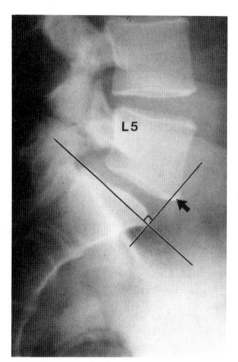

Figure 3.42. Ullmann's Line. Spondylolisthesis of the fifth lumbar segment demonstrated by the intersection of the line with the fifth lumbar body (arrow).

Interpediculate Distance

Synonyms.   Coronal dimension of the spinal canal.
Technique.
   Projection: Anteroposterior cervical, thoracic, and lumbar spines.
   Landmarks: The shortest distance between the inner convex cortical surfaces of the opposing segmental pedicles is measured. (Fig. 3.43)
   Normal Measurements: This varies according to each spinal level and patient age. (34) (Table 3.18)

Table 3.18.
Normal Adult Interpediculate Distances

Spinal Level	Average (mm)	Minimum (mm)	Maximum (mm)
C3	28	25	31
C4	29	26	32
C5	29	26	33
C6	29	26	33
C7	28	24	32
T1	24	20	28
T2	20	17	24
T3	19	16	22
T4	18	15	21
T5	17	14	21
T6	17	14	20
T7	17	14	20
T8	18	15	21
T9	18	15	21
T10	19	15	22
T11	20	18	24
T12	23	19	27
L1	25	21	29
L2	26	21	30
L3	26	21	31
L4	27	21	33
L5	30	23	36

Significance.   This is a useful measurement applied in the evaluation of spinal stenosis, congenital malformation, and intraspinal neoplasms. In stenosis the minimum measurement is exceeded, but for accurate delineation it is best used in combination with other measurements such as the sagittal canal dimension (Eisenstein) and size of the vertebral body (canal/body ratio.) The maximum interpediculate distance may be increased due to pedicular erosion from an expanding spinal cord tumor (*Elseberg-Dyke sign*). (35)

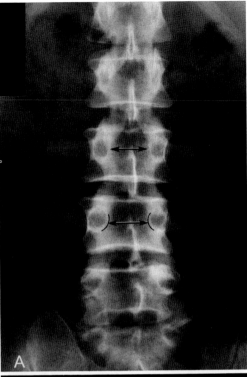
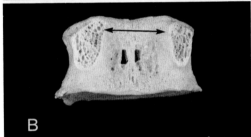
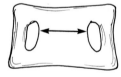

Figure 3.43. A–C. Interpediculate Distance (arrows).

Eisenstein's Method for Sagittal Canal Measurement

Synonyms.   None.
Technique.
   Projection: Lateral lumbar spine.
   Landmarks: For each lumbar level except the fifth, the sagittal canal diameter can be determined by measuring between two points.
   1. Articular process line. A line is drawn to connect the tips of the superior and inferior articular processes at each level.
   2. Posterior body margin. The measurement point is on the posterior body margin at the midpoint between the superior and inferior end plate. (Fig. 3.44)
   3. Sagittal canal measurement. Obtained by determining the distance between the posterior body and articular process line.

For determining the sagittal canal dimension of the fifth lumbar segment the measurement is made between the spinolaminar junction line and posterior body. (36)
Normal Measurements: No single measurement should be less than 15 mm, (36) though some have suggested 14 mm to be minimum value. (37)
Special Considerations: The actual lowest anatomical measurement found on cadaver specimens has been 12 mm. (36)
Significance.   A measurement below 15 mm may indicate the presence of spinal stenosis. This appears to be the single most reliable measurement on plain radiographs in the assessment of spinal stenosis. (36) However, before the definitive diagnosis is made appropriate clinical studies and computerized tomography must be performed. (37)

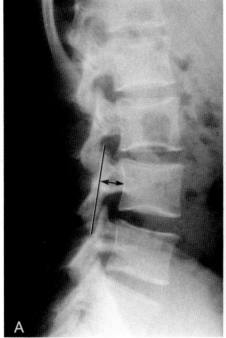
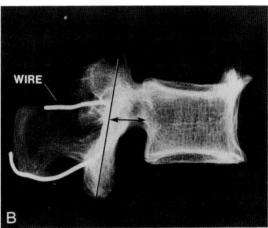
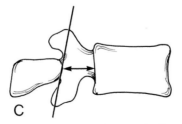

Figure 3.44. A. Eisenstein's Method for Sagittal Canal Measurement (see text). **B and C**. Note that the line will closely approximate the posterior limits of the canal (metal wire).

Canal/Body Ratio

Synonyms.   Spinal index.
Technique.
   Projection: Anteroposterior and lateral lumbar spine.
   Landmarks: Four measurements are made, two per film for each spinal segment. (38,39) (Fig. 3.45)

1. Interpediculate distance (A). The smallest distance between each pedicle.
2. Sagittal canal dimension (B). The method of Eisenstein is applied. A line is drawn from the tips of the superior and inferior articular processes, and adjacent to the midpoint on the posterior body margin the sagittal distance is measured.
3. Transverse body dimension (C). The width of the vertebral body on the anteroposterior film is measured at the midpoint between the end plates.
4. Sagittal body dimension (D). The length of the vertebral body on the lateral film is measured at the midpoint between the endplates.

   Normal Measurements: These four measurements are combined to provide an index of the canal size in relation to vertebral body size. This is derived by:

Interpediculate Dimension × Sagittal Canal Dimension:
Transverse Body Dimension × Sagittal Body Dimension,

i.e.,

$$\text{Canal/Body Ratio} = \frac{A \times B}{C \times D}$$

The normal range will vary according to the lumbar level. (84) (Table 3.19)

Table 3.19.
Normal Lumbar Canal Body Ratios

	Minimum	Maximum
L3	1:3.0	1:6.0
L4	1:3.0	1:6.0
L5	1:3.2	1:6.5

Significance.   The higher the ratio the smaller the spinal canal which is an indicator of possible spinal stenosis; however, this method of spinal canal assessment has been shown not to be reliable. (36)

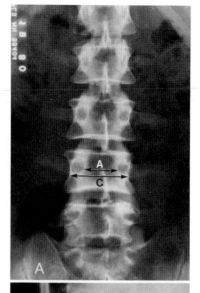
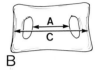
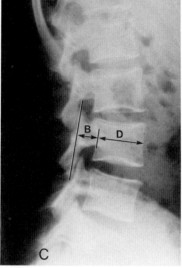
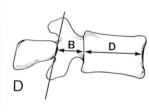

Figure 3.45. CANAL/BODY RATIO. A. Anteroposterior Measurements. Interpediculate distance (A) and transverse body dimension (C). **B. Lateral Measurements.** Sagittal canal dimension (B) and sagittal body dimension (D).

Intercrestal Line

Synonyms. None.
Technique.
Projection: Anteroposterior lumbar spine.
Landmarks: A transverse line is drawn connecting the iliac crests. The relationship of the bodies and discs of the fifth and fourth lumbar segments to this line is then made. (40) (Fig. 3.46)
Normal Measurements: The relative position of these two segments within the pelvis is variable; however, the most stable position appears to be where the line intersects through the bottom half of the fourth lumbar body or disc.
Significance. This line, along with other skeletal parameters, may be a useful indicator in predicting the level where the most biomechanical stress is occurring in the lumbar spine and the level at which degenerative changes are most likely to occur. (40) The criteria for probable L4/L5 degeneration are:
1. A high intercrestal line passing though the upper half of L4.
2. Long transverse processes on L5.
3. Rudimentary rib.
4. Transitional vertebra.

The criteria for L5-S1 degeneration are:
1. An intercrestal line passing through the body of L5.
2. Short transverse processes on L5.
3. No rudimentary rib.
4. No transitional vertebra.

Length of Lumbar Transverse Processes

Synonyms. None.
Technique.
Projection: Anteroposterior lumbar spine.
Landmarks: A vertical line is drawn through the tip of the third lumbar transverse process. This is done bilaterally. The relationship of the fifth lumbar transverse process to this line is then assessed. (40) (Fig. 3.47)
Normal Measurements: Considerable variation in the length of the fifth lumbar transverse occurs.
Significance. If the fifth lumbar transverse process is short then this may be an inherent structural instability factor at the lumbosacral junction. Conversely, a long transverse process can be seen as a stabilizing factor at this level. The length of this transverse process can be used in combination with other parameters to predict segmental instability (see intercrestal line).

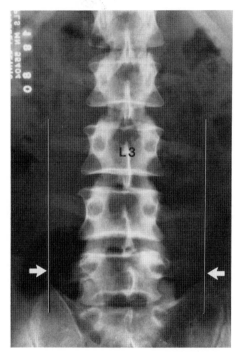

Figure 3.47. Length of the Lumbar Transverse Processes (see text).

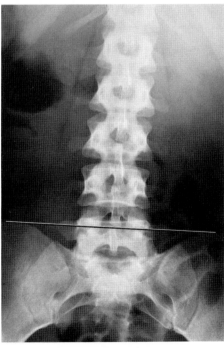

Figure 3.46. Intercrestal Line (see text).

Lower Extremity

Teardrop Distance

Synonyms. Medial joint space of the hip.
Technique.
   Projection: Anteroposterior pelvis, hip.
   Landmarks: The distance between the most medial margin of the femoral head and outer cortex of the pelvic teardrop is measured. (1) (Fig. 3.48)
   Normal Measurements: (Table 3.20)

Table 3.20.
Normal Teardrop Distances

Average (mm)	Minimum (mm)	Maximum (mm)
9	6	11

Significance. If the teardrop distance exceeds 11 mm or there is more than a 2 mm discrepancy from right to left (Waldenstrom's sign), then hip disease should be suspected. This is an especially sensitive sign in early Legg-Calvé-Perthes disease and may also be seen in septic arthritis or other inflammatory diseases.

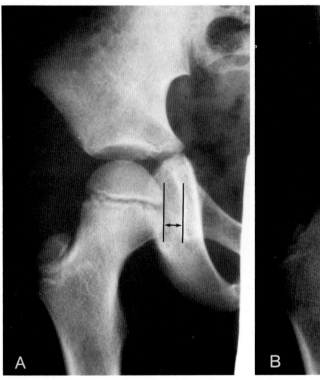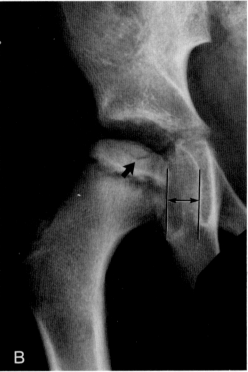

Figure 3.48. TEARDROP DISTANCE. A. Normal. B. Abnormal, Due to Early Legg-Calvé-Perthes Disease. Observe the "crescent" sign in the femoral capital epiphysis (arrow).

Hip Joint Space Width

Synonyms.   None.
Technique.
   Projection: Anteroposterior, hip.
   Landmarks: Three measurements are made of the joint cavity. (2) (Fig. 3.49)
   1. Superior joint space. The space between the most superior point on the convex articular surface of the femur and adjacent acetabular cortex.
   2. Axial joint space. The space between the femoral head and acetabulum immediately lateral to the acetabular notch.
   3. Medial joint space (teardrop distance). The space between the most medial surface of the femoral head and opposing acetabular surface.
   Normal Measurements: Notably, the superior and axial compartments are approximately equal (4 mm), while the medial space is twice as great (8 mm). (2) (Table 3.21)

Table 3.21.
Normal Hip Joint Space Width

	Average (mm)	Minimum (mm)	Maximum (mm)
Superior space	4	3	6
Axial space	4	3	7
Medial space	8	4	13

Significance.   Various disorders may alter normal values; however, changes within the various compartments may be found in specific entities.
   Superior Joint Space: The most common cause for a diminished joint space in this compartment is degenerative joint disease.
   Axial Joint Space: Degenerative arthritis and especially inflammatory arthritis, such as rheumatoid arthritis, will diminish this compartment, often with associated loss of joint space in the other compartments.
   Medial Joint Space: Narrowing is usually due to degenerative or inflammatory arthritis; however, widening of the compartment is a frequent indicator of hip joint effusion or lateral shift of the femur (Waldenstrom's sign).

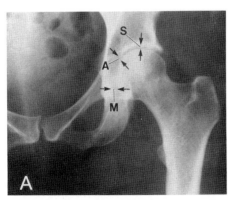
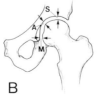

Figure 3.49. A and B. Width of Hip Joint Space: Superior (S), Axial (A), Medial (M). Observe the medial joint space (M) is normally twice the width of the other two compartments (see text).

Acetabular Depth

Synonyms.   None.
Technique.
   Projection: Anteroposterior pelvis.
   Landmarks: A line is drawn from the superior margin of the pubis at the symphysis joint to the upper outer acetabular margin. The greatest distance from this line to the acetabular floor is measured. (3) (Fig. 3.50)
   Normal Measurements: There will be slight variations between males and females. (3) (Table 3.22)

Table 3.22.
Normal Acetabular Depth

	Average (mm)	Minimum (mm)	Maximum (mm)
Male	13	7	18
Female	12	9	18

Significance.   An acetabular depth less than 9 mm is considered to be shallow and dysplastic, which may be a factor in precipitating degenerative joint disease of the hip.

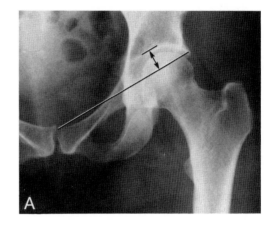
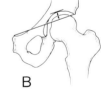

Figure 3.50. A and B. Depth of the Acetabulum (see text).

The Center-Edge Angle

Synonyms.   The CE angle, CE angle of Wiberg.
Technique.
  Projection: Anteroposterior pelvis, hip.
  Landmarks: A vertical line is drawn through the center point of the femoral head. Another line is constructed through the femoral head center to the outer upper acetabular margin. The angle formed is then measured. (4) (Fig. 3.51)
  Normal Measurements: (2,4) (Table 3.23)

Table 3.23.
Normal Center-Edge Angles

Average (deg)	Minimum (deg)	Maximum (deg)
36	20	40

Significance.   A shallow angle may be related to underlying acetabular dysplasia which has been linked to the onset of degenerative joint disease.

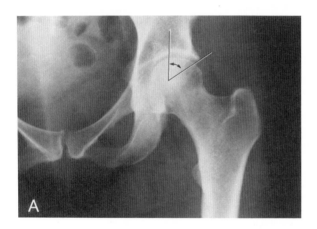

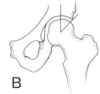

Figure 3.51. A and B. Center-Edge Angle (CE Angle of Wiberg) (see text).

Symphysis Pubis Width

Synonyms.   None.
Technique.
  Projection: Anteroposterior pelvis.
  Landmarks: The measured distance is between the opposing articular surfaces, halfway between the superior and inferior margins of the joint. (Fig. 3.52)
  Normal Measurements: A slight variation exists between males and females. (5) (Table 3.24)
  Special Considerations: If alignment is being assessed, using the inferior margin appears to be the most reliable.

Table 3.24.
Normal Symphysis Pubis Width

	Average (mm)	Minimum (mm)	Maximum (mm)
Male	6	4.8	7.2
Female	5	3.8	6

Significance.   Widening of the symphysis may be due to cleidocranial dysplasia, bladder exostrophy, hyperparathyroidism, post-traumatic diastasis, and inflammatory resorption, such as in ankylosing spondylitis and osteitis pubis.

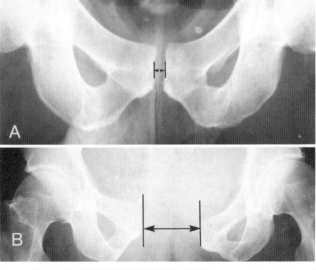

Figure 3.52. WIDTH OF SYMPHYSIS PUBIS (see text). **A. Normal.** **B. Abnormal.** Due to traumatic diastasis.

Measurements of Protrusio Acetabuli

Synonyms. Kohler's Line.
Technique.
  Projection: Anteroposterior pelvis, hip.
  Landmarks: A line is constructed tangentially to the cortical margin of the pelvic inlet and outer border of the obturator foramen. The relationship of the acetabular floor to this line is assessed. (12,13) (Fig. 3.57)
  Normal Measurements: The acetabular floor should not cross this line and usually is laterally to it.
Significance. If the acetabular floor crosses the line then protrusio acetabuli is present. The most common causes include an idiopathic form, rheumatoid arthritis, and Paget's disease.

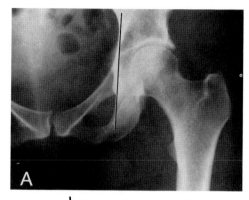

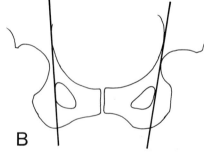

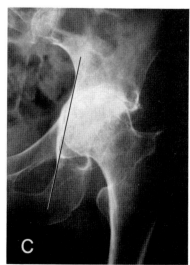

Figure 3.57. A and B. Kohler's Line (see text). **C. Protrusio Acetabuli.** Observe the medial displacement of the acetabulum and femoral head in relation to the line due to rheumatoid arthritis.

Shenton's Line

Synonyms. Makka's line, Menard's line.
Technique.
  Projection: Anteroposterior hip, pelvis.
  Landmarks: A curvilinear line is constructed along the undersurface of the femoral neck and is continued across the joint to the inferior margin of the superior pubic ramus. (11) (Fig. 3.58)
  Normal Measurements: The constructed line should be smooth, especially in the transition zone between the femoral neck and superior pubic ramus. Occasionally, a small portion of the inferior femoral head may just cross the line.
Significance. An interrupted, discontinuous line is useful in the detection of hip dislocation, femoral neck fracture, and slipped femoral capital epiphysis (SFCE).

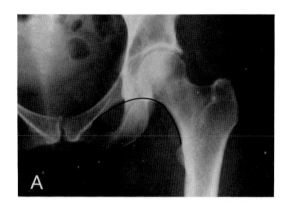

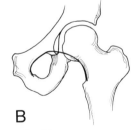

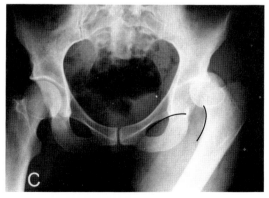

Figure 3.58. A and B. Shenton's Line (see text). **C. Hip Dislocation.** Note the interruption in the smooth arc of Shenton's line.

Iliofemoral Line

Synonyms.   None.
Technique.
  Projection: Anteroposterior pelvis, hip.
  Landmarks: A curvilinear line is constructed along the outer surface of the ilium, across the joint and onto the femoral neck. (14) (Fig. 3.59)
  Normal Measurements: A small portion of the superior femoral head may cause a slight convexity in the line. The most important normal feature is that the line will be bilaterally symmetrical.
Significance.   A discrepancy in symmetry may be due to congenital dysplasia, slipped femoral capital epiphysis, dislocation, and fracture.

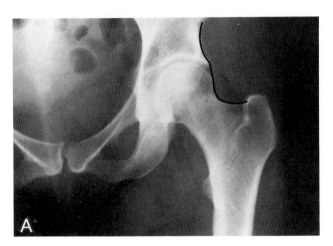

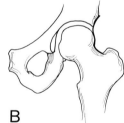

Figure 3.59. A and B. Iliofemoral Line (see text).

Femoral Angle

Synonyms.   Femoral angle of incidence, femoral neck angle, Mickulicz's angle.
Technique.
  Projection: Anteroposterior hip, pelvis.
  Landmarks: Two lines are drawn through and parallel to the midaxis of the femoral shaft and femoral neck. The angle subtended is then measured. (15) (Fig. 3.60)
  Normal Measurements: Slight variation occurs between males and females. (11) (Table 3.29)
  Special Considerations: For accurate depiction of the femoral shaft-neck angle the foot should be medially rotated 15 degrees at the time of radiographic exposure.

Table 3.29.
Normal Femoral Angle

Minimum (deg)	Maximum (deg)
120	130

Significance.   A value less than 120 degrees is designated as coxa vara and above 130 degrees as coxa valga.

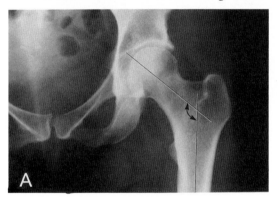

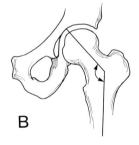

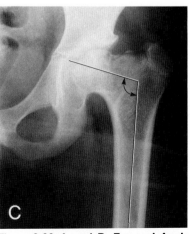

Figure 3.60. A and B. Femoral Angle (see text). **C. Decreased Femoral Angle (Coxa Vara).**

Skinner's Line

Synonyms. None.
Technique.
Projection: Anteroposterior pelvis, hip.
Landmarks: A line is drawn through and parallel to the axis of the femoral shaft. A second line at right angles to the shaft line is constructed tangential to the tip of the greater trochanter. The relationship of the fovea capitus to this trochanteric line is assessed. (16) (Fig. 3.61)
Normal Measurements: The fovea capitus should lie above or at the level of the trochanteric line.
Significance. If the fovea lies below this line then this is due to a superior displacement of the femur relative to the femoral head. The most common causes are fracture and those conditions leading to coxa vara.

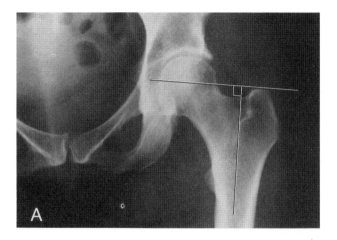

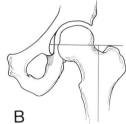

Figure 3.61. A and B. Skinner's Line (see text).

Klein's Line

Synonyms. None.
Technique.
Projection: Anteroposterior and frog-leg, hip, or pelvis.
Landmarks: A line is constructed tangential to the outer margin of the femoral neck. The degree of overlap of the femoral head will be apparent. (17) (Fig. 3.62)
Normal Measurements: Comparison should be made with the opposite side and, normally, there will be the same degree of overlap of the femoral head. In most normal hips the outer margin of the femoral head will be lateral to the line.
Special Considerations: This line can be performed on both the anteroposterior and frog-leg projections.
Significance. If there is a failure of the femoral head overlap in relation to the line or asymmetry from side to side, then slippage of the femoral capital epiphysis should be suspected. (17)

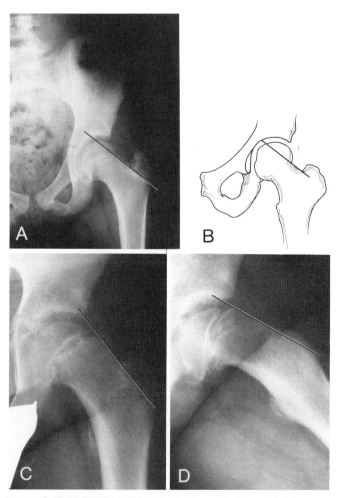

Figure 3.62. KLEIN'S LINE (see text). **A and B. Normal Adolescent Hip. C and D. Slipped Femoral Capital Epiphysis.** Anteroposterior and frog-leg projection of the hip in slipped femoral capital epiphysis. Note the lack of overlap across the line by the femoral head.

Axial Relationships of the Knee

Synonyms. None.
Technique.
   Projection: Anteroposterior knee.
   Landmarks: Four lines and two angles are performed.
   (15) (Fig. 3.63)
      1. Femoral shaft line (A). A line is drawn through and parallel to the midaxis of the femoral shaft.
      2. Tibial shaft line (B). A line is drawn through and parallel to the midaxis of the tibial shaft.
      3. Femoral condyle line (C). A line is drawn through and tangential to the articular surfaces of the condyles.
      4. Tibial plateau line (D). A line is drawn through the medial and lateral tibial plateau margins.
      5. Femoral angle (FA). The angle formed between the femoral shaft and femoral condyle lines.
      6. Tibial angle (TA). The angle formed between the tibial shaft and tibial plateau lines.
   Normal Measurements: Slight variation exists between males and females. (Table 3.30)

Table 3.30.
Normal Axial Relationships of the Knee

	Average (deg)	Minimum (deg)	Maximum (deg)
Femoral Angle	81	75	85
Tibial Angle	93	85	100

Significance. These angles will be altered in fractures and other deformities about the knee.

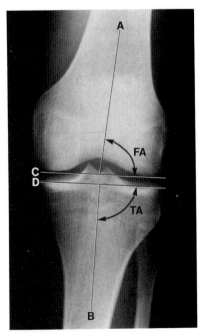

Figure 3.63. AXIAL RELATIONSHIPS OF THE KNEE. Femoral Angle (FA), Tibial Angle (TA) (see text).

Patellar Position

Synonyms. Patella alta evaluation.
Technique.
   Projection: Lateral knee (semiflexed).
   Landmarks:
      1. Patellar length (PL). The greatest diagonal dimension between the superior and inferior poles.
      2. Patellar tendon length (PT). The distance measured is between the insertion points of the posterior tendon surface at the inferior patellar pole and notch at the tibial tubercle. (Fig. 3.64)
   Normal Measurements: Patella length and patellar tendon length are usually equal to each other. A normal variation up to 20 percent, however, is considered insignificant. (18)
Significance. When the patellar tendon length is more than 20 percent greater than the patellar length, patella alta is present. This may be found in association with chondromalacia patellae.

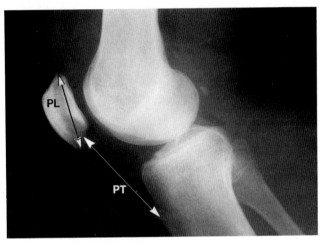

Figure 3.64. Patellar Position (see text).

Axial Relationships of the Ankle

Synonyms.   None.
Technique.
  Projection: Anteroposterior ankle.
  Landmarks: Four lines and two angles are constructed. (15) (Fig. 3.65)
  1. Tibial shaft line (A). A line is drawn through and parallel to the tibial shaft.
  2. Medial malleolus line (B). A line is drawn tangential to the articular surface of the medial malleolus.
  3. Lateral malleolus line (C). A line is drawn tangential to the articular surface of the lateral malleolus.
  4. Talus line (D). A line is drawn tangential to the articular surface of the talar dome.
  5. Tibial angle (I). The angle formed medially between the medial malleolus line and talus line.
  6. Fibular angle (II). The angle formed laterally between the lateral malleolus line and talus line.
  Normal Measurements: Slight variation occurs between males and females. (15) (Table 3.31)

Table 3.31.
Normal Axial Relationships of the Ankle

	Average (deg)	Minimum (deg)	Maximum (deg)
Tibial Angle (I)	53	45	65
Fibular Angle (II)	52	43	63

Significance.   These angles will be altered in fractures of the malleoli, ankle mortise instability, and tibiotalar slant deformities.

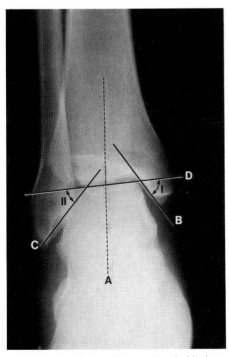

Figure 3.65. Axial Relationships of the Ankle (see text).

Heel Pad Measurement

Synonyms.   None.
Technique.
  Projection: Lateral foot, lateral calcaneus (nonweight-bearing).
  Landmarks: The shortest distance between the plantar surface of the calcaneus and external skin contour is measured. (19) (Fig. 3.66)
  Normal Measurements: Variation between sexes does occur. (20) (Table 3.32)
  Special considerations.   Blacks may have a slightly larger heel pad distance. (21)

Table 3.32.
Normal Heel Pad Measurement

	Average (mm)	Maximum (mm)
Male	19	25
Female	19	23

Significance.   Increased skin thickness, especially of the heel pad, is a frequent accompanying feature of acromegaly.

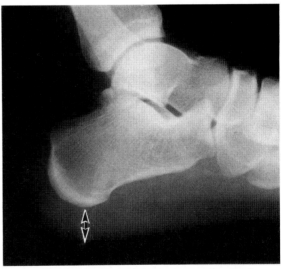

Figure 3.66. Heel Pad Measurement (see text).

Boehler's Angle

Synonyms. Axial relationships of the calcaneus, tuber angle.

Technique.

Projection: Lateral foot, lateral calcaneus.

Landmarks: The three highest points on the superior surface of the calcaneus are connected with two tangential lines. The angle formed posteriorly is then assessed. (Fig. 3.67)

Normal Measurements. The angle formed posteriorly averages between 30–35 degrees in most normal subjects but may range between 28–40 degrees. Any angle less than 28 degrees is abnormal. (22)

Significance. The most common cause for an angle less than 28 degrees is a fracture with displacement through the calcaneus. Dysplastic development of the calcaneus may also disturb the angle.

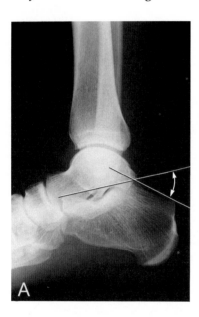

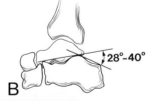

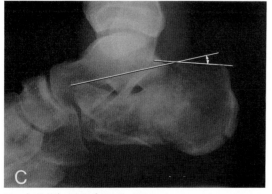

Figure 3.67. BOEHLER'S ANGLE. A and B. Normal Angle. C. Calcaneal Fracture. Observe the decrease in Boehler's angle.

Upper Extremity

Axial Relationships of the Shoulder

Synonyms. Humeral axial angle.

Technique.

Projection: Anteroposterior shoulder with external rotation.

Landmarks: (Fig. 3.68)

1. Humeral shaft line (A). A line is drawn through and parallel to humeral shaft.
2. Humeral head line (B). From the apex of the greater tuberosity a line is drawn toward the medial humeral surface at the point where the diaphyseal cortex changes from a band to line.
3. Humeral angle (HA). The inferior angle between the humeral shaft and head lines.

Normal Measurements: The average humeral angles are 60 degrees for males and 62 degrees for females. (1)

Significance. This relationship may be altered following a fracture, especially in the surgical neck.

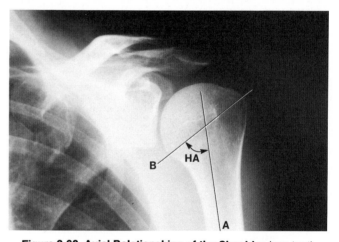

Figure 3.68. Axial Relationships of the Shoulder (see text).

Glenohumeral Joint Space

Synonyms. None.
Technique.
  Projection: Anteroposterior shoulder with external rotation.
  Landmarks: The measurements are made at the superior, middle, and inferior aspects of the joint. These are combined and averaged. Each distance is ascertained between the opposing articular surfaces. (Fig. 3.69)
  Normal Measurements: The average joint space is between 4-5 mm. (2)
Significance. The joint space may be diminished in degenerative arthritis, calcium pyrophosphate dihydrate (CPPD) crystal disease, and post-traumatic arthritis. A widened space is a frequent associated finding of acromegaly and posterior humeral dislocation. (3)

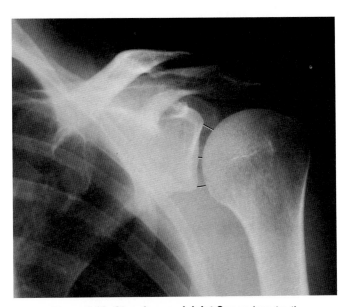

Figure 3.69. Glenohumeral Joint Space (see text).

Acromiohumeral Joint Space

Synonyms. None.
Technique.
  Projection: Anteroposterior shoulder.
  Landmarks: The distance between the inferior surface of the acromion and the articular cortex of the humeral head is measured. (Fig. 3.70)
  Normal Measurements: (4) (Table 3.33)

Table 3.33.
Normal Acromiohumeral Distance

Average (mm)	Minimum (mm)	Maximum (mm)
9	7	11

Significance. A measurement less than 7 mm is indicative of a rotator cuff tear or degenerative tendinitis due to the unopposed action of the deltoid, (4) allowing superior subluxation of the humerus. A measurement greater than 11 mm may indicate post-traumatic subluxation, dislocation, joint effusion, stroke or brachial plexus lesions ("drooping shoulder"). (5)

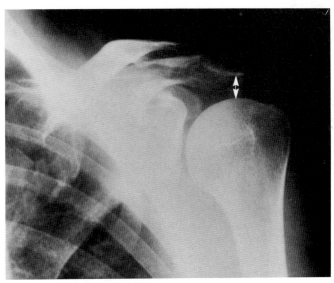

Figure 3.70. Acromiohumeral Space (see text).

Acromioclavicular Joint Space

Synonyms. None.
Technique.
 Projection: Anteroposterior or posteroanterior shoulder.
 Landmarks: The joint space is measured at the superior (S) and inferior (I) borders, and an average of the two values is made. (Fig 3.71)
 Normal Measurements: (2) The average joint space is 3 mm, with sexual variation. There should be no more than 2–3 mm difference between the right and left joint spaces. (Table 3.34)

Table 3.34.
Normal Acromioclavicular Joint Space

	Average (mm)	Minimum (mm)	Maximum (mm)
Male	3.3	2.5	4.1
Female	2.9	2.1	3.7

Significance. A decreased joint space is seen in degenerative joint disease. An increased joint may be due to traumatic separation or resorption due to osteolysis in association with hyperparathyroidism, rheumatoid arthritis or following trauma.

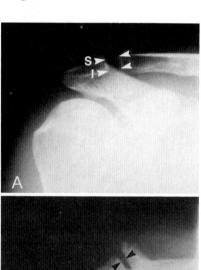

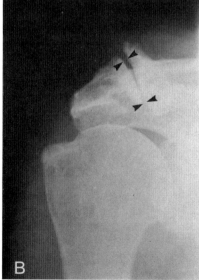

Figure 3.71. ACROMIOCLAVICULAR JOINT SPACE. A. Normal. B. Abnormal. The measurement is abnormally decreased due to degenerative joint disease (arrowheads).

Axial Relationships of the Elbow

Synonyms. None.
Technique.
 Projection: Anteroposterior elbow.
 Landmarks: Three lines and three angles are evaluated. (1) (Fig. 3.72)
  1. Humeral shaft line (A). A line is drawn through and parallel to the humeral shaft.
  2. Ulnar shaft line (B). A line is drawn through and parallel to the ulnar shaft.
  3. Humeral articular line (C). A transverse line is drawn tangentially through the most distal surfaces of the trochlea and capitellum.
  4. Carrying angle (CA). The angle formed between the humeral and ulnar shaft lines.
  5. Humeral angle (HA). The angle formed between the humeral shaft and articular lines.
  6. Ulnar angle (UA). The angle formed between ulnar shaft line and humeral articular line.
 Normal Measurements: Slight variations occur between males and females. (Table 3.35)
 Special Considerations: The elbow must be fully extended with no rotation at the humerus.

Table 3.35.
Axial Relationships of the Elbow

	Average (deg)	Minimum (deg)	Maximum (deg)
Carrying Angle	169	154	178
Humeral Angle	85	72	95
Ulnar Angle	84	72	99

Significance. These angles may be altered from fractures or other deformities at the elbow.

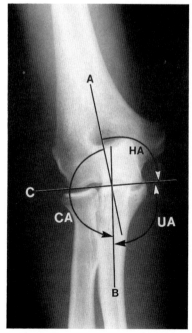

Figure 3.72. AXIAL RELATIONSHIPS OF THE ELBOW. Carrying Angle (CA), Humeral Angle (HA), Ulnar Angle (UA) (see text).

Radiocapitellar Line

Synonyms. None.
Technique.
Projection: Lateral elbow.
Landmarks: A line is drawn through the center of and parallel to the long axis of the radius and is extended through the elbow joint. (Fig. 3.73)
Normal Measurements: This line should pass through the center of the capitellum in all stages of flexion of the elbow. (6)
Significance. This assists in determining the presence of radial head subluxation (pulled elbow) or dislocation.

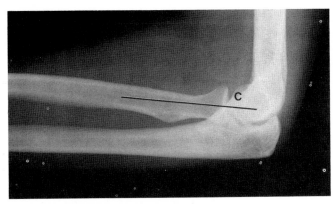

Figure 3.73. RADIOCAPITELLAR LINE. The radial shaft line passes through the center of the capitellum (C) (see text).

Axial Relationships of the Wrist

Synonyms. None.
Technique.
Projection: Posteroanterior and lateral wrist.
Landmarks:
Posteroanterior relationships. (Fig. 3.74A)
  1. Radioulnar articular line (A). A tangential line is drawn from the tip of radial styloid to the base of ulnar styloid.
  2. Radial shaft line (B). A line is drawn through and parallel to the shaft of the radius.
  3. Radioulnar angle (I). The ulnar side angle between the two lines is measured.
Lateral relationships. (Fig. 3.74B)
  1. Radius articular line (A). A line is drawn across the most distal points on the articular surface of the radius.
  2. Radial shaft line (B). A line is drawn through and parallel to the shaft of the radius.
  3. Radius angle (II). The palmar angle is measured between these two lines.
Normal Measurements: (1) (Table 3.36)

Table 3.36.
Normal Axial Angles at the Wrist

	Average (deg)	Minimum (deg)	Maximum (deg)
PA Radioulnar Angle	83	72	95
Lateral Radius Angle	86	79	94

Significance. These lines and constructed angles aid in the assessment of radioulnar deformities, especially those due to displaced fractures.

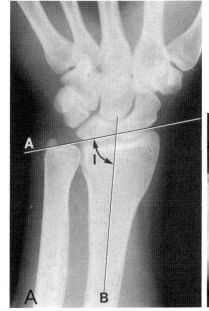
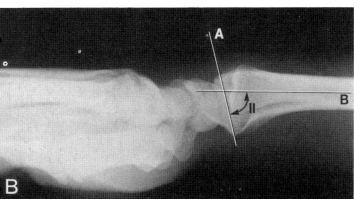

Figure 3.74. AXIAL RELATIONSHIPS OF THE WRIST. A. Posteroanterior. B. Lateral (see text).

Metacarpal Sign

Synonyms. None.

Technique.

Projection: Posterior-anterior hand.

Landmarks: A line is drawn tangentially through the articular cortex of the fourth and fifth metacarpal heads. (Fig. 3.75)

Normal Measurement. The line should pass distal to or just touch the third metacarpal head. (7)

Significance. If the line passes through the third metacarpal head this is a frequent sign of gonadal dysgenesis (Turner's syndrome). A fracture deformity may also produce a positive sign.

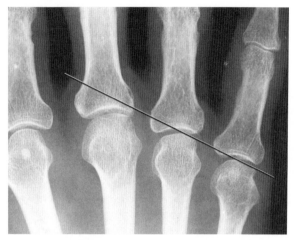

Figure 3.75. METACARPAL SIGN. Normal fourth and fifth metacarpal relationships (see text).

Table 3.37.
Lines and Angles of the Skull

Name	Figure Number	Landmarks	Normal Measurements			Significance
			Average	Minimum	Maximum	
Vastine-Kinney	3.2	Pineal gland to inner skull margins: frontal, occipital, vault, and foramen magnum.	Consult standard tables			Intracranial mass or localized atrophy when pineal displaced.
Sella Turcica Size	3.3	Horizontal: Widest diameter. Vertical: Fossa floor—clinoids.	11 mm 8 mm	5 mm 4 mm	16 mm 12 mm	Pituitary and extrapituitary masses enlarge the fossa.
Basilar Angle	3.4	Nasion—center sella turcica. Basion—center sella turcica.	137 deg	123 deg	152 deg	Basilar impression and platybasia widen the angle (>152 deg).
McGregor's Line	3.5	Hard palate—occiput. Note relative odontoid apex.	Below line		Males: 8 mm Females: 10 mm	Basilar impression when odontoid more than maximum distance above.
Chamberlain's Line	3.6	Hard palate—opisthion	Below line to 4.3 mm above		7 mm	Basilar impression when odontoid more than maximum distance above.
MacRae's Line	3.7	Basion—opisthion.	Occipital bone at or below line			Basilar impression when occipital bone above the line.
Digastric Line	3.8	Right and left digastric grooves: (a) Line—odontoid distance. (b) Line—C1/OCC joint distance.	11 mm 12 mm	1 mm 4 mm	21 mm (Odontoid not above the line) 20 mm	Basilar impression when odontoid is above the line.
Height Index of Klaus	3.9	Tuberculum sellae—IOP. Odontoid to line distance.	40–41 mm	30 mm	None	Basilar impression if less than 30 mm.
Boogard's Line	3.10A	Nasion—opisthion. Basion—opisthion.			Basion below line	Basilar impression if basion above the line.
Boogard's Angle	3.10B	Dorsum sella—basion. Angle between lines.	122 deg	119 deg	135 deg	Basilar impression if angle greater than 135 deg.
Anterior Atlanto-occipital dislocation	3.11	Basion—C1 posterior arch. Opisthion—C1 anterior arch. Ratio of these distances.	Ratio less than one			Atlanto-occipital dislocation where the ratio is equal to or greater than one.

Table 3.38.
Lines and Angles of the Cervical Spine

Name	Figure Number	Landmarks	Normal Measurements			Significance
			Average	Minimum	Maximum	
Atlantodental interspace (ADI)	3.12	C1 anterior tubercle—odontoid.	(a) Adult (b) Child	1 mm 1 mm	3 mm 5 mm	Transverse ligament rupture or instability. Trauma, Down's, and inflammatory arthritis may increase the measurement.
Method of Bull	3.13	Hard palate—opisthion. C1 anterior arch—C1 posterior arch. Posterior angle measured.			13 deg	Odontoid malposition if greater than 13 degrees.
George's Line	3.14	Alignment of posterior body margins.	Aligned			A to P vertebral malpositions when line not smooth.
Posterior Cervical Line	3.15	Spinolaminar junction lines.	Aligned			A to P vertebral malpositions when line is not smooth, especially at C1 and C2.
Sagittal Canal Dimension	3.16	Posterior body—spinolaminar junction.	See Table 3.7	12 mm		Spinal stenosis when less than 12 mm. Intraspinal tumor when enlarged.
Atlantoaxial Alignment	3.17	C1 lateral mass—C2 articular pillar margin alignment.	Aligned			Jefferson's or odontoid fractures or alar ligament instability when margins overlap.
Gravity Line	3.18	Vertical line from odontoid apex.	Passes through C7 body			AP displacement is a gross indicator of gravitational stress at the cervicothoracic junction.
Lordosis						
(a) Depth	3.19A	Odontoid apex—post-C7 body. Greatest distance to line.	12 mm	7 mm	17 mm	Role unclear. Decreased following trauma, muscle spasm, spondylosis, and patient tucking the chin at time of exposure.
(b) Jochumsen	3.19B	C1 anterior tubercle—anterior C7 body. Distance to anterior C5 body	3–8 mm	1 mm	9 mm	
(c) Angle	3.19C	C2 and C7 end plates, then intersecting perpendiculars.	40 deg	35 deg	45 deg	
(d) Drexler	3.19D	Cummulative total of individual disc angles.	40 deg	16 deg	60 deg	
Stress Lines	3.20	C2 and C7 posterior bodies, and note location of intersection. (a) Flexion (b) Extension	 C5–C6 joint C4–C5 joint			Stress point during these movements often altered by muscle spasm, fixation, and spondylosis.
Prevertebral Soft Tissues	3.21	Anterior bodies—posterior air shadow margins.	See Table 3.9			Soft tissue masses (tumor, infection, hematoma) increase the measurements.
		(a) Retropharyngeal (RPI) (C2–C3)		7 mm		
		(b) Retrolaryngeal (RLI) (C4–C5)		20 mm		
		(c) Retrotracheal (RTI) (C5–C7)		20 mm		

Table 3.39.
Lines and Angles of the Thoracic Spine

Name	Figure Number	Landmarks	Normal Measurements			Significance
			Average	Minimum	Maximum	
Method of Cobb	3.22	End vertebral end plate lines then intersecting perpendiculars and the angle measured.				Scoliosis evaluation.
Risser-Ferguson	3.23	Centers of end and apical segments joined and the angle measured.				Scoliosis evaluation.
Thoracic Kyphosis	3.24	T1 superior end plate—T12 inferior end plate, then intersecting perpendiculars and the angle measured.	See Tables 3.10, 3.11			Kyphosis evaluation (Scheuermann's, fractures, etc.)
Thoracic Cage Dimension	3.25	Posterior sternum—anterior T8 body.	Male: 14 cm Female 12 cm	11 cm 9 cm	18 cm 15 cm	Straight back syndrome when the distance is less than 13 cm in males and 11 cm in females.

Table 3.40.
Lines and Angles of the Lumbar Spine

Name	Figure Number	Landmarks	Normal Measurements			Significance
			Average	Minimum	Maximum	
Intervertebral Disc Height (a) Hurxthal method	3.26A	End plate: End plate distance.	Variable			Decreased disc height (degeneration, surgery, infection).
(b) Farfan method	3.26B	Anterior height divided by disc diameter, posterior height divided by disc diameter, then averaged.	Variable			Decreased disc height (degeneration, surgery, infection).
Intervertebral Disc Angles	3.27	At each disc end plate lines are drawn and the angles are measured.	See Table 3.14			Altered in various mechanical pathologies.
Lordosis	3.28	L1 end plate—S1 end plate; perpendiculars and angle formed.	50–60 deg			Altered in various mechanical pathologies.
Lumbosacral Lordosis	3.29	Centers of L3, L5, and S1 bodies found and joined.	146 deg	124 deg	162 deg	Altered in various mechanical pathologies
Sacral Inclination	3.28	Posterior surface of S1 to vertical line angle.	46 deg	30 deg	72 deg	Altered in various mechanical pathologies.
Lumbosacral Angle	3.29	End plate of S1 to horizontal line angle.	41 deg	26 deg	57 deg	Altered in various mechanical pathologies.
Lumbosacral Disc Angle	3.30	Angle between opposing end plates of L5 and S1.	—	10 deg	15 deg	Altered in various mechanical pathologies.
Gravity Line	3.34	A perpendicular line is drawn from the center point of the L3 body.	Intersects sacral base			Altered in various mechanical pathologies.
Macnab's Line	3.35	A line along the inferior end plate.	Through or above superior articular process			Extension malposition, normal variant.

Table 3.40—
 continued

Name	Figure Number	Landmarks	Normal Measurements			Significance
			Average	Minimum	Maximum	
Hadley's "S" Curve	3.36	A line along the inferior surface of the TVP, AP and across the joint.	Smooth across joint			Facet subluxation.
Van Akkerveeken's Measurement	3.37	End plate lines at opposing segments. Measure from the posterior body to point of intersection.	Equal measurements		1.5 mm difference	Nuclear, annular and posterior ligament damage if more than 1.5 mm difference.
Flexion/Extension	3.38	Amount of displacement on flexion/extension (see text).				Flexion instability: Posterior ligamentous failure. Extension instability: Anterior ligamentous failure. Rotation instability: Posterior joint ligamentous failure.
Lateral Bending Instability	3.39	Body alignment.	Aligned			Disc ligament failure if displaced.
		Pedicle position.	Smooth, progressive alteration			Posterior joint ligament laxity.
		Spinous position.	Toward concavity			Posterior joint ligament laxity.
	3.40	Intersegmental wedging.	Gradually decrease away from the sacrum			Disc herniation at level failing to laterally flex (lateral bending sign).
Meyerding's Grading	3.41	Sacral base divided into quarters. Relative position of the posterior body of L5 is made.	—			Grading severity of spondylolisthesis.
Ullmann's Line	3.42	End plate line through S1, perpendicular from sacral promontory.	L5 behind the line			Detection of subtle spondylolisthesis when L5 body crosses perpendicular line.
Interpediculate Distance	3.43	Shortest distance between inner surfaces of opposing pedicles.	See Table 3.18			Widened in intraspinal tumors, Narrowed in spinal stenosis.
Eisenstein's Method	3.44	Tips of superior and inferior articular processes joined. Distance between posterior midbody and this line (except at L5).	Variable	15 mm		Spinal stenosis suspected when less than 15 mm.
Canal/Body Ratio	3.45	Canal size (AP, lateral) divided by body size.				
		(a) L3 and L4		1:3.0	1:6.0	>1:6.0 denotes a small canal.
		(b) L5		1:3.2	1:6.5	>1:6.5 denotes a small canal.
Intercrestal Line	3.46	Iliac crests joined. Relative position of L4 and L5 bodies and discs.				May predict level of most stress and subsequent degeneration.
Transverse Process	3.47	Vertical line through L3 TVP. L5 TVP length assessed relative to this line.				May predict level of most stress and subsequent degeneration.

Table 3.41.
Lines and Angles of the Lower Extremities

Name	Figure Number	Landmarks	Normal Measurements			Significance
			Average	Minimum	Maximum	
Teardrop Distance	3.48	Femoral head—teardrop distance.	9 mm	6 mm	11 mm	Early Perthes or other inflammatory joint disease may widen the space more than 11 mm or create a 2 mm difference from the normal side.
Hip Joint Space Width	3.49	Femoral head—acetabulum distance.				Various joint diseases decrease these distances:
		(a) Superior	4 mm	3 mm	6 mm	Degenerative joint disease.
		(b) Axial	4 mm	3 mm	7 mm	Rheumatoid arthritis.
		(c) Medial	8 mm	4 mm	13 mm	Degenerative and rheumatoid arthritis.
Acetabular Depth	3.50	Superior pubis—outer acetabulum. The distance from the line of the furthest surface is measured.	Male: 13 mm Female: 12 mm	7 mm 9 mm	18 mm 18 mm	A shallow acetabulum exists when the measurement is less than 9 mm.
Center-Edge Angle	3.51	From the center of the femoral head, vertically, and acetabular edge, lines are drawn. The angle between is measured.	36 deg	20 deg	40 deg	A shallow acetabulum may precipitate degenerative joint disease.
Symphysis Pubis Width	3.52	The distance between opposing articular surfaces, halfway between the superior and inferior margins.	Male: 6 mm Female: 5 mm	4.8 mm 3.8 mm	7.2 mm 6.0 mm	Diastasis and inflammatory joint disease may widen the joint.
Presacral Space	3.53	Soft tissue density between the rectum and anterior sacral surface.	Child: 3 mm Adult: 7 mm	1 mm 2 mm	5 mm 20 mm	Soft tissue mass (tumor, infection, hematoma), if exceeds maximum distance.
Acetabular Angle	3.54	Y-Y line drawn. Second line from medial to lateral acetabular surfaces.	20 deg	12 deg	29 deg	Congenital hip dislocation widens the angle. Down's syndrome decreases the angle.
Iliac Angle	3.55	Y-Y line drawn. Second line from iliac wing to iliac body.				Combined with acetabular angles to derive iliac index.
Iliac Index	3.56	Sum of right and left iliac and acetabular angles, divided by 2.	68 deg	Below 68 deg		Down's syndrome probable between 60–80 deg, and very possible below 60.
Protrusio Acetabuli	3.57	Pelvic inlet—outer obturator. Acetabulum should be lateral to the line.				Protrusio acetabuli (Paget's disease, etc.) when acetabulum is medial to the line.
Shenton's Line	3.58	Smooth curvilinear line along medial femoral neck and superior obturator border.				Femur dislocation or fracture if line is interrupted.
Iliofemoral Line	3.59	Smooth curvilinear line along ilium and onto femoral neck. Should be bilaterally symmetrical.				Asymmetry may denote hip joint abnormality.
Femoral Angle	3.60	Lines through the axis of the femoral shaft and neck.		120 deg	130 deg	Coxa vara: Less than 120 deg. Coxa valga: Greater than 130 deg.
Skinner's Line	3.61	Femoral shaft line. Perpendicular second line tangential to the tip of the greater trochanter.	Passes through or below fovea capitus			Hip joint abnormality (fracture, varus, etc.) if the line passes above the fovea capitus.

**Table 3.41—
continued**

Name	Figure Number	Landmarks	Normal Measurements			Significance
			Average	Minimum	Maximum	
Klein's Line	3.62	Tangential line to outer femoral neck. Head just overlaps laterally.				Slipped epiphysis suspected if head does not intersect line.
Axial Relationships of the Knee	3.63	(See text) (a) Femoral angle (b) Tibial angle	81 deg 93 deg	75 deg 85 deg	85 deg 100 deg	Deformities (traumatic, congenital, arthritic) at the knee will alter these angles.
Patellar Position	3.64	Patella length (PL)—patella tendon (PT) ratio.	PL:PT 1:1 (+20%)			Chondromalacia patellae factor if the ratio is more than 20% altered (patella alta).
Axial Relationships of the Ankle	3.65	(See text) (a) Tibial angle (b) Fibular angle	53 deg 52 deg	45 deg 43 deg	65 deg 63 deg	
Heel Pad	3.66	Shortest distance between the calcaneus and plantar skin surface.	Male: 19 mm Female: 19 mm		25 mm 23 mm	Acromegaly produces skin overgrowth exceeding the maximum measurement.
Boehler's Angle	3.67	Three superior points joined on the calcaneus. Posterior angle is measured.	30–35 deg	28 deg		Calcaneal fractures may reduce the angle to less than 28 deg.

Table 3.42.
Lines and Angles of the Upper Extremities

Name	Figure Number	Landmarks	Normal Measurements			Significance
			Average	Minimum	Maximum	
Axial Relationships of the Shoulder	3.68	Humeral shaft—humeral head angle.	60–62 deg			Humeral deformities (fractures, congenital, etc.) will alter these values.
Glenohumeral Joint Space	3.69	Average humeral head—glenoid distance (superior, middle, inferior).	4–5 mm			Degenerative and crystal arthritis diminish the space. Posterior dislocation may widen it.
Acromiohumeral Joint Space	3.70	Acromion—humeral head.	9 mm	7 mm	11 mm	Rotator cuff tear decreases distance. Subluxation and dislocation increases distance.
Acromioclavicular Joint Space	3.71	Average acromion—clavicular distance (superior, inferior).	Male: 3.3 mm Female: 2.9 mm	2.5 mm 2.1 mm	4.1 mm 3.7 mm	Degenerative arthritis decreases distance. Separation and resorption widens distance.
Axial Relationships of the Elbow	3.72	(See text) (a) Carrying angle (b) Humeral angle (c) Ulnar angle	169 deg 85 deg 84 deg	154 deg 72 deg 72 deg	178 deg 95 deg 99 deg	Elbow deformities (fractures, congenital, etc.) will alter these values.
Radiocapitellar Line	3.73	Radius axis line through the elbow joint.	Passes through capitellar center			Radius subluxation/dislocation if line misses the capitellar center.
Axial Relationships of the Wrist	3.74	(See text) (a) PA view: Radioulnar angle (b) Lateral view: Radius angle	83 deg 86 deg	72 deg 79 deg	95 deg 94 deg	Wrist deformities (traumatic, congenital, etc.) will alter these values.
Metacarpal Sign	3.75	Tangential line through the fourth and fifth metacarpal heads. Third head should be proximal to this line.				Turner's syndrome, postfracture deformity.

REFERENCES

Introduction

1. Phillips RB: An evaluation of the graphic analysis of the pelvis on the AP full spine radiograph. *ACA J Chiro* 139:December, 1975.
2. Howe JW: Some Considerations in spinal x-ray interpretations. *J Clin Chiro Archives*, ed 1, 1971.
3. Howe JW: Facts and fallacies, myths and misconceptions in spinography. *J Clin Chiro Archives*, ed 2, 1972.

Geometric Distortion

1. Ball RP, Golden R: Roentgenographic obstetrical pelvicephalometry in erect posture. *AJR* 49:731, 1943.
2. Brown GH: Automatic compensation in roentgenographic pelvicephalometry. *AJR* 78:1063, 1957.

Skull

1. Vastine JH, Kinney KK: The pineal shadow as an aid in the localization of brain tumors. *AJR* 17:320, 1927.
2. Dyke CG: Indirect signs of brain tumor as noted in routine roentgen examinations. Displacement of the pineal shadow. *AJR* 23:598, 1930.
3. Pawl RP, Walter AK: Localization of the calcified pineal body on lateral roentgenograms. *AJR* 105:287, 1969.
4. Camp JD: The normal and pathologic anatomy of the sella turcica as revealed at necropsy. *Radiology* 1:65, 1923.
5. Silverman FN: Roentgen standards for size of the pituitary fossa from infancy through adolescence. *AJR* 78:451, 1957.
6. DiChiro G, Nelsen KB: The volume of the sella turcica.*AJR* 87:989, 1962.
7. Fisher RL, DiChiro G: The small sella turcica. *AJR* 91:996, 1964.
8. Poppel MH, Jacobson HG, Duff BK, et al: Basilar impression and platybasia in Paget's disease. *Radiology* 61:639, 1953.
9. McGregor M: The significance of certain measurements of the skull in the diagnosis of basilar impression. *Br J Radiol* 21:171, 1948.
10. Hinck VC, Hopkins CE, Savara BS: Diagnostic criteria of basilar impression. *Radiology* 76:572, 1961.
11. Chamberlain WE: Basilar impression (platybasia). A bizarre developmental anomaly of the occipital bone and upper cervical spine, with striking and misleading neurologic manifestations.*Yale J Biol Med* 11:487, 1939.
12. Macrae DL, Barnum AS: Occipitalization of the atlas. *AJR* 70:23, 1953.
13. Fischgold H, Metzger J: Etude radio-tomographique de l'impression basilaire. *Rev Rhum* 19:261, 1952.
14. Klaus E: Rontgendiagnostik der platybasie und basilaren impression. Weitere erfahrungen mit einer neuen untersuchungsmethode. *Fortschr Geb Roentgen* 86:460, 1957.
15. von Torklus D, Gehle W: *The Upper Cervical Spine*, London, Butterworths, 1972.
16. Powers B, Miller MD, Kramer RS, et al: Traumatic anterior atlanto-occipital dislocation. *Neurosurg* 4 (1):12, 1979.

Cervical Spine

1. Hinck VC, Hopkins CE: Measurement of the atlanto-dental interval in the adult. *AJR* 84:945, 1960.
2. Locke GR, Gardner JI, VanEpps EF: Atlas-dens interval (ADI) in children. A survey based on 200 normal cervical spines. *AJR* 97:135, 1966.
3. Yochum TR, Rowe LJ: *Aspects of Manipulative Therapy*, ed 2, New York, Churchill Livingstone, chap 3, 1985.
4. Bull JW, Nixon WLB, Pratt RTC: The radiological criteria and familial occurrence of primary basilar impression. *Brain* 78:229, 1955.
5. George AW: A method for more accurate study of injuries to the atlas and axis. *Boston Med Surg J* 181:13, 1919.
6. Litterer WE: A history of George's line. *ACA J Chiro* 39: December 1983.
7. Swischuk LE: Anterior displacement of C2 in children: Physiologic or pathologic. *Radiology* 122:759, 1977.
8. Hinck VC, Hopkins CE, Savara BS: Sagittal diameter of the cervical spinal canal in children. *Radiology* 79:97, 1962.
9. Wolf BS, Khilnani M, Malis L: The sagittal diameter of the bony canal and its significance in cervical spondylosis. *J Mount Sinai Hosp NY* 23:283, 1956.
10. Yousefzadeh DK, El-Khoury GY, Smith WL: Normal sagittal diameter and variation in the pediatric cervical spine.*Radiology* 144:319, 1982.
11. Shapiro R, Youngberg AS, Rothman SLG: The differential diagnosis of traumatic lesions of the occipito-atlanto-axial segment. *Radiol Clin North Am* 11 (3):505, 1973.
12. Fox MG, Young OG: Placement of the gravital line in antero-posterior standing posture. *Research Quart* 25:277, 1954.
13. Borden AGB, Rechtman AM, Gershon-Cohen J: The normal cervical lordosis. *Radiology* 74:806, 1960.
14. Jochumsen OH: The curve of the cervical spine. *ACA J Chiro* S49: August, 1970.
15. Diagnostics. *J Clin Chiro* 2 (4):88, 1969.
16. Drexler L: *Rontgenanatomische Untersuchringen uber Form und Krumning der Halswirbelsaule in den Verscchiedenen Lebensaltern*, Stuttgart, Hippokrates, 1962.
17. Fineman S, Borrelli FJ, Rubinstein BM, et al: The cervical spine: Transformation of the normal lordotic pattern into a linear pattern in the neutral posture. A roentgenographic depiction. *J Bone Joint Surg (Am)* 45:1179, 1963.
18. Juhl JH, Miller SM, Roberts GW: Roentgenographic variations in the normal cervical spine. *Radiology* 78:591, 1962.

19. Jackson R: *The Cervical Syndrome*, ed 4, Springfield, CC Thomas, 1977.
20. Penning L: Prevertebral hematoma in cervical spine injury: Incidence and etiologic significance. *AJR* 136:553, 1981.

Thoracic Spine

1. Cobb JR: Outline for the study of scoliosis. *Am Acad Orthop Surg* 5:261, 1948.
2. Keim HA: *The Adolescent Spine*, New York, Grune & Stratton, 1976.
3. George K, Rippstein J: A comparative study of the two popular methods of measuring scoliotic deformity. *J Bone Joint Surg (Am)* 43 (6):809, 1961.
4. Risser JC, Ferguson AB: Scoliosis: Its prognosis. *J Bone Joint Surg (Am)* 18:667, 1936.
5. Ferguson AB: *Roentgen Diagnosis of Extremities and Spine*, New York, Paul B. Hoeber, 1949.
6. Fon GT, Pitt MJ, Thies AC: Thoracic kyphosis. Range in normal subjects. *AJR* 134:979, 1980.
7. Twigg HL, deLeon AC, Perloff JK, et al: The straight back syndrome. Radiographic manifestations. *Radiology* 88:274, 1967.
8. Yochum TR, et al: The "straight-back" syndrome. *ACA J Chiro, Radiology Corner*, September 1982.

Lumbar Spine

1. Pope MH, Hanley EN, Malteri RE, et al: Measurement of the intervertebral joint space. *Spine* 2 (4):282, 1977.
2. Hurxthal LM: Measurement of anterior vertebral compressions and biconcave vertebrae. *AJR* 103:635, 1968.
3. Farfan HF: *Mechanical Disorders of the Low Back*, Philadelphia, Lea & Febiger, 1973.
4. Busche-McGregor M, Naimen J, Grice AS: Analysis of the lumbar lordosis in an asymptomatic population of young adults. *J Can Chiro Assoc* 25:58, 1981.
5. Banks SD: The use of spinographic parameters in the differential diagnosis of lumbar facet and disc syndromes. *J Manip Physiol Ther* 6 (3):113, 1983.
6. Hildebrandt RW: *Chiropractic Spinography. A Manual of Technology and Interpretation*, ed 2, Baltimore, Williams & Wilkins, 1985.
7. Hansson T, Bigos S, Beecher P, et al: The lumbar lordosis in acute and chronic low back pain. *Spine* 10 (2):154, 1985.
8. Adams MA, Hutton WC: Mechanical factors in the etiology of low back pain. *Orthopedics* 5 (11):1461, 1982.
9. Drum D: The posterior gravity line syndrome, recurrent low back pain of postural origin. *J Can Chiro Assoc* 12:5, 1968.
10. Kraus H: The effects of lordosis on the stress in the lumbar spine. *Clin Orthop* 117:56, 1976.
11. Saraste H, Brostrom LA, Aparisi T, et al: Radiographic measurement of the lumbar spine. *Spine* 10 (3):236, 1985.
12. Ferguson AB: *Roentgen Diagnosis of Extremities and Spine*, New York, Paul B. Hoeber, 1949.
13. Ferguson AB: The clinical and roentgenographic interpretation of lumbosacral anomalies. *Radiology* 22:548, 1934.
14. Meschan I, Farrer-Meschan RMF: Important aspects in the roentgen study of the normal lumbosacral spine. *Radiology* 70:637, 1958.
15. Hellems HK, Keats TE: Measurement of the normal lumbosacral angle. *AJR* 113:642, 1971.
16. Jessen AR: An in depth study of the lumbosacral angle. *ACA J Chiro* 65: September 1971.
17. Splittoff CA: Lumbosacral junction. Roentgenographic comparisons of patients with and without backaches. *JAMA* 152 (17):1610, 1953.
18. von Lackum HL: The lumbosacral region. An anatomical study and some clinical observations. *JAMA* 82 (14):1109, 1924.
19. Adams MA, Hutton WC: The effect of posture on the role of the joints in resisting intervertebral compressive force. *J Bone Joint Surg (Br)* 62:358, 1980.
20. Jayson MIV: Compression stresses in the posterior elements and pathologic consequences. *Spine* 8 (3):338, 1983.
21. Cox JM: *Low Back Pain. Mechanism, Diagnosis, and Treatment*, ed 4, Baltimore, Williams & Wilkins, 1985.
22. *Basic Chiropractic Procedural Manual*, Des Moines, American Chiropractic Association, 1973.
23. Macnab I: *Backache*, Baltimore, Williams & Wilkins, 1977.
24. Hadley LA: Intervertebral joint subluxation, bony impingement, and foraminal encroachment, with nerve root changs. *AJR* 65:377, 1951.
25. Hadley LA: *Anatomico-Roentgenographic Studies of the Spine*, ed 5, Springfield, CC Thomas, 1981.
26. van Akkerveeken PF, Obrien JP, Park WM: Experimentally induced hypermobility in the lumbar spine. *Spine* 4:236, 1979.
27. Morgan FP, King T: Primary instability of lumbar vertebrae as a common cause of low back pain. *J Bone Joint Surg (Br)* 39:6, 1957.
28. Dupuis PR, Yong-Hing K, Cassidy JD, Kirkaldy-Willis WH: Radiologic diagnosis of degenerative lumbar spinal instability. *Spine* 10 (3):262, 1985.
29. Weitz EM: The lateral bending sign. *Spine* 6 (4):388, 1981.
30. Meyerding HW: Spondylolisthesis. *Surg Gynecol Obstet* 54:371, 1932.
31. Ullmann HJ: A diagnostic line for determining subluxation of the fifth lumbar vertebra. *Radiology* 2:305, 1924.
32. Capener N: Spondylolisthesis. *Br J Surg* 19:374, 1932.
33. Garland LH, Thomas SF: Spondylolisthesis. Criteria for more accurate diagnosis of true anterior slip of the involved vertebral segment. *AJR* 55:275, 1946.
34. Hinck VC, Clark WM Jr, Hopkins CE: Normal interpediculate distances (minimum and maximum). *AJR* 97:141, 1966.
35. Elseberg CA, Dyke CG: Diagnosis and localization of tumors of spinal cord

by means of measurements made on x-ray films of vertebrae, and correlation of clinical and x-ray findings. *Bull Neurol Inst NY* 3:359, 1934.

36. Eisenstein S: Measurements in the lumbar spinal canal in two racial groups. *Clin Orthop Rel Res* 115:42, 1976.
37. Weisz GM, Lee P: Spinal canal stenosis. Concept of spinal reserve capacity: Radiologic measurements and clinical applications. *Clin Orthop Rel Res* 179:134, 1983.
38. Jones RAC, Thompson JLG: The narrow lumbar canal. *J Bone Joint Surg (Br)* 50:595, 1968.
39. Williams RM: The narrow lumbar spinal canal. *Australas Radiol* 19:356, 1975.
40. MacGibbon B, Farfan H: A radiologic survey of various configurations of the lumbar spine. *Spine* 4 (3):258, 1979.

Lower Extremity

1. Eyring EJ, Bjornson DR, Peterson CA: Early diagnostic and prognostic signs in Legg-Calvé-Perthes disease. *AJR* 93:382, 1965.
2. Armbruster JG, Guerra J, Resnick D, et al: The adult hip. An anatomic study. *Radiology* 128:1, 1978.
3. Murray RO: The aetiology of primary osteoarthritis of the hip. *Br J Radiol* 38:810, 1965.
4. Wiberg G: Studies on dysplastic acetabula and congenital subluxation of the hip joint—with special reference to the complication of osteoarthritis. *Acta Chir Scand* (Suppl 58):1, 1939.
5. Vix VA, Ryu CY: The adult symphysis pubis: Normal and abnormal. *AJR* 112:517, 1971.
6. Chrispin AR, Fry IK: The presacral space shown by barium enema. *Br J Radiol* 36:319, 1963.
7. Eklöf O, Gierup J: The retrorectal soft tissue space in children: Normal variations and appearances in granulomatous colitis. *AJR* 108:624, 1970.
8. Caffey J: Contradiction of congenital dysplasia—Predislocation hypothesis of congenital dislocation of hip through study of normal variation in acetabular angles at successive periods in infancy. *Pediatrics* (7):632, 1956.
9. Caffey J, Ross S: Pelvic bones in infantile mongoloidism: Roentgenographic features. *AJR* 80:458, 1958.
10. Astley R: Chromosomal abnormalities in childhood, with particular reference to Turner's syndrome and mongolism. *Br J Radiol* 36:2, 1963.
11. Kohler A, Zimmer EA: *Borderlands of the Normal and Early Pathologic in Skeletal Roentgenology*, ed 3, New York, translated by SP Wilk, Grune & Stratton, 1968.
12. Kohler A: *Roentgenology. The Borderlands of the Normal and Early Pathological in the Skiagram*, ed 2, edited by A Turnbull, London, Balliere, Tindall & Cox, 1935.
13. Hubbard MJS: The measurement of progression in protrusio acetabuli. *AJR* 106:506, 1969.
14. Martin HE: Geometrical-anatomical factors and their significance in the early x-ray diagnosis of hip joint disease in children. *Radiology* 56:842, 1951.
15. Keats TE, Teeslink R, et al: Normal axial relationships of the major joints. *Radiology* 87:904, 1966.
16. Sante LR: *Principles of Roentgenological Interpretation*, ed 8, Ann Arbor, Edwards Bros, 1949.
17. Klein A, Joplin RJ, Reidy JA, et al: Roentgenographic features of slipped capital femoral epiphysis. *AJR* 66:361, 1951.
18. Insall J, Salvati E: Patella position in the normal knee joint. *Radiology* 101:101, 1971.
19. Steinbach HL, Russell W: Measurement of the heel pad as an aid to diagnosis of acromegaly. *Radiology* 82:418, 1964.
20. Kho KM, Wright AD, Doyle FH: Heel pad thickness in acromegaly. *Br J Radiol* 43:119, 1970.
21. Puckette SE, Seymour EQ: Fallibility of the heel pad thickness in the diagnosis of acromegaly. *Radiology* 88:982, 1967.
22. Boehler L: Diagnosis, pathology, and treatment of fractures of os calcis. *J Bone Joint Surg (Am)* 13:75, 1931.

Upper Extremity

1. Keats TE, Teeslink R, Diamond AE, et al: Normal axial relationship of the major joints. *Radiology* 87:904, 1966.
2. Petersson CJ, Redlund-Johnell I: Joint space in normal glenohumeral radiographs. *Acta Orthop Scand* 54:274, 1983.
3. Arndt JH, Sears AD: Posterior dislocation of the shoulder. *AJR* 94:639, 1965.
4. Alexander C: The acromio-humeral distance in health and disease. *Proc Coll Radiol Aust* 3:102, 1959.
5. Lev-Toaff AS, Karasick D, Rao VM: Drooping shoulder—non traumatic causes of glenohumeral subluxation. *Skel Radiol* 12:34, 1984.
6. Storen G: Traumatic dislocation of the radial head as an isolated lesion in children. Report of one case with special regard to roentgen diagnosis. *Acta Chir Scand* 116:144, 1959.
7. Archibald RM, Finby N, deVitto F: Endocrine significance of short metacarpals. *J Clin Endocrinol* 19:1312, 1959.

Scoliosis

LINDSAY J. ROWE
TERRY R. YOCHUM

General Considerations

The term "scoliosis" is usually credited to Hippocrates. (1) Its derivation is from the Greek word "skolios," meaning twisted or crooked. Within the disciplines of orthopedics and radiology scoliosis describes any lateral deviation of the spine from the midsagittal plane. A review of the past and present literature available on this subject reveals a voluminous amount of information and sophisticated research. This chapter is not an encyclopedic compilation of this data but represents a presentation of the fundamental concepts, principles, and knowledge, particularly in relation to the role, evaluation, and clinical application of the radiological examination.

Classification and Terminology

A standard vocabulary and classification system is utilized in the literature and is essential for accurate communication and description. (2,3)

CLASSIFICATION

Etiology
An etiological classification for scoliosis is the most accepted method of categorizing lateral deviations of the spinal column. (2) (Table 4.1)

Location
Curvatures are described by the region of the spine in which the apex vertebra is located. (Table 4.2) (Fig. 4.1)

TERMINOLOGY

Numerous terms are commonly employed in the description of scoliotic deviations, vertebral abnormalities, and related findings. These have been standardized by the Terminology Committee of the Scoliosis Research Society. (3)

Scoliosis
Adolescent Scoliosis. .Spinal curvature presenting at or about the onset of puberty and before maturity (10–25 years).
Adult Scoliosis. Spinal curvature existing after skeletal maturity.

Table 4.1.
Etiological Classification of Scoliosis

STRUCTURAL SCOLIOSIS

I. IDIOPATHIC
  A. *INFANTILE*
    1. *Resolving*
    2. *Progressive*
  B. *JUVENILE* (3–10 years)
  C. *ADOLESCENT* (>10 years)
II. NEUROMUSCULAR
  A. *NEUROPATHIC*
    1. *Upper Motor Neuron*
      (a) Cerebral palsy
      (b) Spinocerebellar degeneration
        (1) Friedreich's disease
        (2) Charcot-Marie-Tooth disease
        (3) Roussy-Levy disease
      (c) Syringomyelia
      (d) Spinal cord tumor
      (e) Spinal cord trauma
      (f) Other
    2. *Lower Motor Neuron*
      (a) Poliomyelitis
      (b) Other viral myelitides
      (c) Traumatic
      (d) Spinal muscular atrophy
        (1) Werdnig-Hoffmann
        (2) Kugelberg-Welander
      (e) Myelomeningocele (paralytic)
    3. *Dysautonomia (Riley-Day)*
    4. *Other*
  B. *MYOPATHIC*
    1. *Arthrogryposis*
    2. *Muscular Dystrophy*
      (a) Duchenne (pseudohypertrophic)
      (b) Limb-girdle
      (c) Facioscapulohumeral
    3. *Fiber Type Disproportion*
    4. *Congenital Hypotonia*
    5. *Myotonia Dystrophica*
    6. *Other*
III. CONGENITAL
  A. *FAILURE OF INFORMATION*
    1. *Wedged Vertebra*
    2. *Hemivertebra*
  B. *FAILURE OF SEGMENTATION*
    1. *Unilateral* (Unsegmented Bar)
    2. *Bilateral*
  C. *MIXED*
IV. NEUROFIBROMATOSIS
V. MESENCHYMAL DISORDERS
  A. *MARFAN'S*
  B. *EHLERS-DANLOS*
  C. *OTHERS*
VI. RHEUMATOID DISEASE
VII. TRAUMA
  A. *FRACTURE*
  B. *SURGICAL*
    1. *PostLaminectomy*
    2. *PostThoracoplasty*
  C. *IRRADIATION*
VIII. EXTRASPINAL CONTRACTURES
  A. *POSTEMPYEMA*
  B. *POSTBURNS*
IX. OSTEOCHONDRODYSTROPHIES
  A. *DIASTROPHIC DWARFISM*
  B. *MUCOPOLYSACCHARIDOSES* (e.g., Morquio's syndrome)
  C. *SPONDYLOEPIPHYSEAL DYSPLASIA*
  D. *MULTIPLE EPIPHYSEAL DYSPLASIA*
  E. *OTHER*
X. INFECTION OF BONE
  A. *ACUTE*
  B. *CHRONIC*
XI. METABOLIC DISORDERS
  A. *RICKETS*
  B. *OSTEOGENESIS IMPERFECTA*
  C. *HOMOCYSTINURIA*
  D. *OTHERS*
XII. RELATED TO LUMBOSACRAL JOINT
  A. *SPONDYLOLYSIS AND SPONDYLOLISTHESIS*
  B. *CONGENITAL ANOMALIES OF LUMBOSACRAL REGION*
XIII. TUMORS
  A. *VERTEBRAL COLUMN*
    1. *Osteoid Osteoma*
    2. *Histiocytosis X*
    3. *Other*
  B. *SPINAL CORD* (See Neuromuscular)

NONSTRUCTURAL SCOLIOSIS

I. POSTURAL SCOLIOSIS
II. HYSTERICAL SCOLIOSIS
III. NERVE ROOT IRRITATION
  A. *HERNIATION OF NUCLEUS PULPOSUS*
  B. *TUMORS*
IV. INFLAMMATORY (e.g., Appendicitis)
V. RELATED TO LEG LENGTH DISCREPANCY
VI. RELATED TO CONTRACTURES ABOUT THE HIP

Cervical Curve. Spinal curvature which has its apex from C1 to C6.

Cervicothoracic Curve. Spinal curvature which has its apex at C7 or T1.

Compensatory Curve. A curve which can be structural above or below a major curve that tends to maintain normal body alignment.

Congenital Scoliosis. Scoliosis due to congenitally anomalous vertebral development.

Curve Measurement.

Cobb Method: Select the upper and lower end vertebrae; erect perpendiculars to their transverse axes. They intersect to form the angle of the curve. If the vertebral end plates are poorly visualized, a line through the bottom or top of the pedicles may be used.

Risser-Ferguson Method: The angle of a curve is formed by the intersection of two lines drawn from the center of the superior and inferior end vertebral bodies to the center of the apical vertebral body.

Double Major Scoliosis. A scoliosis with two structural curves.

Double Thoracic Curve (Scoliosis). A scoliosis with

a structural upper thoracic curve, a larger, more deforming lower thoracic, and a relatively nonstructural lumbar curve.

Fractional Curve.   A compensatory curve that is incomplete because it returns to the erect. Its only horizontal vertebra is its caudad or cephalad one.

Full Curve.   A curve in which the only horizontal vertebra is at the apex.

Genetic Scoliosis.   A structural spinal curvature inherited according to a genetic pattern.

Hysterical Scoliosis.   A nonstructural deformity of the spine that develops as a manifestation of a conversion reaction.

Idiopathic Scoliosis.   A structural spinal curvature for which no cause is established.

Infantile Scoliosis.   Spinal curvature developing during the first three years of life.

Juvenile Scoliosis.   Spinal curvature developing between skeletal age of three years and the onset of puberty (3–10 years).

Kyphoscoliosis.   Lateral curvature of the spine associated with either increased posterior or decreased anterior angulation in the sagittal plane in excess of the accepted norm for that region. In the thoracic region 20–40 degrees of kyphosis is considered normal.

Lordoscoliosis.   Lateral curvature of the spine associated with an increase in anterior curvature or a decrease in posterior angulation in the sagittal plane in excess of normal for that region. In a thoracic spine, where posterior angulation is normally present, less than 20 degrees would constitute lordoscoliosis.

Lumbar Curve.   Spinal curvature which has its apex from L1 to L4.

Lumbosacral Curve.   Spinal curvature which has its apex at L5 or below.

Major Curve.   Term used to designate the larger (est) curve (s), usually structural.

Minor Curve.   Term used to refer to the smaller (est) curve (s).

Myogenic Scoliosis.   Spinal curvature due to disease or anomalies of the musculature.

Neurogenic Scoliosis.   Spinal curvature due to disease or anomalies of nerve tissue.

Nonstructural Scoliosis (Functional).   A curve which has no structural component and which corrects or overcorrects on recumbent sidebending roentgenograms.

Osteogenic Scoliosis.   Spinal curvature due to abnormality of the vertebral elements and/or adjacent ribs, acquired or congenital.

Primary Curve.   The first or earliest of several curves to appear, if identifiable.

Structural Curve.   A segment of the spine with a fixed lateral curvature. Radiographically, it is identified in supine lateral sidebending films by the failure to correct. They may be multiple.

Thoracic Curve.   Scoliosis in which the apex of the curvature is between T2 and T11.

Thoracogenic Scoliosis.   Spinal curvature attributable to disease or operative trauma in or on the thoracic cage.

Thoracolumbar Curve.   Spinal curvature which has its apex at T12 or L1.

Vertebral and Other Related Terms

Angle of Inclination. With the trunk flexed 90 degrees at the hips, the angle between the horizontal and a plane across the posterior ribcage at the greatest prominence of a rib hump.

Apical Vertebra.   The most rotated vertebra in a curve; the most deviated vertebra from the vertical axis of the patient.

Body Alignment, Balance, Compensation.   1) The alignment of the midpoint of the occiput over the sacrum

Table 4.2.
Classification of Scoliosis by Location

Classification	Apex Vertebra
Cervical	C1-C6
Cervicothoracic	C7-T1
Thoracic	T2-T11
Thoracolumbar	T12-L1
Lumbar	L2-L4
Lumbosacral	L5-S1

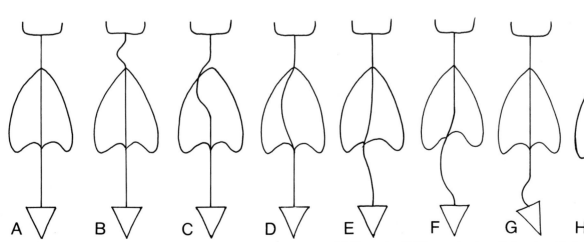

Figure 4.1. CLASSIFICATION OF SCOLIOSIS ACCORDING TO LOCATION. A. Normal Spine. B. Cervical. C. Cervicothoracic. D. Midthoracic. E. Thoracolumbar. F. Lumbar. G. Lumbosacral. H. Double Lumbar and Thoracic.

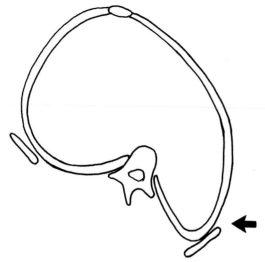

Figure 4.2. RIB HUMP DUE TO SCOLIOSIS. Note the posterior vertebral body rotation on side of the rib hump (arrow) usually most prominent on the convex surface at the apex of the curve.

in the same vertical plane as the shoulders over hips. 2) In radiology, when the sum of the angular deviations of the spine in one direction is equal to that in the opposite direction.

End Vertebra. The most cephalad vertebra of a curve whose superior surface or the most caudad one whose inferior surface tilts maximally toward the concavity of the curve.

Gibbus. A sharply angular kyphosis.

Iliac Epiphysis (Apophysis). The epiphysis along the wing of the ilium.

Iliac Epiphysis (Apophysis Sign, Risser's Sign). In the anteroposterior roentgenogram of the spine, when the excursion of ossification in the iliac epiphysis (apophysis) reaches its ultimate medial migration vertebral growth may be complete.

Kyphosis. A change in the alignment of a segment of the spine in the sagittal plane that increases the posterior convex angulation.

Pelvic Obliquity. Deviation of the pelvis from the horizontal in the frontal plane. Fixed pelvic obliquities can be attributable to contractures either above or below the pelvis.

Rib Hump. The prominence of the ribs on the convexity of a spinal curvature, usually due to vertebral rotation, best exhibited on forward bending. (Fig. 4.2)

Skeletal Age (Bone Age). The age obtained by comparing an anteroposterior roentgenogram of the left hand and wrist with the standards of the Gruelich and Pyle Atlas.

Clinical Features

STRUCTURAL SCOLIOSIS

A structural scoliosis is a lateral curvature that is fixed and which fails to correct on recumbent lateral bending x-ray studies. Many disorders are related to this type of spinal disorder. (Table 4.1)

Idiopathic Scoliosis

This is the most common form of lateral spinal deviation, accounting for up to 80 percent of scolioses. (4) The etiology is unknown, although many factors have been implicated. These include connective tissue disease, diet, enzymes, muscular imbalance, vestibular dysfunction, and inheritance. (5)

Of all causes, an inherited genetic defect appears to play a significant role. (6,7) The age of onset distinctively occurs within the growth period and allows for an age-based classification—infantile, juvenile, and adolescent.

Infantile Idiopathic Scoliosis. These occur between birth and three years of age. The majority will disappear (resolving infantile idiopathic scoliosis), but occasionally will progress (progressive infantile idiopathic scoliosis). (8) This progressive form is rare in the United States, is slightly more common in males, and is usually a left convex thoracic curve.

Juvenile Idiopathic Scoliosis. The onset is between 3 and 10 years of age, with no sexual prevalence.

Adolescent Idiopathic Scoliosis. The curvature develops in the period after the age of 10 until skeletal maturity. This is the most common form of idiopathic scoliosis. Females are predominantly affected, with a ratio of 9 to 1 over males. (9) The critical time period for progression, which may be rapid, is between the ages of 12 and 16. (Fig. 4.3) Once spinal growth has ceased, as determined by fusion of the iliac apophysis, progression is unlikely, although superimposed degenerative changes later in adult life may allow the curvature to increase on an average of 15 degrees (10) and occasionally creating nerve entrapment syndromes. (11)

A frequent finding in a developing scoliosis is a lateral wedged deformity of the vertebral body which will persist into adult life. This is a result of impaired growth at the discovertebral junction on the concave side of the curvature due to excessive compressive forces (Hueter-Volkmann principle). (Fig. 4.4) The most frequent curve pattern is the right convex thoracic type. Three other curves which are frequently present include a right thoracolumbar, a left lumbar, and a combined form of left lumbar and right thoracic. (4,12)

There is a ten times greater incidence of congenital heart disease than in the general population when the idiopathic curve is more than 20 degrees. (13)

Congenital Scoliosis

Congenital scoliosis is distinguished by anomalies of the vertebrae or ribs. The most frequently observed anomalies include hemivertebrae, block vertebrae, spina bifida, bridging vertebral bars, joint deformities, fusion of ribs, and other rib malformations. (14) (Fig. 4.5) This curve is typically a short "C" curve and may be rapidly progressive in the growing years. Occasionally, anterior vertebral body defects may allow superimposed kyphosis (kyphoscoliosis). (15) There is a frequent association in congenital scoliosis with anomalies of the genitourinary system. (16)

Neuromuscular Scoliosis

A large spectrum of neuropathic and myopathic disorders may produce a progressive spinal deformity. (Table 4.1) The most common neuropathy associated with sco-

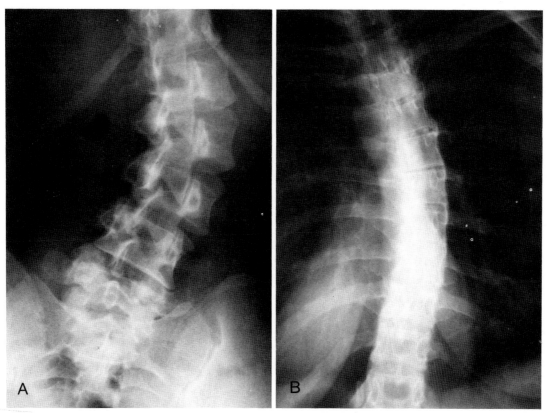

Figure 4.3. IDIOPATHIC SCOLIOSIS. A. No abnormality was observed in this 25-year-old female until 12 years of age, when her deformity was first detected. Despite bracing, her scoliosis progressed and has remained unchanged until this present radiograph.

B. This 23-year-old female was radiographed for evaluation of midthoracic pain. Until this examination she had been unaware of her scoliotic deviation.

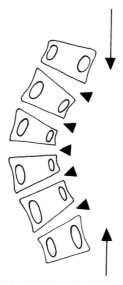

Figure 4.4. HUETER-VOLKMANN PRINCIPLE. Excessive compressive axial loading at the discovertebral junction (arrowheads) due to scoliosis during the period of bone growth may produce permanent wedge-shaped vertebral bodies.

liosis is poliomyelitis. (17) The scoliotic pattern produced is distinctively a long "C" shaped curve frequently extending from the sacrum to the lower cervical region. The convex side is orientated towards the unaffected muscle group. Intersegmental rotation may be severe in these curves, and rapid progression in the curvature angle frequently occurs between the ages of 12 and 16. Cerebral palsy produces the same type of long "C" shaped curve. Other neurologic disorders associated with scoliosis include syringomyelia, spinal cord tumor, trauma, and dysautonomia.

Myopathic scoliotic curves are relatively infrequent. The most frequent cause is from muscular dystrophy of Duchenne. An increasing lordosis usually precedes the onset of the scoliotic deformity. (18) The scoliosis which forms is often rapidly progressive and severe, requiring fusion and Harrington rod implantation. Once the patient has been confined to a wheelchair, the formation of a scoliosis is almost inevitable. (19)

Neurofibromatosis

Neurofibromatosis is a congenital and inherited disorder affecting neuroectodermal and mesodermal tissues. von Recklinhausen first described the relationship in 1882 between the formation of nerve and skin tumors, and his name has since become synonomous with the disease. (20) Scoliosis was first associated with neurofibromatosis in 1921 by Weiss. (21) The classic triad of diagnostic findings include: 1) multiple, soft, elevated cutaneous tumors (fibroma molluscum); 2) cutaneous pigmentation (café au lait spots); and 3) neurofibromas of peripheral nerves. In addition, various skeletal lesions may be

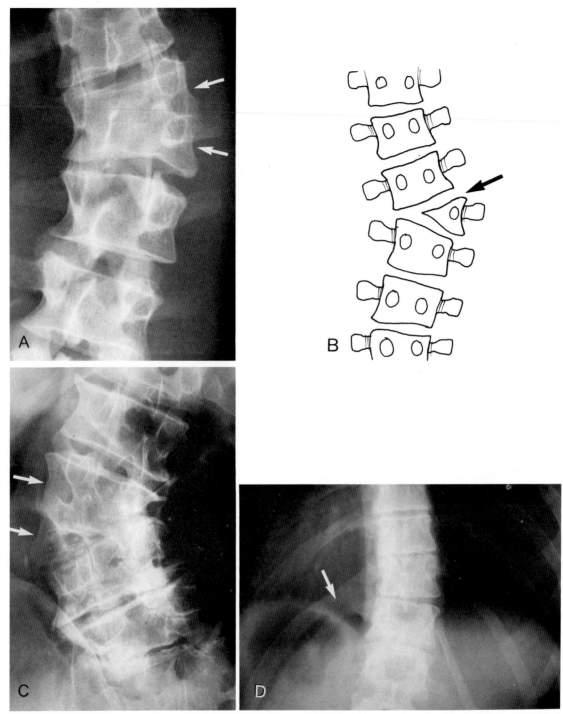

Figure 4.5. CONGENITAL SCOLIOSIS. A–C. Hemivertebrae. The presence of an additional portion of a vertebral body (arrows) produces a structural malformation, leading to the scoliotic deformity.

D. Rib Synostosis. A localized lack of rib separation (arrow) precipitates this thoracolumbar scoliosis.

present in up to 50 percent of these patients, including erosions, intraosseous cystic defects, deformity, pseudarthrosis, growth aberrations, and cranial abnormalities. (22)

Scoliosis is the most common bony abnormality and is present in approximately 50 percent of patients. (22,23) Varying degrees of scoliosis occur, from mild to severe deforming angulations. (Fig. 4.6) The most conspicuous features, when present, consist of a short angular deform-

ity with dysplasia of the vertebral bodies. Kyphosis is the most common superimposed deformity. Additional findings suggestive of a neurofibromatosis-induced scoliosis include enlarged foramina, posterior and lateral vertebral body scalloping, deformed ribs ("twisted ribbons"), and an adjacent smooth soft tissue mass due to either a neurofibroma or protruding meningocele. Notably, the scoliosis frequently progresses and requires surgical fusion and stabilization.

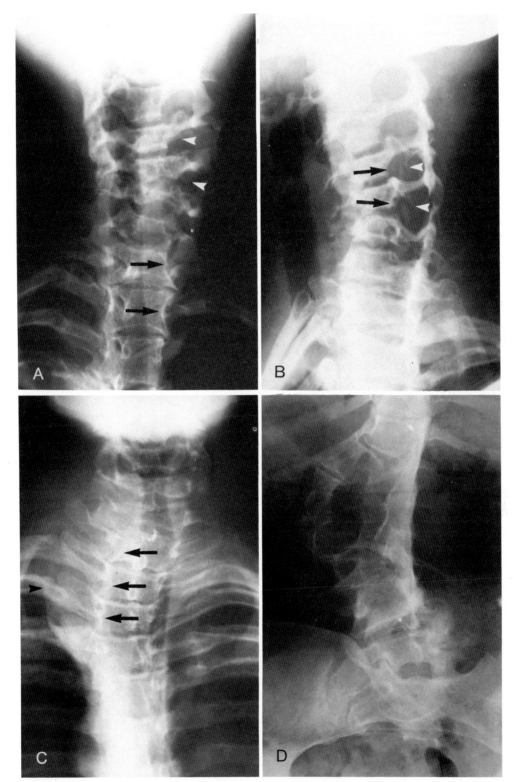

Figure 4.6. NEUROFIBROMATOSIS. A and B. Cervical Spine. Note the lower cervical curvature, scalloped vertebral bodies (arrows), and widened foramina (arrowheads). (Courtesy of William E. Litterer, DC, DACBR, Elizabeth, New Jersey) **C. Upper Thoracic Spine.** Observe the upper thoracic curvature, lateral body scalloping (arrows), and the paraspinal mass (arrowhead) of an associated meningocele. (Courtesy of Clayton F. Thomsen, DC, Sydney, Australia) **D. Lumbar Spine.** A bizarre distortion of the lumbar bodies, posterior arches, and intervertebral foramina accompany the scoliosis. (Courtesy of Lawrence A. Cooperstein, MD, Pittsburgh, Pennsylvania)

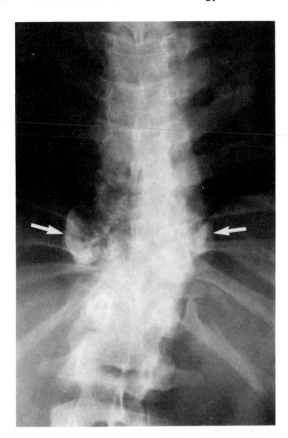

Figure 4.7. TUBERCULOUS SPONDYLITIS (POTT'S DISEASE) PRODUCING A STRUCTURAL SCOLIOSIS. Tuberculous infection of the thoracolumbar vertebrae has precipitated collapse and a lateral scoliosis. The abnormal rib angulation is due to the associated gibbus deformity. Note the flocculent soft tissue calcification within the accompanying cold abscess (arrows).

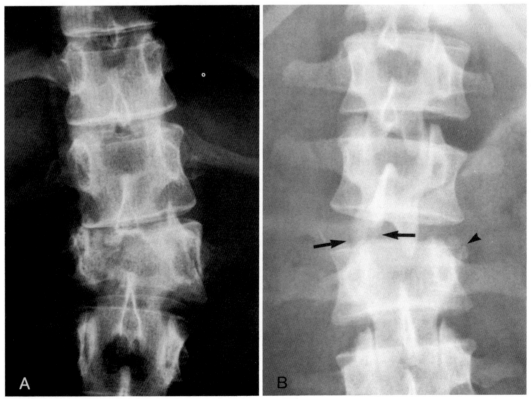

Figure 4.8. TRAUMATIC SCOLIOSIS. A. A traumatic anterior and lateral vertebral body fracture of the first lumbar segment has created an accompanying scoliosis. **B.** A complete facet luxation at the L2/ L3 interspace (arrows) has produced a minor scoliosis. Observe the superior end plate compression fracture of L3 (arrowhead).

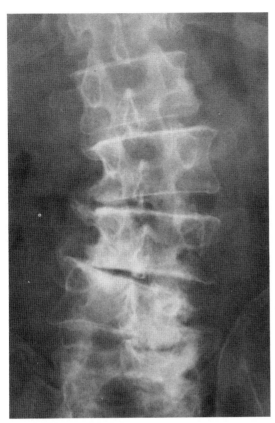

Figure 4.9. DEGENERATIVE DISC AND APOPHYSEAL JOINT DISEASE PRODUCING SCOLIOSIS. Severe discopathic alterations at the second, third, and fourth lumbar discs with associated facet arthrosis has produced lateral listhesis and lateral flexion at these levels. These degenerative changes have resulted in a mild structural scoliosis. Such degenerative changes predispose to spinal stenosis.

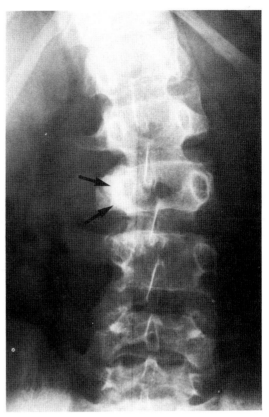

Figure 4.10. SCOLIOSIS DUE TO OSTEOID OSTEOMA. Observe the localized sclerotic focus adjacent to the pedicle (arrows). These tumors are painful and characteristically induce a rotatory scoliosis with the lesion usually being located on the concave side. (Courtesy of Jack Edeiken, MD, Houston, Texas)

Other Causes

Infection. Infectious processes such as tuberculosis may precipitate spinal deformity, due to collapse, and bony destruction. (Fig. 4.7) The most distinctive deformity is a sharp angular kyphosis (gibbus), although varying degrees of scoliosis may also occur.

Radiation. Irradiation to the growing spine may produce vertebral abnormalities in up to 75 percent of patients. (24) These changes consist of growth arrest lines, end plate irregularities, altered vertebral shape, and scoliosis. The most common childhood disorders to be irradiated are Wilm's tumor and neuroblastoma. The treatment field is usually lateral to but includes the spine and results in one side absorbing more radiation. This may produce two types of deformity: (1) a mobile flexion curve or (2) a fixed rotatory scoliosis due to unilateral shortened laminae and pedicles. (25) In both curves the convexity is away from the side of irradiation.

Trauma. Injuries to the spine which produce fracture or dislocation may also induce a lateral spinal curvature which may be permanent. (Fig. 4.8)

Degenerative Joint Disease. Advanced discopathy and facet arthrosis may result in a scoliotic deviation, especially when the changes are extensive unilaterally. (Fig. 4.9)

Miscellaneous Disorders. Many other conditions precipitate a structural scoliosis, including tumors, connective tissue diseases, and surgery. (Fig. 4.10, 4.11)

NONSTRUCTURAL SCOLIOSIS

Curvatures that have no structural alteration and correct on recumbent lateral bending x-ray studies are classified as nonstructural and have a number of possible etiologies. (Table 4.1) These include such conditions as leg length inequality, antalgia from discal herniations ("sciatic scoliosis"), and inflammatory bowel disease. (Fig. 4.12, 4.13)

COMPLICATIONS ASSOCIATED WITH SCOLIOSIS

Complications of a scoliotic curve are numerous. These occur with and without treatment.

Nontreatment-Related Complications

Cardiopulmonary complications. In more severe thoracic curvatures restricted ribcage movement and lung volume ultimately produces pulmonary hypertension with subsequent right (cor pulmonale) and left-sided congestive heart failure. (26) Congestive heart failure is the single most common direct cause of death in the scoliotic patient. Altered lung ventilation also predisposes to pulmonary infection and dyspnea.

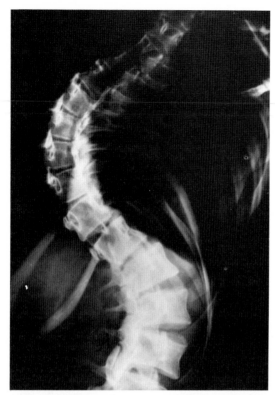

Figure 4.11. SCOLIOSIS ASSOCIATED WITH MARFAN'S SYN-DROME. A severe double lumbar and thoracic curve is typical of this connective tissue defect.

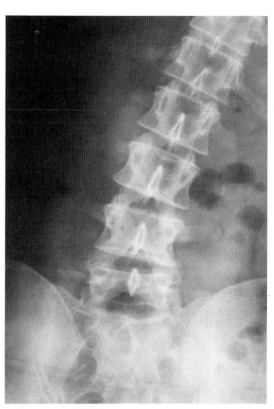

Figure 4.13. ANTALGIC SCOLIOSIS. Note the acute lateral flexion at the fourth lumbar segment and the failure of the vertebrae to rotate despite the lateral spinal deviation. This patient exhibited classic clinical signs of fourth lumbar disc protrusion.

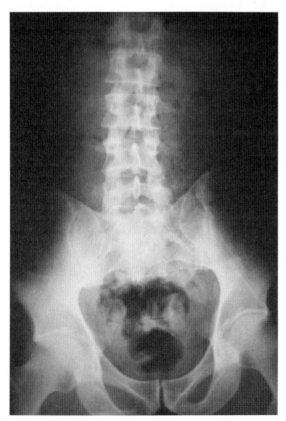

Figure 4.12. SCOLIOSIS SECONDARY TO SHORT LEG SYN-DROME. On this upright radiograph observe the pelvic unleveling and compensatory mild midlumbar rotatory curvature convex to the low side of the pelvic unleveling.

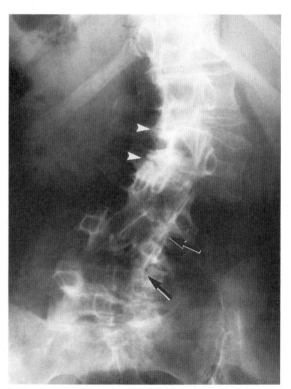

Figure 4.14. COMPLICATING DEGENERATIVE ARTHRITIS. There is severe facet arthrosis (arrows), discal degeneration, and spondylophytes (arrowheads) accompanying this idiopathic lumbar curve. These degenerative changes have occurred at the regions of maximal stress.

Degenerative Spinal Arthritis. Loss of disc height, osteophytes, and intersegmental instability frequently accompany the adult scoliosis and occasionally even the adolescent. (10,27) Distinctively, these degenerative changes are most pronounced on the concave side of the curve and extend to involve other stressed articulations, including costotransverse, sacroiliac, and hip joints. (Fig. 4.14) Secondary spatial compromise of the central and lateral spinal recesses may result in nerve root entrapment syndromes. (11)

Curvature Progression. The most rapid and severely deforming time period for scoliosis is in the adolescent growth spurt (12–16 years), where the curve may increase at the rate of 1 degree a month. (27) In the adult, progression does occur but is relatively less, in the range of 10–15 degrees. (10,27)

Fatigue and Joint Dysfunction Syndromes. Altered biomechanical spinal stresses frequently produce asymmetrical muscle and joint loadings. Muscular and ligamentous strain ensue, spinal joints become inflamed and altered in their normal kinematics, which all contribute to produce significant pain, discomfort, and disability. (28) These symptoms are frequently the most immediately debilitating feature in a scoliosis patient.

Radiation Exposure. A considerable amount of concern has focused on the long-term effects of repeated radiologic examinations. The average patient undergoing conservative therapy with bracing over three years has an average of 22 radiographs taken. The chance of an increased risk of malignancy in scoliosis patients appears to be minimal in comparison with the natural incidence in the general population (.2% for breast carcinoma; 5% for leukemia). (29–31)

Treatment-Related Complications

Nonsurgical and surgical measures utilized in the treatment of scoliosis may produce a wide gamut of complications.

Nonsurgical Complications. The majority of deleterious side effects arise from the use of external braces and supports. Psychologically, the patient undergoes a good deal of mental stress. In long-term bracing superficial skin irritations may be a persistent problem, either due to sweating or allergy. It is rare for pressure sores to occur. Occasionally, nerve compression may occur, with numbness and paresthesias, especially of the anterior femoral cutaneous nerve and, less commonly, the brachial plexus. With curvature correction, compression of the duodenum under the superior mesenteric artery may create obstruction with nausea and vomiting (cast syndrome). (32) Milwaukee braces, which used a chin rest, frequently produced lower facial and dental abnormalities but is a rare finding today. (33)

Surgical Complications. During the operative procedure cardiac arrest and spinal cord injury are the most feared complications. Early postoperative problems include respiratory distress, infection, and loosening of the fixation device. Later, following release from the hospital, infection may still supervene. However, the most frequent complications are pseudarthrosis of the fusion and instrumentation failure.

Radiological Assessment

The radiological examination is the most definitive and important diagnostic modality in the scoliotic patient. (34) The role of the radiograph is multiple: 1) determination of etiology; 2) evaluation of the curvature, including site, magnitude and flexibility; 3) bone maturity; 4) monitoring progression or regression; and 5) an aid in the selection of appropriate treatment. A wide variety of methods and technical factors exist in obtaining a judicial balance between practical clinical information and avoiding unnecessary radiation exposure. (Table 4.3)

STANDARD RADIOGRAPHIC TECHNIQUES
Projections

Erect Anteroposterior and Lateral Views. These are the absolute minimum required for accurate assessment of any scoliosis. Preferably, the AP view should be done by a single exposure on a 14″ x 36″ cassette, to allow for total and continuous curvature evaluation. However, if such equipment is not available, sectional projections can likewise be utilized just as effectively. The disadvantages of the single exposure full spine is the irradiation of unnecessary body parts, sacrifice of bone detail for pathology, and expense of the necessary equipment to do the views adequately. Wherever possible, a long focal-film distance should be utilized, usually 84 inches.

Lateral Bending Views. These are primarily projections to evaluate curvature flexibility. The patient laterally

Table 4.3.
Radiological Examinations in Scoliosis

Projection	Indications-Information
Standard Techniques	
Erect AP	Curve analysis, contributing etiologies
Erect Lateral	Sagittal curvatures (kyphosis, lordosis)
Lateral Bending	Flexibility
Left Hand, Wrist	Skeletal age
Supplementary Techniques	
Chest	Cardiopulmonary status
Contrast Studies	
Angiogram	Vascular compromise, neoplasm
Gastrointestinal	Duodenal obstruction
Genitourinary	Kidney anomalies, obstruction
Myelogram	Cord integrity, anomalies, stenosis
Derotated	Anatomy, anomalies
Erect PA	Reduction of radiation dose
Flexion, Extension	Sagittal curve flexibility
Lumbosacral Spot	
AP	Anomalies
Lateral	Spondylolisthesis
Obliques	Fusion and instrumentation status
Supine	Flexibility
Tangential	Efficacy of rib hump surgery
Tomography	Anatomy, abnormalities
Traction	Flexibility in neuromuscular disease

flexes as much as possible and the exposure is made. This must be done both to the right and left.

Left Hand and Wrist.   A spot AP radiograph is taken of the left hand and wrist in patients under 20 years of age. This is compared with the Greulich and Pyle Atlas to ascertain the skeletal age, which is important in planning the treatment regime. (35)

Technology

Film Identification.   The films are usually viewed as if observing the patient from the posterior, so the markers should be reversed for simplifying interpretation. In addition to the traditional identification by name, age, institution, date, and file number, further information may be helpful. Where lateral bending studies are being taken it is important to show the direction of bending and identify it as a lateral bending study. It likewise is vital to identify whether the views are being taken erect or recumbent.

Equipment.   In producing a quality radiograph for scoliosis mensuration it is desirable to utilize a machine capable of exposures at 84 inches. A minimum capacity for such exposures would be a 125-kilovolts peak (kVp), 300-milliamperes (mA) machine. A grid ratio of no less than 10 to 1, in combination with rare earth screens, produces acceptable images while reducing the radiation dose. (33) Similarly, the use of split screens for compensating in differing body thicknesses should be avoided in preference for balancing filtration at the collimator. (36) Technique factors will vary according to each patient, but a minimum kilovoltage of 90 is recommended. (37)

Sectional AP films should be taken when the patient measures more than 24 cm. Gonadal protection must be applied in all instances of scoliosis evaluation, both in the AP and lateral projections. In repeated examinations the majority of the pelvis, except for the sacral base, should not be exposed. Lateral collimation on AP films should be as close as practical, without compromising necessary rib and curvature details.

SUPPLEMENTARY RADIOGRAPHIC TECHNIQUES

Projections

Numerous specialized projections are available to provide additional information. (Table 4.3)

Chest.   Specific evaluations of the lungs and heart should be periodically obtained to establish any alteration in cardiopulmonary status, especially cor pulmonale and congestive heart failure.

Contrast Examinations.   Occasionally, these studies may be employed to better evaluate certain body systems. Myelography may be employed to evaluate spinal cord integrity, congenital anomalies, and stenosis. Intravenous pyelograms are often used in congenital deformities of the spine due to the increased frequency of renal anomalies and possible obstructive uropathy. Gastrointestinal studies are used where abdominal symptoms may suggest duodenal obstruction by the superior mesenteric artery as the curvature is corrected. (32) Angiograms are rarely used except where vascular compression or vascular neoplasm in the cord is suspected.

Derotated View.   Used only in severe kyphoscoliotic curves (over 100 degrees). By rotating the patient, the effects of segmental rotation are reduced, which allows for better evaluation for underlying anomalies. (38)

Flexion-Extension.   These are analogous to the lateral flexion views for flexibility evaluation. Their main purpose is to demonstrate the degree of mobility within the curvature in the sagittal plane.

Posterior-Anterior.   Various studies have shown significant reductions in radiation doses to radiosensitive structures such as the thyroid, breasts, and active bone marrow by performing the frontal film in a posterior-anterior position. (36,39–42) As an example, this projection reduces the dosage to the breast by a factor of approximately 3, from 60mRad (0–60Gy) to 20mRad (0–20Gy). However, inherent in the placement of the vertebrae further from the film is the magnification, loss of geometric sharpness, and a change in the measured Cobb's angle, therefore making AP comparisons dubious. (40,41)

Lumbosacral Spot Views.   Due to technical underexposure the details of the lumbosacral region are frequently obscured. An anterior-posterior view with a cephalad tube tilt of 20–30 degrees will show the junctional region clearly. Additionally, a lateral, erect view may demonstrate a spondylolisthesis frequently seen in conjunction with scoliosis, especially if rotation is evident on the frontal radiograph. (43,44)

Oblique.   The object of these films is usually to assess the status of a previous bone graft or corrective instrumentation. Additional information is also obtained, such as the integrity of the pars interarticularis and paraspinal soft tissues.

Supine.   When compared with the erect radiographs the effect of gravity on the curve can be observed and once again provide data on the curvature flexibility. An additional bonus is the improved structural detail which is obtained in this position.

Tangential ("Rib Hump" View).   This is only used when cosmetic surgery is contemplated for the posterior rib hump. The patient faces the bucky and flexes forward with the x-ray beam directed tangentially across the back. If the vertebrae are seen to be rotated under the ribs, no surgery is performed, since they will maintain the hump even if the ribs are removed. (42)

Tomography.   The depiction of obscured anatomical details and deformity is best examined by sequential tomography. This is only utilized in selective instances.

Traction.   This is only used in patients with neuromuscular disease who are unable to perform lateral bending studies unassisted. A supine view is taken with traction applied to the head and feet and is compared to the neutral AP film.

Technology

Segmented Field Radiography. (45) A standard AP full spine is taken at the initial visit. Transitional and end levels are located from which the Cobb angles are constructed. Subsequent examinations which may follow with treatment only take collimated, small field views of these same transitional and end levels, with the Cobb method applied again. This technique reduces the radiation dose considerably.

Specialized Shields and Filters. (36) Numerous shields have been developed to reduce doses to radiosensitive organs such as the breast, thyroid, and gonads. These are especially useful on lateral radiographs because of the higher level of exposure necessary to produce this film. Additional filtration is also instrumental in substantially decreasing the absorbed dose and obtaining a better quality image. (46)

SCOLIOSIS MENSURATION

Four basic spinal parameters are evaluated in scoliosis: 1) curvature; 2) rotation; 3) flexibility; and 4) skeletal maturation.

Curvature Measurement

The two most popular measuring methods are the Cobb-Lippman and Risser-Ferguson systems. The Cobb method is the most accepted standard for quantifying scoliotic deviation. (47)

Cobb-Lippman Method. This procedure was introduced by Lippman in 1935 and popularized later by Cobb. (2) (Fig. 4.15, 4.16) A line is drawn along the superior border of the cephalad end vertebra. A similar line is drawn along the inferior surface of the caudad end vertebra. If the end plates are not visible, the bottom or tops of the pedicles can be used. Perpendicular lines are then erected from each horizontal line and the angle of their intersection measured. Seven groups are categorized according to the Cobb angle. Group 1: 0–20 degrees; Group 2: 21–30 degrees; Group 3: 31–50 degrees; Group 4: 51–75 degrees; Group 5: 76–100 degrees; Group 6: 101–125 degrees; and Group 7: 126 degrees and above.

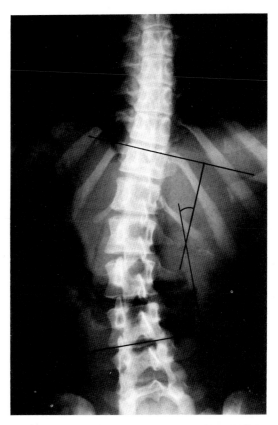

Figure 4.16. COBB METHOD OF MENSURATION.

The Cobb method gives larger measurements than the Risser technique by an average of 25 percent, or about 10 degrees. (47,48) With larger curves this percentage difference increases, and some have advocated using the Risser method to reduce this discrepancy, but this practice is to be discouraged. The Cobb procedure also has the distinction of being more easily applied and reproducible by different observers. (49) In double curvatures both curves should be measured.

Risser-Ferguson Method. Ferguson first introduced his methodology in the early 1920's and later published his findings along with Risser in the 1930's and 1940's. (48,50,51) (Fig. 4.15) In this procedure the centers of the end and apical vertebral bodies are identified. These points are then connected and the angle of intersection measured.

Rotation

Rotation is invariably present in scoliosis and is intimately associated with the degree of external cosmetic deformity, especially in the thoracic spine.

Spinous Method. Cobb first described an evaluation based on the position of the spinous tip to the vertebral body. (2) Spinous processes are prone to malformation and displacement and are frequently difficult to identify. Consequently, these structures should not be used to assess rotation.

Pedicle Method. This is the most accepted method of determining rotation described by Nash and Moe in 1969. (52) (Fig. 4.17) The movement of the pedicle on the convex side of the curve is graded between 0 and 4.

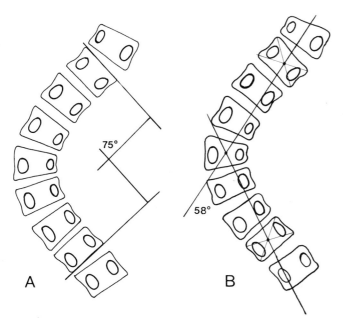

Figure 4.15. CURVATURE MENSURATION. A. Cobb Method. The end vertebrae are located and lines are drawn on their appropriate end plates. Perpendiculars are erected to these end plate lines and the intersecting acute angle measured. **B. Risser-Ferguson Method.** A dot is placed in the center of each end vertebra as well as in the apical segment. These are then joined and their intersecting acute angle measured.

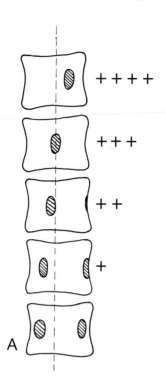

Figure 4.17. ROTATION ASSESSMENT: PEDICLE METHOD. A. Diagrammatic Representation.

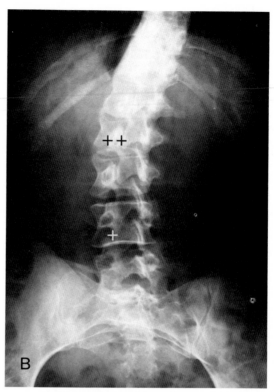

B. Radiographic Depiction. (Courtesy of William E. Litterer, DC, DACBR, Elizabeth, New Jersey)

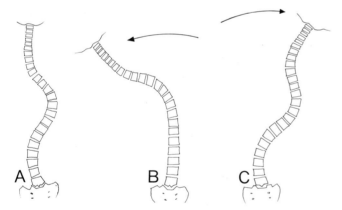

Figure 4.18. FLEXIBILITY EVALUATION BY LATERAL BENDING. A. Erect, Neutral Position. The presence of a left lumbar and right thoracic curvature is evident. **B. Left Lateral Bending**. Note the left lumbar curve disappears, indicating it to be nonstructural. **C. Right Lateral Bending**. The right thoracic curve remains unchanged, indicating it to be structural. ***Comment***: When there is failure of a curvature to correct on lateral bending this can be interpreted as being irreversible but also nonprogressive.

Flexibility

Flexibility is defined as the degree of mobility within a scoliosis. This is an important parameter to assess since it shows not only the correctability but also that it may continue to progress. To the surgeon a lack of flexibility is a contraindication to spinal fusion. The radiographic assessment of flexibility is primarily evaluated by a supine lateral bending radiograph into the convex side of the scoliosis. The Cobb method is applied and the degree of correction induced is the measure of flexibility. (Fig. 4.18)

Skeletal Maturation

Ascertaining skeletal maturity is vital in the application of treatment and determining prognosis. While potential growth remains there is the possibility for curvature progression. Three observations are used in this determination: 1) comparison of the left hand and wrist with the Greulich and Pyle Atlas; 2) vertebral ring epiphyses; and 3) the iliac epiphysis.

Left Hand and Wrist. This is compared with the Greulich and Pyle Atlas. In general, scoliotic female individuals are more mature than normal between 11 and 12 years of age and less mature between 15 and 17. (53,54) Practically interpreted, this means that the growth period in scoliotic females is lengthened. (55)

Vertebral Ring Epiphyses. These are normal traction epiphyses at the peripheral body margins. Although they do not contribute to vertical vertebral body growth, once they have fused to the body rim this very closely parallels arrest in spinal growth. (Fig. 4.19) The recognition of this fusion is the most accurate indicator of completed spinal growth and can be interpreted as a strong inhibiting factor to future scoliotic progression.

Iliac Epiphysis (Risser's Sign). The recognition of the iliac crest epiphysis as an indicator of spinal maturity was first noted by Risser in 1948 (56) and later reconfirmed. (57,58)

In the majority of individuals the apophysis appears

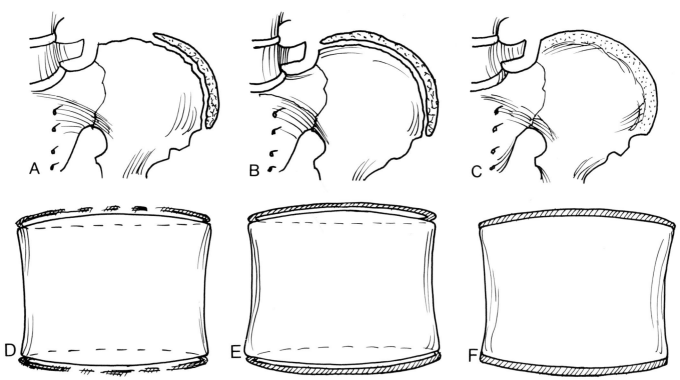

Figure 4.19. RADIOGRAPHIC DETERMINATION OF SPINAL MATURITY. A–C. Iliac Epiphysis. D–F. Vertebral Body Epiphysis. The two most reliable signs of maturation are the status of the iliac and vertebral body epiphyses. When they are both fused and no longer visible spinal maturation is complete and curvature progression is less likely.

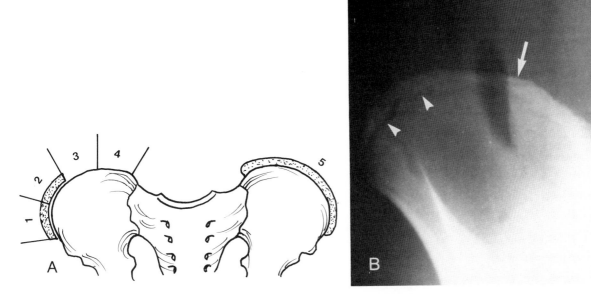

Figure 4.20. ILIAC EPIPHYSIS: RISSER'S SIGN. A. Grading System. The epiphysis first appears at the anterior superior iliac spine and gradually progresses posteromedially before fusing to the ilium. Five grades are utilized, one for each quarter ossified (1+, 2+, 3+, 4+), and 5+ when complete osseous fusion has occurred. **B. Radiographic Depiction.** A 4+ Risser's sign (arrow). The radiolucent line (arrowheads) represents the cartilaginous growth plate.

laterally near the anterior superior iliac spine and progresses medially toward the posterior superior iliac spine ("capping"). This gradual extension in excursion is graded by quarters: 1+, 25 percent; 2+, 50 percent; 3+, 75 percent; and 4+, 100 percent. When the epiphysis is fused to the ilium it is graded 5+. (Fig. 4.20)

The process of "capping" usually begins in boys at the age of 16 and in girls at the age of 14. From the time of appearance to complete excursion to the posterior superior iliac spine, a time period of 1 year has usually elapsed. It then will take 2–3 years for complete osseous union to occur. This pattern of formation and closure parallels the formation and progression of the scoliosis. In the pre-adolescent (10–15 years), prior to the appearance of the iliac epiphysis, it is usual for the curve to show the greatest rate of progression. (57) Once the epiphysis becomes visible curve progression slows and eventually ceases when the epiphysis fuses.

Clinical Radiological Correlation

Application of the radiographic information is vital in the diagnosis, treatment, and management of scoliosis. Specific applications include the selection of therapy, monitoring patient response, and long-term assessment.

THERAPY SELECTION

This is based on combining all facts together. The major objectives in selecting a therapeutic regime hinge on curve progression and its effect on cosmetic appearance and body function. Approximately 25 percent of all curves will show some degree of progression. (59) Indicators of likely progression include curvature pattern, age, onset of menarche, and an absent (0) or early (1+) Risser sign. (59) Double curvatures appear more likely to progress, especially the lumbar component. In addition, other factors such as the magnitude of the curve, flexibility, and family history should be considered.

The major therapeutic decision is between three alternatives—close observation, bracing, and surgery. (60) In minor curves under 20 degrees there is general agreement

that the patient does not require bracing; (61,62) however, in view of possible rapid progression during the growth period (10–15 years) these patients must be frequently and carefully examined for signs of increasing deformity. Radiographic examination every 3 months should be done as part of this monitoring process. If more than a 5-degree increase is demonstrated, bracing should be contemplated. (61) Additionally, if rotation and a rib hump is prominent, bracing is also indicated. The use of exercises has not been shown to decrease scoliosis, but they do have value in improving posture, flexibility, muscular tone, and psychological awareness. Chiropractic spinal manipulation frequently decreases the associated musculoskeletal symptoms.

Indications for bracing include curves which are flexible, skeletally immature, between 20 and 40 degrees, and which are progressive in nature. (47,59,61) The most commonly utilized brace is the Milwaukee brace. (63) Its purpose is not to correct a curve but to prevent further progression. The brace functions by exerting longitudinal traction between the occiput and pelvis, with pressure pads appropriately placed to limit rotation and lateral displacement. Physiologically, the cumulative effect is to decrease the curvature and the segmental torsion. Additionally, this aids in decreasing the compressive forces on the discovertebral growth plate and helps prevent the lateral wedged deformities of the vertebral bodies. The wearing of the brace should be for 23 hours per day, until skeletal maturity, and be combined with a specific exercise regime. (61,62) A weaning period of from 6 to 12 months

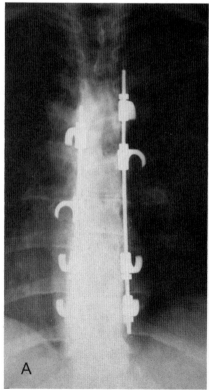
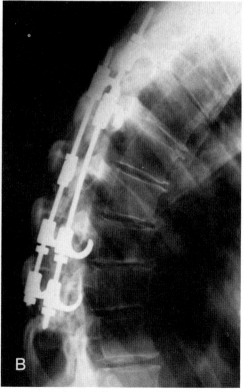

Figure 4.21. A and B. Harrington Rod Procedure. Two rods are placed on either side of the spine and anchored to the bone by hooks. These effectively fuse the spinal segments and prevent progression of the curve. (Courtesy of William E. Litterer, DC, DACBR, Elizabeth, New Jersey)

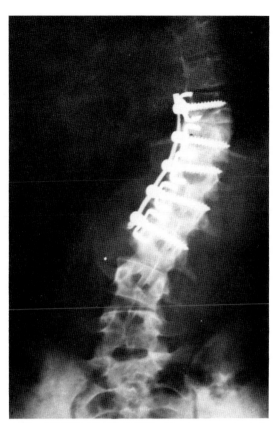

Figure 4.22. DWYER PROCEDURE. The intervertebral discs are removed, screws are inserted, and the connecting wire is shortened to compress the vertebrae together and reduce the flexibility for progression of the curvature. (Courtesy of William E. Litterer, DC, DACBR, Elizabeth, New Jersey)

is usually necessary, with gradually increased hours without the brace. Radiographs should be obtained every three months during this period to evaluate for stability or progression. If progression is evident, the bracing time must again be increased.

Surgical intervention may be done where an underlying abnormality can be treated, rapid progression is occurring in an immature spine, or the curve is over 40 degrees, although these criteria are not definitive. (62,64) Occasionally, milder deformities may be surgically stabilized for cosmetic reasons. The most common surgeries performed include the insertion of Harrington rods and the Dwyer procedure of wire cable and screws. (65) (Fig. 4.21, 4.22)

Response Monitoring and Long-Term Assessment

In both the braced and unbraced scoliotic patient careful and frequent examination should be performed. A radiographic study should be done every 3–4 months, until skeletal maturity, as demonstrated by closure of the iliac epiphysis. Once a brace has been removed, an annual examination for five years is suggested to observe and monitor any delayed tendency for progression. If the curve does show progression, surgical stabilization may be indicated. In surgical cases the x-ray will aid in the placement of stabilizing instruments and graft material. During the postoperative period the degree of correction, the integrity of the fusion, and any complicating infection can be assessed. Over an extended time period the radiographic examination can be used to evaluate superimposed degenerative changes and progressive spinal changes.

CAPSULE SUMMARY. Scoliosis

GENERAL CONSIDERATIONS
Scoliosis: from Greek word "skolios," meaning twisted or crooked. Lateral deviation of the spinal column.

CLASSIFICATION AND TERMINOLOGY
Scolioses are classified according to etiology (Table 4.1) and location. Specific standardized terminology is utilized in the discipline.

CLINICAL FEATURES
Structural scoliosis is a fixed deformity which does not correct on lateral bending.

Idiopathic scoliosis is the most common scoliosis. Three different types—infantile, juvenile, adolescent.

Adolescent idiopathic scoliosis: 10 years of age until skeletal maturity. Females: 9 to 1, usually right thoracic, wedged vertebrae (Hueter-Volkmann principle); most rapid growth between 12 and 16.

Congenital scoliosis: structural anomalies, short curve, high incidence of genitourinary anomalies.

Neuromuscular scoliosis: nerve or muscle disease, long curve convex to weak side.

Neurofibromatosis: mesoectodermal dysplasia. Scoliosis common, often short and angular kyphosis, and with vertebral dysplasia.

Others: infection, radiation, trauma, degenerative joint disease, neoplasm.

Nonstructural scoliosis: deformity fully corrects on lateral bending, leg deficiencies, and antalgia.

Complications of scoliosis: cardiopulmonary disease, degenerative arthritis, curve progression, pain, radiation-induced abnormalities, psychological, nerve palsies, infections, pseudoarthrosis, and instrumentation failure.

RADIOLOGICAL ASSESSMENT
Standard projections: erect AP and lateral full spine, right and left lateral bending, left hand and wrist.

Supplementary projections: many. (Table 4.3)

Technology: 84 inches TFD, compensating filtration, rare-earth screens.

Measurements: curvature–Cobb method; rotation–pedicle method; flexibility–lateral flexion; skeletal maturation–left hand and wrist, vertebral ring epiphyses, iliac epiphysis (Risser's sign).

Therapy selection: indicators of progression include double curvatures, young age, onset of menarche, absent or early Risser sign.

No treatment: under 20 degrees, but must be monitored carefully every three months. Greater than 5 degrees increase should be braced.

Bracing: flexible, immature, 20–40-degree curves which are progressive; usually, Milwaukee brace. Evaluated every 3 months, until maturity, then weaned gradually.

Surgery: abnormality, progression, more than 40 degrees; Harrington rods, Dwyer procedure.

REFERENCES

1. Hippocrates: *The Genuine Works of Hippocrates*, London, F. Adams, 1849.
2. Cobb JR: Outline for the study of scoliosis. *Am Acad Orthop Surgeons Lect* 5:261, 1948.
3. Terminology Committee, Scoliosis Research Society: A glossary of scoliosis terms. *Spine* 1:57, 1976.
4. Keim HA: Scoliosis. *CIBA Clinical Symposia* 30 (1):1, 1978.
5. Wynne-Davies, R: Genetic and environmental aspects. *J Bone Joint Surg (Br)* 50:24, 1968.
6. MacEwan DG, Cowell HR: Familial incidence of idiopathic scoliosis and its implication in patient treatment. *J Bone Joint Surg (Am)* 52:405, 1970.
7. Riseborough T, Wynne-Davies RA: Genetic survey of idiopathic scoliosis in Boston, Massachusetts. *J Bone Joint Surg (Am)* 56:974, 1973.
8. Lloyd-Roberts GC, Pilcher MF: Structural idiopathic scoliosis in infancy. A study of the natural history of 100 patients. *J Bone Joint Surg (Br)* 47:520, 1965.
9. Hoppenfield S: *Scoliosis. A Manual of Concept and Treatment*, Philadelphia, JB Lippincott, 1967.
10. Collis DK, Ponsetti IV: Long term followup of patients with idiopathic scoliosis not treated surgically. *J Bone Joint Surg (Am)* 51:425, 1969.
11. Epstein JA, Epstein BS, Lavine LS: Surgical treatment of nerve root compression caused by scoliosis of the lumbar spine. *J Neurosurg* 41:449, 1974.
12. Ponsetti IV, Friedman B: Prognosis in idiopathic scoliosis. *J Bone Joint Surg (Am)* 32:381, 1950.
13. Reckles LN, Peterson HA, Bianco AJ, et al: The association of scoliosis and congenital heart disease. *J Bone Joint Surg (Am)* 57:449, 1975.
14. Winter RB, Moe JH, Eilers VE: Congenital scoliosis. *J Bone Joint Surg (Am)* 50:1, 1968.
15. Winter RB, Moe JH, Wang JF: Congenital kyphosis. *J Bone Joint Surg (Am)* 55:223, 1973.
16. MacEwan GD, Hardy JH, Winter RB: Evaluation of kidney anomalies in congenital scoliosis. *J Bone Joint Surg (Am)* 54:1451, 1972.
17. Kilfoyle RM, Foley JJ, Norton PL: Spine and pelvic deformity in childhood and adolescent paraplegia. A study of 104 cases. *J Bone Joint Surg (Am)* 47:659, 1965.
18. Spencer GE Jr: Orthopedic considerations in the management of muscular dystrophy. *Curr Pract Orthop Surg* 5:279, 1973.
19. Siegel IM: Scoliosis in muscular dystrophy. *Clin Orthop* 93:235, 1973.
20. von Recklinghausen FD: *Über die Multiplen Fibrome der Haut und ihre Beziehungen zu den Neuromen*, Virchow, Festschr R, 1882.
21. Weiss RS: Curvature of the spine in von Recklinghausen disease. *Arch Dermatol Syphilis* 3:144, 1921.
22. Hunt JC, Pugh DG: Skeletal lesions in neurofibromatosis. *Radiology* 76:1, 1961.
23. Scott JC: Scoliosis and neurofibromatosis. *J Bone Joint Surg (Br)* 47:240, 1965.
24. Neuhauser EBD, Wittenhoy MH, Berman CF, et al: Irradiation effects of roentgen therapy on the growing spine. *Radiology* 59:737, 1952.
25. Rutherford H, Dodd GD: Complications of radiation therapy: Growing bone. *Semin Roentgenol* 9:15, 1974.
26. Samuelson, S: Cor pulmonale resulting from deformities of the chest. *Acta Med Scand* 142:399, 1952.
27. Risser JC: Scoliosis: Past and present. *J Bone Joint Surg (Am)* 46 (1):167, 1964.
28. Diakow PRP: Pain: A forgotten aspect of idiopathic scoliosis. *J Can Chir Assoc* 28 (3):315, 1984.
29. Nash CL, Gregg EC, Brown RH, et al: Risk of exposure to X rays in patients undergoing long term treatment for scoliosis. *J Bone Joint Surg (Am)* 61:371, 1979.
30. Drummond D, Ranallo F, Lonstein J, et al: Radiation hazards in scoliosis management. *Spine* 8 (7):741, 1983.
31. Rao PS, Gregg EC: A revised estimate of the risk of carcinogenesis from X rays to scoliosis patients. *Invest Radiol* 19 (1):58, 1984.
32. Skandalaikis JE, Akin JT, Milsap JH, et al: Vascular compression of the duodenum. *Contemp Surg* 10:33, 1977.
33. Alexander RG: The effects on tooth position and maxillofacial vertical growth during treatment of scoliosis with the Milwaukee brace. *Am J Orthod* 52:161, 1966.
34. Young LW, Oestreich AE, Goldstein LA: Roentgenology in scoliosis: Contribution to evaluation and management. *AJR* 108:778, 1970.
35. Greulich WW, Pyle SI: *Radiographic Atlas of Skeletal Development of the Hand and Wrist*, ed 2, Stanford, Stanford University Press, 1959.
36. Gray JE, Hoffman AD, Peterson HA: Reduction of radiation exposure during radiography for scoliosis. *J Bone Joint Surg (Am)* 65 (1):5, 1983.
37. Davies WG: Radiography in the treatment of scoliosis and in leg lengthening. Part II - Radiography in scoliosis. *Radiography* 26 (311):349, 1960.
38. Archer BR, Whitmore RC, North LB, et al: Bone marrow dose in chest radiography: The posteroanterior vs. anteroposterior projection. *Radiology* 133:211, 1979.
39. Stagnara P: Examen du scoliotique. In *Deviations Laterales du Rachio: Scoliosis*, Encyclopedic Medicochirurgicale, Paris, Appareil Locomotor 7, 1974.
40. DeSmet AA, Fritz SL, Asher MA: A method for minimizing the radiation exposure from scoliosis radiographs. *J Bone Joint Surg (Am)* 63:156, 1981.
41. Schock CC, Brenton L, Agawal KK: The effect of PA versus AP x rays on the apparent scoliotic angle. *Orthop Trans* 4:32, 1980.
42. Lodin H: Transversal tomography in the examination of thoracic deformities, funnel chest and kyphoscoliosis. *Acta Radiol* 57:49, 1962.
43. Tojner H: Olisthetic scoliosis. *Acta Orthop Scand* 33:291, 1963.
44. Fisk JR, Moe JH, Winter RB: Scoliosis, spondylolysis, and spondylolisthesis. Their relationship as reviewed in 539 patients. *Spine* 3 (3):234, 1978.
45. Daniel WW, Barnes GT, Nasca RJ, et al: Segmented field radiography in scoliosis. *AJR* 144:325, 1985.
46. Merkin JJ, Sportelli L: The effects of two new compensating filters on patient exposure in chiropractic full spine radiography. *J Manip Physiol Therap* 5 (1):25, 1982.
47. Goldstein LA, Waugh TR: Classification and terminology of scoliosis. *Clin Orthop Rel Res* 93:10, 1973.
48. George K, Rippstein J: A comparative study of the two popular methods of measuring scoliotic deformity. *J Bone Joint Surg (Am)* 43 (6):809, 1961.
49. Lusskin R: Curves and angles. A comparison of scoliosis measurements. *Clin Orthop Rel Res* 23:232, 1962.
50. Risser JC, Ferguson AB: Scoliosis: Its prognosis. *J Bone Joint Surg (Am)* 18:667, 1936.
51. Ferguson AB: *Roentgen Diagnosis of the Extremities and Spine*, ed 2, New York, PB Hoebner, 1949.
52. Nash CL, Moe JH: A study of vertebral rotation. *J Bone Joint Surg (Am)* 5 (2):223, 1969.
53. Willner S, Nordwall A: A study of skeletal age and height in girls with idiopathic scoliosis. *Clin Orthop* 110:6, 1975.
54. Low WD, Mok CK, Leong AC, et al: The development of Southern Chinese girls with adolescent idiopathic scoliosis. *Spine* 3:152, 1978.
55. Gross C, Graham J, Neuwirth M, et al: Scoliosis and growth. An analysis of the literature. *Clin Orthop Rel Res* 175:243, 1983.
56. Risser JC: Important practical facts in the treatment of scoliosis. *Am Acad Orthop Surgeons Lect* 5:248, 1948.
57. Risser JC: The iliac apophysis: An invaluable sign in the management of scoliosis. *Clin Orthop Rel Res* 11:111, 1958.
58. Zaoussis AL, James JIP: The iliac apophysis and the evaluation of curves in scoliosis. *J Bone Joint Surg (Br)* 40 (3):442, 1958.
59. Lonstein JE, Carlson JM: The prediction of curve progression in untreated idiopathic scoliosis during growth. *J Bone Joint Surg (Am)* 66 (7):1061, 1984.
60. Farady JA: Current principles in the nonoperative management of structural adolescent idiopathic scoliosis. *Phys Ther* 63 (4):512, 1983.
61. Keim HA: *The Adolescent Spine*, New York, Grune & Stratton, 1976.
62. Calliet R: *Scoliosis: Diagnosis and Treatment*, Philadelphia, FA Davis, 1978.
63. Blount WP, Schmidt AC, Keever D, et al: The Milwaukee brace in the operative treatment of scoliosis. *J Bone Joint Dis (Am)* 40:511, 1958.
64. Hassan I, Bjerkreim I: Progression in idiopathic scoliosis after conservative treatment. *Acta Orthop Scand* 54 (1):88, 1983.
65. Dwyer AF, Newton NC, Sherwood AA: An anterior approach to scoliosis. A preliminary report. *Clin Orthop* 62:192, 1969.

5

The Natural History of Spondylolysis and Spondylolisthesis

TERRY R. YOCHUM
LINDSAY J. ROWE

Definitions

Spondylolysis is an interruption of the pars interarticularis, which may be either unilateral or bilateral. The term spondylolysis is derived from two Greek roots: "spondylos," meaning vertebra, and "lysis," meaning a dissolution; a loosing, setting free, releasing. (Fig. 5.1A and B)

Spondylolisthesis is defined as an anterior displacement of a vertebral body in relation to the segment immediately below. The Greek origin of this word is "spondylos," meaning vertebra, and "olisthesis," referring to slippage or displacement. (Fig. 5.1A and B) Traditionally, and even today, in medical literature the term "spondylolisthesis" is synonymous with forward displacement. Perhaps a more precise term for this anatomical disrelationship should be "anterolisthesis with or without spondylolysis." Spondylolisthesis (anterolisthesis) may occur with a defect in the vertebral arch (spondylolytic spondylolisthesis) or without a defect in the vertebral arch (nonspondylolytic spondylolisthesis). (1)

Prespondylolisthesis is defined as the presence of spondylolysis without forward vertebral displacement. This term is misleading since it implies that displacement will necessarily occur and should therefore be discarded.

Historical Considerations

Spondylolisthesis has been a focal point of academic and clinical interest for over 100 years and, as yet, many questions remain unanswered in regard to the etiology, clinical significance, treatment, and prognosis of this common condition.

The first record of spondylolisthesis was written in 1782 by a Belgian obstetrician, Herbinaux. (2) The original report was of a patient who experienced difficulty in childbirth because of displacement of the fifth lumbar vertebra relative to the first sacral segment. Kilian (3) concluded that such displacements occurred gradually and introduced the term "spondylolisthesis." In 1855, Robert (4) performed experiments on cadavers in which

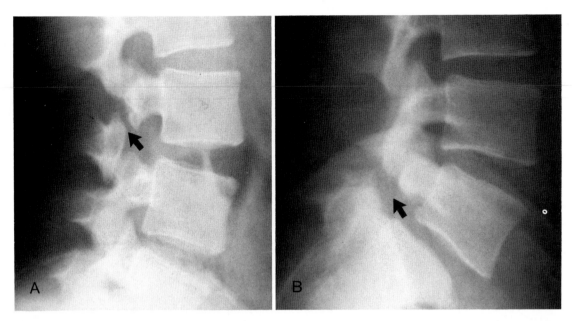

Figure 5.1. SPONDYLOLYSIS AND SPONDYLOLISTHESIS. A. Spondylolysis: Third Lumbar. Observe the pars defects (arrow), but note the absence of anterolisthesis of the third lumbar body. **B. Spondylolisthesis: Fifth Lumbar.** In this case the pars defects (arrow) are accompanied by anterolisthesis of the fifth lumbar body.

he removed all soft tissues around the lumbosacral junction, exposing the pars interarticularis. His studies revealed that no displacement occurred if the neural arch was intact, an observation later challenged. (5,6) In 1858 Lambl (5) demonstrated the defect in the pars interarticularis, which is presently known as "spondylolysis." In 1895 Neugebauer (6) was the first to describe displacement of the L5 vertebral body upon the sacrum occurring without pars interarticularis defects as a result of congenital elongation of the pars interarticularis (Type I: Dysplastic).

Prevalence of Spondylolysis and Spondylolisthesis

Approximately 90 percent of all spondylolistheses involve the fifth lumbar vertebra. (7) The remaining 10 percent are found throughout the other lumbar and cervical vertebrae. (Table 5.1).

Several studies have suggested that there are variations in the prevalence of spondylolysis in different populations. There is a 5 to 7 percent prevalence of pars defects in the white population, with a two to one male predominance. (8) Moreton (9) found a 7.2 percent prevalence of spondylolysis in a pre-employment study of 32,600 asymptomatic young men aged 18 to 35.

Stewart (10) in 1953 studied the skeletal remains of 243 Northern Eskimos and found a 40.3 percent prevalence of pars defects in the specimens. Kettelkamp and Wright (11) reviewed the radiographs of 153 Northern Eskimos and noted the presence of pars defects in 28

percent. In addition to a much higher overall prevalence of spondylolysis compared with other groups, Alaskan Eskimos have demonstrated a proportionately higher percentage of upper lumbar involvement (L1–L3) than has been observed in other series. (10) We suggest that the papoose fashion of carrying their infants places an undue amount of premature stress on the pars interarticularis, perhaps explaining the unusually high prevalence of pars defects in the Northern Eskimos. Therefore, the recent prolonged usage of vertical support and restraining devices for children should be discouraged, as it may be a

Table 5.1.
Common Sites for Spondylolysis and/or Spondylolisthesis (7)

Location	Percentage
L5	90
L4	5
L1,2,3	3
C5,6,7	2

predisposing factor to premature mechanical stress upon the pars interarticularis. The upright walker is discouraged until the child can walk unassisted.

Rowe and Roche (12) report a prevalence of spondylolisthesis of 2.4 percent in the black populations of North America and South Africa. According to Wiltse, (13) there is a 13-fold increase in the prevalence of spina bifida occulta among persons with pars defects when compared to the general population. Spina bifida are not necessarily found at the level of the spondylolysis, nor are they etiologically related. (13)

Etiology of Spondylolysis

The etiology of spondylolysis is controversial, with many suggested mechanisms. (Table 5.2)

Table 5.2.
Hypothesized Mechanisms of Development of Spondylolisthesis (13)

Separate ossification centers.
A fracture which occurs at the time of birth.
An ordinary fracture at that region.
A stress or fatigue fracture.
Displacement secondary to an increased lumbar lordosis.
Displacement secondary to a pinching mechanism of superior and inferior articular processes.
Weakness of regional ligamentous and fascial support structures.
Aseptic necrosis of the pars interarticularis.
Dysplasia of the pars interarticularis.
Pathological changes of the pars interarticularis.

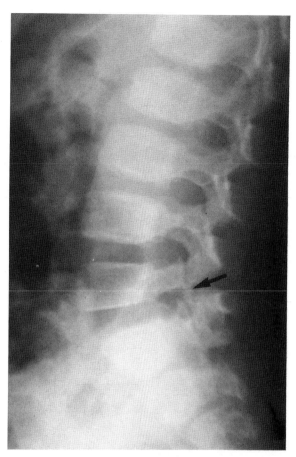

Figure 5.2. SPONDYLOLISTHESIS, THREE-YEAR-OLD PATIENT. Pars defects are visible at the fifth lumbar segment (arrow), with accompanying anterolisthesis. (Courtesy of Victor Y. W. Tong, DC, DACBR, Los Angeles, California)

CONGENITAL

For many years spondylolysis and spondylolisthesis have been referred to as congenital anomalies; (14,15) however, extensive studies of cadavers have not revealed these lesions in the newborn. Batts (16) in 1939, in a study of 200 fetal spines, found no pars interarticularis defects, nor did Rowe and Roche (12) in 509 stillborn and neonatal cadavers. More recently, Fredrickson et al, (17) in 1984, reviewed the lumbar radiographs of 500 newborns and found no evidence of spondylolysis or spondylolisthesis, thus supporting an acquired etiology. The youngest person with a spondylolisthesis was reported by Borkow and Kleiger (14) and was a 4-month-old child who was born after an uneventful pregnancy and delivery. It was reported that shortly after birth the parents noted a deformity in the lower back and brought it to the attention of their physician. Radiological examination revealed a pars defect at the L4 vertebra and a hypoplastic L5 vertebral body was noted. The youngest persons previously reported were 10 and 17 months of age, respectively. (18,19) (Fig. 5.2)

Although some workers attempt to explain spondylolysis as being caused by the nonunion of two separate ossification centers in the pars interarticularis or due to a defect in cartilaginous development, no evidence has been produced to support these theories. (13)

STRESS FRACTURE

Presently, the most commonly proposed etiology leading to a pars interarticularis defect is that of stress fracture.

(20) The most common skeletal location for stress fracture is the pars interarticularis. (20) Wiltse et al (20) has proposed that spondylolysis is a fatigue fracture caused by recurrent mechanical stress. His theory is supported by a recent in vitro study conducted by Cyron and Hutton, (21) in which they subjected 28 human lumbar spines, consisting of the lower three lumbar vertebrae and the sacrum, to repetitive mechanical stress. The lumbar vertebrae were subjected to a loading pattern calculated to simulate walking with a heavy backpack. They found that the pars interarticularis of the lumbar vertebrae was vulnerable to mechanical fatigue failure. (Fig. 5.3A and B) Similar fatigue fracture may occur at the vertebra above a transitional segment. (Fig. 5.4 A–C)

Except for a single case reported at C4 in a gorilla, (22) the defect of spondylolysis has not been reported in mammals other than man. We therefore suggest that the upright posture of man, combined with additional repetitive mechanical stress, would appear to be a significant etiological factor. Rosenberg et al (23) reviewed the radiographs of 143 life-long nonambulatory patients. The condition underlying the nonambulatory status varied but was most commonly cerebral palsy. No case of spondy-

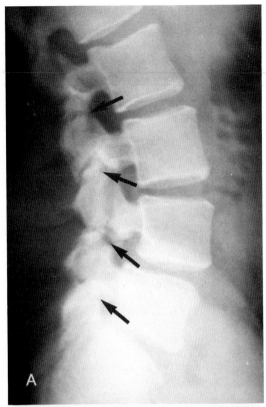

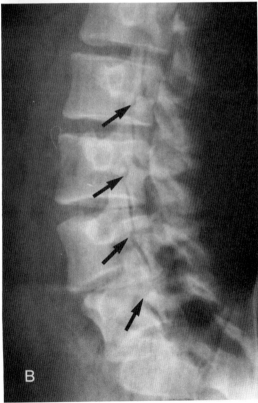

Figure 5.3. SPONDYLOLYSIS AT MULTIPLE LEVELS. A and B. A 22-year-old male power weightlifter had these films taken following an acute low back strain. Observe the multiple pars defects from the fifth to second lumbar levels (arrows). This patient totalled eight pars defects from L2 through L5.

lolysis or spondylolisthesis was detected in this study. These patients had the same prevalence as the general population for other spinal anomalies such as spina bifida occulta, transitional vertebrae, and structural scoliosis. These findings support the hypothesis that ambulation and upright posture, with added repetitive mechanical stress, are intimately related in the etiology of spondylolysis.

Age of onset augments the argument for the stress fracture etiology. Spondylolysis in children can occur shortly after walking begins; however, clinical and radiographic detection occurs most commonly after the age of five and most often between the ages of 10 and 15. (12) There appears to be a meaningful etiological association between the onset of the pars defect, the development of the lumbar lordosis, and repeated infant falls, particularly if premature walking occurs. (24) Parents should be discouraged from prompting their children to walk before the child is prepared to do so. Repetitive lumbar hyperextension has also been implicated as a mechanism in the development of pars interarticularis defects. (19,25)

Increased prevalence of spondylolysis and spondylolisthesis has been noted in persons participating in above average levels of physical activity, particularly activity involving stressful movements of the lumbar spine unique to certain sports. Rossi, (25) in a report to the Italian Olympic Committee in 1978, reviewed 1,430 lumbar spine x-rays of athletes in the 16 to 27 age range. Two hundred and thirty-nine athletes (16.7 percent) were found to have spondylolysis and/or spondylolisthesis. Those athletic activities in which participants had the highest prevalence of spondylolysis and/or spondylolisthesis were diving and gymnastics. The prevalence among persons in those sports was higher than for the general population and supports the assertion that athletic activity resulting in greater spinal mechanical stress is related to the development of spondylolysis and spondylolisthesis. (Fig. 5.5A and B) Similarly, a high percentage of polevaulters develop spondylolysis. (26) Raynal et al (27) examined the radiographs of 4,619 middle-aged manual laborers involved in heavy lifting and found a 9.4 percent prevalence of spondylolysis and spondylolisthesis, which is similar to the prevalence among Japanese athletes of 10.9 percent. (28) Diving, gymnastics, weightlifting and polevaulting all require repetitive hyperextension of the lumbar spine, coupled with jarring, which suggests that hyperextension is a factor in the etiology of spondylolysis and spondylolisthesis. (29)

Accepting the stress fracture etiology presents a challenge. Since all other stress fractures heal with immobilization, why doesn't this one? The answer appears to be that these individuals are not immobilized at the time the spondylolysis occurs. This results in the nonunion of the stress fracture and, thereby, a spondylolysis.

OTHER FACTORS

Rarely, an acute fracture following trauma does occur through the pars area, creating a spondylolysis. Certain disease processes such as osteopetrosis can weaken the bone and thereby allow spondylolysis to occur. (30)

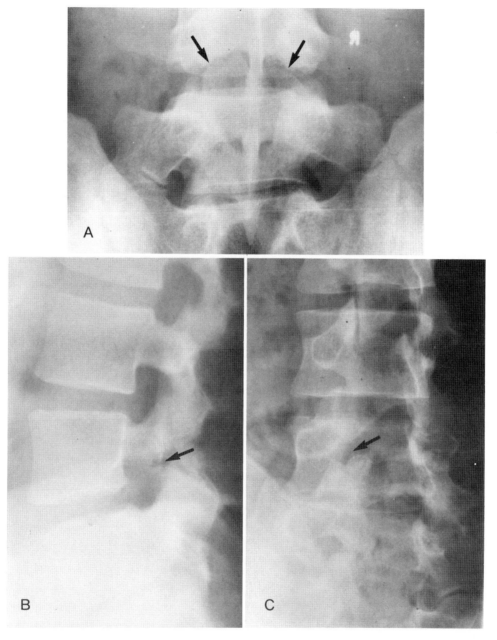

Figure 5.4. SPONDYLOLISTHESIS ASSOCIATED WITH A TRANSITIONAL LUMBOSACRAL SEGMENT. A. AP Angulated View. The bilateral accessory joints are identified. Note the pars defects visible on this angulated (30 degrees cephalad) lumbosacral view (arrows). **B and C. Lateral and Oblique Views**. The pars defects and anterolisthesis are identified (arrows).

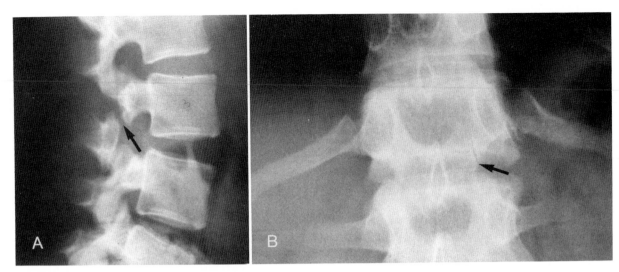

Figure 5.5. PARS INTERARTICULARIS DEFECTS AT UNUSUAL LEVELS. A. Third lumbar (arrow), male polevaulter. **B.** Twelfth thoracic (arrow). (Courtesy of Simon Breen, BAppSc (Chiro), Adelaide, Australia)

Classification of Spondylolisthesis

The most widely used classification of spondylolisthesis is that described by Wiltse, Newman, and Macnab in which five distinct types have been identified. (31)

Type I: Dysplastic: This type includes those spondylolistheses with a congenital abnormality in the upper sacrum or the neural arch of L5 that allows displacement to occur.

Type II: Isthmic: This type has three subtypes which involve alteration to the pars interarticularis as follows:

A. A lytic or stress (fatigue) fracture of the pars, or
B. An elongated but intact pars, or
C. An acute fracture of the pars.

Type III: Degenerative (Pseudospondylolisthesis): Secondary to longstanding degenerative arthrosis of the lumbar zygapophyseal joints and discovertebral articulations, without a pars separation.

Type IV: Traumatic: Secondary to a fracture of part of the neural arch other than the pars interarticularis.

Type V: Pathological: In conjunction with generalized or localized bone disease (e.g., Paget's disease, metastatic bone disease, osteopetrosis, etc.).

TYPE I: DYSPLASTIC

This type of spondylolisthesis involves a congenital malformation of the upper sacrum and/or the neural arch of the L5 vertebra. (32) There is an anterior displacement of the L5 vertebral body upon the sacrum as a result of inadequate bony architecture to withstand the forward vectors of thrust of the lumbar spine on the sacral promontory. Usually, there is an accompanying wide spina bifida occulta involving the sacrum and the L5 vertebra. This type usually progresses to a more severe grade of displacement. (32) This is one of the nonspondylolytic (no pars defects) forms of spondylolisthesis. There is a 4:1

prevalence of isthmic versus dysplastic spondylolisthesis. (32)

TYPE II: ISTHMIC

Subtype A

This subtype is caused by biomechanical stress; the mode of failure is believed to be fatigue fracture of the pars interarticularis. It is the most common type found in persons below the age of 50 and has not been noted in the newborn. (32)

Subtype B

This subtype of spondylolisthesis results from elongation of the pars interarticularis without separation. It is fundamentally the same lesion as Subtype A; however, it is thought to be secondary to repeated minor trabecular stress fractures of the pars. Healing of these fractures occurs, but the pars is elongated as the vertebral body of L5 is displaced anteriorly. Eventually the pars may separate, as displacement progresses, making differentiation from Subtype A difficult. (32)

Subtype C

This subtype includes those spondylolistheses resulting from acute pars fractures following a severe traumatic incident and is a rare presentation. The mechanism of injury usually involves hyperextension of the lower lumbar vertebral column, and displacement seldom occurs. (31)

TYPE III: DEGENERATIVE

Degenerative spondylolisthesis (Type III) has been referred to as a "pseudospondylolisthesis" by Junghans to differentiate spondylolisthesis with an intact neural arch from those with a true defect of the neural arch. (22) Macnab (33) prefers the phrase "spondylolisthesis with an intact neural arch," which is a more accurate description. Thus, degenerative spondylolisthesis is another type of nonspondylolytic spondylolisthesis. Degenerative spondylolisthesis is approximately ten times more common at L4 than at the L3 or L5 vertebrae and is six times more common in females 60 years of age or older, compared with males of the same age. (34) Type III is rare in persons younger than 50 years of age. (29) Degenerative spondylolisthesis is three times more common in blacks than in whites, with no adequate explanations for these sexual and racial disparities. (34) Finally, degenerative spondylolisthesis is four times more likely to be found in association with a sacralized fifth lumbar vertebra. (34) (Table 5.3)

The mechanisms of displacement are thought to involve a combination of zygapophyseal joint arthrosis, disc degeneration, and remodeling of the articular processes and pars. (33) An increase of the "pedicle-facet angle" has been noted in the degenerative type of spondylolisthesis. (1) This angle, formed by the long axis of the pedicle (or vertebral root) at its intersection with the long axis of the articular pillar, indicates the more horizontal alignment of the degenerative zygapophyseal joints as seen on the lateral radiograph and demonstrates the overriding of the articular surfaces. (1) (Fig. 5.6A–C)

Several explanations have been proposed for degenerative spondylolisthesis occuring with such great frequency at the L4 level. Allbrook (35) has stated that the greater mobility of L4 due to the sagittal orientation of the facets at the L4/L5 level may explain the unusual frequency of degenerative spondylolisthesis at the L4 level. Additionally, the firmly attached, normal lumbosacral joint may place increased stress on the L4/L5 intervertebral joints, ultimately leading to hypermobility

Table 5.3.
The Three F's of Degenerative Spondylolisthesis

Female
Four (L4)
Above Forty years

and degeneration of the articular triad. (34) No greater than 25 percent anterior displacement of the L4 vertebral body occurs, and the majority involve 10 to 15 percent displacement. (34)

TYPE IV: TRAUMATIC

Traumatic spondylolisthesis can occur as a result of a recent severe injury creating a fracture of a portion of the neural arch other than the pars interarticularis. (Fig. 5.7A and B) These fractures generally heal when appropriately immobilized. (32) It is common at C2 and is referred to as a Hangman's (Hangee's) fracture. (Fig. 5.8)

TYPE V: PATHOLOGICAL

Generalized or systemic disorders of bone may affect the neural arch of the spine and allow spondylolisthesis to develop. Metastatic carcinoma, osteopetrosis, (30) and Paget's disease are some of the more common disorders which may contribute to the formation of spondylolysis. (Fig. 5.9)

A *sixth* type may be offered which is called "postsurgical" or "iatrogenic spondylolisthesis." This includes two different types of lesions. The first is a stress fracture of the pars at a level immediately above or below a spinal fusion (spondylolisthesis acquisita). (1) (Fig. 5.10) Many of these patients have had anterior interbody fusion for spondylolisthesis. This creates abnormal stress above or below the fusion site. With the advent of posterolateral fusions for spondylolisthesis, this entity is disappearing. The second disorder in this group is caused by removing too much bone in posterior decompression laminectomies, usually for a herniated nucleus pulposus. This unilateral decompression creates spinal instability and abnormal stress upon the neural arch opposite the surgical defect. This abnormal stress may lead to a sclerotic hypertrophied pedicle and lamina or spondylolysis (see Fig. 5.21 A and B).

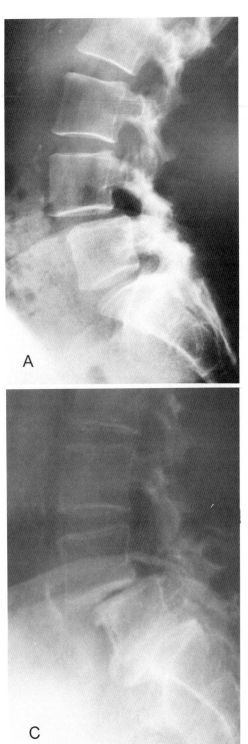

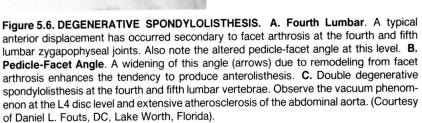

Figure 5.6. DEGENERATIVE SPONDYLOLISTHESIS. A. Fourth Lumbar. A typical anterior displacement has occurred secondary to facet arthrosis at the fourth and fifth lumbar zygapophyseal joints. Also note the altered pedicle-facet angle at this level. **B. Pedicle-Facet Angle.** A widening of this angle (arrows) due to remodeling from facet arthrosis enhances the tendency to produce anterolisthesis. **C.** Double degenerative spondylolisthesis at the fourth and fifth lumbar vertebrae. Observe the vacuum phenomenon at the L4 disc level and extensive atherosclerosis of the abdominal aorta. (Courtesy of Daniel L. Fouts, DC, Lake Worth, Florida).

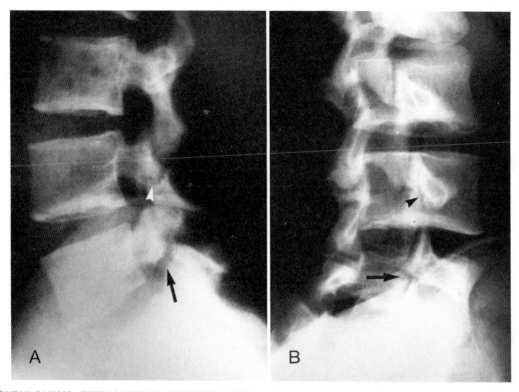

Figure 5.7. SPONDYLOLYSIS: FIFTH LUMBAR SEGMENT, WITH ACUTE UNILATERAL PARS FRACTURE AT THE FOURTH LUMBAR SEGMENT. A 16-year-old male football player was "clipped" from behind. **A. Lateral View.** Note the defect at the fifth lumbar pars (arrow), with no anterolisthesis. The fractured fourth lumbar pars is also identified (arrowhead). **B. Oblique View.** The difference between each defect is apparent—smooth and more horizontal at the fifth (arrow) and irregular and more vertical at the fourth (arrowhead). **Comment**: Despite the considerable force required to fracture the fourth lumbar pars, no anterolisthesis of the fifth segment occurred, demonstrating the usual stability of spondylolytic pars defects. (Courtesy of Barton W. Dukett, DC, Bigelow, Arkansas)

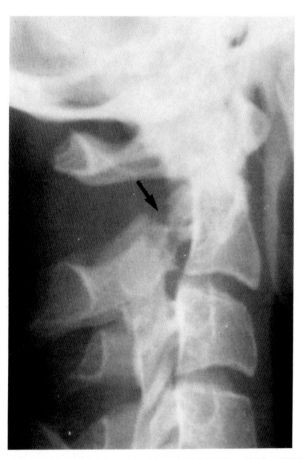

Figure 5.8. TRAUMATIC SPONDYLOLISTHESIS: AXIS (HANG-MAN'S FRACTURE). Note the anterolisthesis of the axis body and fractures through the pedicles of the C2 vertebra (arrow).

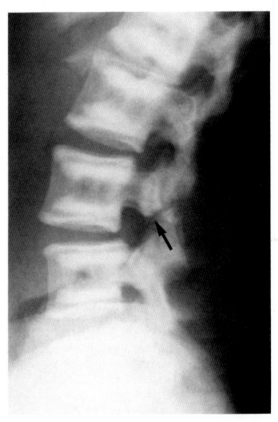

Figure 5.9. PATHOLOGICAL SPONDYLOLISTHESIS: OSTEOPE-TROSIS. In this condition the bones are rendered brittle and prone to fracture; in this case, at the third lumbar pars interarticularis (arrow).

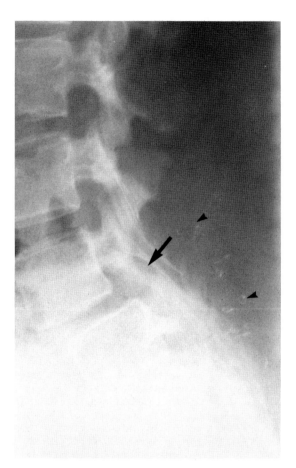

Figure 5.10. SPONDYLOLISTHESIS ACQUISITA. Following a decompressive laminectomy and posterior arthrodesis at the fourth and fifth lumbar vertebrae, pars defects developed at the fourth lumbar vertebra (arrow), which allowed for a Grade 1 spondylolisthesis to occur. Of incidental notation are surgical metallic sutures in the soft tissues of the lumbosacral region (arrowheads).

Clinical Features of Spondylolysis and Spondylolisthesis

PAIN

In addition to their controversial etiology, spondylolysis and spondylolisthesis present a challenging clinical picture. Spondylolysis and/or spondylolisthesis may be found in asymptomatic individuals, and in most cases the lesion has been present since the age of 5 or 6 years. (17) Studies indicate that approximately one half of patients with radiological signs of spondylolisthesis never develop symptoms. (24,31,36,37) Nachemson (32) believes that spondylolysis does not contribute to the cause of pain at all and, according to Schmorl and Junghans (22), pain specifically related to spondylolysis and/or spondylolisthesis does not exist. Additionally, Fredrickson et al, (17) in their extensive prospective study, found that the development of spondylolysis, with or without spondylolisthesis, does not cause pain in most patients. We feel that back pain may often be present with patients developing spondylolysis, but its presence goes unrecognized because

of the young age (2–10 years) of the patient and the failure of the parents to acknowledge the child's complaints which may be simply discarded as "growing pains." The development of spondylolysis in a teenager or young adult is usually painful; (25,26) therefore, why shouldn't it be in the young child? Patients with severe displacement may experience only minimal back pain. There is no correlation between the degree of anterior displacement and the severity of symptoms. (15,38) Of those patients with back pain related to their spondylolisthesis, 25 percent have a recent history of antecedent trauma. (7) These patients have a deep-seated, dull, aching pain which is localized to the area of spondylolysis or spondylolisthesis.

EXAMINATION FINDINGS

Examination of the patient with spondylolisthesis often reveals distinct postural changes consistent with the degree of anterolisthesis. The buttocks are often prominent, assuming a heart-shaped appearance when viewed from the posterior. A hyperlordosis of the lumbar spine and anterior shift of the gravitational weightbearing line is often noted. Patients with advanced displacement often demonstrate a transverse skin furrow which may be seen above the iliac crest bilaterally. An associated spina bifida occulta may be signaled by localized hypertrichosis. Lower lumbar spine palpation of a patient with a spondylolytic spondylolisthesis reveals prominence of the spinous process at the affected vertebral level. (Fig. 5.11A) Conversely, in a patient with a nonspondylolytic spondylolisthesis the spinous process of the affected level will be palpated as a depression ("step defect"). (Fig. 5.11B) A clicking sensation at the level of the involved segment may be felt or heard during active trunk flexion or on straight leg raising. Hamstring tightness has long been thought to be associated with spondylolisthesis, yet its cause is not known. Decreased anterior trunk flexion and reduced straight leg raising may be manifestations of tight hamstring muscles and not evidence of an anterolisthesis. No statistically significant correlation is found between hamstring tightness, low back pain, and the radiographic evidence of pars defects. (39)

Neurological evaluation of the lower extremities is usually unremarkable. However, if leg pain is present it may be nondermatomal and will likely be a referred-pain phenomenon following sclerotomal patterns from irritation of the mesodermal structures, such as the ligaments and muscles. (40) Disc herniations are generally not associated with spondylolisthesis. (17)

DISPLACEMENT

There has been debate in the literature concerning the progression of anterior displacement in spondylolisthesis. Only 2 to 3 percent of patients with spondylolisthesis show progressive displacement. (17) The majority of these occur due to underlying degenerative changes. (22) The presence of a spina bifida occulta has been shown to be associated with an increased risk of anterior displacement. (41)

Progression of the anterior displacement in spondylolisthesis occurs primarily between the ages of 5 and 10,

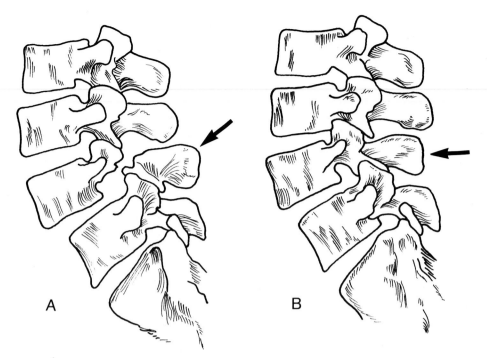

Figure 5.11. SPONDYLOLYTIC VERSUS NONSPONDYLOLYTIC SPONDYLOLISTHESIS: LUMBAR PALPATION. A. Spondylolytic Spondylolisthesis. Bilateral pars defects at the L4 vertebra allow anterior displacement of its body and pedicles. The intact upper lumbar segments (L1–L3) move in unison with the displaced L4 body and pedicles, leaving the rest of the L4 neural arch behind, which will be palpated as the prominent spinous process (arrow). **B. Nonspondylolytic Spondylolisthesis.** Observe the anterior displacement of the intact L4 on L5. Since there are no pars defects, the neural arch of L4 must naturally accompany the anterior displacement of the vertebral body. This results in a palpable depression ("step defect") as the spinous process is drawn forward (arrow).

although some may continue to displace between the ages of 10 and 15. (17) Maximum anterior displacement is usually seen within 18 months to 2 years following the development of spondylolysis, which is usually below 10 years of age. (17) It is rare for greater than 15 percent anterior displacement to occur in the adult patient with pseudospondylolisthesis, unless it is associated with severe degenerative changes and the instability of zygapophyseal joint arthrosis. (42) Very few cases demonstrate further anterolisthesis beyond the age of 18. (17,31)

Taillard (8) has suggested that two anatomical factors are important in the development of a displacement: the "trapezoidal" shape of the fifth lumbar vertebra and the "doming" deformity of the anterior sacral promontory. Fredrickson et al (17) found that a change in the shape of the fifth lumbar vertebra and sacrum occurred at the same time or soon after the displacement was noted. We concur with their opinion that these changes in the shape of the vertebrae are the result of the displacement rather than the cause. (17) Occasionally, a buttressing of new bone will occur at the anterior margin of the sacrum as a protective measure to resist further anterior displacement of the L5 vertebral body and is a good prognostic sign, as progression of the anterior displacement is unlikely. (8) Turek (43) states that severe anterior displacement (Grades 3 and 4) is twice as common in young females and that the most rapid displacement occurs between the ages of 9 and 15. Although the anteriorly placed weight gain which occurs during pregnancy would seem to predispose to displacement, such is not the case. No further displacement of spondylolisthesis or fetal risk has been found to be associated with pregnancy, and most patients have no difficulty during parturition unless the child is presented breech. (17) Schmorl and Junghans (22) have stated that they have not found a case described in the literature that suggests that trauma induced displacement in a known pre-existing spondylolysis.

The information presented concerning the signs and symptoms of patients with spondylolisthesis demonstrates the lack of direct correlation with back pain. Therefore, the clinician must look past the spondylolisthesis in the total evaluation of back pain patients with spondylolisthesis to identify any other causes. Medical authorities who attest to a direct correlation between the presence of spondylolysis and/or spondylolisthesis and back pain have based their conclusions on cases that also included the presence of biomechanical instability and longstanding neurological deficits. (24,31) These represent such a small percentage of the total patients with spondylolisthesis that this conclusion is questioned by the authors, since we feel this does not apply to the majority of spondylolisthesis cases. We concur with Fredrickson et al (17) that a child over 10 years of age with spondylolysis or spondylolisthesis should be permitted to enjoy normal activities during childhood and adolescence without fear of progressive displacement or disabling pain. When spondylolisthesis has been detected below the age of 10, we recommend limitation of gymnastic and sports activities until serial flexion and extension upright lateral lumbar radiographic studies, taken six months apart, demonstrate no evidence of progressive displacement of the involved segment.

ATHLETIC ACTIVITY

There has been a trend in the clinical management of athletes with spondylolisthesis to curb or restrict their athletic activities. This in effect creates a "spondylo invalid," even though only an uncomplicated bilateral pars defect with spondylolisthesis may exist. The current literature does not support this approach to the clinical management of patients with spondylolisthesis. (17, 25,44) Fredrickson et al (17) do not restrict children's activity in any way, and they allow full participation in sports.

Semon and Spengler (44) reviewed the records of 506 college football players from the University of Washington spanning an eight-year period. The medical records of the football players included documentation of practices and games missed because of injury. One hundred and thirty-five players (27%) had low back pain following their games. Because of persistent low back symptoms of pain and stiffness 58 players had roentgenograms of the lumbosacral spine performed, and in 12 persons defects of lumbar spondylolysis were observed. Therefore, spondylolysis was present in 20.7 percent of all players with back pain who were x-rayed. We consider the significant finding in this study to be that those players with low back pain and lumbar spondylolysis had no greater time lost from games and practices than players with low back pain without spondylolysis. Ferguson (45) reported a 50 percent prevalence of pars defects (6 out of 12) in interior linemen on the University of Pittsburgh football team. These players were also performing their football tasks quite adequately, and it may well be the same for many others playing rigorous sports with spondylolysis and spondylolisthesis.

Many coaches and physicians have discouraged individuals with lumbar spondylolysis and/or spondylolisthesis from participating in rigorous sports, despite recent studies which do not support this approach; therefore, it is in the best interest of the patient for the clinician to reconsider seriously the management of these athletes. Semon and Spengler's conclusions are that skeletally mature football players with lumbar spondylolysis and/or spondylolisthesis are able to engage in college and professional-level football without problems. (44) It would seem that the presence of lumbar spondylolysis and/or spondylolisthesis was of modest clinical significance during the 4-year period of active participation in football; (44) however, those patients with spondylolysis and/or spondylolisthesis who demonstrate biomechanical instability, along with persistent symptoms, warrant further clinical consideration.

Radiological Features

Radiological evaluation is the definitive method of confirming the presence of spondylolysis and spondylolisthesis. A complete series of the lumbar spine and sacrum is recommended and should include weightbearing anteroposterior (AP), lateral, and weightbearing or recumbent bilateral 45-degree oblique projections and the anteroposterior angulated view. The likelihood of not identifying pars defects increases significantly when oblique projections are not included in the radiological evaluation.

ANTEROPOSTERIOR NONANGULATED VIEW

Anteroposterior (AP) views of the lumbar spine generally do not yield sufficient information for the radiological evaluation of the pars interarticularis. The pars interarticularis on the AP view projects immediately inferior and slightly medial to the pedicle outline. A pars defect will sometimes be visible as an irregular linear radiolucency approximately paralleling the inferior cortex of the adjacent pedicle. Normally, the L5 pars interarticularis is not easily discernible in this view because of projectional distortion produced by the presence of the lordotic lumbosacral angle. However, when there is significant anterior displacement of the L5 segment, the vertebral body and transverse processes will become superimposed over the sacral base. The subsequent superimposition of densities at the lumbosacral junction creates an appearance termed the "inverted Napoleon's Hat" sign or the "Gendarme's Cap." (46) The inferior border of this density corresponds to the anterior aspect of the L5 vertebral body with the attached transverse processes and has been referred to as the "Bowline of Brailsford." (46) (Fig. 5.12A and B)

According to Ravichandran, (47) a useful radiological sign in detection of spondylolisthesis is the appearance of the rotated spinous process of a single lumbar vertebra. This is found in a vertebral segment not demonstrating lateral flexion of the vertebral body and without scoliosis and is appreciated in the AP lumbar spine film by drawing a line joining the spinous processes of the lumbar vertebrae. When singular rotation is noted, this may suggest an area of spondylolysis. (47)

ANTEROPOSTERIOR ANGULATED VIEW

In the evaluation of spondylolisthesis the anteroposterior (AP) angulated view may be used to more adequately visualize the L5 pars interarticularis. (48) The tube is angled 30 degrees cephalad so that the central ray passes through the lumbosacral disc directed about midway between the pubic symphysis and umbilicus. Defects in the pars interarticularis may be identified as focal areas of radiolucency below the pedicle outline. (Fig. 5.13A and B)

LATERAL VIEW

The lateral view is the most helpful projection in depicting vertebral body anterolisthesis (spondylolisthesis). Comparison of the alignment of the posterior vertebral body margins (George's line) will reveal a distinct misalignment between the involved segments. Also, a line drawn perpendicular to the sacral base from the sacral promontory (Ullmann's line) will show the anteroinferior margin of the L5 vertebral body to touch or be anterior to this line. (Fig. 5.14) Occasionally, a slight change in position of the anterolisthesis may occur when recumbent and upright lateral lumbar films are compared, with the greatest degree of displacement found in the upright radiograph.

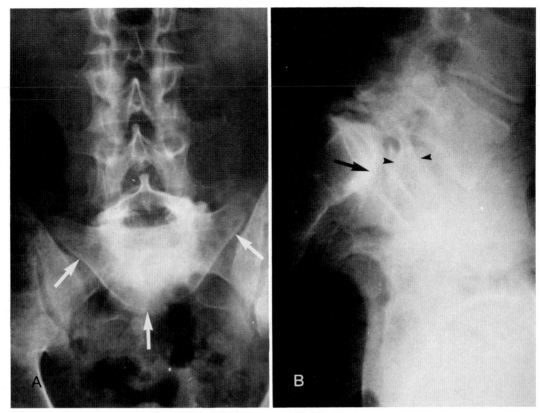

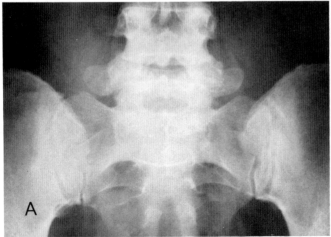

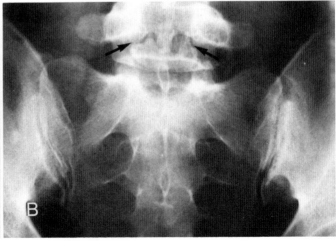

Figure 5.12. SPONDYLOPTOSIS, FIFTH LUMBAR. A 22-year-old Australian Rules football player with mild back pain. **A. AP View.** Note the "inverted Napoleon's hat" sign and the "bowline of Brailsford" (arrows). **B. Lateral View.** The fifth lumbar body has completely slipped over the sacrum. The sacral promontory is dome-shaped (arrow), and the fifth lumbar body is trapezoidal (arrowheads), which is characteristic of Grades 3, 4, and 5 types of spondylolisthesis. (Reprinted with permission: Yochum TR et al:

Reactive sclerosis of a pedicle due to unilateral spondylolysis—A case study. *ACA J Chiro, Radiology Corner,* September 1980) **Comment:** Despite the severity of this spondylolisthesis, the patient quickly responded to conservative care and continued to participate in football without recurrence of back pain. He has been pain free for the past five years. (Courtesy of Bruce F. Walker, DC, and C. Alison Hogg, MD, Melbourne, Australia)

Figure 5.13. ANTEROPOSTERIOR DETECTION OF PARS DEFECTS. A. Normal AP Film. No defects are visible. **B. Angulated AP Film.** The bilateral defects now become visible (30 degrees cephalad tube-tilt) (arrows). (Courtesy of Donald E. Freuden, DC, FACO, Denver, Colorado)

The degree of spondylolisthesis has been described by Meyerding. (49) The sacral base length is divided into four equal quarters, and the posterior aspect of the displaced vertebra is compared to this division and "graded"

accordingly (Fig. 5.15A and B, 5.16A–D); that is, a Grade 1 spondylolisthesis is present when the posterior aspect of the vertebral body lies between the posterior aspect of the sacrum and the first of the four divisions. A Grade 2

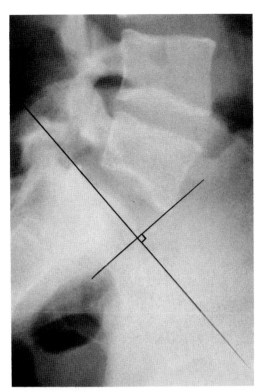

Figure 5.14. ULLMANN'S LINE, FIFTH LUMBAR SPONDYLOLIS-THESIS. A line drawn perpendicular to the sacral base line from the sacral promontory is shown intercepting the fifth lumbar body, indicating a spondylolisthesis.

a thick, bony protruding buttress may also be seen extending forward from the sacral promontory. (8) (Fig. 5.12) This radiographic sign (buttressing) represents a stress response secondary to significant anterolisthesis and usually denotes stability of the spondylolisthetic segment. (8) (Fig. 5.17A and B)

Flexion and extension lateral radiographs will provide better visualization of a defect and allow for evaluation of the intersegmental stability. The pars defect is typically seen just below the pedicle in an oblique plane as a linear radiolucency extending through the junction of the superior and inferior articular processes. The greater the vertebral body anterolisthesis, the easier it is to visualize the pars defects.

In lateral films of the upper lumbar spine, superimposition of the transverse processes over the pars region may simulate pars defects. (50) (Fig. 5.18A)

OBLIQUE VIEW

This is the most diagnostic view for depicting pars abnormalities and must be performed bilaterally. This projection can be performed in either the anterior or posterior oblique position and can be done upright or recumbent. Occasionally, the pars defect may be difficult to see as a result of improper positioning of the patient, superimposed structures such as the iliac crest and abdominal contents, and asymmetry of the pars defects.

Lachapelle (46) describes the appearance of the neural arch and its processes on the oblique film as simulating that of a "Scotty Dog." The anatomical counterparts of the Scotty Dog are outlined in an accompanying table. (51) (Table 5.4) (Fig. 5.18B) A pars defect will appear as an irregular linear radiolucency which has often been called the "collar" or "broken neck" of the Scotty Dog. (1) The bony margin of the defect may be sclerotic, with an irregular margin at the apposing surface of nonunion. (Fig. 5.18B)

An additional sign that may be noted on the oblique film is referred to as the "stepladder sign." (52) This sign is produced by a misalignment of the zygapophyseal joints at the involved level. This sign is demonstrated by drawing lines through the plane of each zygapophyseal joint and is considered positive if any line passes through the joint space below it or lies anterior to it. In such cases a "stepladder" pattern is formed by these lines. (Fig. 5.18C) This sign may not be present in some patients with the degenerative type of spondylolisthesis (Type III).

corresponds to the posterior vertebral body margin positioned between the first and second division, and a Grade 3 between the third and fourth division. Next is a Grade 4, in which the posterior surface of the L5 vertebral body lies between the anterior sacral promontory and the third division. A patient may reach beyond a Grade 4 spondylolisthesis and have complete anterior displacement beyond the sacral promontory; this has been referred to as "spondyloptosis" (24) or a Grade 5 spondylolisthesis and is rare. (Fig. 5.12) A percentage of displacement may alternatively be used to grade the degree of anterolisthesis and is considered more accurate than the Meyerding method.

In the developing child with a Grade 3 or 4 spondylolisthesis of L5 a trapezoid posterior narrowing or wedging of the L5 vertebral body is often seen. Occasionally,

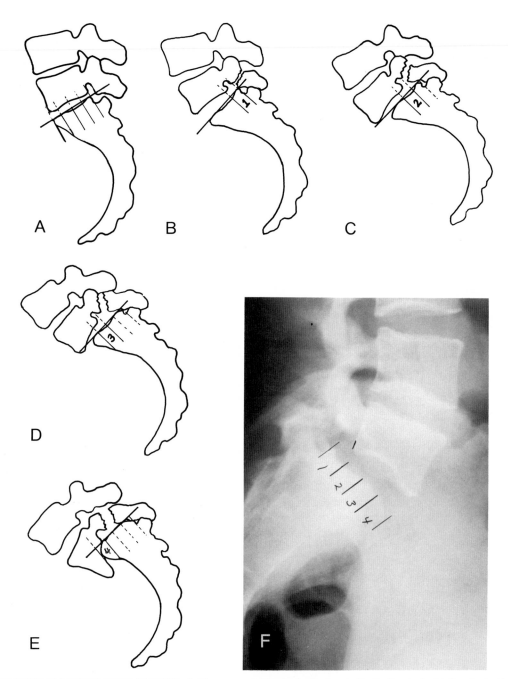

Figure 5.15. MEYERDING CLASSIFICATION SYSTEM. A. The sacral base is divided into four equal segments, and the alignment of the posterior surface of the fifth lumbar body is ascertained. **B.** Grade 1. **C.** Grade 2. **D.** Grade 3. **E.** Grade 4. **F.** An example of a Grade 1 spondylolisthesis.

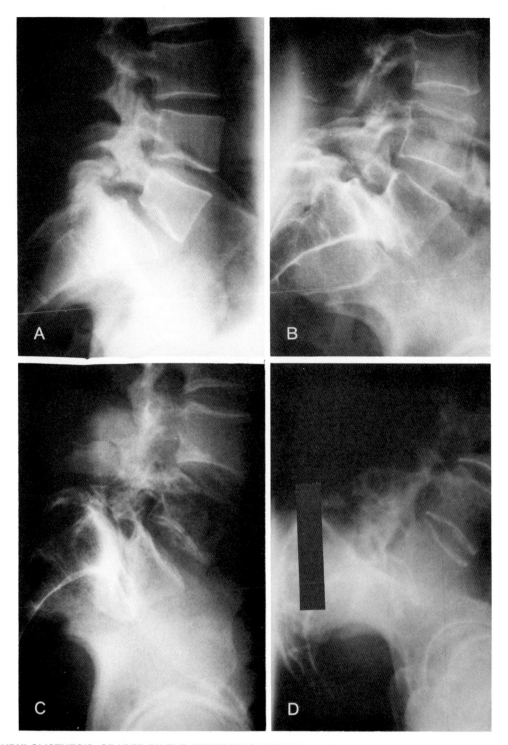

Figure 5.16. SPONDYLOLISTHESIS: GRADED BY THE MEYERDING METHOD. **A.** Grade 1. **B.** Grade 2. **C.** Grade 3. **D.** Grade 4, almost a Grade 5.

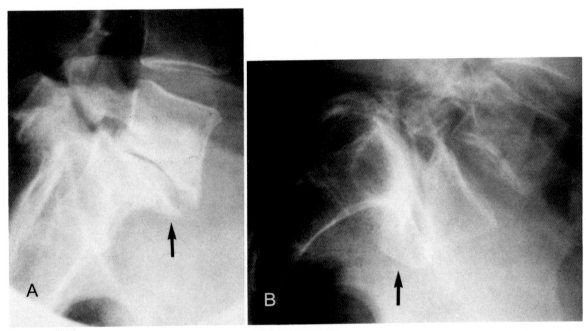

Figure 5.17. SPONDYLOLISTHESIS: BUTTRESSING PHENOMENON OF THE SACRUM. A. Small anterior buttressing bone formation of the sacrum (arrow). **B.** Larger anterior sacral buttress (arrow).

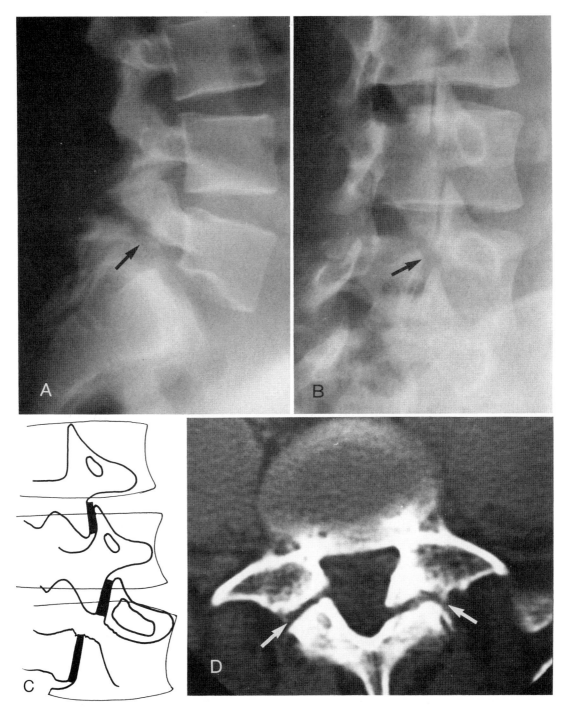

Figure 5.18. CLASSIC SIGNS OF SPONDYLOLISTHESIS. A. Lateral View. Note the pars defects (arrow) and anterior displacement of the L5 vertebra. **B. Oblique View.** The lucent "collar" is clearly visible (arrow). **C. Stepladder Sign.** On an oblique film the alignment of the facet joints changes abruptly at the level of slippage. **D. CT** Scan. The pars defects are readily identified (arrows). Observe the asymmetry of the defects, which is usually present in spondylolysis and may explain why some pars defects are hard to demonstrate on symmetrically positioned oblique lumbar radiographs.

Table 5.4.
Anatomical Counterparts of the Scotty Dog

Eye – Pedicle
Nose – Transverse Process
Ear – Superior Articular Process
Foreleg – Inferior Articular Process
Neck – Pars Interarticularis
Body – Lamina

Unilateral Spondylolysis

Spondylolysis may involve only one pars interarticularis of a single vertebra and may allow a 5 to 10 percent anterolisthesis. Unilateral spondylolysis may result in a compensatory stress hypertrophy of the contralateral pedicle in the region of the pars. (53) This compensatory hypertrophy is manifested radiographically by a contralateral, dense, sclerotic, enlarged pedicle and pars region. (Fig. 5.19) This appearance may mimic osteoid osteoma, osteoblastoma, or osteoblastic metastatic disease, which are common at this site. Agenesis of the pedicle may also show the same stress hypertrophy of the contralateral pedicle and pars region. (Fig. 5.20A and B, 5.21A and B) The key differential sign is the presence of a unilateral pars defect. Regression of the compensatory bone changes may occur, should a stress fracture develop on the same side as the dense pedicle, resulting in bilateral spondylolysis, and thereby equalizing the weightbearing and reducing the stress within the involved spinal motion segment. (37) (Fig. 5.22A–G)

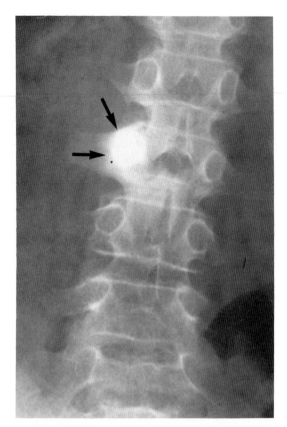

Figure 5.19. OSTEOID OSTEOMA: PEDICLE. Observe the unilateral dense pedicle due to the benign tumor (arrows), osteoid osteoma. (Reprinted with permission: Yochum TR: Osteoid osteoma of the thumb. *ACA Council Roent, Roentgen Brief*, November 1979) (Courtesy of John E. MacRae, DC, DACBR, Toronto, Canada)

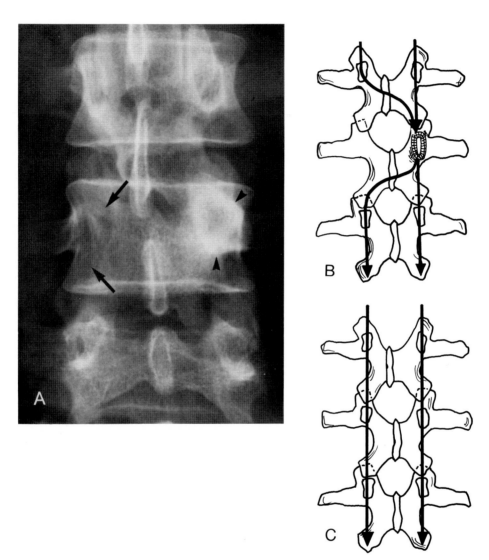

Figure 5.20. AGENETIC PEDICLE: CONTRALATERAL SCLE-ROSIS. A. Note the absence of the pedicle outline (arrows) and the prominence of the contralateral pedicle (arrowheads). **B.** Diagrammatic representation of the redistribution of mechanical forces due to pedicle agenesis. The increased pedicle density and cortical thickness is a stress-induced compensatory change. **C.** Distribution of mechanical forces when the posterior arches are normal. Any disruption in the ring of the neural arch will alter this distribution.

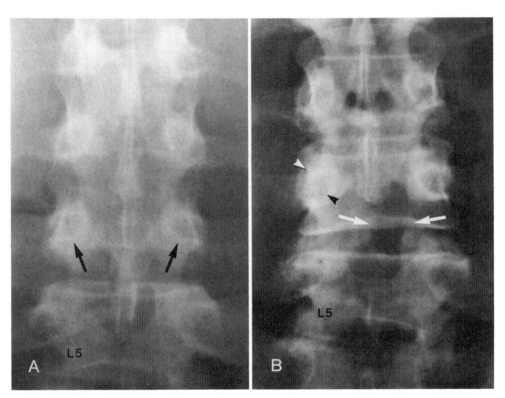

Figure 5.21. PEDICLE STRESS HYPERTROPHY FROM CONTRA-LATERAL LAMINECTOMY. A. Preoperative Film. Note the symmetrically uniform density of both pedicles of the fourth lumbar vertebra (arrows). **B. One-Year Postoperative Film**. Observe the lamina defect (arrows) and the contralateral sclerotic pedicle (arrowheads). (Courtesy of Tyrone Wei, DC, DACBR, Portland, Oregon)

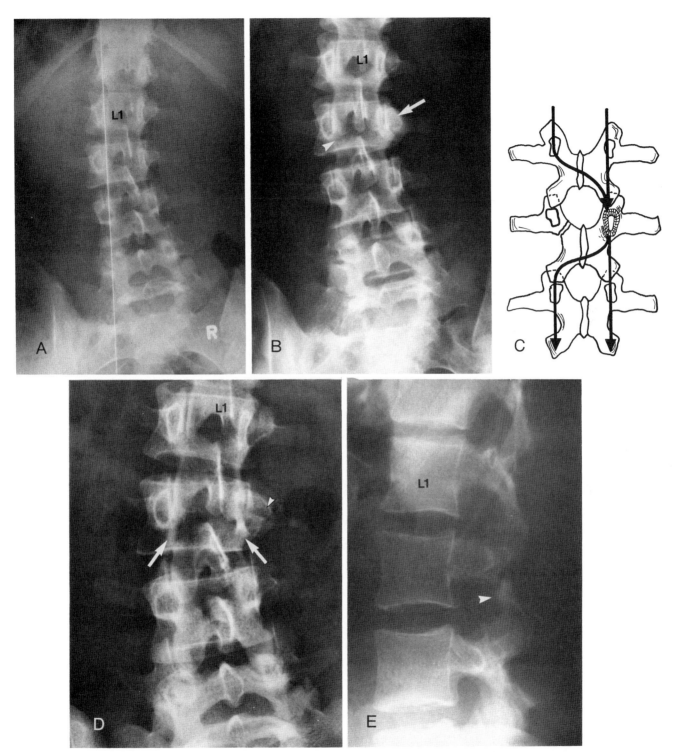

Figure 5.22. SPONDYLOLYSIS: ITS PATHOGENESIS. A young female followed over a 4-year period. **A. Initial Film**. A left rotatory scoliosis is visible, with the second lumbar vertebra showing no pars defects or pedicle abnormalities. **B. Two Years Later**. The scoliosis remains. Observe the second lumbar sclerotic pedicle (arrow) and the left pars interarticularis defect (arrowhead). **C. Diagrammatic Representation.** The mechanism operating to produce the sclerotic pedicle is demonstrated. The hypertrophy is due to the additional stress of the contralateral pars defect. **D. Four Years Later**. The scoliosis persists, but note the resolution of the sclerotic pedicle due to the formation of bilateral pars defects (arrows). Also note the retained hypertrophy of the previously sclerotic pedicle (arrowhead). **E. Lateral Film.** Shows the defect (arrowhead) and no anterolisthesis. **F and G. Oblique Tomograms.** Confirms the bilateral defects (arrows). (Courtesy of Rae Batten, B App Sc (Chiro), Melbourne, Australia) *Comment*: This case demonstrates the important role of stress in the production of a pars defects. (Reprinted with permission: Yochum TR, et al: Reactive sclerosis of a pedicle due to unilateral spondylolysis. *ACA J Chiro, Radiology Corner*, September 1980)

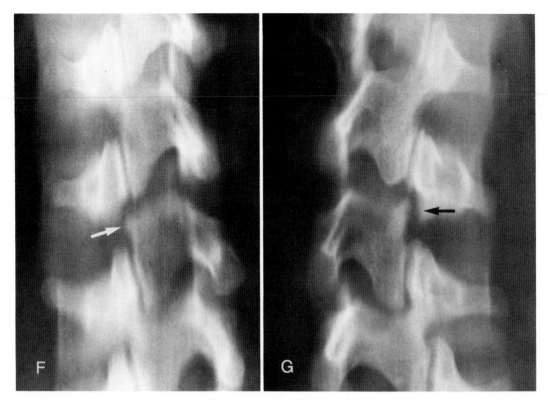

Figure 5.22. F–G

Cervical Spondylolisthesis

Isolated spondylolisthesis in the cervical spine is a rare and unusual disorder. (54) The majority of these cases are discovered incidentally during radiographic studies initiated as a result of antecedent trauma. Cervical spondylolisthesis is most commonly found at the C6 vertebral segment but has also been noted at the C2, C5, and C7 segments. (54) There are only 31 patients with cervical spondylolisthesis reported in the literature. (54) The majority of these cases of cervical spondylolisthesis have occurred in males, suggesting a sex-linked genetic disorder. (55) The most likely etiology for cervical spondylolisthesis is that of congenital dysplasia, (54) which may be manifested radiographically as bilateral hypoplasia of the articular pillars and the pedicles. Some patients may also present with unilateral agenesis of the pedicle, which will allow anterolisthesis of the involved cervical segment to occur. (54) (Fig. 5.23A and B)

It is noteworthy that 50 percent of patients with cervical spondylolisthesis have an associated spina bifida occulta of that particular vertebra. Since spina bifida occulta of the C6 segment is uncommon as an isolated anomaly, its presence should raise some clinical suspicion for associated cervical spondylolisthesis. Flexion and extension radiographs of the cervical spine are recommended to evaluate for motion segment instability. (56) (Table 5.5)

Dysplasia is thought to be the most common cause of cervical spondylolisthesis; there are, however, other conditions which may predispose to anterolisthesis of a cervical body. (54) These include acute fracture, pedicle agenesis, degenerative arthritis, inflammatory arthritides (rheumatoid arthritis, ankylosing spondylitis, psoriatic arthropathy) and pathological bone diseases (infection, neoplasm, and others). (54) It is therefore important to establish the etiology of the anterolisthesis in every patient. (Fig. 5.24A and B)

Table 5.5
Cervical Spondylolisthesis

C6 level anterolisthesis (most common site)
C6 spina bifida
Underdeveloped pillars, pedicles, etc.

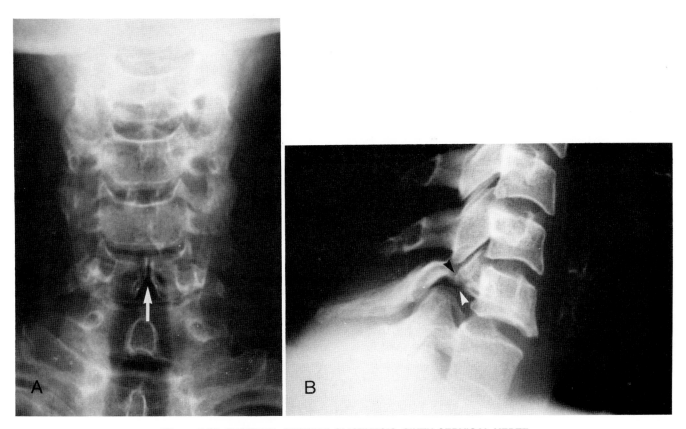

Figure 5.23. CERVICAL SPONDYLOLISTHESIS: SIXTH CERVICAL VERTE-BRA. A. AP View. Note the spina bifida occulta at the sixth cervical segment (arrow). **B. Lateral View**. Almost total agenesis of the sixth articular pillar is apparent (arrowheads), with minimal anterolisthesis of the associated vertebral body. (Courtesy of James F. Winterstein, DC, DACBR, Chicago, Illinois)

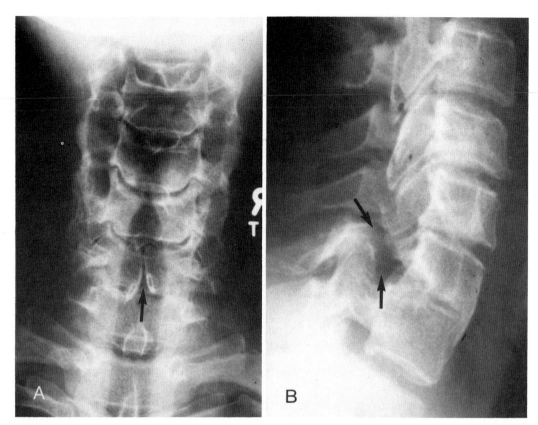

Figure 5.24. CERVICAL SPONDYLOLISTHESIS: MISDIAGNOSIS. A 45-year-old female had x-rays following a motor vehicle accident. A diagnosis of fracture and dislocation at the sixth cervical level was made, and a surgical fusion was performed. **A. AP View**. Note the spina bifida occulta at the sixth cervical segment (arrow). **B. Lateral View**. There is partial agenesis of the sixth cervical articular pillar (arrows). A complete interbody fusion has been performed between the sixth and seventh cervical segments. **Comment**: The findings of a spina bifida and absence of the pillar suggest a congenital rather than a post-traumatic deformity. (Courtesy of Dennis M. Richards, DC, Tweed Heads, New South Wales, Australia)

Treatment and Prognosis of Spondylolisthesis

CONSERVATIVE MANAGEMENT

Considerable controversy exists concerning the treatment and management of patients with spondylolisthesis. The conservative medical approach to treatment includes the following: restriction of physical activities, abdominal and back muscle-strengthening exercises, bedrest, low-back bracing, and non-narcotic analgesics. (44)

An additional conservative approach which has proved beneficial for the treatment and management of patients with symptomatic spondylolisthesis is chiropractic spinal manipulative therapy. (40) Since a large majority of patients with spondylolisthesis have an associated hyperlordosis, most of the symptoms and back pain are associated with a facet syndrome and/or sacroiliac fixation rather than being directly related to the presence of spondylolisthesis. (40,57)

According to Illi, (58) restoration of normal sacroiliac joint mobility may decrease the strain on the lower lumbar spine, thereby giving patients relief from lower back pain which he thought was an indirect effect of the lumbar spondylolisthesis. Cassidy, Potter, and Kirkaldy-Willis (40) performed chiropractic spinal manipulative therapy on patients who had varying degrees of spondylolisthesis. They found that 80 percent of these patients responded favorably to specific manipulation of the sacroiliac joint or the lumbar zygapophyseal joints above the segment with the pars defects, thus avoiding direct manipulation of the area of spondylolisthesis. (40) They concluded that spinal manipulation offers rapid symptomatic relief to many patients with back pain who coincidentally have spondylolisthesis.

INSTABILITY EVALUATION

Instability is defined as excessive mobility of the spondylolisthetic segment. In the context of this discussion the term does not imply altered biomechanical function at other motion segments.

In order to evaluate the stability of the spondylolisthetic segment, lateral lumbar flexion and extension erect stress radiographs should be performed. (Fig. 5.25A–C) Although conflicting views exist among clinical authorities on the definition of motion segment instability, additional displacement of the spondylolisthetic segment of 4-mm or greater is considered to have a poor prognosis with conservative treatment. (59) This 4-mm displace-

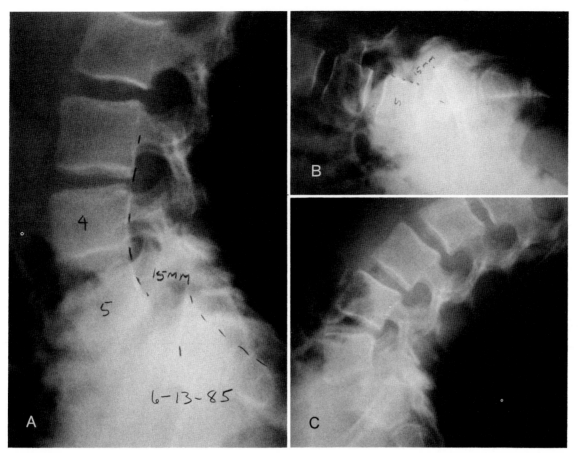

Figure 5.25. SPONDYLOLISTHESIS WITH STABILITY ON ERECT FLEXION AND EXTENSION RADIOGRAPHS. A 9-year-old female gymnast who fell was radiographed and found to have a pre-existing spondylolisthesis. **A. Lateral View.** A 15-mm displacement is evident at the fifth lumbar vertebra. **B and C. Flexion (B) and Exten-** sion (C) Views. These views fail to show any alteration in the degree of displacement of the fifth lumbar vertebra. *Comment*: This case demonstrates the unlikelihood of further progression based on the stability exhibited even after trauma. (Courtesy of Richard Krauss, DC, FACO, Phoenix, Arizona)

ment may occur either anteriorly or posteriorly from the position seen on the erect neutral lateral lumbar film. When vertebral movement of 4-mm or more in either direction is present, the segment may be considered unstable and likely to be symptomatic.

Limitation of physical activity in the growing child under the age of 10 with spondylolysis and/or spondylolisthesis is appropriate. When patients present with back pain several years after the development of their spondylolisthesis, this is unlikely to be the cause of their pain. Since back pain can become a major limiting factor in an athlete's continuing participation in rigorous sports, the clinical management should not be based on the mere presence of spondylolysis and/or spondylolisthesis alone. (44) No evidence presently exists to support the theory that cessation of sports activity will prevent the development of more serious complications of spondylolisthesis; therefore, the management of athletes should be based upon their clinical symptoms rather than the presence of spondylolysis or spondylolisthesis. (60) Athletes with spondylolisthesis should be allowed to continue to participate in sports, since there is no evidence that they are any more susceptible to back injuries than athletes without spondylolisthesis, and since cessation of sports may needlessly create a "spondylo-athletic invalid." (60)

SURGICAL MANAGEMENT

A small percentage of patients with spondylolisthesis will demonstrate biomechanical instability on erect posture radiological stress studies. Instability is defined as an increase in anterolisthesis or retrolisthesis of 4-mm or more noted on standing flexion or extension lateral lumbar radiographs when compared with a neutral lateral view. These patients may require surgical arthrodesis, with bilateral vertebral body or transverse process fusions being the most current surgical approaches. (15,61) Surgical intervention should only be used when patients fail to respond to thorough conservative management and show associated signs of biomechanical instability. Those individuals with progressive neurological deficits should also be considered surgical candidates. Within these specific guidelines, arthrodesis is usually successful in the reduction of the patient's back pain.

Some patients who have undergone successful spinal fusion for spondylolisthesis may develop severe back pain months or years after the spinal surgery. (1) In these cases the development of a stress or fatigue fracture of the pars at the end vertebra or at a neighboring mobile vertebra, as the result of increased stress placed upon these structures, is referred to as spondylolisthesis acquisita. (1)

Diagnosis requires flexion and extension lumbar radiographs and occasionally tomography. This fracture may heal with prolonged immobilization, but it is best treated by extending the fusion mass to include the affected vertebra. (1)

It should be emphasized that a very small percentage of young patients will not limit their physical activities, may be unresponsive to spinal manipulative therapy or other conservative measures, and may require surgical stabilization. However, Wiltse (62) has stated that "to operate on a child simply because he has spondylolisthesis, without other reasons, would be wrong," and we applaud his view.

There is no guaranteed reduction of symptoms as a result of spinal fusion; therefore, the physician and patient should have exhausted all conservative procedures prior to surgical intervention. (63) The detailed surgical treatment and management of spondylolisthesis is beyond the scope of this work, and the reader is referred to the following references: 1, 13, 17, 32, 43, and 62.

Degenerative Spondylolisthesis

The persistently symptomatic patient with spondylolisthesis usually has a degenerative type (Type III) rather than the more common isthmic variety (Type IIA). Most of these patients also have spinal stenosis of a degenerative nature which may respond quite readily to surgical decompression, with or without fusion. (64)

PRE-EMPLOYMENT X-RAY SCREENING

In many countries, including the United States, pre-employment low back radiographs are used to screen employees for potential risk of injury in the workplace. Often, patients are denied employment or promotion because of the radiographic presence of an asymptomatic lumbar spondylolysis and/or spondylolisthesis. (65,66) Based on the performance of the athletes in the previously cited studies, this attitude may not be justified. (25,28,44,45) We found no studies which demonstrate that workers with spondylolysis or spondylolisthesis involved in the heavy labor sector of industry are at any greater risk from back injuries or have any greater loss of work time than those employees without spondylolysis or spondylolisthesis. A plethora of personal opinions exist to the contrary; these opinions, however, cannot be supported by documented clinical case studies or research data. It is our opinion that refusal of employment based on the existence of spondylolysis and/or spondylolisthesis is as antiquated as the procedure of pre-employment x-ray screening, which is now receiving considerably less emphasis. (65,66)

Adults in the work force with coincidental asymptomatic spondylolysis and/or spondylolisthesis should not be discriminated against in employment opportunities until further studies clearly define the true etiology of low back pain in patients with spondylolysis and/or spondylolisthesis.

IMPAIRMENT RATING

A similar injustice in regard to spondylolysis and spondylolisthesis exists within the current *Guides to the Evaluation of Permanent Impairment* published by the American Medical Association. (67) For example, a rating of 20 percent whole person impairment is given persons with a Grade 1 or 2 spondylolysis and spondylolisthesis with aggravation, persistent muscle spasm, rigidity, and pain aggravated by trauma. For Grades 3 and 4 spondylolisthesis with the same clinical presentation a 30 percent whole person impairment is recommended. (67) These ratings seem too high and are based to a large extent on the radiographic presence of spondylolysis and/or spondylolisthesis and neglect clinical assessment of (1) decreased physical range of motion or (2) radiographic stress studies (instability evaluation). Similar neglect of occupational assessment exists in spondylolysis and/or spondylolisthesis patients. The impairment ratings are especially high when compared with the ratings for intervertebral disc lesions in either the operated or nonoperated case. A clinically established disc derangement with residuals only receives 5 percent (position of function), and operated, disc removed without residuals receives 5 percent. (67) Thus, revision of these ratings as they relate to spondylolisthesis is needed.

Summary

Although for many years the true etiology of spondylolysis and/or spondylolisthesis has been unclear, stress fracture has emerged as the most likely cause. Some populations demonstrate an apparent genetic predisposition to spondylolysis. The relationship between spondylolisthesis and back pain appears to encompass an unclearly defined primary cause for the pain. A small percentage of patients may have instability or spinal stenosis (degenerative spondylolisthesis) which eventually may require surgical intervention. Most, however, will respond to conservative care.

Many athletes with spondylolisthesis compete in rigorous sports without any reduction in their performance or any greater prevalence of back pain, as compared with controls. (44,60) Therefore, participation in sports should not be discouraged unless biomechanical instability, spinal stenosis, or neurological deficit is present. The use of pre-employment low back x-rays as a screening measure for industry is antiquated. There is no evidence to support the premise that a patient (over the age of 18 years) with a spondylolysis and/or spondylolisthesis is unable to perform heavy manual labor or is at greater risk of injury. Until data become available to contradict this premise, these patients should not be discriminated against in their employment opportunities. Additionally, the *Guides to the Evaluation of Permanent Impairment* published by the American Medical Association (67) provide too high an impairment rating for patients with spondylolisthesis (Grade 1 through 4) who have persistent back pain which is usually coincidentally associated with their occupations. Therefore, these guides need revision in this area.

CAPSULE SUMMARY. Spondylolysis and Spondylolisthesis

DEFINITIONS

Spondylolysis describes an interruption of the pars interarticularis; this may be either unilateral or bilateral. The term spondylolysis is derived from two Greek roots, "spondylos," meaning vertebra, and "lysis," meaning a dissolution; a loosing, setting free, releasing.

Spondylolisthesis is defined as an anterior displacement of a vertebral body in relationship to the segment immediately below. The Greek origin of this word is "spondylos," meaning vertebra, and "olisthesis," referring to displacement. Spondylolisthesis may be associated with defects in the pars interarticularis (spondylolytic spondylolisthesis) but may occur without them (nonspondylolytic spondylolisthesis).

Prespondylolisthesis represents the presence of spondylolysis without forward vertebral displacement. This term is somewhat confusing since it implies that displacement will necessarily occur. It is suggested that this term be discarded.

GENERAL CONSIDERATIONS

The first recorded article relating to spondylolisthesis was in 1782 by a Belgian obstetrician, Herbinaux.

An historical overview as well as a new perspective of spondylolysis and/or spondylolisthesis is offered.

INCIDENCE

A prevalence of 5–7 percent is found in the white population, with a much higher figure being noted in highly active individuals and athletes.

An explanation regarding the true reason for a 40 percent prevalence in Stewart's studies of the Northern Eskimo is still not available. We offer a hypothesis related to the early upright posture in the infant.

ETIOLOGY

The etiology of this peculiar disorder is now clearly classified, with the majority of these lesions being acquired stress fractures.

A small percentage are dysplastic in origin.

Since this lesion has been reported only in humans (except for one gorilla), the upright posture coupled with inappropriate stresses would appear to be a strong etiological factor.

CLASSIFICATION

Type I: Dysplastic: A congenital abnormality in the upper sacrum or the neural arch of L5, allowing displacement to occur.

Type II: Isthmic:
(a) a lytic or fatigue fracture of the pars
(b) elongated but intact pars
(c) acute fracture of the pars.

Type III: Degenerative: Secondary to longstanding degenerative arthrosis of the zygapophyseal joints and discovertebral articulation.

Type IV: Traumatic: Secondary to fractures in the area of the neural arch other than the pars interarticularis.

Type V: Pathological: In conjunction with generalized or localized bone disease (e.g., Paget's disease, metastatic bone disease, osteopetrosis, etc.).

CLINICAL FEATURES

A very large percentage of the patients with spondylolysis and/or spondylolisthesis never develop back pain.

Those patients who suffer from back pain usually have a separate cause for their symptoms.

Progression of displacement seldom occurs after the age of 18.

It is thought by many that by the age of 10 the greatest degree of displacement has been obtained.

RADIOLOGICAL FEATURES

A Bowline of Brailsford.

The inverted Napoleon's hat sign or the Gendarme's cap.

Meyerding method for determination of the degree of anterolisthesis (Grades 1, 2, 3, and 4).

A trapezoid posterior narrowing of L5 body, creating a doming of the anterior surface of the sacrum.

A radiolucent defect in the pars interarticularis is visualized optimally on oblique lumbar radiographs and referred to as the collar or broken neck of the Scotty Dog.

The stepladder sign is produced by malalignment of the zygapophyseal joints at the involved level of spondylolisthesis.

UNILATERAL SPONDYLOLYSIS

Unilateral spondylolysis often creates compensatory stress hypertrophy of the contralateral pedicle in the pars and pedicle region.

The sclerotic enlarged pedicle and pars region may simulate an osteoid osteoma, osteoblastoma, or an osteoblastic metastatic deposit.

A key differential clue is to search for the unilateral pars defect opposite the sclerotic pedicle.

CERVICAL SPONDYLOLISTHESIS

This is a rare and unusual disorder.

The majority of these lesions present asymptomatically.

It is most commonly found at the C6 vertebral segment; however, it has been noted at C2, C5, and C7.

The defect is nearly always bilateral and is most frequently found in males.

The most likely etiology is congenital agenesis or dysplasia of the pedicle.

Approximately 50 percent of the patients with cervical spondylolysis have an associated spina bifida occulta of the involved vertebra.

This lesion should not be misinterpreted as a fracture, and the presence of spina bifida occulta at C6 confirms its congenital etiology.

TREATMENT AND PROGNOSIS

Medical management is conservative initially, although surgical fusion is still being recommended by many orthopedic surgeons.

A more conservative approach, including chiropractic spinal manipulative therapy, has been found beneficial in managing patients' low back pain with the presence of spondylolysis or spondylolisthesis.

Caution is advised to those patients who consider surgery without exhausting all conservative measures first.

Some innovative thoughts are presented concerning the ability of patients with spondylolisthesis to continue to participate in rigorous sports and function in a work place requiring heavy manual labor.

An injustice in regard to spondylolysis and spondylolisthesis exists within the current *Guides to the Evaluation of Permanent Impairment* published by the American Medical Association. Revision of these ratings as they relate to spondylolisthesis is needed.

REFERENCES

1. Gehweiler JA, Osborne R, Becker, RF: *The Radiology of Vertebral Trauma*, Philadelphia, WB Saunders, 1980.
2. Herbinaux G: *Traite sur divers laborieux, et sur les polypes de la matrice*, Bruxelles, JL DeBoubers, 1782.
3. Kilian HF: Spondylolysteses gravissimae causa nuper detecta. In: Commentatio anatomica obstetricia. Bonnae Lit. C. Geirgii, 1854, cited in *Clin Radiol* 20:315, 1969.
4. Robert: *Monatsschrift fur Geburtskunde und Frauenkrankheiten*, 5:81, 1855.
5. Lambl W: *Beiträge zur geburkskunde und gynackologie*, von FWV Scanzoni, 1858.
6. Neugebauer FL: Neuer beitrag zur aetiologie und causistik der spondylolisthesis. *Arch Gynaekol* 25:182, 1895. Translated in part in *Clin Orthop* 117:4, 1976.
7. McKee BM, Alexander WJ, Dunbar JS: Spondylolysis and spondylolisthesis in children: A review. *J Can Assoc Radiol* 22:100, 1971.
8. Taillard WF: Etiology of spondylolisthesis. *Clin Orthop* 117:30, 1976.
9. Moreton RD: Spondylolysis. *JAMA* 195:671, 1966.
10. Stewart TD: The age incidence of neural arch defects in Alaskan natives, considered from the standpoint of etiology. *J Bone Joint Surg (Am)* 35:937, 1953.
11. Kettlekamp DB, Wright DG: Spondylolysis in the Alaskan eskimo. *J Bone Joint Surg (Am)* 53:563, 1971.
12. Rowe GG, Roche MB: The etiology of separate neural arch. *J Bone Joint Surg (Am)* 35:102, 1953.
13. Wiltse LL: The etiology of spondylolisthesis. *J Bone Joint Surg (Am)* 44:539, 1962.
14. Borkow SE, Kleiger B: Spondylolisthesis in the newborn: A case report. *Clin Orthop* 81:73, 1971.
15. Turner RH, Bianco AJ: Spondylolysis and spondylolisthesis in children and teen-agers. *J Bone Joint Surg (Am)* 53:1298, 1971.
16. Batts M Jr.: The etiology of spondylolisthesis. *J Bone Joint Surg (Am)* 21:879, 1939.
17. Fredrickson BE, Baker D, McHollick WJ, et al: The natural history of spondylolysis and spondylolisthesis. *J Bone Joint Surg (Am)* 66:699, 1984.
18. Kleinberg S: Spondylolisthesis in an infant. *J Bone Joint Surg (Am)* 16:441, 1934.
19. Laurent L, Emola S: Spondylolisthesis in children and adolescents. *Acta Orthop Scand* 31:45, 1961.
20. Wiltse LL, Widell EH, Jackson DW: Fatigue fracture: The basic lesion in isthmic spondylolisthesis. *J Bone Joint Surg (Am)* 57:17, 1975.
21. Cyron BM, Hutton WC: The fatigue strength of the lumbar neural arch in spondylolysis. *J Bone Joint Surg (Br)* 60:462, 1978.
22. Schmorl G, Junghans H: *The Human Spine in Health and Disease.*, ed 2, New York, Grune and Stratton, 1971.
23. Rosenberg NJ, Bargar WL, Friedman B: The incidence of spondylolysis and spondylolisthesis in nonambulatory patients. *Spine* 6:35, 1981.
24. Newman PH, Stone KH: The etiology of spondylolisthesis. *J Bone Joint Surg (Br)* 45:39, 1963.
25. Rossi F: Spondylolysis, spondylolisthesis and sports. *Sports Med* 18:317, 1978.
26. Gainor BJ, Hagen RJ, Allen WC: Biomechanics of the spine in the polevaulter as related to spondylolysis. *Am J Sport Med* 11:53, 1983.
27. Raynal L, Coaard M, Elbanna S: Contribution a l'etude de la spondylolyse traumatique. *Acta Orthop Belg* 43:653, 1977.
28. Kono S, Hayashi M, Kashahara T: A study on the etiology of spondylolysis with reference to athletic activities (Japanese). *J Jpn Orthop Assoc* 49:125, 1975.
29. Schulitz KP, Niethard FU: Strain on the interarticular stress distribution—measurements regarding the development of spondylolysis. *Arch Orthop Trauma Surg* 96:197, 1980.
30. Saha MM, Bhardwaj OP, Gupta A, et al: Osteopetrosis with spondylolysis: Four cases in one family. *Br Radiol* 43:738, 1970.
31. Wiltse LL, Newman PH, Macnab I: Classification of spondylolysis and spondylolisthesis. *Clin Orthop* 117:23, 1976.
32. Moe JH, Winter RB, Bradford DS, Lonstein JE: *Scoliosis and Other Spinal Deformities*, Philadelphia, WB Saunders, 1978.
33. Macnab I: Spondylolisthesis with an intact neural arch - so-called pseudospondylolisthesis. *J Bone Joint Surg (Br)* 32:325, 1950.
34. Rosenberg MJ: Degenerative spondylolisthesis. *Clin Orthop* 117:112, 1976.
35. Allbrook B: Movements of the lumbar spine column. *J Bone Joint Surg (Br)* 39:339, 1957.
36. Pease CN, Najat H: Spondylolisthesis in children. *Clin Orthop* 52:187, 1967.
37. Yochum TR et al: Reactive sclerosis of a pedicle due to unilateral spondylolysis—a case study. *ACA J Chiro, Radiology Corner*, September 1980.
38. Friberg S: Studies on spondylolisthesis. *Acta Chir Scand* 82 (Suppl. 55), 1939.
39. Albanese M, Pizzutillo PD: Family study of spondylolysis and spondylolisthesis. *J Pediatr Orthop* 2:496, 1982.
40. Cassidy JD, Potter GE, Kirkaldy-Willis WH: Manipulative management of back pain in patients with spondylolisthesis. *J Can Chirop Assoc* 22:15, 1978.
41. Blackburne JS, Velikas EP: Spondylolisthesis in children and adults. *Proceedings of the Royal Society of Medicine* 70:421, 1977.
42. Monticelli G, Ascani E: Spondylolysis and spondylolisthesis. *Acta Orthop Scand* 46:498, 1975.
43. Turek SL: *Orthopedic Principals and Their Application*, ed 4, Philadephia, JB Lippincott, 1984.
44. Semon RL, Spengler D: Significance of lumbar spondylolysis in college football players. *Spine* 6:172, 1981.
45. Ferguson RJ, McMasters JH, Stanitski CL: Low back pain in college football linemen. *Am J Sports Med* 2:63; 1974.
46. Zatkin HR: *The Roentgen Diagnosis of Trauma*, Chicago, Year Book Medical Publishers, 1965.
47. Ravichandran G: A radiological sign in spondylolisthesis. *AJR* 134:113, 1980.
48. Libson E, Bloom RA: Anteroposterior angulated view—A new radiographic technique for the evaluation of spondylolysis. *Radiology* 149:315, 1983.
49. Meyerding HW: Low backache and sciatic pain associated with spondylolisthesis and protruded intervertebral disc. *J Bone Joint Surg (Am)* 23:461, 1941.
50. El-Khoury GY, Yousefzadeh DK, Kathol MH, et al: Normal roentgen variant: Pseudospondylolysis. *Radiology* 139:72, 1981.
51. Kohler A: *Borderlands of the Normal and Early Pathologic in Skeletal Roentgenology*, ed 3, New York, Edited by EA Zimmer, Grune and Stratton, 1968.
52. Edeiken J, Hodes PJ: *Roentgen Diagnosis of Diseases of Bone*, Baltimore, Williams & Wilkins, 1973.
53. Wilkinson RH, Hall JE: The sclerotic pedicle: Tumor or pseudotumor? *Radiology* 111:683, 1974.
54. Schwartz AM, Wechsler RJ, Landy MD, et al: Posterior arch defects of the cervical spine. *Skel Radiol* 8:135, 1982.
55. Bellamy R, Lieber A, Smith SD: Congenital spondylolisthesis of the sixth cervical vertebra. *J Bone Joint Surg (Am)* 56:22, 1974.
56. Niemeyer T, Penning L: Functional roentgenographic examination in a case of cervical spondylolisthesis. *J Bone Joint Surg (Am)* 45:1671, 1973.
57. Mooney V, Robertson J: The facet syndrome. *Clin Orthop* 115:157, 1976.
58. Illi FW: *The Vertebral Column: Lifeline of the Body*, Chicago, National College of Chiropractic, 1951.
59. Nachemson A: Lumbar spine instability—A critical update and symposium summary. *Spine* 10:290, 1985.
60. Knight NA, Burleson RJ, Higginbotham JA: Spondylolysis of the L2 vertebra in the female gymnast—A case report. *J Med Assoc State Alabama*, December 1977.
61. Wiltse LL: Etiology of spondylolisthesis. *Clin Orthop* 10:48, 1957.
62. Wiltse LL, Hutchinson RH: Surgical treatment of spondylolisthesis. *Clin Orthop* 35:116, 1964.
63. DeWald RL, Faut MM, Taddonio RF, et al: Severe lumbosacral spondylolisthesis in adolescents and children. *J Bone Joint Surg (Am)* 63:292, 1981.
64. Feffer HL, Weisel SW, Rothman RH, et al: Degenerative spondylolisthesis—To fuse or not to fuse. *Spine* 10:287, 1985.
65. Frymoyer JW, Newberg A, Pope MH, et al: Spine radiographs in patients with low-back pain—An epidemiological study in men. *J Bone Joint Surg (Am)* 66:1048, 1984.
66. Magora A, Schwartz A: Relation between low back pain and X-ray changes (lysis and olisthesis). *Scand J Rehab Med* 12:47, 1980.
67. American Medical Association: *Guides to the Evaluation of Permanent Impairment*, ed 2, Chicago, American Medical Association, 1984.

Diagnostic Imaging of Spinal Stenosis and Intervertebral Disc Disease

JOSEPH W. HOWE
TERRY R. YOCHUM
LINDSAY J. ROWE

Introduction

SPINAL STENOSIS

Back and neck pain are among the most common of human ailments. Low back pain, with or without leg pain, will affect most people at least once in their lifetime. Neck and shoulder pain, headache of cervical origin, and other neck-related problems are not far behind low back pain as to their incidence. Despite the widespread incidence of these complaints and the considerable associated disabilities, they remain enigmas both as to cause and treatment.

A discussion of the complex etiological factors involved and the many mechanisms which interact in the production of spinal-related pain far exceeds the scope of this presentation. One area integrally related to such problems, the several causes of spinal stenosis, is the focus of this chapter.

Definition

The word "stenosis" has been defined as narrowing of a hollow tubular structure, (1) although more sophisticated definitions have been offered. (2) This discussion will consider spinal stenosis to include any narrowing of the spinal canal or the various tunnels through which nerves and other structures communicate with that canal, i.e., the lateral recesses and neural foramina (which are in fact nerve root tunnels). Stenosis of these tubular areas may be from bone, soft tissue, or both. The spinal canal and associated tunnels have characteristics peculiar to each spinal area caused by the specific morphology of each region and their contents. While under most circumstances lesions of the nucleus pulposus are considered as a separate entity from spinal stenosis, using the definition above, for purposes of this presentation, they will be considered as one aspect of the spinal stenosis syndromes.

SCOPE OF THIS PRESENTATION

Since Mixter and Barr, in 1934, (3) most of the emphasis relating to low back and leg pain has been focused upon the intervertebral disc, and particularly toward herniation of the nucleus pulposus. There have been those like Mooney and Robertson (4) who have continued to emphasize the role of the facets. Recently, Kirkaldy-Willis and Hill, (5,6) among others, have redirected attention to other associated factors such as intersegmental dysfunction, lateral recess stenosis, posterior joint problems, and other aspects of spinal degenerative disease which are part of the mosaic of low back and leg pain syndromes. Chiropractors and other manipulators have had historic interest in these conditions and have enjoyed successes in treating many patients with such afflictions. Successes and failures from conservative treatment, orthodox medical treatment, bedrest, surgery, back schools, and other therapeutic approaches have done little to clarify the problem. Instead, there continue to be questions as to relationships of pain and discomfort to the anatomical and pathophysiological circumstances which may or may not be found in those suffering from these complaints. The situation is similar relative to the cervical spine and neck-related symptoms—indeed, to back pain as a whole.

In this chapter we will deal with radiological approaches which attempt to shed light upon some of the factors associated with pain of spinal origin, realizing that 1) there is much that is not known about the subject, 2) there is significant question as to the relationship of many of the findings from radiological studies to the cause of pain, and 3) the various imaging procedures presently available, while some are quite sophisticated, are still not necessarily sensitive for detection of early disease.

COMPUTERIZED TOMOGRAPHY AND MAGNETIC RESONANCE IMAGING

In the material to follow there will be considerable reference to studies done by computed tomography (CT)

and magnetic resonance imaging (MRI). For that reason, a brief review of these modalities is offered. Many of the terms which will be used in the discussions of CT and MRI may not be familiar to some readers. Because of this, a glossary of terms is supplied.

CT and MRI Glossary

Tomography (Body Section Radiography). By moving the x-ray tube and detector synchronously, while the body remains stationary, a thin section (slice) of the body remains in focus, with the remaining structures being blurred. This allows examination of thin sections of the body as though they were removed from adjacent structures.

Scanner. The term used to describe a CT or MRI unit.

Control Console. The part of a CT or MRI unit where the controls and viewing screen (CRT) are located. (Fig. 6.1) The console usually has two CRT's—one to display the image(s), and one which shows the data relating to the patient and examination parameters. There is also a keyboard with standard and special features which allows manipulation of the computer and other controls relating to both the radiological parameters and alteration of the image characteristics. A trackball to control the cursor and other functions is a usual part of the console.

Gantry. The "doughnut" or circular enclosure which houses the x-ray tube or magnet and detectors. In a CT scan, the patient is placed into the gantry on a mechanized table which controls his/her passage through the x-ray beam. For an MRI scan, the patient is stationary in the magnetic field. (Fig. 6.2, 6.3)

Generation (1st, 2nd, 3rd, 4th). The original devices (CT or MRI) are called 1st generation. As significant alterations in the mechanisms and characteristics are developed, each succeeding upgrade is given the next generation number. (Fig. 6.4)

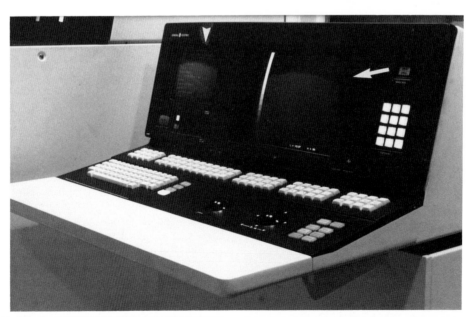

Figure 6.1. CONSOLE OF A COMPUTERIZED TOMOGRAPHIC SCANNER. There are two cathode ray tubes (CRT): one used to display the CT image (arrow), the other to display patient data and examination parameters (arrowhead). A modified typewriter-like key-board and many special function keys are available to manipulate the computer, which controls the x-ray machine within the gantry, the table that is indexed to the gantry, image characteristics, and other functions.

Cathode Ray Tube (CRT). A viewing device on the control console, essentially like a TV screen or the viewer of a personal computer.

Cursor. A small indicator seen on the CRT which can be manipulated from the keyboard and/or trackball. The cursor is used to mark areas, make measurements, and/ or enter data of various kinds onto the image.

Detector Array. The x-ray beam is intercepted by a series of detectors which measure the energy deposited within them. That energy is the product of the number and energy of the individual photons which reach the detector. The configuration of the array of detectors and the characteristics of the x-ray beam are primary differences between the several generations of CT scanners. (Fig. 6.4)

Pixel. Each square in the image matrix is called a pixel (picture element). A pixel represents the end area of a voxel. (Fig. 6.5)

Voxel. The representation of a tiny elongated block of tissue is called a voxel (volume measurement). (Fig. 6.5)

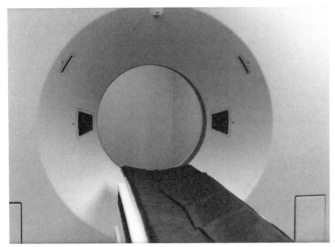

Figure 6.2. GANTRY OF A COMPUTERIZED TOMOGRAPHIC SCANNER. The gantry or "doughnut" houses the x-ray tube and detectors. (Fig. 6.4) The table is padded for patient comfort and can be adjusted in height. It moves in and out of the gantry, being indexed to the gantry so that its movements can be precisely controlled. This allows the location of each tomographic section to be exactly known. Patient placement within the gantry is aided by laser locators which mark the area of the beam.

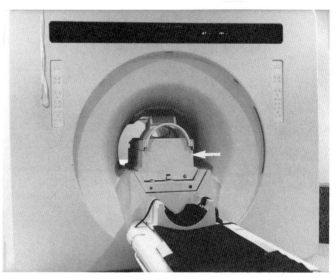

Figure 6.3. GANTRY OF A MAGNETIC RESONANCE SCANNER. This device somewhat resembles a CT gantry but is much larger since it will allow most of a human body to be within its "doughnut." Shown within the bore of the gantry in this illustration is the device used for imaging the head and neck (arrow). The table of an MR scanner does not need to be indexed to the gantry, as is that of a CT unit, since the patient is stationary during an MR examination. It must be adjustable, however, so that the patient may be properly placed.

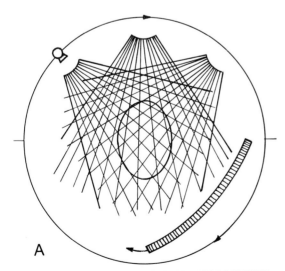

A

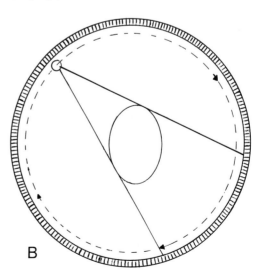

B

Figure 6.4. SCHEMATIC REPRESENTATIONS OF THE GANTRIES OF THIRD AND FOURTH GENERATION CT SCANNERS. A. Third Generation CT Gantry. The x-ray tube and detector array are synchronized and move through an arc for each tomographic section (slice). Collimation to a thin fan beam limits the radiation as closely as possible to the size and thickness of the detector array. Further collimation at the detectors controls scatter to the detectors to enhance image quality. **B. Fourth Generation CT Gantry**. In these scanners the tube moves through an arc for each tomographic section, but the array of detectors is fixed and is circumferential to the gantry. This has the advantage of elimination of moving parts but requires many more detectors.

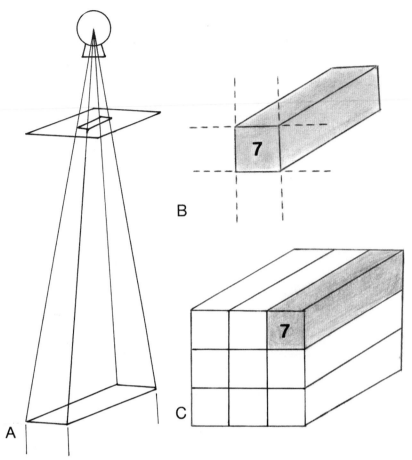

Figure 6.5. IMAGE COMPONENTS.   A. Collimation of the Fan X-Ray Beam. Precise collimation is employed so that a very thin fan beam of x-rays is used to scan thin sections of the body.   **B. Voxels and Pixels**. At each detector the photons intercepted by the detectors represent a small block of tissue, a voxel (volume measurement). The shaded block represents a voxel. Its end, the square containing the number 7, represents a pixel (picture element).   **C. Composite of Voxels and Pixels**. The CT image is formed from the data received by the computer from the detectors and is displayed on the CRT screen as the composite of pixels. Each pixel represents the end section of a voxel, which represents a tissue block.

CT Numbers. Usual radiographic images cannot show density differences of less than 10 percent. CT images, however, can be manipulated to be much more sensitive. A CT image is formed by assigning densities to numbers generated by the computer in response to the data it receives from the detectors. Each pixel is assigned a number in accordance with the flux of photons it receives and the image is formed from the composite of pixels. (Fig. 6.6) A gray scale image on the CRT is generated by assigning specific densities to these numbers.

Hounsfield Units.   These are values assigned to CT numbers. The usual scale of these numbers is from -1000 (air) to +1000 (dense bone), with water representing 0. An extended scale is available on many of the more recent scanners in order to increase the gray scale and thus display a greater range of densities. Differences in scanners and technical parameters makes comparison of these units inexact from one scanner to another, and even from one examination to another on the same scanner.

Windows (Window Width and Window Level).   The range of CT numbers selected for a specific gray scale amplification is called "window width." Window width can be adjusted by increments from full scale to a single unit. "Window level" is another term used which designates a central point within a specific window width. By computer manipulation of window width and level, the densities of structures shown in any CT image can be altered to produce the desired contrast.

Reconstruction (Reformatting).   A CT scan of any body part produces a three-dimensional matrix of CT numbers. Although these are produced from contiguous rows of axial tomographic sections, the computer can select rows of numbers from other planes to form images in those planes. The usual display of images is axial, because this is the plane of the x-ray beam relative to the body. When images are taken from the block of numbers and displayed to represent body planes other than axial or in orientations different than the original x-ray tomographic slices, this is called "reconstruction" or "reformatting." Sophisticated computer programs allow the images to be displayed in many formats. (Fig. 6.7, 6.8)

Digital (Scout) Radiograph.   Prior to the capture of the tomographic sections, the patient is passed through the gantry while the x-ray tube is activated and a digital image similar to a routine radiograph is obtained. (Fig.

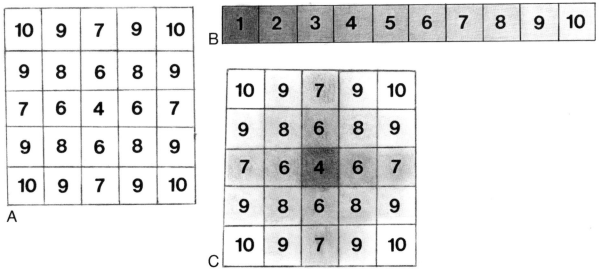

Figure 6.6. IMAGE FORMATION. A. A Matrix of Pixels. The CT image is formed from the pixels described in Figure 6.5. The flux of photons received by the detectors in the array determines the CT number assigned to each pixel. **B. Gray Scale**. The computer then assigns a density to each number as dictated by the window width and level determined by the operator at the console. These represent a gray scale. **C. Formation of an Image**. Using the gray scale determined by window width and level, the pixels, when displayed on the CRT, form an image of the material through which the x-ray beam passed. **Comment**: The above is a much oversimplified explanation of CT image formation.

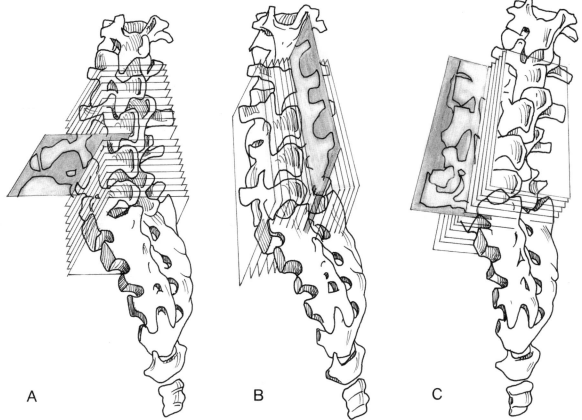

Figure 6.7. REFORMATTING (IMAGE RECONSTRUCTION). A. Axial Images. In CT the x-ray beam passes through the patient axially. The matrix of CT numbers generated represent axial sections of the body, as this figure depicts. Each section is formed by a block of pixels (Fig. 6.6), with the study comprised of a series of these sections. Images are formed by assigning a specific gray scale to the numbers in any axial section. **B. Sagittal Images**. The numerical data can be used to produce sagittal images as well, by choosing sections of numbers in sagittal planes rather than in the original axial planes in which the numbers were collected. **C. Coronal Images**. Using the numbers selected from coronal planes in the matrix will yield coronal images in the same fashion as sagittal images are produced. **Comment**: Just as different planes can be selected and displayed from the CT data, portions of any section can be selected and displayed in differing formats. Size of an image and its orientation (right to left, anterior to posterior, etc.) can be manipulated by the appropriate computer programs.

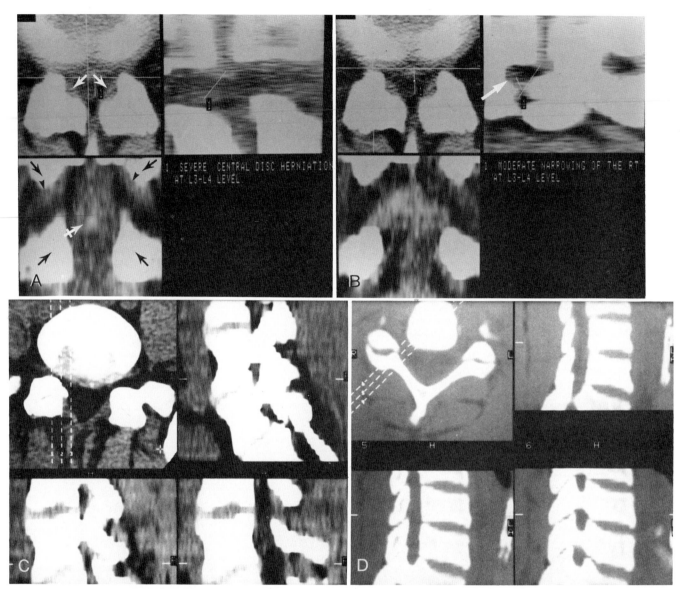

Figure 6.8. REFORMATTED CT IMAGES.   A. Axial, Midsagittal, and Coronal Sections at L3/L4. The image on the upper left is a specific area taken from an axial section at the level of the L3/L4 disc. Note the index lines set by the cursor, which show where the sagittal and coronal sections are located relative to the axial image. The spinal canal is well depicted, and the central disc protrusion is shown at the anterior of the canal (labeled 1). The ligamentum flavum are also well demonstrated at the posterolateral aspects of the canal (arrows). The upper right image is a midsagittal reconstruction. The posterior aspects of the vertebral bodies and disc space are shown at the top, and the disc herniation is well demonstrated. Note how well the midsagittal spinal canal is shown. The image at the lower left is a coronal section. The pedicles of L3 are seen bilaterally above and those of L4 below (arrows). Nerve roots are shown exiting underneath the pedicles (arrowheads). The disc herniation is shown in the central aspect of the canal (crossed arrow).   **B. Axial, Sagittal at IVF, and Coronal Sections at L3/L4.** These are images at the same level as in Figure A. Note the index lines which show the sagittal image to be from the section at the right IVF. The occlusion of the IVF at its inferior aspect is shown. The nerve root at the upper portion of the foramen is well seen (arrow). The axial and coronal sections are the same as in A.   **C. Axial and Sagittal Images at IVF.** These are images from a different patient. Note the index lines which show the locations of the three sagittal sections. In this way, the foramen can be shown throughout its length. Since IVF's are actually tunnels, it may be important to demonstrate stenosis of a portion of the tunnel, which may not be visible from adjacent sections.   **D. Axial and Oblique Images: Cervical Spine.** On the axial image the index lines show where the three oblique sections are located. This demonstrates that reformatting may be done to fit the needs of the examination of a specific patient.   **Comment**: The usual orientation of CT images is as though they are being viewed looking up from the patient's feet from the anterior of the body. This places the anterior of the body at the top of the image, the patient's right, on the reader's left. This format will be used, with a few exceptions, in the CT images in this chapter. Other orientations are used on occasion. Life-size images oriented as though the patient is being viewed from the back are preferred, especially by surgeons.

6.9–6.11) These images allow precise placement of the patient and allow the operator of the scanner to set examination parameters, such as where the tomographic sections will be obtained. Digital radiographs also allow one to see exactly where a specific image was obtained during the scan.

Hard Copy.   By means of a multiformat camera, the images seen on the CRT's of the control console can be

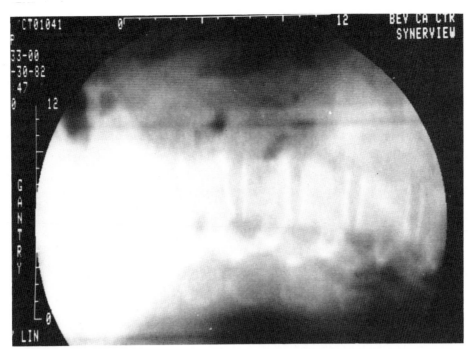

Figure 6.9. DIGITAL SCOUT LATERAL RADIOGRAPH. This image is produced from data acquired from passing the patient through the gantry with the tube activated. It checks on patient placement and, subsequently, index lines can be placed by the computer to indicate section levels, as is shown in Figures 6.10 and 6.11.

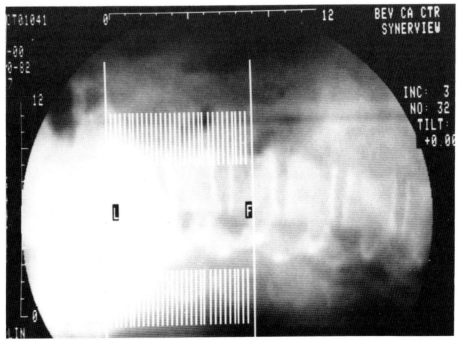

Figure 6.10. DIGITAL SCOUT LATERAL RADIOGRAPH WITH NONANGULATED INDEX LINES. The index lines indicate the location of the sections taken during the CT examination. The images will show identification of the sections so that the observer can determine the exact level of any axial image.

copied onto film. In this way, films are produced which can be viewed in the usual fashion on a viewbox. Such copies may show the images in many different formats.

Partial Volume Averaging. Because of differences in attenuation of the x-ray photons by bone and soft tissue, and because of the curve of the spine (which often causes overlap of vertebrae and the interposed discs), sometimes there are appearances which may be misinterpreted. When overlap occurs and a portion of a vertebra is superimposed over a disc space, the resulting density may give a false impression of disc protrusion. This is called partial volume averaging.

Radio-Frequency (RF). Electromagnetic energy of the wavelength of radio waves. This is the energy applied perpendicular to the magnetic field in MR scanning.

Larmor Frequency. The resonance frequency at

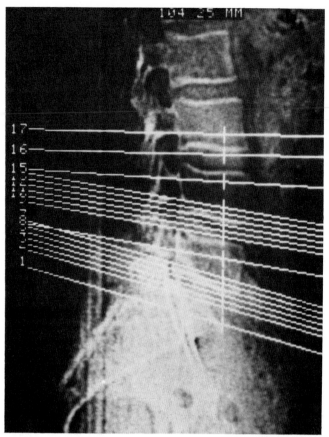

Figure 6.11. DIGITAL SCOUT LATERAL WITH ANGULATED IN-DEX LINES.   The gantry of a CT scanner can be angulated to some degree, allowing scanning through disc spaces, so long as the angle of the disc space to vertical is not greater than the ability to angle the gantry. The index lines indicate the level of each tomographic section.   **Comment**: Few CT studies are now done using only angulated scans through disc spaces, since this leaves areas of the spinal canal unimaged. Usually, angled scans are supplemental to vertical sections, as shown in Figure 6.10.

which a proton will align its axis of rotation parallel to the direction of an external magnetic field.

Surface Coils.   These are electromagnetic devices utilized in body MR imaging to localize the magnetic field, thus producing high quality images of relatively small body parts. They have particular application to spinal imaging.

Nuclear Magnetic Resonance (NMR).   This was the original term used for what is now known as magnetic resonance imaging (MRI) or, simply, magnetic resonance (MR). The word "nuclear" was dropped because, to the public, it implied nuclear radiation. No ionizing radiation is involved in MR imaging.

Computerized Tomography

In 1973 Godfrey N. Hounsfield presented his invention of a new imaging technique that was to revolutionize radiology. (7) The principle was that a thin cross-sectional image, a tomographic section, could be reconstructed from data fed into a computer from a scintillation counter which intercepted a series of pencil-thin x-ray beams projected from multiple angles. The ability to obtain a

cross-sectional picture of the body was not entirely new, having been accomplished by transaxial tomography previously.

The remarkable characteristic of Hounsfield's invention was that it demonstrated a radiographic difference in the various soft tissues, i.e., gray and white matter, cerebrospinal fluid, cerebral edema, even blood clots, could be distinguished from one another. Previously, all soft tissues had the radiographic characteristics of water, so that differentiation of adjacent structures was difficult or impossible, except when fat planes existed between those structures. Further, the computer was able to assign arbitrary densities to the numbers it received from the detectors and the contrast of the image could thus be manipulated so that the information from the same tomographic slice could be displayed in different ways.

Basic Principles.   The basic principle of computed tomography is that the internal structure of an object can be reconstructed from multiple projections of the object. Each tomographic section is received as a block of numbers, the numbers coming from the intensity of x-ray photons interacting with the detectors. Figure 6.5 depicts the concepts of pixels (a single square in the image matrix) and voxels (a tiny elongated block of tissue image, the pixel representing its end area). The image is composed of pixels, each being given a density in accordance with its CT number. Different densities can be assigned to the numbers representing pixels so that the same data can be manipulated to achieve different contrast characteristics. By altering window widths and window levels, and, thus, the gray scale of the image, any given CT "slice" can be shown as an image where bone is accentuated or where the various soft tissue densities are more optimally seen. (Fig. 6.12, 6.13) A further advantage is that, since a three-dimensional matrix of numbers from contiguous slices is generated, by selecting rows of numbers from the different planes the data which was received from axial sections can be reconstructed so as to be displayed as a sagittal or a coronal image as well as an axial view. (Fig. 6.7, 6.8) Rothman and Glenn and associates (8–10) have perfected methods whereby images of curved structures can be reformatted in exacting detail.

Late Generation Scanners.   Figure 6.4 illustrates schematically the gantries of third and fourth generation CT scanners. In these, a fan beam of x-rays is collimated to be very thin, and collimation is also used at the receptor so that the data received is extremely discrete. Third and fourth generation scanners may use a beam as narrow as 1–1.5 mm.

The first and second generation CT scanners were relatively crude by today's standards, but the images they generated excited the radiological world. The third and fourth generation scanners presently in use allow remarkable ability to image many parts of the body, including the spine. These produce such elegant images that a number of invasive radiological procedures have been largely replaced by CT studies. For example, encephalography and ventriculography are now rarely performed. The ability to distinguish the contents of the spinal canal afforded by high-resolution CT has allowed myelography to be used far less often than in the past, and there are

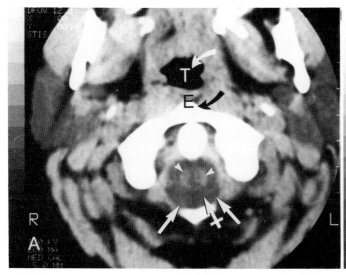

Figure 6.12. AXIAL CT SECTIONS THROUGH C1.   A. Soft Tissue Window. This image depicts the excellent detail of soft tissues which can be shown in addition to outlines of the bony structures. Note how well the dural sac is shown (arrows) and how well the spinal cord is shown (arrowheads), differentiated from the cerebrospinal fluid (CSF) surrounding it (crossed arrow) within the dural sac. Note, also, the detail of paraspinal soft tissues—muscles, fascia (shown by the fat), and the air in the trachea (T) and esophagus (E) (curved arrows) separated by the walls of those structures between the air columns.   **B. Bone Window**. By altering the window width and level, the same numerical data can be displayed with different image characteristics. Compare bone detail in this figure to that seen in A, with sacrifice of soft tissue depiction. Since these two images came from the same set of data, this is actually another manifestation of reformatting.

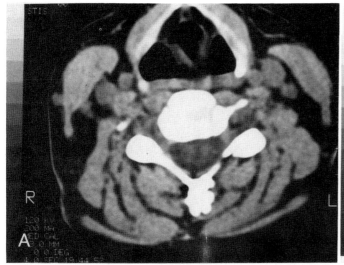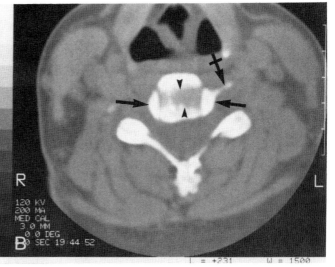

Figure 6.13. MIDCERVICAL AXIAL IMAGES, SOFT TISSUE AND BONE WINDOWS.   A. Soft Tissue Window. The paraspinal and intraspinal soft tissue details are well depicted.   **B. Bone Window**. Bony detail is well shown. Note the uncinate processes (arrows), disc material within the confines of the vertebral end plate margins (arrowheads), and an edge of the anterior horn of the left transverse process (crossed arrow). These were not as well appreciated from the soft tissue image.

many who believe that CT and MRI may in the future negate the myelogram as a diagnostic procedure.

Examination Procedure.   In the performance of a CT scan the patient is placed on a motorized table which allows him to be exactingly positioned within the gantry of the scanner. The table is indexed to the gantry so that movements are precise and the system can be set to automatically move the patient through the gantry. This allows the narrow beam of x-rays to be precisely located for each tomographic section in reference to digital scout radiographs which are performed prior to the tomographic procedure.

At the beginning of the examination the table passes the patient through the gantry to obtain a lateral and/or AP digital radiographic image. The computer is then programmed to obtain the individual sections, make the exposure, then move the patient to the next level. Present-day scanners can accomplish a single sectional scan (slice) in 1–10 seconds, with a usual low back examination taking approximately 30–45 minutes, cooling time for the tube and calculation time for the computer occupying much of that interval.

Figure 6.2 shows the gantry of a scanner, and Figure 6.1 depicts the control panel of that scanner. Figure 6.10

is taken from a hard copy of a CT scan and depicts a digital scout radiograph with index marks to show the location of the several axial sections. Figure 6.14 is a replica of the information panel from a CT scan which gives information about the patient and the examination parameters.

Because of the computer's ability to manipulate the digital data, images can be displayed on the CRT of the control console in many formats—single, multiple, magnified, minified, presented life-size images, oriented as the physician prefers, etc.—and made into "hard copy" films. This allows each institution to create formats to suit its desires; however, lack of standardization makes it necessary for an observer to reorient to different formats when receiving studies from different institutions.

Some experts believe that axial images are all that is necessary for adequate CT examinations. (11) Others strongly maintain that reconstructions in sagittal and coronal planes, or even oblique or curved reconstructions, add greatly to the ability to understand the information recorded by the scans. (8–10)

Two imaging formats have become those most used for low back studies: 1) contiguous or overlapping sections done without gantry angulation; (Fig. 6.10) and 2) angled gantry sections done through the disc spaces. These are usually added to the nonangulated slices (Fig. 6.11) but occasionally are done without the nonangled sections. Coronal and/or sagittal reconstructions are added to bone and soft tissue window axial images at most CT installations.

Radiation Dosage. The amount of radiation dosage a patient receives from CT scanning varies according to patient size and the technical parameters used. Because of the very thin beams used, only a small volume of tissue is irradiated with each slice; therefore, radiation is minimal.

Some scanning techniques use overlapping slices, while others use adjacent nonoverlapping slices. Occasionally, noncontiguous slices are used, but this seldom applies to spine examinations. Fairly high kVp is standard, usually in the 110–120 range. (8,12) Milliamperage varies with different techniques and in patients of different sizes. Filtration to remove low-energy photons which would not contribute to the image is also used.

For a patient of average size, an average CT scan of the lumbar spine (30–40 slices) results in a skin dose of about 2.2 rads. (13) This compares to an average exposure at skin entrance of approximately 2.3–3.2 rads for a standard five-view lumbosacral radiographic series. (14) These figures must be taken as approximations, since many factors (amount of filtration used, mAs and kVp values, screen and film speed) vary in different radiographic facilities.

Magnetic Resonance Imaging (MRI)

In this chapter we will touch only briefly on the subject of this relatively new and very exciting imaging technique. MRI has the potential to be as revolutionary to diagnostic imaging as has been CT. Although in many aspects its potential is still being developed, MRI has already become the imaging method of choice for many neurological studies. MR images of the brain and spinal cord are exquisite, and because soft tissues are not obscured by artifacts from bone or metal, areas where CT has difficulty showing clear detail (e.g., the base of the brain) are very well demonstrated by MRI. A syrinx within the cord can be nicely demonstrated without the necessity for contrast medium. Lesions such as those from multiple sclerosis and amyotrophic lateral sclerosis are discernible via MRI. Disc degeneration as well as protrusion can be shown in earlier stages than by other imaging methods. (15)

There are those who now believe MRI to be superior to CT for spinal imaging as well as for imaging the brain. Further development of this modality holds promise for

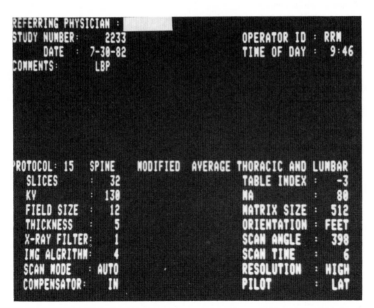

Figure 6.14 INFORMATION PANEL FROM CT STUDY. This data is made part of hard copies of CT studies and shown on one panel of those films. Patient identification, parameters relating to the examination, and other pertinent material is given.

increased ability to discriminate various disease processes. With the passage of time, it is possible that MRI may allow recording of chemical changes, blood flow, and other dynamic phenomena, which could have immense diagnostic yield.

Basic Principles and Examination Procedure. A discussion of the physics of MRI exceeds the scope of this presentation. The reader is referred to several dissertations on that subject which can lead to understanding the formation of these images. (15,16) Since a few MR images will be presented herein, a cursory explanation relating to MRI is as follows.

Briefly, the patient is placed within the gantry of the MR unit on a table which, as in CT, allows precise placement. (Fig. 6.3) The gantry houses a very strong magnet which, when activated, brings the nuclei of atoms having magnetic properties from the usual random alignment of their magnetic poles (Fig. 6.15A) into a defined orientation with the strong external magnetic field (Fig. 6.15B). A specific radio-frequency (RF) electromagnetic field is then applied perpendicular to the external magnetic field. The RF field at the appropriate resonance (Larmor) frequency causes the nuclei to absorb energy and change their orientation to the external magnetic field. (Fig. 6.15C) When the RF field is removed, the net magnetization realigns itself to the external magnetic field and then decays to its natural equilibrium state. (Fig. 6.15D) This induces a current in the receiver coil of the gantry which is proportional to the nuclear density and the rate of realignment. This data is then manipulated by the computer to produce an image. (Fig. 6.16)

Magnetic Resonance Images

As in CT, each MR image is a tomographic slice. MRI, however, produces images in specified sagittal, coronal, or axial planes rather than just axial images. Because of this, there is no need for reformatting into the other planes; however, the images in each specific plane must be produced separately, not from the data of a single set of slices.

At present, the atoms imaged by MR are mainly hydrogen. In human tissues these are mainly found in water. The concentration of water in the various tissues allows discrimination between them. Soft tissue structures containing variable percentages of water (muscles and organs) are well depicted and very easily discriminated from one another by MRI. The cortex of bone contains very little water and gives a weak MR signal, although bone marrow, because of its fat and water content, produces an excellent image. It was originally thought that MRI would be of little value in imaging bone lesions, but with increasing resolution and tissue discrimination it is finding greater utilization (e.g., imaging of ischemic necrosis in hips, temporomandibular joint disease). Bone tumors are especially well demonstrated, and their soft tissue extensions can be appreciated particularly well.

In spinal imaging the vertebrae are well seen, due to the abundance of marrow, the cortex of the bone noted as having almost no magnetic signal. Cerebrospinal fluid (CSF) is easily distinguished from neural tissues. Discs, because of their water content, demonstrate a signal dif-

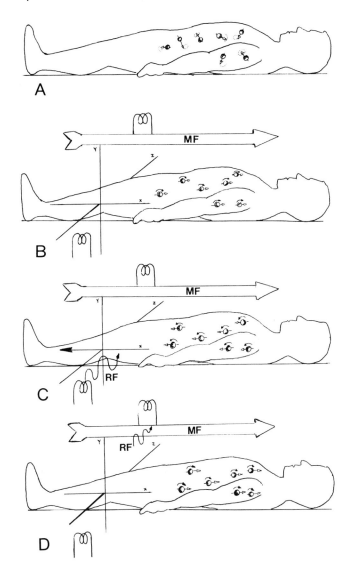

Figure 6.15. SCHEMATIC REPRESENTATION OF ATOMIC RESPONSE TO MAGNETIC RESONANCE IMAGING PROCEDURE. A. Random Proton Alignment. Atoms have magnetic properties due to the electrical charges of the protons in their nuclei and the electrons in their orbital shells. Protons are in a constant state of spin, which is eccentric and elliptical, referred to as precession. The magnetic field (MF) of the earth, to which we are all constantly exposed, is relatively weak, and thus does not significantly affect alignment of the protons within the body. Their orientation, therefore, under usual circumstances is random, as illustrated in Figure A. **B. Proton Alignment Within a Strong Magnetic Field**. During a magnetic resonance scan, the strong electromagnet housed in the gantry is activated and the protons within the patient, who is within the gantry, align themselves with the magnetic field (MF) created. **C. Superimposition of a Radiofrequency Field**. When a radiofrequency (RF) electromagnetic field is superimposed at the appropriate (Larmor) frequency, the atoms are excited to a higher energy state and their orientation is altered in a specific fashion. **D. Realignment of Protons**. When the RF field is removed, the protons realign themselves to the positions brought on by the original high magnetic field (MF). The energy changes brought about by these phenomena induce changes in the receiver coil of the gantry. The computer takes the data from the receiver coil and manipulates it to form images. **Comment**: The above is a very simplistic explanation of a complicated series of events and must be considered in that context.

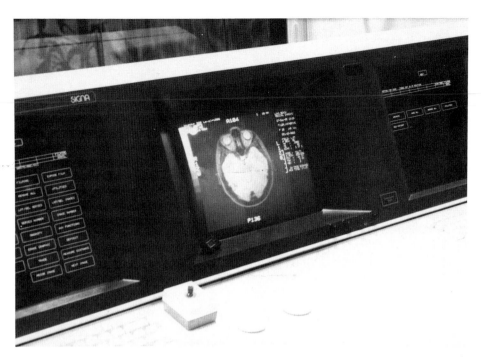

Figure 6.16. CONSOLE OF A MAGNETIC RESONANCE SCANNER. The console of an MR scanner, like that of a CT scanner, displays the images on a CRT. Console configurations vary somewhat among scanners from different manufacturers but will contain a keyboard and other controls to modify examination and display parameters as well as allow recording of pertinent data input from the operator.

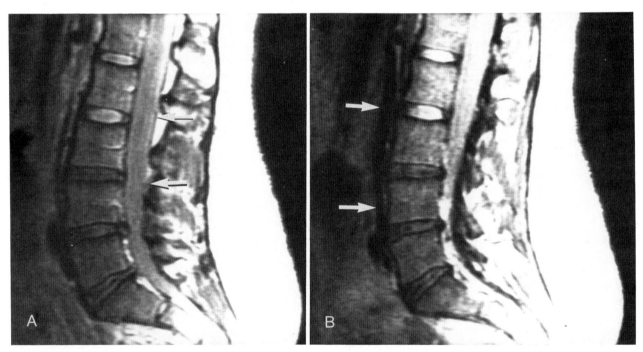

Figure 6.17. LUMBOSACRAL SAGITTAL MAGNETIC RESONANCE IMAGES. A. Midsagittal Image. Note the ability to distinguish the dural sac (arrows) within the spinal canal. Note, also, the differing densities of the disc images at different levels. At L1/L2 and L2/L3 the bright disc images represent the normal, the water content being high enough to give the bright image. At L3/L4, L4/L5, and L5/S1 the darker appearances of the discs indicate degeneration. At L4/L5 and L5/S1 the posterior protrusion of disc material into the spinal canal is well depicted. **B. Image Lateral to Midsagittal Plane**. This is an image done in a sagittal plane to the left of the midsagittal portion of the spinal canal. Note that the dural sac is not as well shown, since this image plane is lateral to it. The disc protrusions at the three lowest interspaces are seen, showing them to extend laterally to the plane of this section. Again, as in A, the difference in image density of the discs is appreciated, allowing diagnosis of degenerative disease at those three levels. The dark linear shadow anterior to the spine on both images is the aorta (arrows). It is better seen in B, which is left of midline, as is the aorta. (Courtesy of Joel B. Levine, MD, Keith R. Burnett, MD, and Lance Sieger, MD, Long Beach, California)

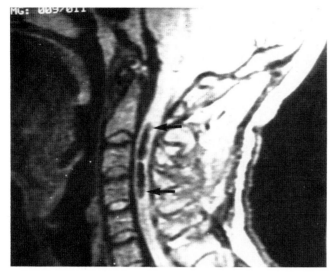

Figure 6.18. SAGITTAL MAGNETIC RESONANCE IMAGE: CERVICAL SPINE. A syrinx is shown in the spinal cord extending from the midbody of C2 caudally to the lower aspect of the C4 vertebral body (arrows). Using these imaging parameters, the cavity within the cord shows dramatic difference, as compared to the adjacent cord. Note how well the cancellous bone in the vertebral bodies is shown because of the marrow content. The cortex of the vertebrae is depicted by the black margins on the segments. (Courtesy of Joel B. Levine, MD, Keith R. Burnett, MD, and Lance Sieger, MD, Long Beach, California)

ferent from other structures. Indeed, disc degeneration can be visualized much earlier with MRI due to the loss of water content. (Fig. 6.17) Protrusion of disc material into the spinal canal with impingement against the dural sac is also well demonstrated by MRI. Cord lesions and other abnormalities within the spinal canal can be appreciated from MR images without the use of contrast media. (Fig. 6.18)

Radiation Dosage. Magnetic resonance imaging does not utilize ionizing radiation. The only known detrimental side effect from the energies to which a patient is subjected in MR imaging is that excessively long procedures may generate increases in internal body temperature which can be harmful. Much research has been done and continues to be carried on to assess possible detrimental long-term effects on the genetic pool from the high-powered magnetic field. (17) Since we are constantly in fields of magnetism from the earth and RF radiation is inescapable anywhere on earth, it is not expected that MRI will result in significant biological damage to those examined. Along with the excellent quality of MR images and the possibilities for insights into chemical changes as the modality is developed, the nonionizing aspects of MRI hold especially exciting prospects for the future.

The Spinal Canal: Characteristics and Morphology

IMAGING METHODS

Plain Film Radiography

Routine radiography remains the initial imaging examination for patients suffering from low back pain.

Certainly, it offers the ability to appreciate alterations of bony structures, but only relatively late in pathological processes. The importance of anatomical variation and anomalies in low back pain is given differing emphasis by different authors, (1–5) and discussion of those arguments will not be attempted in this chapter.

In Chapter 3 the routine radiographic representation of the spinal canal was depicted and measurement mechanisms relating to it were presented. Of the several methods for measuring the sagittal dimension of the spinal canal, Eisenstein's (6) procedure is probably the best, since the points chosen for measurement are more easily located than in other methods. However, at best, due to inherent magnification and inability to precisely locate landmarks, routine radiography allows only rough estimation of the size of the spinal canal and almost no idea of its configuration.

Likewise, the visualization of neural foramina (more properly from an anatomical viewpoint called nerve root tunnels) is suboptimal from routine radiography. The bony margins of these foramina (hereafter abbreviated as IVF's), despite their tunnel-like characteristics, are fairly well seen on lateral views of the thoracic spine and lumbosacral spine, except at L5/S1, where their orientation is oblique. The cervical IVF's are properly visualized only on oblique films. Nonetheless, only portions of their margins are depicted. Because these so-called foramina are actually canals or tunnels, there may be stenosis within them somewhere along their course which cannot be appreciated from the two-dimensional visualization offered by routine radiography. Conventional (plain film) tomography does allow better ability to appreciate the bony confines of the spinal canal and IVF's but at high radiation levels. It is not capable of depicting their soft tissue contents.

Myelography

Myelography, fluoroscopic and radiographic studies done with a radiographic contrast medium present in the subarachnoid space have been utilized since the early 1920's to visualize the dural sac within the spinal canal. (7) At first, air was the contrast medium used, and it has continued to be used occasionally, especially in Europe. Sicard and Forestier, (8) after accidental injection of lipiodol into the subarachnoid space, used it to localize spinal cord tumors. The use of lipiodol myelography became popular following Mixter and Barr's publication in 1934 on disc herniation. (9)

Disadvantages of the use of lipiodol were quickly discovered, and the use of other media followed, with pantopaque becoming the medium of choice in the United States. (7) Although pantopaque had far fewer adverse side effects than previously used media, complications in patients after its use were occasionally encountered. Pantopaque, an oil-based medium, is absorbed very slowly (approximately 1 cc/year); (7) therefore, that which cannot be removed after examination remains in the subarachnoid space for many years, with long-term side effects (particularly arachnoiditis) being documented.

The density of pantopaque in usual concentration also results in suboptimal visualization of nerve roots and has other disadvantages. Metrizamide (Amipaque), a water-soluble contrast medium, has now become the medium of choice in the United States, since its introduction in 1968. Because metrizamide is absorbed from the cerebrospinal fluid (CSF) in approximately 6 hours and excreted by the kidneys, the problems of long-term retention and other problems which attended the necessity of removing as much as possible of nonsoluble media are avoided. Use of metrizamide is accompanied by a greater incidence of acute side effects than was the case with pantopaque, due to passage of the water-soluble medium into the intracranial space and its miscibility with CSF. The long-term effects, however, are relatively few. (7)

Two new nonionic contrast media, Iohexol and Iopamidol, were released for use in myelography in December 1985. Testing of these substances has shown them to be less toxic than metrizamide because of more optimal osmolality and their ability to offer as good or better imaging characteristics. (7,10) Metrizamide and other aqueous media offer a distinct advantage over oily media in that, due to their lesser radiodensity, the spinal cord, cauda equina, and nerve roots are much better visualized.

While myelography allows the dural (thecal) sac to be visualized, other structures within the spinal canal are appreciated from this procedure only when they affect the sac. Tumors, discal protrusions, and other abnormal structures within the canal which impinge upon or constrict the sac can be discovered by this means. Intradural abnormalities, of course, affect the myelographic appearance. Significant spinal canal stenosis, by constricting the thecal tube, can be myelographically demonstrated, but alterations in the IVF's and far lateral disc protrusions which do not impinge on the column of contrast medium are beyond its efficacy.

Computerized Tomography

Axial visualization of the spine afforded by CT, and especially the opportunity to discriminate the soft tissues within the spinal canal and paraspinally, has allowed greatly increased ability to appreciate many aspects of spinal anatomy. Through CT, the spinal canal and IVF's can be seen in their entirety, along with their contents. (Fig. 6.19, 6.20) The ability to alter window widths and levels therein also allows appreciation of anatomy that is not possible from other radiographic methods.

Because the images are derived from digital matrices, exact measurements can be made via CT, although their significance may be questioned in light of clinical findings. Reformatting, showing tomographic anatomy in sagittal and coronal planes, also allows appreciation of relationships of structures, particularly of nerve roots to adjacent bony structures or discs. Stenosis of the spinal canal and/or nerve root tunnels from anatomic variation or from pathology can be appreciated. Bulging of disc material, or herniation, and thickening of ligamentum flavum are other findings well demonstrated by CT and, by means of reformatting, are particularly well appreciated. (Fig. 6.8)

CT metrizamide myelography (CTMM) is occasionally used to enhance the subarachnoid space when noncontrast CT is equivocal and is used almost routinely in cervical spine CT. Two mechanisms are in use: (1) CT examination following routine myelography (this may be

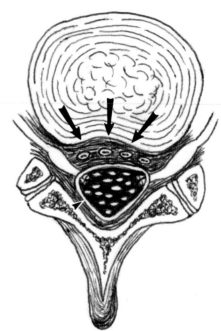

Figure 6.19. SCHEMATIC AXIAL VIEW OF A LUMBAR VERTEBRA. This is the representation of a normal lumbar vertebra at the disc interspace and the contents of the spinal canal and IVF's, as viewed axially. It should be used for reference when observing axial CT and MR images. Note: 1) the concave posterior border of the disc (arrows); 2) the epidural veins embedded in the fat posterior to the vertebral body; 3) the dural sac (arrowhead) containing the nerve roots comprising the cauda equina; and 4) the nerve roots exiting the dural sac and passing through the IVF's with 5) the ganglia within the foramina. The relationships of the facet articular structures and the posterolateral aspects of the discs to the IVF's are also depicted.

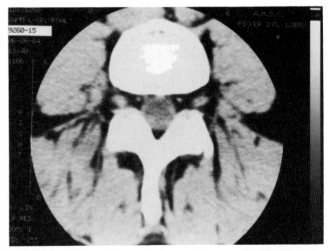

Figure 6.20. CT AXIAL IMAGE AT THE L4/L5 INTERSPACE. This is a soft tissue windowed image. Compare the features to those of the schematic in Figure 6.19. The posterior disc border is not as concave as the schematic depicts, but it is normal. The epidural veins and fat are well seen, as is the dural sac. The ganglia are seen within the IVF's.

done immediately or may be delayed 3–4 hours after completion of the myelogram; and (2) alternatively, introduction of a small amount (usually about 2 ml) of metrizamide, followed by CT examination, is done rather than routine myelography. (11) (Fig. 6.21)

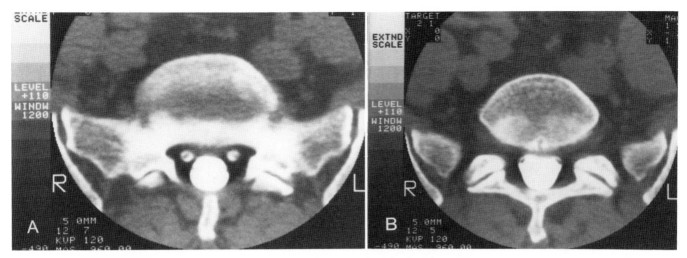

Figure 6.21. COMPUTERIZED TOMOGRAPHIC METRIZAMIDE MYELOGRAPHY. A. Axial Section at S1. The dural sac is shown, opacified by metrizamide. The opaque nodules anterolateral to the sac are nerve roots with their dural sleeves filled with contrast medium ("Panda bear" appearance). **B. Axial Section at the Lum-** bosacral Junction. At this level the dural sac has a more triangular shape than below and is somewhat larger. The dark nodules at the anterolateral aspects of the opacified sac are nerve roots just before their exit from the sac, displacing some of the contrast medium. **Comment**: Both images show normal findings.

Magnetic Resonance Imaging (MRI)

MRI is capable of providing images in axial, sagittal, or coronal planes. This ability and the exquisite soft tissue detail produced by this imaging method promises that MRI may become one of the optimal ways to assess the adequacy or inadequacy of spinal canal dimensions. High-resolution images rival or exceed myelography in the ability to appreciate the contents of the canal. (12) Cerebrospinal fluid is differentiated from the cord or cauda equina, which allows visualization similar to, or perhaps better than, that which can be gained by myelography. Additionally, the contents of the canal can be differentiated from one another rather than simply appearing as indentations into a column of contrast material, as in myelography. The spinal nerve roots, dorsal ganglia, and spinal nerves peripheral to the IVF's can all be seen, along with other paraspinal structures. Note that not only is disc protrusion into the spinal canal shown, but loss of water content due to degeneration of that disc makes its signal different from the others visualized. MRI will show disc degeneration before it can be demonstrated by other diagnostic methods. (13) (Fig. 6.22) Formerly, it was said that MR could not image bone, but with surface coil technology and improvement in resolution and other imaging parameters the collagen and marrow of bone are well seen, although the calcium in the cortex and trabeculae is not. (14)

Discography

Although this method of radiographic examination is infrequently used in recent years, it is presented here because it will occasionally be encountered. Its use is almost entirely reserved for the lumbar spine. The following description of procedure is adapted from Shapiro. (7) In discography a contrast medium is injected directly into the disc itself. (Fig. 6.23A and B) A long needle, usually 21-gauge, is inserted through the soft tissues to the level of the ligamentum flavum, at which time a smaller gauge needle is passed through the larger needle and into the

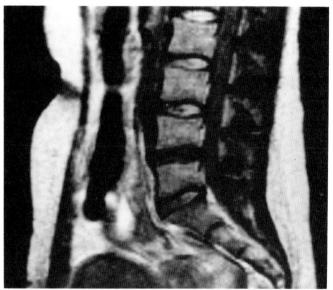

Figure 6.22. MAGNETIC RESONANCE IMAGE, DISC DEGENERATION AT L4/L5. The difference in density of the disc image at L4/L5 as compared to those at other interspaces indicates degeneration of that disc. With these particular image characteristics, the density of the degenerated disc and that of the adjacent dural sac makes it impossible to determine whether or not disc protrusion is present. Altering the image characteristics could allow such determination. (Courtesy of Joel B. Levine, MD, Keith R. Burnett, MD, and Lance Sieger, MD, Long Beach, California)

disc. The procedure is nearly always done under fluoroscopic control, and radiographic confirmation of the position of the needle must be done before the contrast medium is injected. In a normal disc, 0.5–1 ml of contrast medium is accepted with difficulty. There is usually little or no pain upon injection of a normal disc. When a pathological disc is injected, the patient's clinical pain may be reproduced. The contrast medium may escape into the extradural space through a tear in the annulus or may distend the interspace. Two to three milliliters of

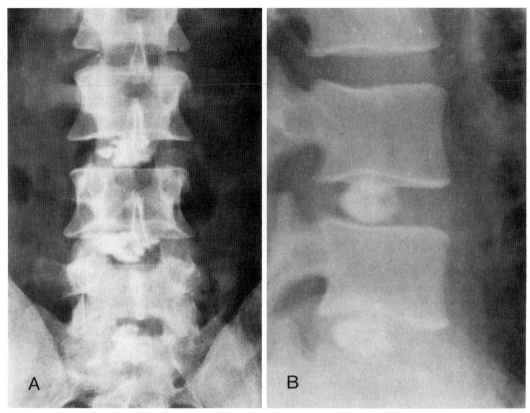

Figure 6.23. NORMAL DISCOGRAM.   A. AP Lumbar Spine.   B. Lateral Lumbar Spine. Observe the opacification of the nucleus pulposus of the third, fourth, and fifth lumbar discs.

contrast medium is usually sufficient to demonstrate degeneration or rupture of the disc. The discs at L2/L3, L3/L4, L4/L5, and L5/S1 are injected. The needles may or may not be left in place for the radiographs following injection.

The advantage of discography is that the disc itself is visualized directly. Shapiro (7) uses it only after a negative or equivocal myelogram in a patient with findings strongly suggestive of herniated disc with few or no neurological findings or poor neurological localization. There is definitely more pain involved in discography than in myelography. It is also a more complicated procedure. Discography does not give information relative to the spinal canal, except when a disc rupture is demonstrated or when contrast medium escapes or is extravasated into the extradural space. As time passes, due to the ready availability of CT and the increasing use of MRI, discography will undoubtedly be used even less.

Extradural Venography

The radiographic demonstration of the extradural veins has been used to demonstrate lumbar disc herniation. The procedure known as extradural venography is usually performed by catheterization of a femoral vein, the catheter passed via the ascending lumbar vein to the appropriate radicular vein(s). (7) Radiographs taken after injection of the contrast medium may demonstrate interruption of the usual venous pattern within the spinal canal.

Claims regarding the accuracy of epidural venography vary considerably, false positive rates being claimed as high as 30 percent or as low as 0.3–1 percent. (7) Because of the location of the anterior internal vertebral veins (just posterior to the vertebral bodies and anterior to the dural tube), a posteriorly or posterolaterally protruding disc may compress them, resulting in radiographic demonstration, when they are opacified by contrast medium, of narrowing or attenuation or even complete occlusion. These are valveless veins, and there is much intercommunication, so that above and below the obstructive disc the veins will be well filled. Intravenous contrast medium injected during CT examination has also been used. The veins are enhanced by this procedure, and their appearance may be altered by disc herniation, especially central herniation.

ANATOMY

Lumbosacral Spine

Spinal Canal

Boundaries.   In the lumbar spine the spinal canal is bounded anteriorly by the vertebral bodies and discs, the posterior longitudinal ligament (PLL) covering these, in part. The PLL is widest and thinnest where it attaches to the posterior aspects of the intervertebral discs, blending with the oblique fibers of the annulus fibrosis. It forms a narrow band behind the vertebral bodies, running like a bowstring between the discs. The lateral boundaries of the spinal canal are the pedicles and the articular processes which form the facet joints. Posteriorly, its walls are the ligamentum flavum and the laminae. The parietal layer of the dura mater is the external cover of the spinal canal.

The shape of the canal is determined by the variations in morphology of the ligaments and bony structures at each motion unit. In general, the canal is ovoid in the upper lumbar spine, with the shorter pedicles, thicker laminae, and more prominent facet structures of the lower segments bringing it to an increasingly triangular configuration caudally. The transverse diameter of the canal increases caudally while the anteroposterior diameter decreases. By CT measurements, the normal sagittal (AP) diameter of the normal lumbar canal varies from 15–25 mm. (14)

Contents. The contents of the spinal canal, in addition to the thecal sac, include epidural fat, the internal vertebral venous plexuses at the anterior of the canal bordering the dural sac, arteries, nerves, and lymphatics. The epidural fat serves as a radiographic landmark which allows visualization of nerve roots and the anterior and anterolateral borders of the dura. Fat also lies between the two plates of the ligamentum flavum, allowing it to be well seen. A thin membrane, the plica mediana dorsalis, runs in the midline behind the dural sac and prevents completely free diffusion of solutions within the epidural space. It is sometimes seen on high resolution CT scans. The volume of the thecal sac varies considerably, determined by its contents and the amount of epidural tissue.

Lateral Recesses

Boundaries. The small, cone-shaped, extradural spaces extending anterolaterally from the borders of the dural tube to the medial portions of the IVF's are called the lateral recesses. These recesses are also known as the radicular or nerve root canals, since they transmit the nerve roots contained in their dural sleeves. In the lower lumbar spine these recesses form acute angles at the bases of the pedicles. The lateral recesses can only be appreciated via axial views. (Fig. 6.24)

Contents. The nerve roots lie anteriorly in the thecal sac just before they emerge and, upon leaving the tube, pass through the lateral recesses closely underlying the inferior aspect of the pedicles which form the roofs of the IVF's through which they pass. About 3–4 mm of fat is usual in the lateral recesses, outlining the nerves in transit.

Neural Foramina

Boundaries. The IVF's are contiguous with the lateral recesses. In the lumbar spine the lower portion of the IVF is narrower because of the normal slight bulge of the disc which forms its anterior border. The major portion of the anterior wall is the inferior aspect of the superior vertebral body; the remainder is the disc. The floor and roof of the foramen are formed by the pedicles of the inferior and superior vertebrae, respectively. The posterior wall is mainly the superior articular process of the inferior vertebra.

Contents. The lumbar spinal ganglia are thicker than those in other spinal areas and lie in the upper portion of the IVF's. The nerve roots and ganglia are surrounded by

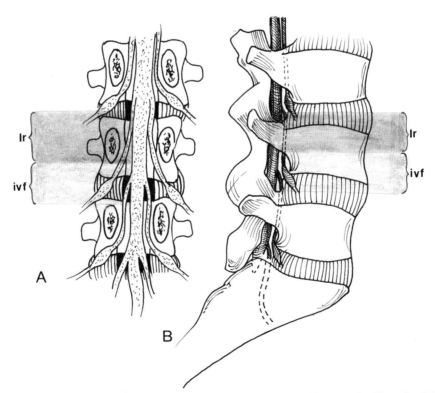

Figure 6.24. SCHEMATIC REPRESENTATIONS OF THE LUMBO-SACRAL SPINE INDICATING AREAS OF THE LATERAL RE-CESSES. A. AP View. The dural tube, nerve roots (as they exit the tube and pass beneath the pedicles), and their relationships to the vertebral bodies and discs are shown. The areas of the lateral recesses (lr) and intervertebral foramina (ivf) are shaded. **B. Lateral View.** The IVF's are plainly seen. The shaded area labeled as "lr" denotes the area of the lateral recesses. ***Comment:*** These schematics show the designated areas. Axial views are necessary to really see the lateral recesses.

fat and connective tissue. Just beyond the ganglia, the nerve roots join to form the spinal nerves which pass out through the foramina, then divide into the dorsal and ventral rami. The sinuvertebral nerves and segmental arteries also course through the upper part of the foramina. The lower portion of the IVF's are occupied by intervertebral veins.

Cervical Spine
Spinal Canal (Cervicocranial Area)
Boundaries.   The cruciform ligament residing behind the dens of C2 forms the central anterior aspect of the upper cervical spinal canal. Its transverse portion is usually called the transverse ligament and secures the dens to the anterior arch of the atlas. Its superior portion extends to the margin of the foramen magnum, covering the apical and alar ligaments which attach the dens to the skull base. Inferiorly, its attachment is to the C2 body. The broad tectorial membrane, an anterior layer of the posterior longitudinal ligament (PLL), in turn covers all of the anterior aspect of the canal in this area. The PLL begins at the foramen magnum, and its posterior layer spans several vertebrae.

The lateral margins of the spinal canal are the occipital condyles and lateral masses of the atlas at those levels, and the wide, thin, elastic posterior atlanto-occipital membrane forms the posterior wall of the canal at that level. This membrane is pierced by the first cervical nerves and the vertebral arteries. Below C1, the pedicles and laminae of C2 form the lateral and posterior borders of the canal, with the ligamentum flavum beginning at the C2 laminae and passing caudally to cover the posterior aspect of the canal.

The shape of the upper cervical spinal canal is roughly triangular and decreases in size from the foramen magnum to C2. Its sagittal diameter at C1 ranges from about 19–32 mm, averaging 25 mm. In the upper cervical spine the canal is nearly round in cross-section.

Contents.   The space between the dura mater and the margins of the spinal canal contains neural, vascular, and connective tissues. The spinal cord is continuous, with the medulla oblongata at the foramen magnum. The dural tube in the upper cervical area is significantly smaller than the spinal canal and is surrounded by a moderate amount of fat, except at its very cranial aspect anteriorly, where it approximates the anterior ligaments. Epidural venous sinuses are subdivided by septa of fibrous tissue and fat. The nerve roots in this area run almost horizontally. They leave the spinal canal through the posterior atlanto-occipital membrane between the occiput and C1 and between the C1 posterior arch and C2 laminae behind the lateral mass articulations.

Spinal Canal (C3–C7)
Boundaries.   The vertebral bodies and discs form the anterior boundaries of the canal and are covered in part by the posterior longitudinal ligament (PLL). Laterally, the pedicles, articular pillars, facet joints, and, posteriorly, the ligamentum flavum and neural arch, border the canal. The shape of the canal becomes increasingly triangular from C3 caudally. Its dimensions are relatively consistent from C3 through C7. The sagittal diameter averages 18 mm but ranges from 15–24 mm. (15)

Contents.   The cord and dural tube are elliptical in the cervical region, with the transverse diameter greater than the anteroposterior dimension. There is little epidural fat in this spinal region, which makes identification of the theca more difficult on noncontrast CT than is true in the lumbosacral spine. Wide epidural venous sinuses are present at the lateral aspects of the canal. As the nerve roots emerge from the dural sac, their course is progressively more anterior, oblique, and downward from C3 caudally.

Lateral Recesses
Boundaries.   As in the lumbar spine, the extradural spaces from the dural tube anterolaterally to the IVF's are called the lateral recesses.

Contents.   These primarily contain the spinal nerve roots in their periradicular dural sheaths. Because of this, they are also referred to as root or radicular canals.

Neural Foramina
Boundaries.   Especially in the cervical region, these so-called foramina are really fibro-osseous tunnels. They pass anterolaterally from the spinal canal, continuous from the lateral recesses. They lie between the vertebral bodies and the facet joints. Their anterior borders are the uncinate processes of the inferior vertebra. These processes articulate with grooves in the body of the upper vertebra to form the neurocentral joints (uncovertebral joints or joints of Luschka). The floor of the foramen is the subjacent pedicle. The gutter of the transverse process continues the floor of the tunnel anterolaterally. The facet joint with its ligamentous covering forms the posterior aspect of the foramen. The foraminal roof is the superior pedicle.

Contents.   The IVF's contain the cervical nerve roots which join to become the spinal nerves lateral to the dorsal root ganglia. These lie in the upper portion of the IVF. Also, there is some fat and connective tissue, and a few small arteries and veins. The vertebral arteries pass through the transverse foramina of C6 cephalically to C2 and are closely apposed to the spinal nerves which course through the gutters of the transverse processes as high as C3.

Thoracic Spine
Spinal Canal
Boundaries.   The vertebral bodies, discs, and posterior longitudinal ligament form the anterior wall of the canal. The lateral portions of the canal are the pedicles which arise from the upper portions of the bodies. The posterior articulations, laminae, and the associated capsular ligaments and ligamentum flavum comprise the posterior boundaries of the canal. The upper portion of the thoracic canal is somewhat elliptical and flattened in the sagittal plane, similar to the lower cervical canal. The lower thoracic canal becomes more triangular in shape, transitioning to the lumbar configuration. Most of the thoracic canal, however, is round and has approximately equal anteroposterior and transverse dimensions.

Contents.   In general, the contents of the epidural space are similar to those in the other spinal regions. There are a few notable differences, mainly appreciable via CT and MRI. There is abundant posterior and lateral epidural fat but, as in the cervical region, little anteriorly.

Anterior and posterior venous plexuses link with intercostal and azygos veins. Even without contrast media, CT demonstrates the azygos system in axial views. In the thoracic spine the nerve roots descend in the subarachnoid space for varying distances from their cord segments before exiting the dural sac. In the upper thorax the cord segment is two levels above the corresponding IVF, while in the lower thorax this becomes three levels. The dorsal and ventral nerve roots leave the dural sac separately, each arising from a number of rootlets. The roots emerge from the thecal sac at the inferomedial border of the pedicles, forming short, cone-shaped pouches.

In the thoracic spine the dural tube is significantly larger than the spinal cord. The thoracic cord is round in cross-section. CT myelography will often identify an anterior median fissure in the cord. The lumbar enlargement of the cord can be demonstrated in the lower part of the thoracic canal, and extending from this and below it are many vertically aligned nerve roots which become the cauda equina below the termination of the cord.

Lateral Recesses

Boundaries and Contents.   As in the other spinal regions, the area from the lateral aspect of the dural tube to the IVF is designated the lateral recess. These contain the nerve roots in their dural sleeves. Large venous sinuses also occupy the recesses and extend into the IVF's.

Neural Foramina

Boundaries.   The thoracic IVF's are laterally directed and lie at the level of the inferior portions of the vertebral bodies. Most of their anterior borders are the bodies with the discs at their extreme inferior aspects. The superior margins of the pedicles below are the foraminal floors. Posteriorly, the IVF's are bounded by the facet joints and their covering ligaments.

Contents.   The nerve roots are surrounded by abundant fat and join to form the spinal nerves just lateral to the dorsal ganglia, in the medial portions of the IVF's. The nerves divide into ventral and dorsal rami as they exit the IVF's. The upper six thoracic roots and nerves are larger than the lower six. Both groups, however, are smaller in cross-section than those in either the cervical, lumbar, or sacral regions. They are therefore difficult to discern on axial CT sections. The venous sinuses which are present in the lateral recesses extend into the foramina.

For further material relating to correlation of spinal anatomy with CT, the reader is referred to two elegant presentations by Rauschning. (16,17)

Diagnostic Imaging in the Stenotic Syndromes

DEGENERATIVE DISC DISEASE AND DISC HERNIATION

Pathology

Beginning in the second decade of life, physiological changes in intervertebral discs begin to occur which progress throughout life. (1) Biomechanical changes occur within the nucleus pulposus which lessen water-binding capability, leading to disintegration of large molecule proteoglycans. This is accompanied by increase in collagen content. Around age 60, the water content of the nucleus has decreased to approximately 70 percent from the 90 percent found in youth. (2,3) This aging process brings about decreasing turgor of the nucleus and lessened ability to absorb and redistribute compressive forces. Along with the nuclear changes, the annulus loses elasticity and fissures develop which are predominantly radial but may also be concentric. Increased pigmentation accompanies the cartilaginous degeneration and neovascularization develops. Accompanying these changes, the disc bulges concentrically, usually accompanied by some loss of height. Eventually, the nucleus and annulus are indistinguishable. The likelihood of herniation of the nucleus pulposus therefore diminishes with age and is unlikely after the fifth decade of life. (4)

The annulus is narrowest posteriorly and posterolaterally, predisposing those areas to the greatest changes. While annular defects may heal by fibrosis, in younger individuals the intradiscal nuclear pressure may cause herniation of nuclear material through the annular layers, progressively, until there is herniation to a position underlying the posterior longitudinal ligament. Further extrusion of the nuclear material through the posterior longitudinal ligament may occur, resulting in a free fragment. (2)

Because of a lack of standardization of terminology in the literature, the following terms will be used throughout this discussion in relation to the varying degrees of disc herniation:

Bulging Annulus (Disc Bulge).   Concentric or eccentric outward protrusion of the annulus fibrosis without herniation of nuclear material. This is usually diffuse and symmetrical, but it may occasionally be asymmetrical. (Fig. 6.25, 6.26)

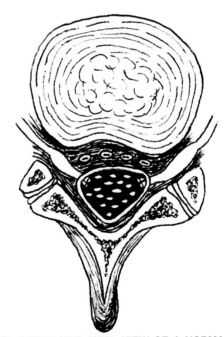

Figure 6.25. SCHEMATIC AXIAL VIEW OF A NORMAL LUMBAR VERTEBRA.   This is the same figure as 6.19. It is presented here to compare to Figures 6.26–6.28.

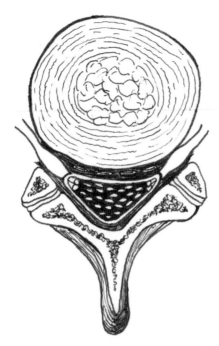

Figure 6.26. SCHEMATIC LUMBAR VERTEBRA: DISC BULGE.
Compare to Figure 6.25. The posterior border of the disc usually becomes convex as degeneration of the annulus fibrosus allows bulging. Bulging is usually concentric and relatively symmetrical. Note that the epidural fat and veins at the posterior of the disc are preserved and serve as an inherent contrast medium to differentiate the disc from the dural sac.

Herniated Nucleus Pulposus (HNP) or Disc Protrusion. Herniation of nuclear material through a defect or defects in the annulus fibrosis. This material may have violated the outer annular fibers but remains attached. These are primarily posterior or posterolateral and are contained by the posterior longitudinal ligament. (Fig. 6.27) CT depiction shows a smooth focal protrusion.

Disc Extrusion or Free Fragment or Disc Prolapse. When herniated material passes through or around the posterior longitudinal ligament into the epidural space, it becomes an extruded or free fragment. (Fig. 6.28) These may move up or down in the spinal canal or into a lateral recess, and they may be quite large. Such fragments have also been called *sequestered* discs.

Imaging in the Diagnosis of Disc Disease

The diagnostic imaging modalities used in assessment of disc disease include *plain film radiography, myelography, computerized tomography (CT), computerized tomographic metrizamide myelography (CTMM), magnetic resonance imaging (MRI), and, rarely, discography and epidural venography.* Following the presentation of imaging findings in the stages of disc herniation, there is a discussion of the relative efficacy of the several imaging methods.

Bulging Annulus. Quite commonly, especially with increasing age, the annulus will bulge or protrude beyond the margins of the vertebral bodies. This is usually symmetrical but is occasionally asymmetrical. Bulges are seldom of clinical significance, since neurological structures

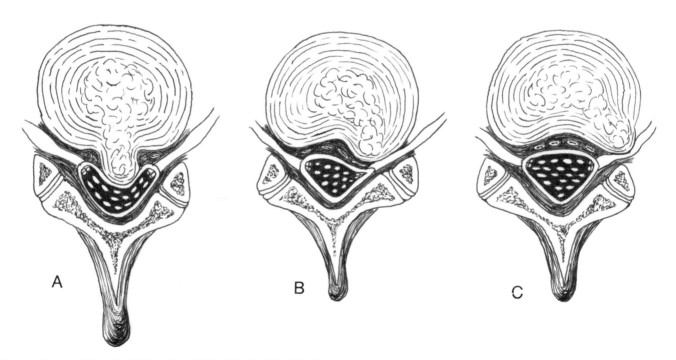

Figure 6.27. SCHEMATIC OF TYPES OF DISC HERNIATION. A. Central Herniation. Posterior protrusion will obliterate the epidural fat, if sufficiently large, and will distort the dural sac as it impinges against it. **B. Posterolateral Herniation.** As the disc herniates posterolaterally, it will usually deform the dural sac as it impinges against it. The epidural fat is obliterated in the area of the herniated nucleus pulposus (HNP). Although such herniation represents outward protrusion of the nucleus pulposus, the outer annular fibers

may be intact and the posterior longitudinal ligament is not violated. **C. Far Lateral Herniation.** Herniation which is lateral to the dural sac may stenose the IVF, as shown in this drawing. These herniations will not be shown by myelography, since the contrast medium is contained within the subarachnoid space. Depending on the size of the herniation, the epidural fat may or may not be obliterated.

are not compromised. Disc bulges are best appreciated by CT (Table 6.1) but are discernible by all imaging modalities except plain film radiography. They may be misconstrued as herniations by one not familiar with CT or myelographic interpretation.

Lumbar Spine.   In the lumbar spine a bulging disc will usually be seen on CT as a generalized extension of

the disc margin beyond that of the adjacent vertebral bodies. This usually results in convexity of the midportion of the posterior disc margin in contrast to the central concavity that characterizes the normal disc border. (Fig. 6.25, 6.26) There are occasions, however, when the concavity remains despite the bulge. (5) Bulging of the annulus is usually concentric and symmetrical but may be asymmetrical, in which case the appearance may simulate a small herniation of the nucleus pulposus. Intradiscal gas (nitrogen), known as the vacuum phenomenon, is occasionally seen in bulging discs. (Fig. 6.29) Intradiscal gas is usually found with degeneration of the nucleus pulposus but may be present in a nondegenerated disc. (6) CT allows even better visualization of vacuum phenomenon than does radiography.

MRI is the most sensitive imaging mechanism in the diagnosis of disc disease and will allow appreciation of degeneration before bulging is demonstrable, as well as depict bulging or further protrusion of disc material. MR demonstrates disc degeneration by an obvious difference in density of degenerated as compared to normal discs. (Fig. 6.22)

Thoracic Spine.   In the thoracic spine bulging discs may also be seen by CT or MRI and, as in the lumbar spine, the bulge is usually symmetrical. Because of the rigidity of the thoracic spine, disc degeneration progresses more slowly than in the lumbar spine. Vacuum phenomena are uncommon in the thoracic spine. Thoracic disc degeneration is most common at T9/T10, T10/T11, and T11/T12, occurring predominantly in males. (7,8)

Cervical Spine.   As in the other spinal areas, a bulging

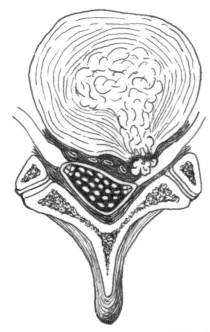

Figure 6.28. SCHEMATIC OF EXTRUDED DISC (FREE FRAGMENT, DISC PROLAPSE, SEQUESTERED DISC).   When the herniated nuclear material violates the posterior longitudinal ligament, it becomes detached from the annulus and is a free fragment. Such fragments may migrate either upward or downward within the spinal canal and symptoms will vary accordingly. Because of migration of free fragments, it is important that CT scans not skip the canal at the midportion of vertebral bodies as may occur when only the disc spaces are scanned.

Table 6.1.
Common Computerized Tomographic Signs of Disc Bulge

1. Generalized extension of disc margin beyond that of adjacent vertebral bodies (usually concentric and symmetrical).
2. Convexity of midportion of posterior disc margin.
3. Vacuum phenomenon (most common in lumbar spine).

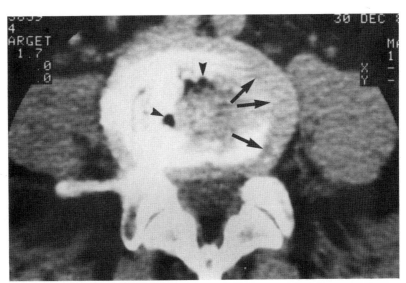

Figure 6.29. DISC BULGE, INTRADISCAL GAS.   The bulging of the disc in this image is nearly circumferential (arrows). The bulging material can be differentiated from the more opaque appearance of the vertebral body. Within the disc material gas is seen (arrowheads). Such intradiscal gas is referred to as the "vacuum phenomenon."

disc will present as a simple protrusion of disc material beyond the vertebral body margin, midline at the anterior of the spinal canal. Protrusions beyond 2 mm indicate herniation rather than simple bulge. The uncinate processes and neurocentral joints provide a relative barrier to posterolateral disc protrusion. Not uncommonly, calcification or gas may be seen in the nucleus or annulus, usually indicating degeneration. Bulging cervical discs are rarely demonstrable by conventional myelography. They are usually of little clinical significance, unless the spinal canal is small, although they frequently progress to herniation. (9)

Herniated Nucleus Pulposus (HNP).   Actual herniation or prolapse of nuclear material through the annulus, but not to the extent of total extrusion of a free fragment, is a relatively common cause of low back pain, especially sciatica. HNP may be suspected from plain films when there is antalgic distortion of spinal contours. CT, MRI, and myelography are definitive for this diagnosis. (Table 6.2)

Lumbar Spine.   Because the annulus is thinner and the posterior longitudinal ligament is less substantial than the anterior longitudinal ligament, protrusion of nuclear material through the annulus most commonly occurs posterolaterally or posteriorly. (10,11) Herniated nuclear

material beneath the PLL (subligamentous herniation) produces focal protrusion which is well demonstrated by CT or MRI. On CT the identification of disc herniation is made easier by the abundant epidural fat at the anterior of the dural sac. (Fig. 6.30–6.36) Deformity of the dural sac by HNP is common and is afforded clinical significance. At L5/S1, where the epidural space is greater, HNP may not cause dural impingement, making its significance less certain. (Fig. 6.36) Central herniation, unless large enough to compress the cauda equina, will probably not be accompanied by radiculopathy or bladder or bowel dysfunction, although low back pain may be associated,

Table 6.2.
Common Computerized Tomographic Signs of Herniated Nucleus Pulposis

1. Smooth focal protrusion at disc margin. The soft tissue density of the herniated material is nearly always greater (CT Hounsfield numbers) than the thecal sac. This permits its recognition even when superimposed upon a portion of the sac.
2. Deformity or obliteration of epidural fat at the anterior aspect of the spinal canal.
3. Deformity of the dural sac and/or nerve root displacement.
4. Calcification in the herniated (protruding) portion of the disc.
5. Homolateral nerve root swelling.

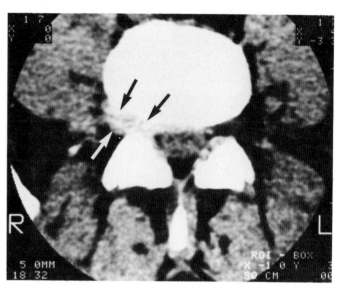

Figure 6.31. FAR LATERAL HERNIATED NUCLEUS PULPO-SUS.   This image shows a large far lateral HNP (arrows). The dural sac is not distorted, but the IVF is filled with the herniated material.

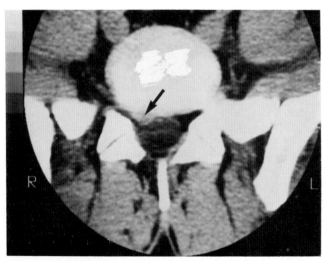

Figure 6.30. POSTEROLATERAL HERNIATED NUCLEUS PULPO-SUS.   The discrete HNP is well demonstrated (arrow). The dural sac is slightly deformed by the HNP, and the epidural fat in the area of the herniation is obliterated.

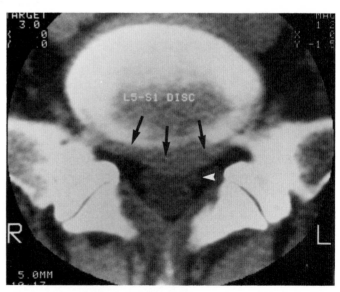

Figure 6.32. CENTRAL TO PARAMEDIAN HERNIATED NUCLEUS PULPOSUS.   A massive HNP is shown which occupies the central portion of the spinal canal anteriorly and extends laterally both to the right and left (arrows). The dural sac is somewhat deformed by the impinging HNP, and the nerve root on the left is slightly displaced (arrowhead).

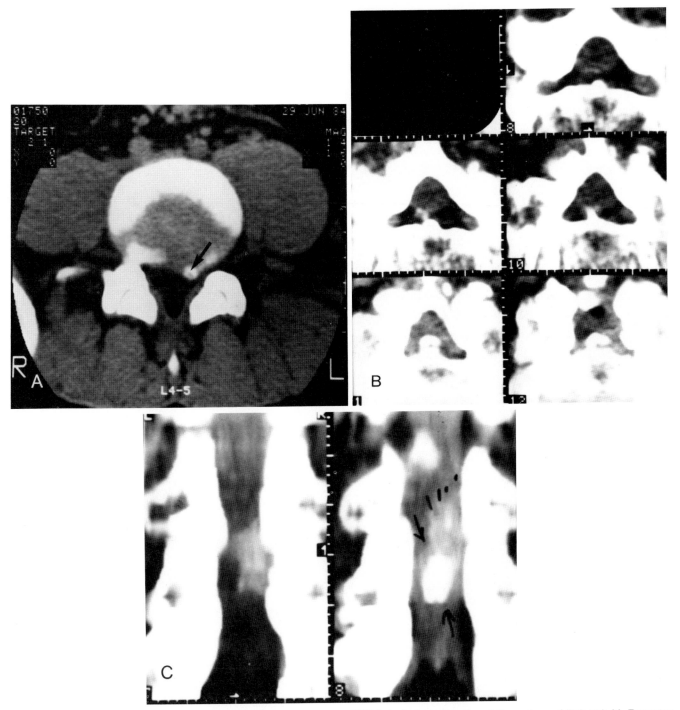

Figure 6.33. POSTEROLATERAL HERNIATION WITH CALCIFICATION. A. Axial Image. There is calcium within the posterolateral HNP (arrow). **B. Multiple Adjacent Images**. A small HNP containing calcium is seen in adjacent sections in another patient. This has some characteristics of a free fragment. **C. Coronal Reconstructions**. These are from the same scan as Figure B. The area of the HNP is indicated. (Fig. B and C courtesy of Deborah M. Forrester, MD, Los Angeles, California) *Comment*: Figure B is formatted with the anterior of the vertebra down and with the patient's right side on the right of the image. These are life-size reconstructions oriented as surgeons prefer.

because the meninges, posterior longitudinal ligament, and outer aspect of the annulus have sensory innervation. (8,12)

HNP is demonstrated myelographically by impingement of the protrusion against the dural sac, which may obliterate one or more dural root sleeves. (Fig. 6.37, 6.38)

Far lateral disc herniations are demonstrable via CT (Fig. 6.31, 6.36) but because they do not impinge upon the opacified dural sac are not at all visible by myelography. Axial MRI should also allow visualization of far lateral HNP. (Fig. 6.39A and B) Herniation of nuclear material through the vertebral end plate was described by Schmorl and Junghanns. (13) The cartilagenous defects in the vertebral bodies resulting from these herniations are usually rimmed by sclerosis and have long been known as Schmorl's nodes. They are very well demonstrated by MRI and CT. (Fig. 6.40, 6.41) Their clinical significance in the adult is doubtful.

Thoracic Spine. HNP in the thoracic spine is rare but has been known to cause spinal cord compression because of the relatively small spinal canal. (14) The lack of fat at

the anterior of the spinal canal may make CT depiction of thoracic HNP more difficult than is the case in the lumbar spine. Myelography or CTMM may be of particular value in this spinal region. MRI can be used to demonstrate disc degeneration and/or herniation in all spinal areas. Calcification is common in herniated thoracic discs. (15) Such calcification is usually not visible in MRI studies due to signal averaging from adjacent structures. Its presence may be implied from areas showing a total lack of signal which will appear as blackness.

Cervical Spine. In the cervical spine disc herniation is most common at C6/C7 or C5/C6. (16–18) Cervical HNP is usually found in the third and fourth decades. It is much less common than lumbar HNP, probably because there is less compressive force involved, although the stress resulting from intersegmental mobility is greater. The uncinate processes provide at least some resistance to herniation by buttressing the interspace posterolaterally. There is little epidural fat in the mid and lower cervical spinal canal. The abundance of such fat anteriorly and anterolaterally in the lumbar canal provides a natural radiographic contrast material which aids in CT depiction of HNP. The lack of fat in the cervical canal to offer such contrast and the relatively similar densities of the dural sac and herniated nuclear material makes noncontrast CT diagnosis of cervical disc herniation difficult.

Conventional myelography and CTMM allow excellent depiction of the dural sac, spinal cord, and nerve roots in their dural sleeves in the cervical region. (Fig. 6.42) Myelographic procedures, therefore, are of particular value in the cervical region. As in other spinal areas, MR images offer excellent visualization of disc degeneration and herniation. (Fig. 6.43) Calcification may or may not be present in protruding cervical discs and, if present, is usually not imaged by MRI, but it is well demonstrated via CT.

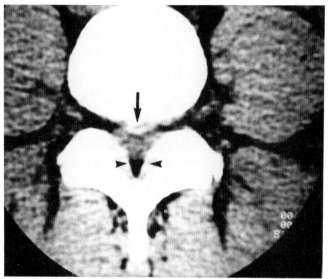

Figure 6.34. CENTRAL HERNIATION IN A PATIENT WITH A SMALL SPINAL CANAL. The central HNP (arrow) is not particularly large, but the spinal canal is small and there is also hypertrophy of the ligamentum flavum (arrowheads), creating further narrowing of the spinal canal. The dural sac is compromised, and the anterior epidural fat is obliterated.

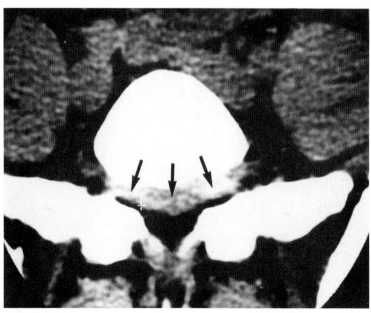

Figure 6.35. MASSIVE DISC HERNIATION. The HNP extends across the entire anterior aspect of the spinal canal and into both IVF's (arrows). The cursor (white cross) indicates the extent of protrusion at the right posterolateral aspect. (Courtesy of Joel B. Levine, MD, Keith R. Burnett, MD, and Lance Sieger, MD, Long Beach, California)

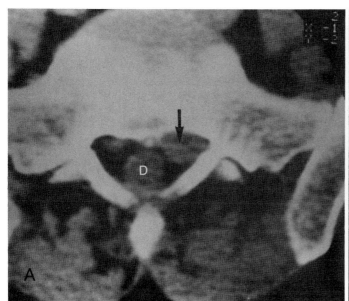

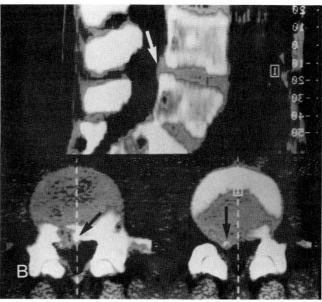

Figure 6.36. POSTEROLATERAL DISC HERNIATION. A. Large Posterolateral HNP. Although the size of this herniation is quite large (arrow), it does not appear to affect the dural sac (D); it probably extends into the lateral recess. Sagittal and coronal reformatted images would help to determine such involvement. (Courtesy of William E. Litterer, DC, DACBR, Elizabeth, New Jersey). **B. Iso-** dense (Blink Mode) Images of a Posterolateral HNP. These images utilized the isodense or blink mode program, wherein all structures of the same density are outlined. It gives excellent depiction of the herniated material (arrows) on the two axial images and the sagittal reconstruction.

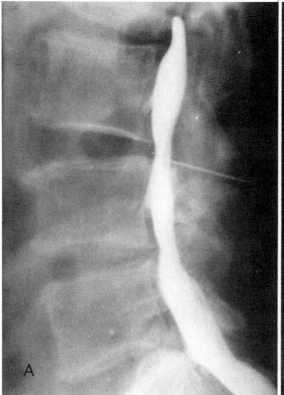

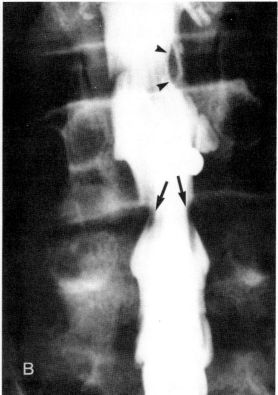

Figure 6.37. MYELOGRAPHIC DEPICTION OF HERNIATED DISC. A. Lateral View. A lateral view from a pantopaque myelogram shows the protrusion of disc material slightly indenting the myelographic column at the posterior of the L3/L4 and L4/L5 interspaces. **B. AP View**. The AP view shows indentation of the con- trast column bilaterally at L4/L5 (arrows) and on the left at L3/L4 (arrowheads). These findings suggest a large HNP at L4/L5, with a left posterolateral HNP at L3/L4. Note that the lateral view does not allow as good an appreciation of the herniations as does the AP in this case.

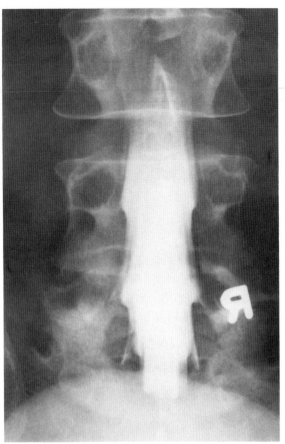

Figure 6.38. NORMAL LUMBAR METRIZAMIDE MYELOGRAM. This AP metrizamide myelogram is presented for comparison with

Chronic cervical disc herniation may lead to posterior spondylotic ridging. (19)

Differential Diagnosis of Disc Herniation

Neoplasms which occur within or extend into the spinal canal may simulate the mass caused by HNP. Among the neoplasms which might need differentiation are lymphoma, metastases, and chordoma or ependymoma. (20) A neural tumor extending into an IVF may simulate herniated disc. (21) The differentiation of recurrent or residual disc herniation from postsurgical fibrosis is a particularly difficult problem. (22,23)

Another entity which is difficult to differentiate from HNP via CT is the presence of a conjoined nerve root. (Fig. 6.44, 6.45) Partial volume averaging from spondylolisthesis or simply from a vertebral body projectionally overlapping a disc space may be misinterpreted as massive disc herniation. (20,24) (Table 6.3)

Disc Extrusion

When material from the nucleus pulposus herniates through or around the posterior longitudinal ligament and sequestrates as a free fragment, it poses a clinical diagnostic challenge. Movement of these fragments may

Figure 6.37. It shows the normal configuration of the myelographic column within the subarachnoid space. Also note the difference in radiodensity of the metrizamide column as compared to the column of pantopaque seen in Figure 6.37. Metrizamide, having less density, allows better depiction of the nerve roots and, because of its lesser viscosity, fills the dural root sleeves of the nerve roots to a degree which pantopaque will not.

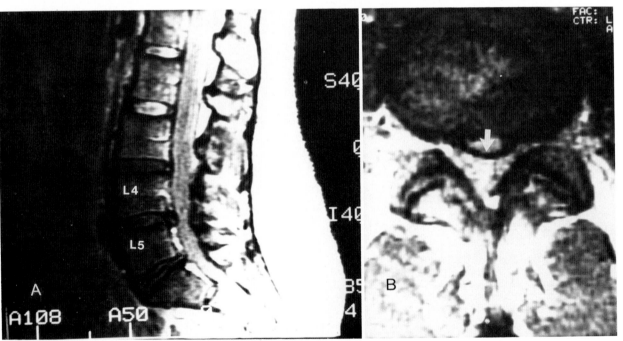

Figure 6.39. MAGNETIC RESONANCE IMAGES: LUMBAR DISC HERNIATION. A. Midsagittal Section. Disc degeneration at L3/L4, L4/L5, and L5/S1 is shown by the darker appearance of the disc material compared to the normal interspaces above. Posterior herniation is seen at L4/L5. Note how well the dural tube is depicted within the spinal canal. **B. Axial Section at L4/L5.** The HNP is shown (arrow) centrally in the spinal canal. Stenosis of the right IVF is also suggested. (Courtesy of Joel B. Levine, MD, Keith R. Burnett, MD, and Lance Sieger, MD, Long Beach, California)

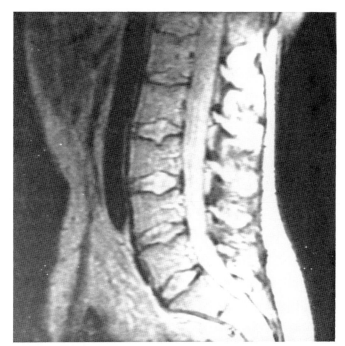

Figure 6.40. SCHMORL'S NODES: MAGNETIC RESONANCE IMAGE. This midsagittal MRI shows the herniation of nuclear material into the vertebral bodies at several levels. These represent Schmorl's nodes. (Courtesy of Joel B. Levine, MD, Keith R. Burnett, MD, and Lance Sieger, MD, Long Beach, California)

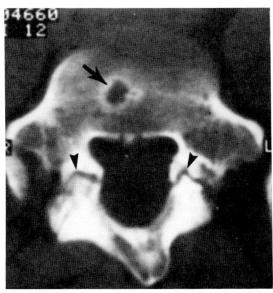

Figure 6.41. SCHMORL'S NODE IN A PATIENT WITH SPONDYLOLYSIS. This axial CT section shows a well-demonstrated Schmorl's node (arrow), with sclerotic margins and bilateral spondylolysis (arrowheads).

be attended by symptoms which differ as the fragment lodges in different locations. Free fragments are relatively rare and occur almost exclusively in the lumbar spine. In some cases the disc margin shows no deformity, despite the extruded fragment. Once free in the epidural space, the free fragment may migrate cranially or caudally. For this reason, it is important that CT scans include more

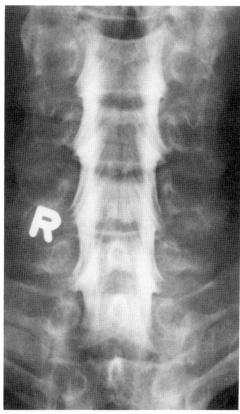

Figure 6.42. NORMAL CERVICAL METRIZAMIDE MYELOGRAM. The cord is well seen within the column of contrast medium. Nerve roots are also well visualized. This film is from a normal study. A single film does not represent an adequate study, multiple views being necessary.

than just sections through the disc interspaces. A free fragment lying adjacent to a nerve root may simulate a dilated root sheath. CTMM may be necessary to distinguish a free fragment from other abnormalities. (24)

Spondylosis (Spondylosis Deformans)

Degeneration of the annulus fibrosis may result in osteophytic buildup along the margins of the vertebral end plate. (13) These osteophytes occur predominantly at the anterior and anterolateral aspects of the vertebral bodies at the attachments of the anterior longitudinal ligament (ALL). The spurs thus formed may be marginal, called "claw spurs," or nonmarginal, called "traction spurs." (13,25,26) (Fig. 6.46) Occasionally in the lumbar and thoracic spinal areas posterior osteophytes may develop which encroach upon the spinal canal, lateral recesses, or IVF's. In the cervical spine, more commonly than in the other spinal regions, chronic disc herniation leads to posterior spondylotic changes, with ridges which narrow the spinal canal. This is an important mechanism of spinal canal stenosis in the cervical spine. The bony excrescences of spondylosis are osteophytes and are properly referred to as spondylophytes. Spondylosis is well demonstrated by CT as well as by conventional radiography. MRI, with sophisticated surface coils, now coming into use, is beginning to allow such bony changes to be appreciated.

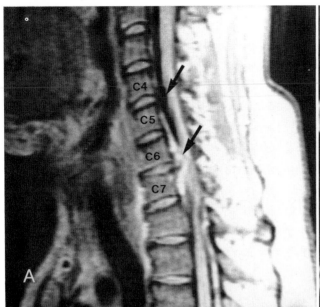
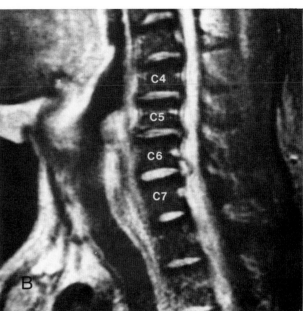

Figure 6.43. CERVICAL DISC HERNIATION: MAGNETIC RESONANCE IMAGE. A. The disc herniation at C4/C5 and C6/C7 are well seen protruding into the spinal canal and distorting the dural tube (arrows). **B.** With different imaging parameters, the herniations are even better seen, but the dural tube is not as well visualized. In this image the spondylosis is better appreciated than in image A. This image shows more extensive disease than can be determined from Figure A. (Courtesy of Joel B. Levine, MD, Keith R. Burnett, MD, and Lance Sieger, MD, Long Beach, California)

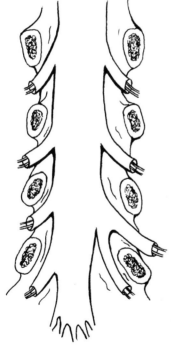

Figure 6.44. SCHEMATIC REPRESENTATION OF CONJOINED NERVE ROOT. Occasionally, two nerve roots will exit the dural sac in one dural sleeve (sheath). They separate as depicted here, or, less commonly, may pass out together through one IVF. This anomaly most commonly involves the L5 and S1 roots. It is not, in and of itself, a cause of symptoms.

Roles of Various Imaging Modalities in Diagnosis of Disc Disease

Plain Film Radiography.   Plain films remain the first imaging study to be done in investigation of spinal disease. Spondylosis, disc space narrowing, vacuum phenomena, and other late manifestations of degenerative disc disease are appreciable through routine radiography. In addition to the fact that these are *late manifestations* of disease, their severity shows little relationship to symptoms or objective findings, and they are common in asymptomatic individuals.

There are those who have advocated that postural deviations in the low back such as antalgia, especially when there are accompanying intersegmental misalignments, may be evidence of lumbar HNP and may even indicate the disposition of the herniation. (27–32) The course of the lumbar nerve roots and their relationships to the discs is the basis of this idea. (Fig. 6.47) Lateral bending AP (Fig. 6.48) and flexion/extension lateral films of the low back have been used to demonstrate abnormal intersegmental mobility, which is a possible manifestation of disc herniation. (28–30,32) The efficacy and accuracy of radiographic bending studies in this regard deserves further investigation.

Computed Tomography, Myelography, CT Metrizamide Myelography.   CT has become the imaging method of choice in diagnosis of disc herniation, particularly in patients who have not undergone prior spinal surgery. (23,33) MRI appears to be challenging CT, as to efficacy, in diagnosis of disc herniation. Conventional myelography is less frequently used, except where CT findings are uncertain. CTMM is often favored rather than conventional myelography where CT findings are equivocal, especially in post-surgical circumstances where differentiation of recurrent disc herniation from scar tissue is important. Use of intravenous contrast material may enhance fibrosis and aid in differentiation of scar tissue from recurrent HNP in evaluation of failed low back surgery.

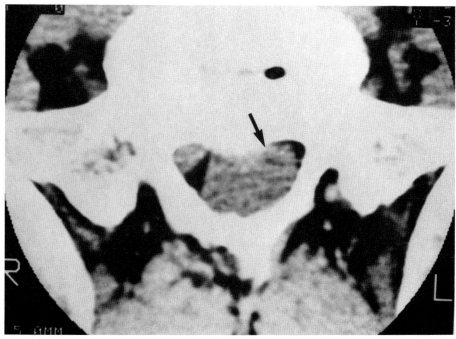

Figure 6.45. AXIAL CT SECTION OF CONJOINED NERVE ROOT. The density in the area of the lateral recess is a conjoined nerve root (arrow). Such a conjoined nerve root may be misinterpreted on CT study as disc herniation. It may also be associated with HNP or spinal stenosis. Metrizamide myelography or computed tomographic metrizamide myelography (CTMM) may be necessary for adequate differentiation.

Table 6.3.
Differential Diagnosis of Disc Herniation Via Computerized Tomography

1. Conjoined nerve root.
2. Partial volume averaging (projectional overlap in axial images, especially found in spondylolisthesis).
3. Postsurgical fibrosis.
4. Ossification of the posterior longitudinal ligament (OPLL).
5. Tumors:
    Metastasis
    Neurofibroma, neurolemmoma, ependymoma,
      other neural tumors
    Lymphoma

In 1984 a Volvo award winning paper showed by its data that myelography was more accurate than CT in determination of HNP. (34) That paper has been criticized (35) because the data was collected several years ago, when CT was relatively new to its authors. Also, the method of CT examination used (sections taken through disc spaces only) is no longer advocated, since it does not image the entirety of the canal and free fragments may be missed. Many other papers have concluded that CT is at least as accurate, or more so, than myelography in diagnosis of HNP. (36–39) Figures vary as to the accuracy of CT versus myelography in diagnosis of lumbar disc herniation, 96 percent for CT, and 90–93 percent for

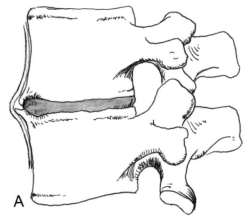

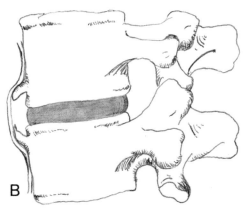

Figure 6.46. SCHEMATIC REPRESENTATION: CLAW SPURS AND TRACTION SPURS. A. Claw Spurs. These marginal osteophytes occur when degeneration of the annulus fibrosus causes new bone to proliferate at the junction of the annulus with the vertebral bodies. Claw spurs project nearly perpendicularly from the vertebral body margin. **B. Traction Spurs.** These are nonmarginal osteophytes and occur at the attachments of the anterior longitudinal ligament (ALL) to the vertebral bodies. It is postulated that these are caused by excessive intersegmental mobility and instability, and they are the result of traction on the ligamentous bony interface.

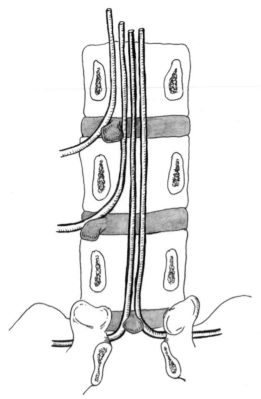

Figure 6.47. SCHEMATIC REPRESENTATION: RELATIONSHIPS OF NERVE ROOTS TO VARIOUS DISC HERNIATIONS. At L3/L4 a posterolateral focal disc herniation is depicted. Herniation in this area may impinge upon the nerve root exiting through the L3/L4 IVF, but it is more likely to affect the root exiting at the next caudal IVF. At L4/L5 a far lateral focal HNP is shown which affects the nerve root exiting through the L4/L5 IVF. At L5/S1 a central herniation is shown that can affect nerve roots bilaterally which exit at IVF's below the herniation. **Comment**: Although in this drawing these are shown at specific interspaces, any type can occur at any disc level. The depiction in this figure is done in this way only to illustrate the various locations separately.

myelography being claimed in two studies. (35,36) A paper presented at the Radiological Society of North America in November 1985 (35) claimed *prospective* accuracy for CT versus myelography as 87 and 85 percent, respectively, for lumbar herniated discs, while *retrospectively*, CT was judged as 92 percent accurate, with myelography 85 percent. CT is more useful than myelography for determining the nature of an epidural lesion. It is also able to determine the presence of lateral herniations which are not visible via myelography.

In the thoracic and cervical spinal areas noncontrast CT is less rewarding than in the lumbar spine. CTMM is recommended in these areas if results from noncontrast CT are equivocal.

Magnetic Resonance Imaging. The role of MRI in assessment of disc herniation is still developing. As images improve, and especially with the greater use of surface coil technology and better axial imaging, MR studies are suggested by some as having the potential to surpass CT in this regard. (40,41)

Discography and Epidural Venography. These modalities are less often used than those discussed above.

Discography allows direct visualization of the discs but is both complicated to perform and painful to the patient. With the availability of CT and MRI, its use will undoubtedly diminish even further. Epidural venography also is infrequently performed and is likely to be even less used as time passes. Both of these are invasive procedures and have less yield than is expected for the noninvasive modalities of CT and MRI.

SPINAL STENOSIS

True spinal stenosis implies bony constriction of the spinal canal and tunnels compressing their contents, (23,42) but soft tissue intrusions into those areas are also capable of causing neural compression. For purposes of brevity, this discussion will consider both true stenosis and constriction from soft tissues. Different authors use varying nomenclatures relative to the types of stenosis encountered. (23,43,44) (Table 6.4) Based on spinal anat-

Table 6.4.
Pathoetiological Classification of Spinal Stenosis*

CONGENITAL/DEVELOPMENTAL STENOSIS
Idiopathic
Achondroplasia
Hypochondroplasia
Morquio's mucopolysaccharidosis
Dysplasias associated with atlantoaxial laxity (subluxation): metatropic dwarfism, spondyloepiphyseal dysplasia, Kniest's disease, multiple epiphyseal dysplasia, chondrodystrophia punctata
Down's syndrome (C1/C2 instability)
Hypophosphatemic vitamin D resistant rickets

ACQUIRED STENOSIS
Degenerative:
  Spondylosis and arthrosis
  Soft tissue stenosis
  Isolated intervertebral disc resorption
  Degenerative spondylolisthesis
Combined:
  Any possible combinations of congenital or developmental stenosis, degenerative stenosis, and protrusions of intervertebral disc material
Spondylolysis:
  Without spondylolisthesis
  With spondylolisthesis
Iatrogenic:
  Postlaminectomy
  Postfusion (anterior or posterior)
Miscellaneous:
  Ankylosing spondylitis
  Calcification or ossification of the posterior longitudinal ligament (OPLL)
  Diffuse idiopathic skeletal hyperostosis (DISH)
  Calcification or ossification of the ligamentum flavum
  Conjoined lumbar nerve root (relative stenosis of neural canal)
  Paget's disease of bone
Metabolic:
  Epidural lipomatosis (Cushing's syndrome or long-term steroid therapy)
  Acromegaly
  Fluorosis
  Calcium pyrophosphate dihydrate deposition disease (CPPD)

* Adapted from Dorwart RH, Vogler JB III, and Helms CA: Spinal stenosis. *Radiol Clin North Am* 21:301, 1983.

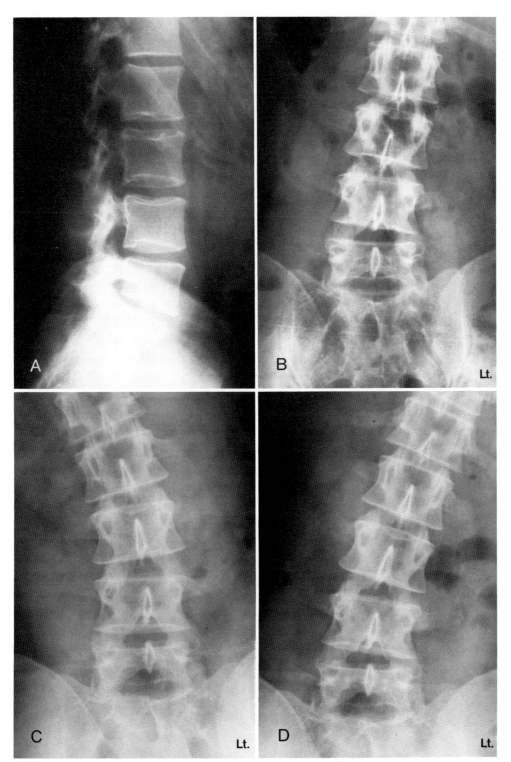

Figure 6.48. ERECT PLAIN FILMS: ANTALGIA, LATERAL BEND-ING STUDY.   A. Lateral View. This film shows a diminished lumbar curve which correlates with the significant paraspinal muscle spasticity exhibited by the patient clinically.   **B. Neutral AP View**. The lateral inclination of the spine cephalically is accompanied by lateral flexion misalignment of L4 to the left upon L5. This is thought by some to suggest an antalgic response to disc herniation, especially when it accompanies flattening of the normal anterior lumbar convexity.   **C. Right Lateral Bending AP View**. Note that, upon bending the body toward the right, there is very limited lateral flexion of L4 to the right upon L5. Above L4 intersegmental lateral flexion occurs at each motion segment, but there is little coupled vertebral rotation associated.   **D. Left Lateral Bending AP View**. This maneuver is better accomplished than the contralateral motion. There is also better intersegmental mobility above L4, more appropriate, but limited, coupled rotation being demonstrated.   ***Comment***: According to Weitz, (32) disc herniations can be located with accuracy via lateral bending studies of this nature. The findings from this study suggest a right posterolateral herniation at L4/L5 if there was right sciatic pain or a left paramedian herniation and if the sciatic pain was on the left.

omy, three regions of stenosis are herein discussed—central, lateral recess, and intervertebral foraminal.

Central Stenosis

Etiology. Narrowing of the central spinal canal may be either congenital (developmental) or acquired. (Table 6.4) Congenital stenosis may be due to achondroplasia or anomaly, or may be idiopathic. Acquired central stenosis is usually due to the several manifestations of degenerative disc disease, facet disease, ligamentum flavum hypertrophy, post-surgical scar formation, or spondylolisthesis (especially degenerative spondylolisthesis), or may be caused by trauma, either as an acute or late manifestation.

Congenital Central Stenosis. The classical manifestation of congenital stenosis is in achondroplasia, where the lumbar canal, instead of increasing in dimension caudally, does the opposite. Achondroplastics may also suffer from stenosis due to spinal curvature. In achondroplasia, thoracolumbar and lumbar stenosis is most common, but the cervical spine may be abnormal. (45)

Congenital idiopathic stenosis is characterized by short, thick pedicles with decreased interpediculate distance. (17) Usually, symptoms in these patients do not develop until trauma (especially hyperextension injury), degeneration with osteophytes or disc protrusion, or hypertrophy of the ligamentum flavum are superimposed. (46) Laminar hypertrophy with "whiskering" bony proliferation, periarticular swelling, and fibrosis, as well as degenerative hypertrophy of the facetal structures and degenerative (nonspondylolytic) spondylolisthesis, are all acquired causes of central stenosis and may also occur in patients with idiopathic stenosis to produce symptoms. (23)

Acquired Central Stenosis. Disease of discs and/or facets, ligamentum flavum hypertrophy, spondylolisthe-sis (especially nonspondylolytic), trauma and its late manifestations, post-surgical scarring, and other problems discussed above as complicating congenital stenosis may stenose a canal which is not congenitally narrow, especially one which is at the lower range of normal. An uncommon cause of acquired central stenosis is ossification of the posterior longitudinal ligament (OPLL). (47–49) (Fig. 6.49)

Ossification of the posterior longitudinal ligament may occur in up to 50 percent of patients who have diffuse idiopathic skeletal hyperostosis (DISH). (50) Intraspinal tumors, dural cysts, cord and cauda equina abnormalities are soft tissue abnormalities which may cause symptoms resembling those of central stenosis.

Measurements. Measurements of the spinal canal are not as helpful in determination of stenosis as is evaluation of the contents. The thecal sac may not be compromised, even in a small canal. Conversely, even in a relatively large canal, a large thecal sac may be present and there may be symptoms of stenosis. (43) The dimensions of the canal in each spinal area were given earlier in this chapter, in the descriptions of spinal canal morphology.

CT window settings affect measurements, especially when done from axial sections. Sagittal reformatting allows better measurements and can allow the smallest portion of the canal to be measured, wherever it may be. (23) CTMM is especially helpful in questionable causes. Myelography remains, for the present, the "gold standard" in this regard.

Cervical Spine. At the cervicocranial junction stenosis of the spinal canal may attend anomalies such as os odontoideum, occipitalization of C1, and absence of the transverse ligament; however, in these patients symptoms are usually not present unless trauma or disease is superimposed. Trauma may rupture the transverse ligament,

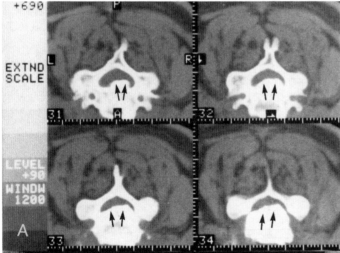

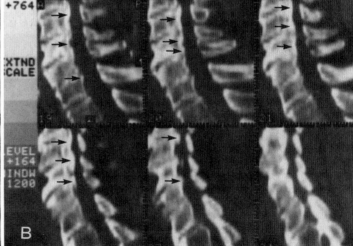

Figure 6.49. OSSIFICATION OF THE POSTERIOR LONGITUDINAL LIGAMENT (OPLL).   A. Sequential Axial CT Sections. These films demonstrate the ossification which severely stenoses the spinal canal. The extent and configuration of the ossification can be appreciated from the sections at consecutive levels (arrows). **B. Sequential Oblique CT Reformatted Images**. These represent sequential slices, beginning near the center of the spinal canal on the upper left and progressing toward the IVF's. Note the ossified posterior longitudinal ligament (arrows). (Reprinted with permission: Foreman SM: Ossification of the posterior longitudinal ligament. *J Manip Physiol Ther* 8:251, 1985).   *Comment*: The images in Figure A are presented with the vertebral bodies at the bottom of the image and the patient's right at the image right.

or it may be damaged by inflammatory disease such as rheumatoid arthritis, resulting in atlantoaxial subluxation, causing stenosis of the high cervical canal. Ankylosing spondylitis and the seronegative spondyloarthropathies are also associated with atlantoaxial subluxation. (51)

Basilar invagination from any cause may also be associated with cervicocranial stenosis. Paget's disease, which has both bone-softening and bony-expansion characteristics, or other diseases causing bone hypertrophy such as fluorosis, may rarely be causes of stenosis. (43,52) (Fig. 6.50, 6.51)

Posterior bony ridging from spondylosis may narrow the cervical canal (Fig. 6.52), as may ligamentum flavum hypertrophy. These may be symptom-producing only on extension, especially if the ridges are small and the canal relatively large. With a congenitally or developmentally tight canal, even small ridges may cause myelopathy.

Thoracic Spine. Thoracic stenosis is less common than is stenosis in either the cervical or lumbar spinal areas. It can, however, occur from spondylosis, ossification of the posterior longitudinal ligament, ligamentum flavum ossification, or, rarely, with disc herniation. In both the cervical and thoracic areas, the lack of epidural fat makes stenosis less evident than is the case in the lumbar spine.

Lumbar Spine. In the lumbar spine 10–20 percent of the normal population may have a trefoil or three-leaf clover configuration of the spinal canal. (52–54) (Fig. 6.53) Unless this is accompanied by compromise of the neural structures, it should not be considered as evidence of stenosis. Absence of epidural fat in areas where it should be present is suggestive of stenosis. (55)

Lumbar stenosis may result from spondylosis with posterior ridging, facet hypertrophy, ligamentum flavum hypertrophy (Fig. 6.54), disc degeneration with bulging or herniation, spondylolisthesis (especially degenerative),

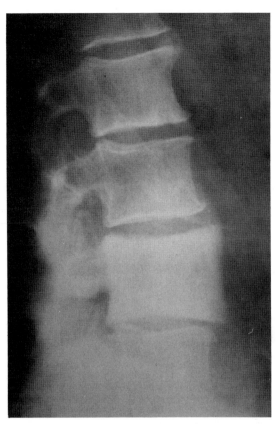

Figure 6.51. PAGET'S DISEASE AFFECTING A VERTEBRA WITH ENLARGEMENT. The gross enlargement of the "ivory" vertebra affects pedicles as well as the vertebral body. The spinal canal appears to be narrowed by the vertebral enlargement.

or combinations of these. Of course, these are more problematic if the canal is congenitally small. Stenosis can also be found in any spinal area from post-surgical fibrotic scarring. This may be very difficult to differentiate from recurrent disc herniation.

Symptomatology. In the cervical spine central stenosis may cause spinal cord compression (with or without myelopathy) or radicular manifestations. With cord involvement, the symptoms may be remote. In the lumbar spine cauda equina compression results. Symptoms may be bizarre. Pain may occur in one or both legs and may involve one dermatome in one leg and a different dermatome in the other leg. Neurogenic claudication, where the patient has to rest after walking because of leg pain, is typical; however, after resting a few minutes, a similar walk may be pain free. Various sensory symptoms—paresthesia, hypesthesia, a feeling of cold when the leg is not cold—have all been noted. (29,30,56) The symptoms only slightly resemble vascular claudication. (29,56)

Lateral Recess Stenosis

Etiology. Facet hypertrophy or degenerative marginal changes of articular processes are particularly likely to cause lateral recess stenosis. (Fig. 6.55) Posterolateral disc herniation is another major cause of lateral stenosis. The combination of posterolateral disc herniation and facet hypertrophy is not uncommon. Post-surgical fibrosis is likely to be found in the lateral recess. Ligamentum

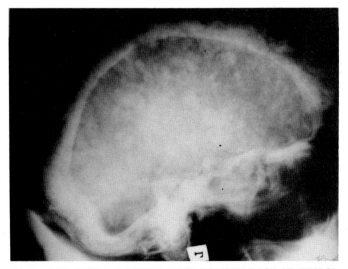

Figure 6.50. SKULL: PAGET'S DISEASE WITH BASILAR INVAGINATION. The "cottonwool" appearance of the skull is typical of advanced Paget's disease in the combined stage. The bone softening accompanying the disease has produced considerable basilar invagination, which is a cause of stenosis of the upper cervical spinal canal.

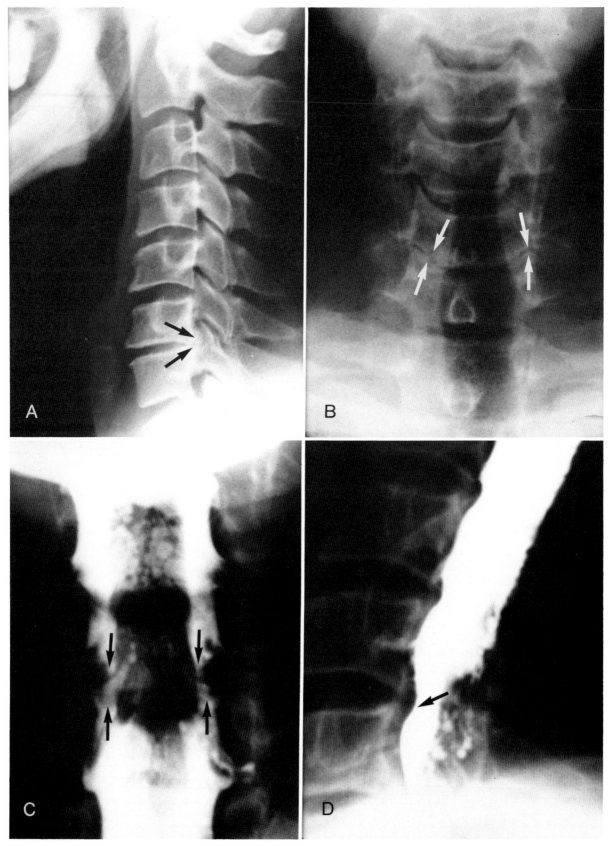

Figure 6.52.

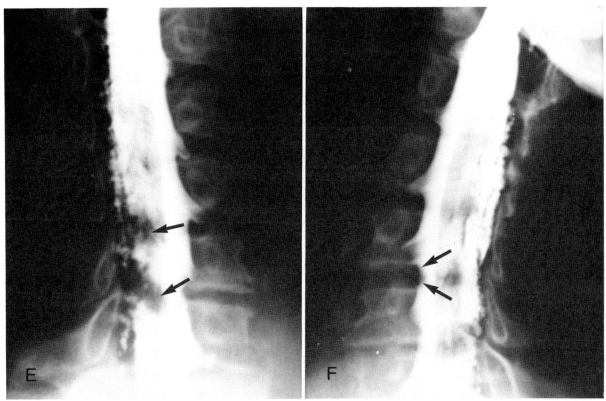

Figure 6.52. CERVICAL SPINE: POSTERIOR SPONDYLOTIC RIDGING. A. Plain Film Lateral View. The cervical curve is flattened and nearly reversed from C3 through C5. The disc space at C6/C7 is narrowed posteriorly, and posterior spondylotic new bone is apparent at those end plates (arrows). **B. Plain Film AP View.** The uncinate processes of C7 are flattened, and the C6/C7 uncovertebral joints are obscured, with sclerosis of the components (arrows). **C. AP Myelogram.** Defects in the column of myelographic medium are seen (arrows), corresponding to the spondylotic ridges. **D. Lateral Myelogram.** Indentation of the myelographic column is noted at the affected interspace (arrow). Lesser indentations at the posterior aspect of other interspaces are not significant. **E. Oblique Myelogram.** The spondylotic ridges are shown by the deviation in the column of contrast medium (arrows). **F. Oblique Myelogram.** The opposite oblique film does not show the myelographic defects as well, but a small defect connotes a ridge (arrows).

flavum hypertrophy can also cause narrowing of the lateral recesses. Patients with short pedicles or a trefoil canal in the lumbar area are particularly at jeopardy relative to lateral recess stenosis when any degenerative situation occurs. In the cervical spine, uncovertebral (neurocentral or Luschka joint) arthrosis or uncinate hypertrophy may stenose the lateral recess. Lateral recess stenosis frequently coexists with central stenosis.

Types of Lateral Recess Stenosis. The lateral recess or nerve root tunnel is narrowest at the superior border of the pedicle, where the superior articular process is angled forward. This is the area where facet hypertrophy is most likely to constrict the recess. (43) Stenosis in the recess has been subcategorized into *lateral stenosis, subarticular stenosis,* and, further, may be either *dynamic* or *fixed.*

Lateral Stenosis. In this subcategory, a nerve root is compressed as it enters its neural foramen, the compression occurring because of superior migration of the superior articular process or osteophyte formation at the superior aspect of the facet.

Subarticular Stenosis. Subarticular stenosis occurs when the superior facet entraps the nerve root just below the disc in patients with short pedicles, and there is indentation of the recess by the subarticular portion of the lamina. (57)

Dynamic Stenosis. In any spinal region increased intersegmental motion secondary to the unstable phase of degeneration may cause what has been called "dynamic stenosis." (30,58,59) This may be recurrent and may be relieved by conservative treatment and/or bedrest.

Fixed Stenosis. This term is best used in lateral recess stenosis when spinal degeneration has reached the stage of stabilization, or it can apply during the unstable phase if the stenosis is so severe that it is unable to be relieved by a change in vertebral position. (59)

Symptomatology. Since the recess contains the nerve root, the symptoms in any spinal area will be radicular in nature. In dynamic stenosis the symptoms are characteristically intermittent.

Foraminal Stenosis

Etiology. It needs to be restated that the neural foramina are really tunnels, especially in the cervical region. The varying morphology of the IVF's in each spinal area needs to be held in mind as the possibility of foraminal stenosis is considered. Stenosis in a foramen may result

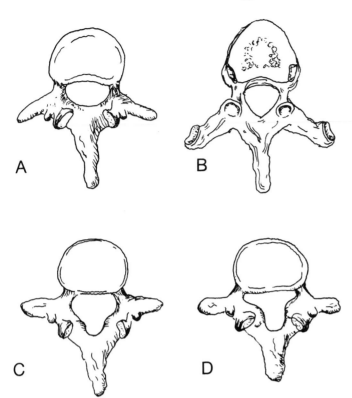

Figure 6.53. NORMAL SPINAL CANAL CONFIGURATIONS. A. Oval. B. Triangular. C. Deltoid. D. Trefoil (Three-Leaf Clover). While these configurations are normal, the possibility of lateral recess stenosis from posterolateral or far lateral disc herniation or of central stenosis with central disc herniation and/or ligamentum flavum hypertrophy can be better appreciated with certain canal shapes.

from bony overgrowth, lateral disc herniation, disc extrusion (free fragment), or from post-operative fibrosis.

Cervical Spine. In the cervical spine uncovertebral arthrosis is apt to constrict the foramen. Marginal osteophytes from the facets are particularly problematical, since they protrude into the upper portion of the foramen where the nerve structures lie. Fibrous or bony changes in the gutter of the cervical transverse processes which form the floors of the foramina may cause foraminal stenosis, which is very difficult to appreciate except by reformatted oblique CT sections sequentially along the tunnel. (23)

Thoracic Spine. Foraminal stenosis in the thoracic spine is uncommon but possible from either degenerative disease of the facet or the costovertebral articulations.

Lumbar Spine. Lumbar foraminal stenosis is usually well appreciated from axial CT images, but reformatted sagittal views are often helpful in its appreciation, particularly by those less skilled in CT interpretation. Because of their orientation in the lumbar spine, especially at L5/S1, plain films of the low back should not be relied upon to assess the possibility of IVF stenosis.

Symptomatology. Symptoms from IVF stenosis are radicular. Clinically, there may be few to no symptoms found, even in radiographically advanced disease. On the other hand, well-demonstrated symptoms may be found in patients with few to no radiographic changes.

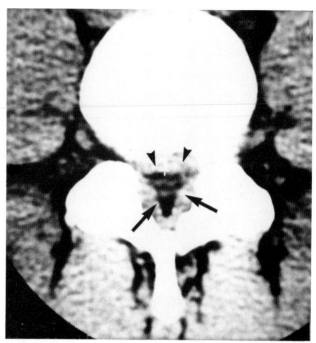

Figure 6.54. STENOSIS FROM LIGAMENTUM FLAVUM HYPERTROPHY. The thickened ligamentum flavum (arrows) narrow the spinal canal significantly. There is also a posterior disc bulge (arrowheads). The dural sac is compromised by the stenosis from both of these abnormalities.

Spondylolisthesis

This entity is thoroughly covered in Chapter 5 of this book. Rarely, nerve root compression may result from displacement of the pars in isthmic spondylolisthesis. (Fig. 6.56) IVF stenosis may be caused by degenerative osteophytes from the facets or from lateral bulging of the annulus fibrosis. Degenerative spondylolisthesis can cause central stenosis. (23,60) This is most common at L4/L5 and is most frequently found in women in the 6th decade. (60) Degenerative spondylolisthesis is the most common cause of direct symptoms from spondylolisthesis. Spondylolisthesis may also be iatrogenic following laminectomy, especially when accompanied by facetectomy. (See Chapter 5, Fig. 5.21A and B) Retrolisthesis may rarely cause central or lateral recess stenosis. Retrolisthesis may be due to degenerative disease or may follow surgery. (23,60)

TREATMENT OF THE STENOTIC SYNDROMES

Surgical

Surgical treatment of the several stenotic syndromes should be considered only after an adequate trial of conservative therapy has been unproductive. This includes chiropractic manipulation, exercises, supports, bedrest, various physical therapy modalities, and medication. (29,30,55,56)

Conservative therapy should be continued as long as pain can be tolerated. (61) Neurological changes alone are rarely indications for surgery. (62) In the opinion of several authors, as few as 5 percent of those with low back pain should have surgery. (30,63,64) A noted au-

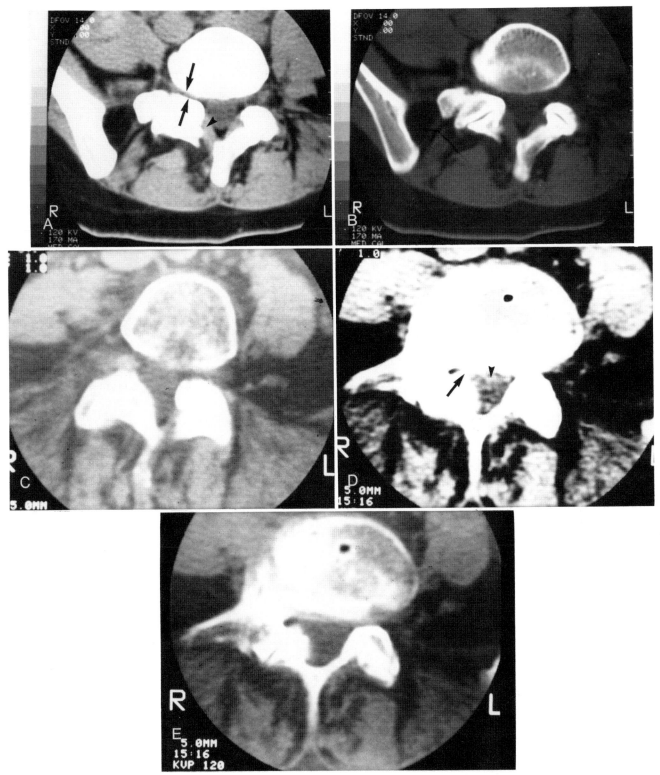

Figure 6.55. LUMBAR SPINE: LATERAL RECESS STENOSIS.   A. Axial CT Section, Soft Tissue Window. The right facet is hypertrophied due to arthrosis. Note the narrowing of the area of the lateral recess and the IVF narrowing (arrows). Also note the thickened ligamentum flavum on the right (arrowhead).   **B. Bone Window**. The bone-windowed image allows better appreciation of the facet degeneration. Observe the difference in the width of the right IVF as compared to its apparent width in Figure A. Differences in window width alter CT measurements, as these sections illustrate.   **C. Axial CT Section, Bone Window: Same Patient, Different Level**. This illustrates severe stenosis of the central canal, the lateral recesses bilaterally, and the IVF's by considerable hypertrophy of arthrotic facet structures.   **D. Axial CT Section, Soft Tissue Window: Same Patient, Different Level**. Right lateral recess stenosis results from facet hypertrophy (arrow). The central canal is also narrowed by the facet disease. Mild disc herniation is also seen (arrowhead), its significance increased by the facet-related stenosis.   **E. Axial CT Section, Bone Window: Same Patient, Different Level**. The bony findings are enhanced by the different window width.

thority on treatment of low back pain, from a retrospective study, expressed the opinion that 80 percent of surgical cases should not have been surgically treated. (64)

Although it is not within the scope of this presentation to discuss surgical approaches to disc herniation or stenosis, several illustrations of the results of surgical procedures are presented. (Fig. 6.57–6.62)

Chemonucleolysis

Chemonucleolysis, injection of discs with chymopapain (a proteolytic agent derived from papaya), has been used again in the USA since late in 1982, after having been used in clinical trials in the 1960's and early 1970's, then withdrawn from use in 1974. (65)

Reports as to effectiveness vary. According to a multi-

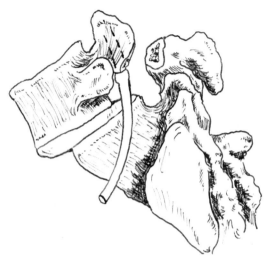

Figure 6.56. SCHEMATIC REPRESENTATION: NERVE ENTRAPMENT IN SPONDYLOLISTHESIS. With anterior subluxation in spondylolisthesis, the nerve root may become entrapped under the pars, as depicted in this drawing.

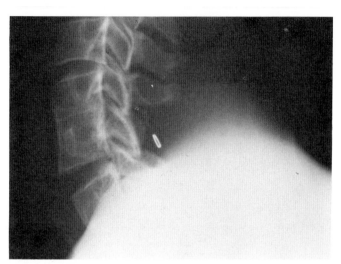

Figure 6.58. CERVICAL LAMINECTOMY WITH INTERBODY FUSION. Total laminectomy has been performed at C7, with surgical fusion of the C6 and C7 vertebral bodies. Note the metal surgical clip in the soft tissues adjacent to the laminectomy.

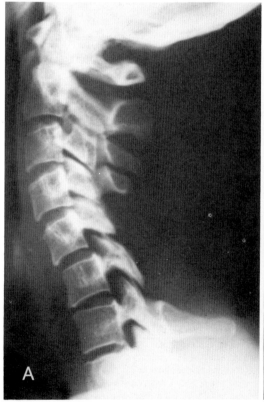

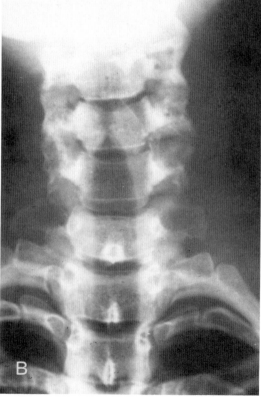

Figure 6.57. CERVICAL SPINE, C5 AND C6: TOTAL LAMINECTOMY. A. Lateral View. Note the total absence of laminae and spinous processes at C5 and C6. There is flexion misalignment of both the C5/C6 and C6/C7 motion segments, which may be the result of post-surgical instability. **B. AP View.** The absence of the laminae and spinous processes is not as evident because of the superimposed tracheal air column.

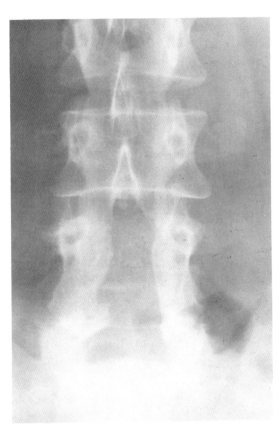

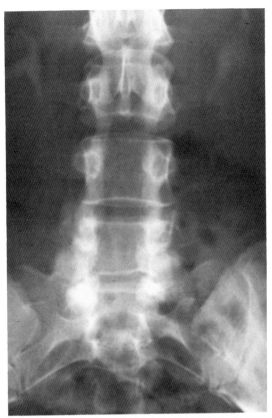

Figure 6.59. LUMBAR TOTAL LAMINECTOMIES. Laminae and spinous processes have been removed at both L4 and L5. Fusion has not been performed.

Figure 6.60. EXTENSIVE LUMBOSACRAL TOTAL LAMINECTO-MIES. The laminectomies were done at L4, L5, and S1. There is no evidence that surgical fusion was attempted.

center study involving 1,498 patients, successful results were achieved in 79.9–88.9 percent of cases, depending on criteria employed in tabulation. (66) Another study claimed 70–75 percent good results. (65) Major complications have occurred in a significant number of cases, anaphylaxis being the most serious, with neurotoxicity from dural puncture also notable. (65–68) A preoperative fluorescence enzyme immunoassay test has been developed as an objective screening method for identifying patients most likely to tolerate chymopapain in order to minimize risks. This has shown good predictive values for both positive and negative findings based on substantial post-marketing surveillances. (69)

Early studies showed demonstrable decrease in size of herniations via CT. (70) As more cases of chymopapain failure are scanned, it is important to know of the CT changes following the injection. The disc margin loses definition, and soft tissue infiltrate appears around the nerve roots in the first weeks after injection. The infiltrate gradually disappears after a few weeks, although blurring of the disc margin may persist for months. The first objective change in the injected disc is a decrease in attenuation value of the disc, probably due to chemical changes within the disc. (23) Because of the severity of chymopapain complications, another enzyme, collagenase, is being utilized by some surgeons, with reportedly fewer resultant problems. (71)

Actual resorption of the herniated nuclear material may take up to six months. There is good correlation between relief of symptoms and objective decrease in size of the herniation. Failure of the therapy is indicated when there is no change in the CT appearance of the disc. One complication is early disc space narrowing due to a volume loss of the disc, which leads to premature discogenic spondylosis. Chemonucleolysis is not an indicated treatment for free fragments, but a few have been shown to disappear after this therapy. (23)

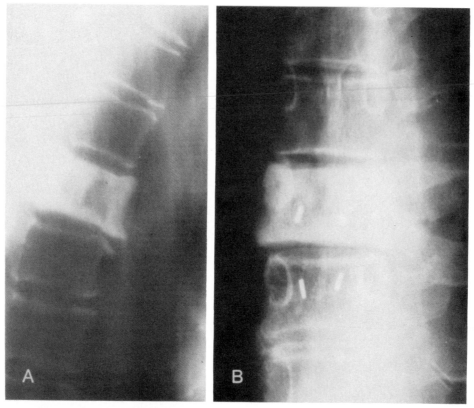

Figure 6.61. THORACIC LAMINECTOMY, PAGETIC VERTE-BRA. A. Lateral View. Enlargement of T8 due to Paget's disease has caused stenosis of the spinal canal. **B. AP View.** Total lami-nectomies at T8, T9, and T10 have been performed. Metal surgical clips are seen in the area of the surgery.

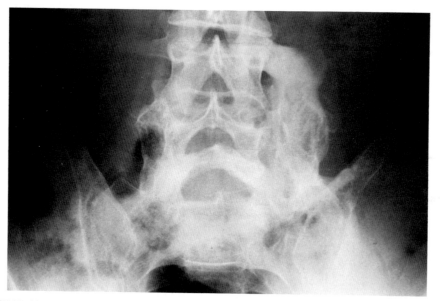

Figure 6.62. LUMBOSACRAL SPINE: EXTENSIVE SURGICAL FU-SION. Fusion has been performed from L3 through S1. Note the extensive bony overgrowth associated with the bone grafts, fusing transverse processes and articular processes.

CAPSULE SUMMARY. Diagnostic Imaging in the Stenotic Syndromes

DEGENERATIVE DISC DISEASE AND DISC HERNIATION
PATHOLOGY
Physiological changes in the intervertebral disc, beginning in the second decade, progress throughout life with degenerative changes resulting. As the nucleus pulposis and annulus fibrosis degenerate, a bulging, herniation of the nucleus, or even nuclear extrusion may occur.

IMAGING IN THE DIAGNOSIS OF DISC DISEASE
Plain film radiography, myelography, computerized tomography, computerized tomographic metrizamide myelography, magnetic resonance imaging, and, rarely, discography and epidural venography may be used in the diagnosis of disc disease.

BULGING ANNULUS
Lumbar Spine. Computed tomography is presently the optimum imaging method to assess disc bulge. MRI will allow diagnosis of disc degeneration before other imaging methods. Intradiscal gas is occasionally found in bulging discs.

Thoracic Spine. Disc degeneration progresses more slowly in the thoracic spine. It is most common at T9/T10, T10/T11, and T11/T12, and is predominantly found in males.

Cervical Spine. Cervical disc protrusions beyond 2 mm indicate herniation. The uncovertebral joints provide a relative barrier to posterolateral disc protrusion. Simple cervical disc bulges are rarely clinically significant unless the spinal canal is small.

HERNIATED NUCLEUS PULPOSUS
Lumbar Spine. Lumbar HNP is most commonly posterior or posterolateral. HNP does not violate the posterior longitudinal ligament. CT identification is made easier by the abundance of epidural fat found in the lumbar spinal canal. The most common location for HNP in the lumbar spine is L4/L5 and L5/S1. Central HNP may cause back pain, although it may not be accompanied by radiculopathy. Myelography demonstrates HNP, which impinges upon the dural sac and/or one or more nerve roots. Far lateral HNP is not demonstrable by conventional myelography but is well seen by CT. Axial MRI may also demonstrate far lateral herniations. Schmorl's nodes represent herniation of nuclear material through end plates into vertebral bodies.

Thoracic Spine. Although thoracic HNP is rare, it may cause spinal cord compression. Myelography or CTMM may be of greater value in the thoracic spine than in the lumbar spine. MRI is also valuable. Intradiscal calcification is common in thoracic HNP.

Cervical Spine. Cervical HNP is less common than is lumbar HNP. It is most common at C6/C7 or C5/C6. Because there is little epidural fat in the cervical spinal canal, myelography or CTMM are especially valuable for demonstration of HNP in this spinal region. MR images demonstrate cervical HNP very well. Chronic cervical disc protrusion may lead to posterior spondylotic ridging.

DIFFERENTIAL DIAGNOSIS OF DISC HERNIATION
Intraspinal neoplasms, conjoined lumbar nerve roots, and partial volume averaging associated with spondylolisthesis in CT studies may be difficult to differentiate from HNP.

DISC EXTRUSION
This is also known as sequestration of the disc, disc prolapse, and free disc fragment. When nuclear material violates the posterior longitudinal ligament and becomes a free fragment in the spinal canal, the fragment may move, causing varying symptoms. CTMM may be necessary to make this diagnosis.

SPONDYLOSIS
Osteophytic buildup along vertebral end plate margins may result from annular degeneration. These may form marginal "claw" spurs, or nonmarginal "traction" spurs. Posterior osteophytes may be the cause of spinal canal, lateral recess, or foraminal stenosis. Plain films indicate the presence of spondylosis, but CT is necessary to determine whether or not there is underlying stenosis present.

ROLES OF VARIOUS IMAGING MODALITIES IN DIAGNOSIS OF DISC DISEASE
Plain Film Radiography. Although this is the first imaging study in patients with spinal disease, it shows only relatively late manifestations of such diseases. Their severity may have little relationship to symptoms or objective findings. Lateral bending and flexion/extension lumbar studies have been noted by some authors to be indicators of disc herniation.

Computerized Tomography, Myelography, and CT Metrizamide Myelography. CT has become the imaging method of choice in diagnosis of HNP in patients who have not undergone previous surgery. Myelography is less frequently used, except when CT is equivocal. CTMM is often favored rather than conventional myelography. CTMM is especially of value in the cervical and thoracic spines.

Magnetic Resonance Imaging. The role of MRI is still developing. It has promise of becoming the most efficacious imaging method for disc disease.

Discography and Epidural Venography. These invasive modalities are not frequently used in diagnosis of disc disease, although both offer some characteristics that are helpful in such diagnosis.

SPINAL STENOSIS
CENTRAL STENOSIS ETIOLOGY
Congenital Central Stenosis. This may result from achondroplasia, several other dysplasias, congenital diseases, or may be idiopathic. Usually, patients with congenital stenosis do not become symptomatic until trauma or degeneration are superimposed.

Acquired Central Stenosis. This may be caused by degenerative disease of discs and/or facets, ligamentum flavum hypertrophy, spondylolisthesis, trauma, post-surgical scarring, ossification of the posterior longitudinal ligament, or other diseases of the vertebrae or joints.

CENTRAL STENOSIS MEASUREMENTS
Measurements of the canal are not as helpful in determination of stenosis as is evaluation of the contents. CT sagittal reformatting allows the best measurements at the present state of the imaging art. Myelography remains the "gold standard" in determination of effects on the thecal sac.

Cervical Spine. At the cervicocranial junction, anomalies, diseases affecting the transverse ligament of the atlas, bone-softening diseases, or trauma may cause stenosis. In the mid and lower cervical spine, spondylosis, arthrosis, inflammatory diseases, ossification of the posterior longitudinal ligament (OPLL), and HNP may result in stenosis of the canal.

Thoracic Spine. Stenosis is less common in the thoracic spine than in the lumbar or cervical regions, although the same disease processes that cause stenosis in the other regions may do so in the thorax as well.

Lumbar Spine. A trefoil canal may be present in 10–20 percent of the normal population. This is not, of itself, evidence of stenosis, but any of the usual causes of stenosis are of greater significance in such people. All the causes of stenosis noted to affect the other spinal regions are important in the lumbar spine. Post-surgical scarring is more frequently encountered in the lumbar canal.

Symptomatology. Cervical stenosis may cause spinal cord compression with remote symptoms. Lumbar stenosis is accompanied by cauda equina compression, sometimes with bizarre symptoms. Neurogenic claudication, paresthesias, hypesthesia, and other symptoms have been related.

LATERAL RECESS STENOSIS ETIOLOGY

Degenerative facetal disease, posterolateral disc herniation, ligamentum flavum hypertrophy, or a combination of these are the most common causes of lateral recess stenosis. A lumbar trefoil canal is particularly in jeopardy. Uncinate hypertrophy is a cause of cervical lateral recess stenosis. Lateral recess and central canal stenosis frequently coexist.

Types of Lateral Recess Stenosis. *Lateral stenosis* results when there is superior migration of a superior articular process or when an osteophyte at the superior of a superior process compresses a nerve root. In *subarticular stenosis* the nerve is entrapped just below the disc. Either of these can be classified as *dynamic* or *fixed* stenotic situations, depending upon whether changes in vertebral position does or does not relieve the symptoms.

Symptomatology. Symptoms are radicular in nature.

FORAMINAL STENOSIS ETIOLOGY

Bony overgrowth, lateral disc herniation, disc extrusion, or post-surgical scarring are the most common causes of foraminal stenosis.

Cervical Spine. Uncovertebral arthrosis is the most common cause of cervical IVF occlusion. CT is more helpful in proper assessment than is plain film radiography.

Thoracic Spine. IVF stenosis is uncommon in the thoracic spine but may occur from facet or costovertebral arthrosis.

Lumbar Spine. Axial CT images usually allow adequate visualization of lumbar IVF stenosis, but reformatted sagittal views are often very helpful.

Symptomatology. Radicular symptoms result from IVF stenosis. Even with what appears radiographically to be severe disease, there may be surprisingly few symptoms. The opposite may be true.

SPONDYLOLISTHESIS

Rarely, nerve root compression results from displacement in isthmic spondylolisthesis. Degenerative spondylolisthesis may cause central stenosis and is the most common cause of direct symptoms from spondylolisthesis. Iatrogenic (post-laminectomy) spondylolisthesis may also be encountered. Retrolisthesis may be degenerative or post-surgical. Refer to Chapter 5 for thorough discussion of spondylolisthesis.

TREATMENT OF STENOTIC SYNDROMES

Surgical. Surgery should be considered only after an adequate trial of conservative therapy, including bedrest, chiropractic manipulation, physical therapy, medication, exercises, and supports have been unproductive. Neurological changes alone are rarely indications for surgery. There is controversy, even among surgeons, as to the efficacy of this treatment.

Chemonucleolysis. This is also a controversial treatment method. Although some good results have been shown from chemonucleolysis, the severity of complications—anaphylaxis, which on a few occasions has resulted in death, and neurotoxicity, which may be severe—raises a question as to the advisability of this approach.

REFERENCES

Introduction

1. Arnoldi CC, Brodsky AE, Cauchoix J, Crock HV, Domisse GF, Edgar MA, Gargano FP, Jacobson RE, Kirkaldy-Willis WH, Kurihara A, Langenskiold A, MacNab I, McIvor GWD, Newman PH, Paine KWE, Russin LA, Sheldon J, Tile M, Urist MR, Wilson WE, Wiltse LL: Lumbar spinal stenosis and nerve root entrapment syndromes, definition and classification. *Clin Orthop* 115:4, 1976.
2. Verbiest H: Fallacies of the present definition, nomenclature, and classification of the stenoses of the lumbar spinal canal. *Spine* 1:217, 1976.
3. Mixter WJ, Barr JS: Rupture of the intervertebral disc with involvement of the spinal canal. *N Engl J Med* 211:210, 1934.
4. Mooney V, Robertson J: The facet syndrome. *Clin Orthop* 115:149, 1976.
5. Kirkaldy-Willis WH, Hill RJ: A more precise diagnosis for low-back pain. *Spine* 4:102, 1979.
6. Kirkaldy-Willis WH: *Managing Low Back Pain*, New York, Churchill Livingstone, 1983.
7. Hounsfield GN: Computerized transverse axial scanning (tomography). *Br J Radiol* 46:10, 1973.
8. Rothman SLG, Glenn WV Jr: *Multiplanar CT of the Spine*, Baltimore, University Park Press, 1985.
9. Glenn WV Jr, Rothman SLG, Rhodes ML, et al: An overview of lumbar computed tomography/multiplanar reformations: What are its elements and how do they fit together. In Post MJD: *Computed Tomography of the Spine*, Baltimore, Williams & Wilkins, 1984.
10. Glenn WV Jr, Rothman SLG, Rhodes ML: Computed tomography/multiplanar reformatted (CT/MRP) examinations of the lumbar spine. In Gennant HK, Chafetz N, Helms CA: *Computed Tomography of the Lumbar Spine*, San Francisco, University of California, 1982.
11. Gennant HK: Computed tomography of the lumbar spine: Technical considerations. In Gennant HK, Chafetz N, Helms CA: *Computed Tomography of the Lumbar Spine*, San Francisco, University of California, 1982.
12. Gennant HK, Chafetz N, Helms CA: *Computed Tomography of the Lumbar Spine*, San Francisco, University of California, 1982.
13. Burton CV: The practical present and the anticipated future of computed tomography. In Post MJD: *Computed Tomography of the Spine*, Baltimore, Williams & Wilkins, 1984.

14. Rosenstein M: Organ doses in diagnostic radiology. *BRH Publication FDA 76-8030*, Washington, DC, US Govt Printing Office, 1976.
15. Tuddenham WJ (editor): Nuclear Magnetic Resonance. *Radiographics* 4 (special edition), 1984.
16. Partain CL, James AE Jr, Rollo FD, et al: *Nuclear Magnetic Resonance (NMR) Imaging*, Philadelphia, WB Saunders, 1983.
17. Budinger TF, Cullander C: Health hazards in nuclear magnetic resonance in vivo studies. *Radiographics* 4:74, 1984.

The Spinal Canal: Characteristics and Morphology

1. Schmorl G, Junghanns H: *The Human Spine in Health and Disease*, American ed 2 (Translated and edited by Besemann EF), New York, Grune & Stratton, 1971.
2. Hadley LA: *Anatomico-Roentgenographic Studies of the Spine*, Springfield, IL, Charles C. Thomas, 1964.
3. MacNab I: *Backache*, Baltimore, Williams & Wilkins, 1977.
4. Farfan HF: *Mechanical Disorders of the Low Back*, Philadelphia, Lea & Febiger, 1973.
5. Cox JM: *Low Back Pain: Mechanism, Diagnosis, and Treatment*, ed 4, Baltimore, Williams & Wilkins, 1985.
6. Eisenstein S: Measurement of the lumbar spinal canal in two racial groups. *Clin Orthop* 115:43, 1976.
7. Shapiro R: *Myelography*, ed 4, Chicago, Year Book Medical Publishers, 1984.
8. Sicard JA, Forrestier J: Methode generale d'exploration radiologique par l'huile iodee (Lipiodol). *Bull et mem soc med hop Paris* 46:463, 1922.
9. Mixter WJ, Barr JS: Rupture of the intervertebral disc with involvement of the spinal canal. *N Engl J Med* 211:210, 1934.
10. Keiffer SA: *Thoracic and Cervical Spine Myelography: Technical Considerations and Selection of Contrast Media*. Presented at the NYU Medical Center Symposium on Diseases of the Spine, New York, 1985.
11. Lin JP: *Myelography of the Lumbar Spine*. Presented at the NYU Medical Center Symposium on Diseases of the Spine, New York, 1985.
12. Han JS, Bick RJ, Anderson P, et al: *MR Imaging of Remote Spinal Injury*. Presented at the 71st scientific assembly and annual meeting of the Radiological Society of North America, Chicago, 1985.
13. Lesh P, Maravilla KR, Sory C, et al: *MR imaging of the Lumbar Spine: Correlation with CT, Diskography, and Pathological Sections in Cadaver Specimens*. Presented

at the 71st scientific assembly and annual meeting of the Radiological Society of North America, Chicago, 1985.

14. Markisz JA, Kazam E, Knowles RJR, et al: *Role of MR Imaging in the Diagnosis and Evaluation of Bone Disease: Comparison with Bone Scan, CT, and Radiographic Study.* Presented at the 71st scientific assembly and annual meeting of the Radiological Society of North America, Chicago, 1985.

15. Dorwart RH, Sauerland EK, et al: Normal lumbosacral spine. In Newton TH, Potts DG: *Computed Tomography of the Spine and Spinal Cord,* San Anselmo, Clavadel Press, 1983.

16. Rauschning W: Detailed sectional anatomy of the spine. In Rothman SLG, Glenn WV Jr: *Multiplanar CT of the Spine,* Baltimore, University Park Press, 1985.

17. Rauschning W: Correlative multiplanar computed tomographic anatomy of the normal spine. In Post MJD: *Computed Tomography of the Spine,* Baltimore, Williams & Wilkins, 1984.

Imaging In Degenerative Disease and Stenosis

1. Coventry MB, Ghormley RK, Kernohan JW: The intervertebral disc: Its microscopic anatomy and pathology. Part 1. Anatomy, development, and physiology. *J Bone Joint Surg (Am)* 27:105, 1945.

2. DePalma AF, Rothman RH: *The Intervertebral Disc,* Philadelphia, WB Saunders, 1970.

3. Morris JM: *Surgical Management of Lumbar Disc Disease.* Presented at the University of California course on CT of the lumbar spine, San Francisco, 1981.

4. Coventry MB, Ghormley RK, Kernohan JW: The intervertebral disc: Its microscopic anatomy and pathology. Part 2. Changes in intervertebral disc concomitant with age. *J Bone Joint Surg (Am)* 27:233, 1945.

5. Williams AL, Haughton VM, Meyer GA, et al: Computed tomographic appearance of the bulging annulus. *Radiology* 142:403, 1982.

6. Gershon-Cohen J, Schraer H, Sklaroff DM, et al: Dissolution of the intervertebral disc in the aged normal: The phantom nucleus pulposis. *Radiology* 62:383, 1954.

7. Tovi D, Strang RR: Thoracic intervertebral disc protrusions. *Acta Chir Scand Suppl* 267:1, 1960.

8. Coin CG: Computed tomography of cervical disc disease (herniation and degeneration). In Post MJD: *Computed Tomography of the Spine,* Baltimore, Williams & Wilkins, 1984.

9. Naylor A: Intervertebral disc prolapse and degeneration. *Spine* 1:108, 1976.

10. Coventry MB, Ghormley RK, Kernohan JW: The intervertebral disc: Its microscopic anatomy and pathology. Part 3. Pathologic changes in the intervertebral disc. *J Bone Joint Surg (Am)* 27:460, 1945.

11. Harris RI, McNab I: Structural changes in the lumbar intervertebral discs. *J Bone Joint Surg (Br)* 36:304, 1954.

12. Hirsch C, Schajowicz F: Studies in structural changes in the lumbar annulus fibrosis. *Acta Orthop* 22:184, 1953.

13. Schmorl G, Junghanns H: *The Human Spine in Health and Disease,* American ed 2 (Translated and edited by Besemann EF), New York, Grune & Stratton, 1971.

14. Love JG, Kiefer EJ: Root pain and paraplegia due to protrusions of thoracic intervertebral disks. *J Neurosurg* 7:62, 1950.

15. Post MJD: *Radiologic diagnosis of cervical disc herniation.* Presented at the academy of orthopedic surgeons course on the intervertebral disc, Philadelphia, 1979.

16. Spurling RG, Segerberg LH: Lateral intervertebral disc lesions in the lower cervical region. *JAMA* 151:354, 1953.

17. Epstein BS: *The Spine: A Radiological Text and Atlas,* ed 4, Philadelphia, Lea & Febiger, 1976.

18. Epstein BS, Epstein JA, Jones MD: Cervical spinal stenosis. *Rad Clin N Am* 15:215, 1977.

19. Williams AL, Haughton VM, Syvertsten A: Computed tomography in the diagnosis of herniated nucleus pulposis. *Radiology* 135:95, 1980.

20. Williams AL, Haughton VM: Disc herniation and degenerative disc disease. In Newton TH, Potts DG: *Computed Tomography of the Spine and Spinal Cord,* San Anselmo, Clavadel Press, 1983.

21. Yang WC, Zappula R, Malis L: Neurolemmoma in lumbar intervertebral foramen. *J Comput Asst Tomogr* 5:904, 1981.

22. Haughton VM, Williams AL: *Computed Tomography of the Spine,* St. Louis, CV Mosby, 1982.

23. Rothman SLG, Glenn WV Jr: *Multiplanar CT of the Spine,* Baltimore, University Park Press, 1985.

24. Meyer JD: Computed tomographic myelography in degenerative disc disease and spinal stenosis. In Latchaw RE: *Computed Tomography of the Head, Neck and Spine,* Chicago, Year Book Medical Publishers, 1985.

25. MacNab I: *Backache,* Baltimore, Williams & Wilkins, 1977.

26. Greive GP: *Common Vertebral Joint Problems,* New York, Churchill Livingstone, 1981.

27. Herlin L: *Sciatic and Pelvic Pain Due to Lumbosacral Nerve Root Compression,* Springfield, IL, Charles C. Thomas, 1966.

28. Howe JW: Preliminary observations from cineroentgenological studies of the spinal column. *ACA J Chiro* 4:S65, 1970.

29. Cox JM: *Low Back Pain: Mechanism, Diagnosis, and Treatment,* ed 4, Baltimore, Williams & Wilkins, 1985.

30. Kirkaldy-Willis WH: *Managing Low Back Pain,* New York, Churchill Livingstone, 1983.

31. Ben-Eliyahu DJ, Rutili MM, Przybysz JA: Lateral recess syndrome: Diagnosis and chiropractic management. *J Manip Physiol Ther* 6:25, 1983.

32. Weitz EM: The lateral bending sign. *Spine* 6:388, 1981.

33. Firooznia H: *CT Diagnosis of Disc Disease.* Presented at the NYU Medial Center, Symposium on Diseases of the Spine, New York, 1985.

34. Bell GR, Rothman RH, Booth RE, et al: A study of computer-assisted tomography II: Comparison of metrizamide myelography and computed tomography in the diagnosis of herniated lumbar disc and spinal stenosis. *Spine* 9:552, 1984.

35. Heithoff KB, Moyle JW, Dowdle J, et al: *Cooperative Study of the Efficacy of Metrizamide Myelography and CT in the Study of Lumbar Disc Disease and Spinal Stenosis.* Presented at the 71st scientific assembly and annual meeting of the Radiological Society of North America, Chicago, 1985.

36. Gado MH, Chandra-Schur B, Patel J, et al: *An Integrated Approach to the Diagnosis of Lumbar Disc Disease by Computed Tomography and Myelography.* Presented at the 67th scientific assembly and annual meeting of the Radiological Society of North America, Chicago, 1981.

37. Haughton VM, Eldevik OP, Magnaes B, et al: A prospective comparison of computed tomography and myelography in the diagnosis of herniated lumbar discs. *Radiology* 142:103, 1982.

38. Raskin FP, Keating JW: *The Relative Accuracy of CT in Myelography for Lumbar Disc Disease: A Collaborative Study (100 Cases).* Presented at the 19th meeting of the American Society of Neuroradiology, Chicago, 1981.

39. Glenn WV Jr, Brown BM, Murphy RM, et al: *Computed Tomography in the Evaluation of Lumbar Disc Disease.* Presented at the 67th scientific assembly and annual meeting of the Radiological Society of North America, Chicago, 1981.

40. Lesh P, Maravilla KR, Sory C, et al: *MR Imaging of the Lumbar Spine: Correlation with CT, Discography, and Pathological Sections in Cadaver Specimens.* Presented at the 71st scientific assembly and annual meeting of the Radiological Society of North America, Chicago, 1985.

41. Han JS, Bick RJ, Anderson P, et al: *MR Imaging of Remote Spinal Injury.* Presented at the 71st scientific assembly and annual meeting of the Radiological Society of North America, Chicago, 1985.

42. Verbiest H: Fallacies of the present definition, nomenclature, and classification of the stenoses of the lumbar spinal canal. *Spine* 1:217, 1976.

43. Helms CA, Vogler JB III: Spinal stenosis and degenerative lesions. In Newton TH, Potts DG: *Computed Tomography of the Spine and Spinal Cord,* San Anselmo, Clavadel Press, 1983.

44. Dorwart RH, Vogler JB III, Helms CA: Spinal stenosis. *Radiol Clin North Am* 21:301, 1983.

45. Pyeritz RE, Sack GH Jr, Udvarhelyi GB: Cervical and lumbar laminectomy for spinal stenosis in achondroplasia. *Johns Hopkins Med J* 146:203, 1980.

46. Ehni G: Stenosis and cervical myelopathy. *J Neurosurgery* 52:290, 1980.

47. Minagi H, Gronner AT: Calcification of the posterior longitudinal ligament: A cause of cervical myelopathy. *AJR* 105:365, 1969.

48. Hyman RA, Merten CW, Liebeskind AL, et al: Computed tomography in ossification of the posterior longitudinal spinal ligament. *Neuroradiology* 13:227, 1977.

49. Foreman SM: Ossification of the posterior longitudinal ligament: A cause of spinal stenosis syndrome. *J Manip Physiol Ther* 8:251, 1985.

50. Resnick D, Guerra J Jr, Robinson CA, et al: Association of diffuse idiopathic skeletal hyperostosis (DISH) and calcification and ossification of the posterior longitudinal ligament. *AJR* 131:1049, 1978.

51. Resnick D, Niwayama G: *Diagnosis of Bone and Joint Disorders,* Philadelphia, WB Saunders, 1981.

52. Buehler MT: Spinal stenosis. *J Manip Physiol Ther* 1:103, 1978.

53. Epstein JA, Epstein BS, Lavine L: Nerve root compression associated with narrowing of the lumbar spinal canal. *J Neurol Neurosurg Psychiatry* 25:165, 1962.

54. Eisenstein S: The trefoil configuration of the lumbar spinal canal: A study of South African skeletal material. *J Bone Joint Surg (Br)* 62:73, 1980.

55. Kirkaldy-Willis WH, Paine KWE, Cauchoix J, et al: Lumbar spinal stenosis. *Clin Orthop* 99:30, 1974.

56. Cox JM: Pedicogenic stenosis: Its manipulative implications. *J Manip Physiol Ther* 2:35, 1979.

57. Heithoff KB: High resolution computed tomography and stenosis: An evaluation of the causes and cures of the failed back surgery syndrome. In Post MJD: *Computed Tomography of the Spine,* Baltimore, Williams & Wilkins, 1984.

58. Kirkaldy-Willis WH, Heithoff KB, Bowen CT, et al: Pathological anatomy of lumbar spondylosis and stenosis, correlated with the CT scan. In Post MJD: *Radiographic Evaluation of the Spine: Current Advances with Emphasis on Computed Tomography,* New York, Masson, 1980.

59. Kirkaldy-Willis WH, Heithoff KB, Tchang S, et al: Lumbar spondylosis and stenosis: Correlation of pathological anatomy with high resolution computed tomographic scanning. In Post MJD: *Computed Tomography of the Spine,* Baltimore, Williams & Wilkins, 1984.

60. Rothman SLG, Glenn WV Jr: Spondylolysis and spondylolisthesis. In Newton TH, Potts DG: *Computed Tomography of the Spine and Spinal Cord,* San Anselmo, Clavadel Press, 1983.

61. Ehheverria T, Lockwood R: Lumbar spinal stenosis. *NY J Med* 872, 1979.

62. Wiltse LL, Kirkaldy-Willis WH, McIvor GW: The treatment of spinal stenosis. *Clin Orthop* 115:483, 1976.

63. Finneson BE: A lumbar disc surgery predictive score card. *Spine* 3:186, 1978.

64. Finneson BE: A lumbar disc surgery predictive score card: A retrospective evaluation. *Spine* 4:141, 1979.

65. Shields CB, Arpin EJ: Update on chymopapain. *Neurol Clin* 3:393, 1985.

66. McDermott DJ, Agre K, Brim M, et al: Chymodiactin in patients with herniated lumbar intervertebral disc (s). *Spine* 10:242, 1985.

67. Dyck P: Paraplegia following chemonucleolysis: A case report and discussion of neurotoxicity. *Spine* 10:359, 1985.

68. Dabezies EJ, Murphy CP: Dural puncture using the lateral approach for chemonucleolysis. *Spine* 10:93, 1985.

69. Tsay Y-G, Jones R, Calenoff E, et al: A preoperative chymopapain sensitivity test for chemonucleolysis candidates. *Spine* 9:764, 1984.

70. Heithoff KB, Burton CV, Salib RM: Computed tomographic evaluation in chemonucleolysis. In Gennant HK: *Spine Update 1984: Perspectives in Radiology, Orthopedic Surgery, and Neurosurgery*, San Francisco, Radiology Research and Education Foundation, 1983.

71. Brown MD: *Intradiscal Therapy: Chymopapain or Collagenase*, Chicago, Year Book Medical Publishers, 1983.

Principles of Radiological Interpretation

LINDSAY J. ROWE
TERRY R. YOCHUM

"In radiography, as in photography, microscopy, and many other observations, the appearance which seems the most obvious does not always correspond with the real condition."

Anonymous

General Considerations

Conventional radiographic procedures (plain film) are the most frequently utilized imaging modality in the evaluation of the skeletal system. This chapter will outline the essentials of skeletal imaging, anatomy, physiology, and interpretation.

Technical Considerations

Numerous methods of investigating the skeletal system are available. (Table 7.1) Each modality has its own area of specific use and of deriving specialized information. Usually, a number of these are used in combination to provide the necessary information in arriving at an accurate diagnosis.

Table 7.1.
Skeletal Imaging Modalities

	Biomechanics	Pathology
CONVENTIONAL IMAGING		
Plain film radiography	+	+++
Specialized projections (angulation, stress)	+++	+++
Tomography	+	+++
Xeroradiography	−	+++
CONTRAST IMAGING		
Arthrography	+	+++
Angiography	−	+++
Lymphangiography	−	+++
Myelography—discography	+	+++
Sinography	−	+++
RADIOISOTOPIC IMAGING		
Bone scan	−	+++
ADVANCED IMAGING		
Ultrasound	+	++
Cineroentgenology	+++	+
Computerized tomography (CT)	+	+++
Magnetic resonance imaging (MRI)	?	+++

+++   High sensitivity
 ++   Sensitive
  +   Low sensitivity
  −   No application
  ?   Unknown application

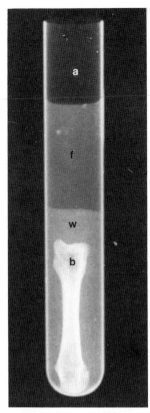

Figure 7.1. NORMAL RADIOGRAPHIC DENSITIES. There are four naturally occurring radiodensities as shown in this x-ray of a test tube: air (a), fat (f), water (w), and bone (b). Note the distinctive difference in density of each component.

PLAIN FILM RADIOGRAPHY

This is the most widely utilized imaging method and is usually the screening procedure applied in the initial examination. No contrast media is used to enhance various body structures. The visualization of these components is dependent on the natural contrast between the five radiographic densities—air, fat, water, bone, and metal. (Fig. 7.1, 7.2) There are distinct limitations in diagnostic sensitivity, with up to 30–50 percent loss of bone density and a lesion size of at least 1–5 cm often necessary before being visible on a radiograph. (1–3) In this context the patient may have extensive histologic disease and have a normal appearing radiograph. (Fig. 7.3) A basic premise in plain film evaluation is the absolute necessity of having a minimum of two views, preferably perpendicular to each other. (Fig. 7.4) These should be supplemented with additional projections, such as oblique, angulated, or stress studies, as clinically indicated. (4) (Fig. 7.5, 7.6)

TOMOGRAPHY

Tomography is derived from the Greek word "tome," meaning to cut or slice to a designated layer. Essentially, tomography is a method enabling examination of anatomic structures and abnormalities in detail (not technically possible with conventional radiography) by examining a selective tissue level in the body. To produce a tomographic image a fulcrum is selected at the required level in the patient between the x-ray tube and film cassette, which move in opposite directions during the exposure. (Fig. 7.7) The effect is to produce a sharp, in-focus image at the level of the fulcrum while blurring out those structures above and below. Numerous films are taken at varying fulcrum levels to totally evaluate the structure in question. This procedure is especially useful in skeletal evaluations in complex structures such as the skull and spine, as well as in delineating the site, characteristics, and extent of a bony abnormality. (Fig. 7.8)

XERORADIOGRAPHY

Although xeroradiography is used mainly for examination of the breast (mammography), there are some applications in skeletal imaging. (Fig. 7.9) The system is different from conventional radiography in that it uses an electrically charged selenium plate as the "cassette." When x-rays strike the plate, the charge is lost. A fine blue powder is blown onto the plate and adheres to the charged regions. The powder is then fused by heat onto paper to produce the image. The selenium plate is then washed and recharged, ready for the next use. The major advantage of the procedure is the exquisite edge enhancement between different densities of bone and soft tissue. It is especially useful in the detection of foreign bodies. However, the x-ray exposure required is several times greater than by conventional methods.

CONTRAST EXAMINATIONS

The major contrast examinations which may be used in the evaluation of skeletal disease include arthrography, angiography, lymphangiography, myelography, and sinography.

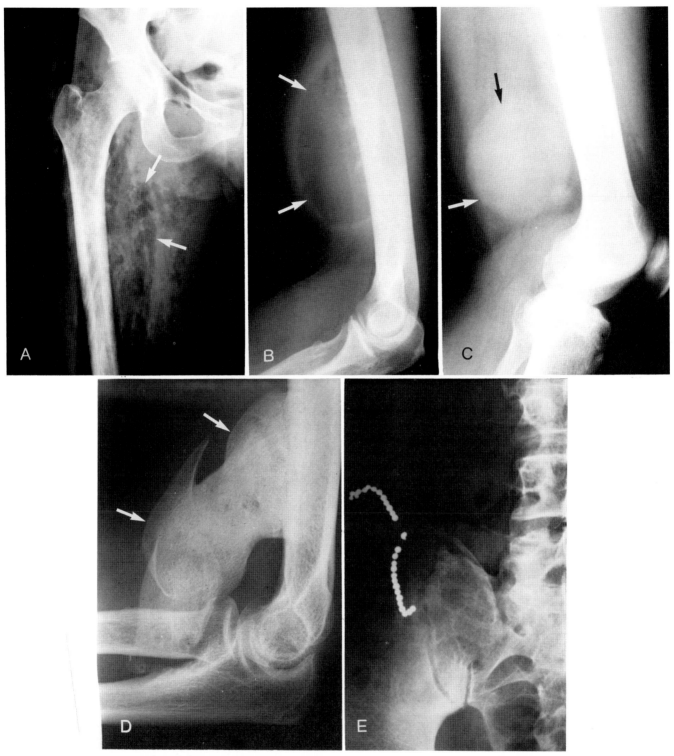

Figure 7.2. EXAMPLES OF RADIOGRAPHIC DENSITIES.   A. Air Density. Observe the radiolucent densities within the soft tissues of the thigh in this patient with gas gangrene (arrows).   **B. Fat Density.** A well-demarcated radiolucent mass is present within the soft tissues of the anterior arm (arrows). This appearance is characteristic of the benign fatty tumor lipoma.   **C. Water Density.** Posterior to the distal femoral shaft is a round, well-circumscribed mass of the same density as the surrounding muscle (arrows). The diagnosis was malignant synovial sarcoma. (Courtesy of C. H. Quay, MD, Melbourne, Australia).   **D. Bone Density.** A smooth bony growth extends from the anterior arm (arrows). Observe the smooth cortical margin and internal trabecular pattern characteristic of post-traumatic myositis ossificans.   **E. Metal Density.** Numerous round metallic densities appear aligned in an "S" shaped configuration in the right lower quadrant of the abdomen. These represent ingested shot pellets lodged in the appendix.

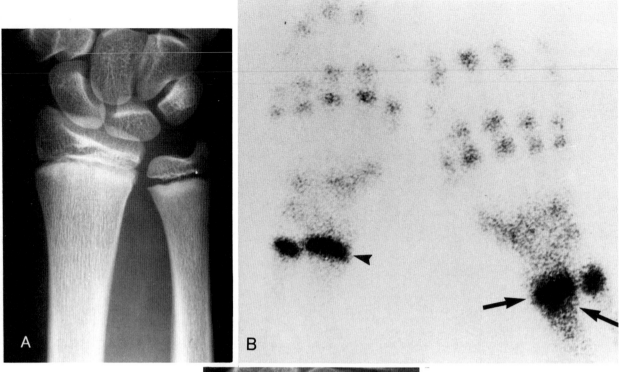

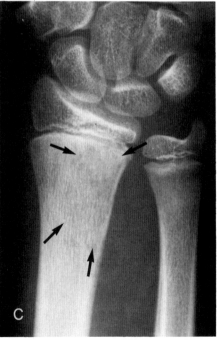

Figure 7.3. LIMITATIONS OF PLAIN FILM EXAMINATIONS.
A. Initial Anteroposterior View: Wrist. Despite swelling, pain, and a slight fever, the radius shows no radiographic abnormality.
B. Radioisotope Bone Scan at Initial Presentation. Note the increased area of blackness ("hot spot") in the corresponding symptomatic radius (arrows) as compared to the normal side (arrowhead).
C. Ten Days Later: Anteroposterior View, Wrist. Observe the motheaten-type radiolucencies within the radial metaphysis (arrows).

These are early plain film findings in osteomyelitis. ***Comment:*** This study demonstrates the sensitivity of the bone scan to increased bone activity, even when the plain film is normal. Plain films require at least 30 to 50 percent destruction of bone before one can demonstrate the lesion, while bone scans will be positive with 3–5 percent destruction. Additionally, the need to re-x-ray when signs and symptoms persist is demonstrated. (Courtesy of David P. Thomas, MD, Melbourne, Australia)

Arthrography

Contrast opacification of joint cavities is a useful procedure in the evaluation of joint disease. Air is often combined with the injected water soluble media to provide a double contrast arthrogram which provides better evaluation of the articular surfaces, menisci, and synovium. (Fig. 7.10) The most common joint examined by

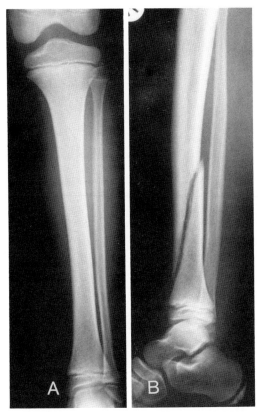

Figure 7.4. DEMONSTRATION OF MINIMUM RADIOGRAPHIC PROCEDURE. A. Anteroposterior View: Tibia and Fibula. No abnormality is evident. **B. Lateral View: Tibia and Fibula.** An oblique fracture line is seen in the tibia which was not visible on the AP view. *Comment:* No radiographic study is complete without a minimum of two views perpendicular to each other.

this procedure is the knee. Other joints less frequently injected include the shoulder, hip, and wrist. In addition, tendon sheaths (tenography) and bursae (bursography) are examined by the same method.

Angiography

The introduction of a water soluble contrast agent into an artery (arteriogram) or vein (venogram) in skeletal disease is utilized mainly in the evaluation of bone tumors and traumatic skeletal injuries. In bone tumors the size and aggressiveness of the lesion can be assessed by the degree of neovascularity, speed of media removal, and local structure invasion. Traumatic injuries may tear, distort, obstruct, dilate, or produce anomalous connections in vessels, which will only be demonstrated by angiography.

Lymphangiography

In selected individuals, especially those with lymphoma or metastatic disease, evaluation of the lymphatic system by an injection of an oil-based medium may be performed. The procedure requires the injection of a blue-green dye between one or more webs of the toes, followed 1 hour later by an incision on the dorsum of the foot to identify a large lymphatic channel. Once identified, the channel is cannulated and an oil-based medium is injected

slowly over 1–3 hours. Approximately 24 hours later the contrast medium will be identifiable within the lower extremity, inguinal, iliac, and para-aortic nodes. The media may remain visible for many months. The lymph nodes are assessed according to location, size, shape, and configuration for evidence of abnormality. The major disorders evaluated with lymphangiography include lymphoma, metastasis, and lymphatic obstruction.

Myelography

Contrast examination of the spine and spinal cord is achieved by injection into the subarachnoid space, usually in the lumbar spine at the second or third lumbar level. This procedure aids in the diagnosis of disc, vertebral, or cord disease. (Fig. 7.11) Injection of an opaque medium into the intervertebral nucleus pulposus (discography) has been used to evaluate discal pathology.

Sinography

This is a selective technique applied in the evaluation of bone infections which are associated with a draining external sinus. The sinus is catheterized and the contrast media injected to show the origin and extent of the infection.

RADIONUCLIDE IMAGING

The principle of nuclear imaging hinges on the selective uptake of certain compounds by different organs of the body. Tissues which can be imaged include the brain, heart, lung, kidneys, and skeleton. In bone imaging (bone scan) the most common isotope used is Technetium-99m phosphate and, less frequently, Gallium-67. Only 3–5 percent bone destruction is necessary to be visible on a bone scan, representing up to ten times an increased sensitivity factor over plain film radiography in the detection of bone abnormalities.

The procedure is performed by injecting 15–20 millicuries of Technetium-99m intravenously and waiting various time periods from 30 minutes to 2 hours for concentration in bony areas of increased blood flow and osteoblastic activity. An imaging device—the gamma camera—is placed over the patient and records the bone-emitted gamma rays as the isotope undergoes degeneration. These rays are transformed into light, and an image is transposed onto a polaroid or radiographic film. Views are taken of the entire body in the posteroanterior and anteroposterior planes in combination with selected spot projections over questionable locations. Regions of increased uptake will show as dark spots ("hot spots"). Normally, the isotope will collect more in the long bone metaphyses, thyroid, sternum, costochondral junctions, spine, and sacroiliac joints. (5) (Fig. 7.12) The isotope half-life is 6 hours and is readily excreted by the kidneys.

The indications for a bone scan include the detection of skeletal metastases, tumors, infection, arthritis, fractures, and avascular necrosis. This is especially useful in diagnosing occult, stress, and recent fractures, in addition to those whose plain films are normal but have pain of undetermined origin. (Fig. 7.13) Diagnostically, the image obtained is quantitative only—it is a measure of activity. Therefore, the scan of a neoplasm may appear identical

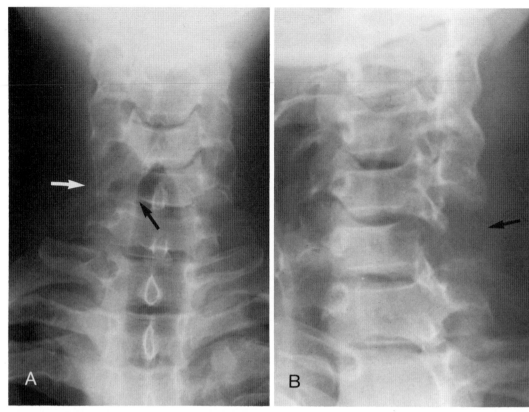

Figure 7.5. USE OF SUPPLEMENTARY SPINAL RADIOGRAPHS. A. Anteroposterior View: Lower Cervical Spine. A subtle destructive lesion is present in the sixth cervical pedicle and articular pillar (arrows). **B. Oblique View: Lower Cervical Spine.** The destruction is now clearly depicted (arrow). This is a characteristic lesion of osteolytic metastatic carcinoma. ***Comment:*** Cervical pedicles, foramina, and articular pillars require oblique films for proper visualization and evaluation. Lumbar obliques serve the purpose of demonstrating abnormalities of the pedicle, facets, and pars region.

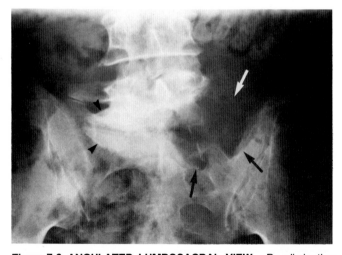

Figure 7.6. ANGULATED LUMBOSACRAL VIEW. By eliminating the sacral base angle greatly improved depiction of the sacrum, sacroiliac joint, and the fifth lumbar body and disc is obtained. Observe the osteolytic destruction of the sacral ala (arrows) from metastatic carcinoma and the large degenerative osteophytes on the contralateral side (arrowheads). ***Comment:*** This is an excellent projection to evaluate for pathology in any patient with low back pain.

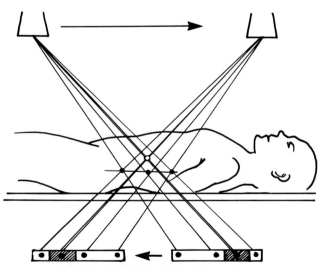

Figure 7.7. PRINCIPLES OF TOMOGRAPHY. The film and x-ray tube move synchronously in opposite directions. Note that the fulcrum (open circle) during the motion remains in clear focus, while areas above and below will be blurred and rendered almost invisible.

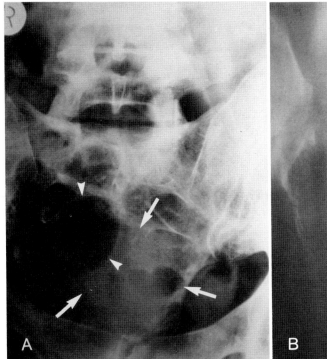
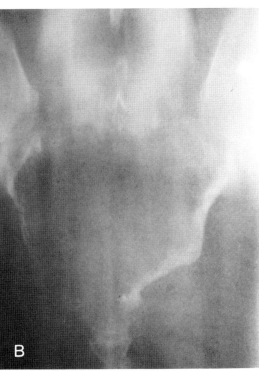

Figure 7.8. DEMONSTRATION OF TOMOGRAPHY. A. Antero-posterior View: Sacrum. Close scrutiny of the lower sacrum reveals destruction of the sacral foramina, cortices, and trabecular patterns (arrows). Note the obscuring gas shadow (arrowheads).

B. Tomography, Anteroposterior View: Sacrum. The degree of sacral destruction is now more clearly depicted. The overlying confusing gas shadows are eliminated by this form of study. Diagnosis: chordoma. (Courtesy of David P. Thomas, MD, Melbourne, Australia)

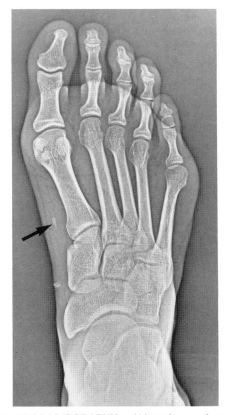

Figure 7.9. XERORADIOGRAPHY. Although seen here in a black and white reproduction, the image is a light blue and is mounted on paper. Observe the exquisite bone and soft tissue detail, as well as the foreign body glass artifact (arrow).

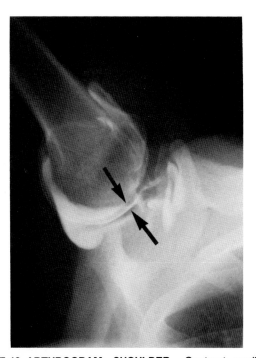

Figure 7.10. ARTHROGRAM: SHOULDER. Contrast media has been placed into the glenohumeral joint and adjacent bursa. Note the lucent zone paralleling the surface of the humeral head (arrows), representing the articular cartilage.

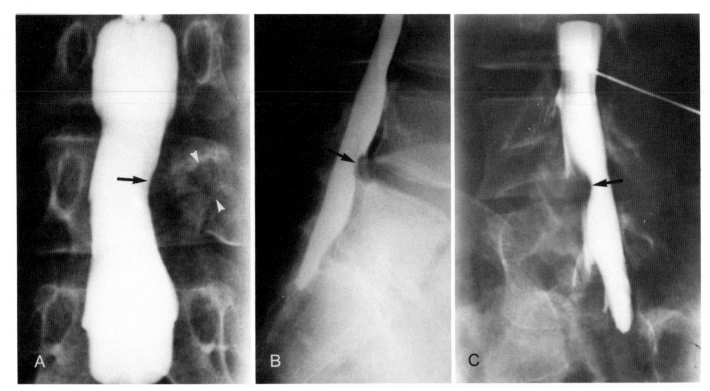

Figure 7.11. MYELOGRAM.   A. Neoplasm: Fourth Lumbar Pedicle. Note the destruction of the pedicle and adjacent vertebral body (arrowheads), with adjacent displacement of the contrast column from the soft tissue mass (arrow). These are characteristic findings of osteolytic metastatic carcinoma.   **B and C. Disc Protrusion: Fourth Lumbar Disc.** Observe the smooth indentation in the myelographic column (arrow).

to infection, with only further correlation providing the definitive diagnosis.

Ultrasound

Diagnostic ultrasound has received little attention as to its practicability in the evaluation of skeletal disease; however, some limited use in the evaluation of spinal stenosis and soft tissue abnormalities has been delineated. (6)

Cineroentgenology

The use of dynamic motion studies has been mostly derived from videoflouroscopy, especially of the spine. Due to the high levels of radiation this is an elective procedure. Information obtained includes aberrant or diminished mobility. (7,8)

COMPUTERIZED TOMOGRAPHY

Although computerized tomography (CT) has had its greatest impact in the evaluation of the central nervous system, various uses have been found in skeletal imaging. Following its introduction in 1973 by Hounsfield, many technical advances have occurred to improve resolution and diagnostic capability. (9,10) The essential components of a CT system include a circular scanning gantry which houses the x-ray tube and image sensors, a table for the patient, an x-ray generator, and a computerized data processing unit. The patient lies on the table and is placed inside the gantry. The x-ray tube is rotated 360 degrees around the patient while the computer collects the data

and formulates a transverse image or "slice." Each cross-sectional slice represents a thickness of between 0.5–1.3 cm of body tissue. In order to produce an optimal examination multiple sequential slices are obtained, with an average dose of 1–3 rads. (11) A more recent development in computer technology has allowed for sagittal and coronal reconstructions to be made. Skeletal applications include assessment of neoplasms, trauma, infections, metabolic disease, and spinal syndromes. (Fig. 7.14)

MAGNETIC RESONANCE IMAGING

The most recent method of body imaging to become available is magnetic resonance imaging (MRI) or what was originally called nuclear magnetic resonance (NMR). Acute interest presently is focused on this modality due to its inherent advantages in observing body physiochemistry and possessing no known complications. (12) Instead of using x-rays, the patient is placed in a magnetic field which produces vibrations within atoms that can be measured and formed into an image. Those structures which have a high water content produce the highest image details, such as the liver, spleen, muscles, and heart. The nucleus pulposus is readily identified in normal or degenerative conditions. When bone is examined it is actually the marrow which forms the image, due to the low levels of osseous water. The skeletal applications of this technique are just beginning to be explored, although startling information is being accrued in the spine and spinal cord. (13) (Fig. 7.15)

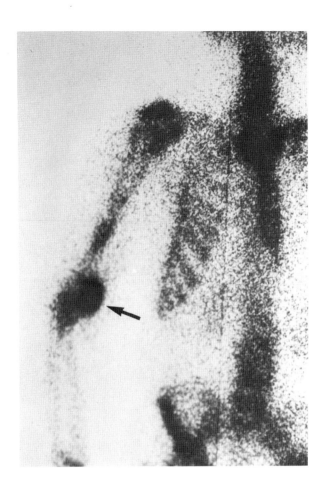

Figure 7.12. NORMAL RADIOISOTOPIC BONE SCAN. Note the normal increased uptake in the metaphysis of the humerus, sternum, costochondral junctions, lumbar spine, ilium, and sacroiliac joints. The dense region in the elbow is the site of the intravenous injection of the isotope (arrow). *Comment:* Bone scans are evaluated for asymmetry in uptake since, normally, metabolically active regions will concentrate the isotope. (Courtesy of Thomas E. Hyde, DC, North Miami, Florida)

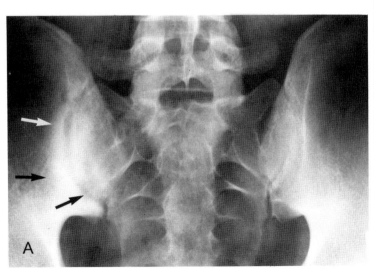

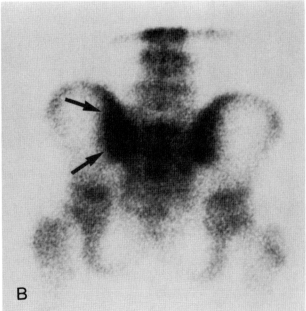

Figure 7.13. ABNORMAL RADIOISOTOPIC BONE SCAN. A. Anteroposterior View: Sacroiliac Joints. Unilateral sacroiliitis (arrows) is evidenced by loss of the sacral and iliac articular margins, with prominent reactive sclerosis. **B.** Observe the increased isotopic uptake ("hot spot") over the corresponding sacroiliac joint (ar-

rows). *Comment:* Although the diagnosis is not definitive on these findings, the scan confirms the presence of increased bone activity. The diagnosis following aspiration of the joint was infection due to *Staphylococcus aureus*. (Courtesy of Gerald A. Fitzgerald, MD, Sydney, Australia)

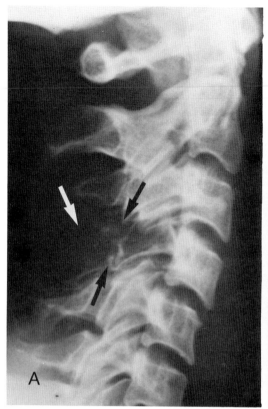

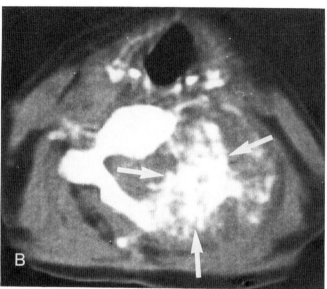

Figure 7.14. COMPUTERIZED TOMOGRAPHY (CT). A. Neutral Lateral: Cervical Spine. Lytic destruction of the fourth cervical spinous, lamina, and articular pillar is observed (arrows). The diagnosis was aneurysmal bone cyst (ABC).

B. Computerized Tomogram. A selected image of the lesion confirms the anatomical location of the tumor in the posterior arch (arrows). Additional information is gained about its size, internal matrix, and soft tissue extension.

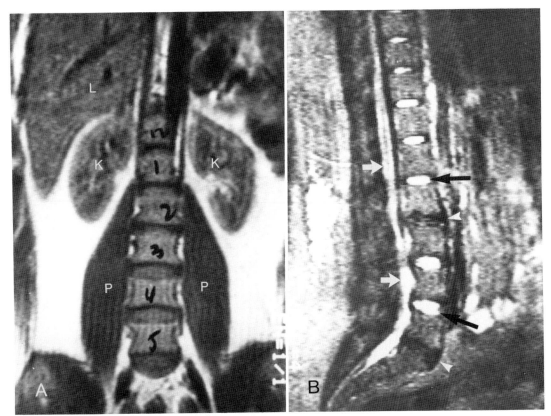

Figure 7.15. MAGNETIC RESONANCE IMAGING (MRI). A. Anteroposterior View. Exquisite detail of the liver (L), kidneys (K), and psoas muscle (P) is obtained. **B. Lateral View.** Note the intense white appearance of the normally hydrated nucleus pulposus (black arrows) as compared to the dehydrated degenerated discs (arrowheads). Additionally, the vertical white structure posteriorly represents the cerebrospinal fluid surrounding the spinal cord (white arrows). **Comment:** MRI is currently primarily dependent on the presence of the hydrogen proton, in particular, to produce an image. The bone marrow is visible due to its high water content. (Courtesy of Steven P. Brownstein, MD, Springfield, New Jersey)

Skeletal Anatomy and Physiology

SKELETAL DEVELOPMENT

Bone is derived from mesodermal tissue. The first bone to ossify in the body is the clavicle. Two processes of bone formation occur—intramembranous and enchondral.

Intramembranous Ossification

Initially, a model is formed from condensed mesenchymal cells. These cells then differentiate into two forms: 1) fibroblasts, producing collagen fiber membranes; and 2) osteoblasts, producing osteoid. Subsequently, bone is formed in this fibrous membrane. There is no preformed stage of cartilage. Bones formed by this process include the parietal and temporal bones, squama, and tympanic parts of the temporal bone, upper occipital squamosa, vomer, medial pterygoid, and upper face. The clavicles and mandible are also membranous bones but later develop secondary cartilaginous centers. In normal bones the width of bone is largely controlled by this method, due to the activity of the periosteum (appositional bone growth).

Enchondral Ossification

From the condensed mesenchymal model cartilage cells form (chondroblasts and chondrocytes) and produce a cartilage cast of the definitive bone. Subsequently, this cartilage template is transformed to bone as peripheral capillaries penetrate and induce the formation of osteoblasts. This peripheral collar of new bone then extends bidirectionally along the long axis of the bone. A similar but separate process occurs within epiphyseal centers. This process is responsible for the formation of all tubular bones, vertebrae, skull, ethmoids, and inferior conchae. This method of ossification is primarily used to lengthen long bones after birth, until skeletal maturity.

BONE STRUCTURE

The anatomic structure of bone includes various divisions—epiphysis, physis, zone of provisional calcification, metaphysis, and diaphysis. (Fig. 7.16) In addition, two types of bone are identifiable—cortical and medullary. These are encased by an outer covering of invisible periosteum.

Epiphysis

The end of a growing bone is called an epiphysis. Initially, composed of cartilage, there is gradual ossification which eventually fuses with the shaft at the end of the growth period. Its function is primarily to produce and support the articular cartilage. Pathologically, an epiphysis is prone to dysplasia, ischemia, arthritic deformation, and special neoplasms such as chondroblastoma and giant cell tumor. Apophyses of bone should also be

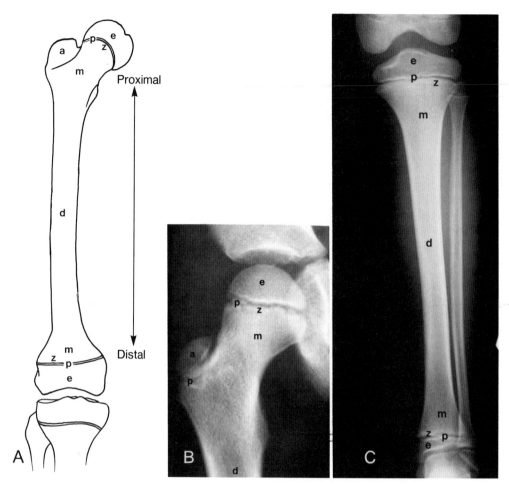

Figure 7.16. GROWING BONE, ANATOMICAL DIVISIONS. A. Diagrammatic Representation. B and C. Radiograph. Observe the epiphysis (e), physis (p), zone of provisional calcification (z), metaphysis (m), diaphysis (d), and apophysis (a).

thought of as epiphyses despite their function as muscle attachments.

Physis

The cartilage growth plate between the epiphysis and metaphysis is known as the physis. Alternate terms include the epiphyseal plate, epiphyseal growth plate, and bone growth center. There are layers of progressively maturing cartilage and developing bone. Adjacent to the physis a stable zone of resting cells is found, followed by sequential zones of proliferation and hypertrophy. These layers are responsible for providing longitudinal growth of a long bone and remain radiolucent during skeletal development. Altered hormonal or vascular dynamics may decrease or increase growth-producing abnormalities of length such as dwarfism and giantism.

Zone of Provisional Calcification (ZPC)

At the junction of the physis and metaphysis a thin line of increased density is identifiable. This represents the region of calcification of the physis cartilage and is the precursor to bone formation. Calcium disorders such as rickets will disturb the appearance of this line. Residuals of intermittent growth arrest from systemic disease may be seen later in life as transverse, opaque metaphyseal lines (growth arrest lines).

Metaphysis

Between the zone of provisional calcification and diaphysis lies the metaphysis. The metaphysis is the most metabolically active region of a bone and as a result is the most common site for tumors and infections of bone. In this location calcified cartilage is transformed into definitive weightbearing stress trabeculae (primary trabeculae) and supporting transverse or oblique trabeculae (secondary trabeculae). Additionally, as part of this process the constricting tubulation of the bone occurs by periosteal resorption. Abnormalities of tubulation result in overconstriction or overexpansion of the metaphysis (Erlenmeyer flask deformity). (Fig. 7.17)

Diaphysis

This lies between both metaphyses and is the longest part of the bone. It is also known as the shaft of the bone. The most notable feature of the diaphysis is the thickened cortex and decreased medullary space. Its main function is to provide mechanical strength and contain the bone marrow. Abnormalities of the diaphysis include marrow diseases such as multiple myeloma, Ewing's sarcoma, non-Hodgkin's lymphoma, adamantinoma, and infection.

Cortex

The densest and strongest of all bone is the cortex. It

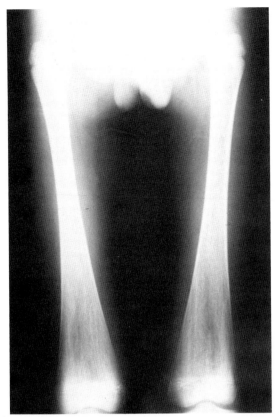

Figure 7.17. ERLENMEYER FLASK DEFORMITY. A lack of the normal metaphyseal/diaphyseal constriction is characteristic of this deformity due to a lack of metaphyseal remodeling. Although present in a number of disorders, this is most notable in Gaucher's disease.

is constructed of densely packed compact lamellar bone and osteons and is interconnected by the Haversian canal systems. Externally, it is enveloped by the periosteum and lined internally with endosteum. Its thickness and integrity is a strong radiological indicator in the diagnosis of bone tumors, infections, and other disorders.

Medulla

The internal cavity of bone is traversed by thin, interconnecting trabeculae (spongiosa) and contains the bone marrow. In children red marrow predominates in all bones. Adults only exhibit red marrow in the axial skeleton, epiphyses, and metaphyses.

Periosteum

A thin membrane of tissue envelops the diaphysis and metaphysis of bone and is called the periosteum. Epiphyseal periosteum does not exist. In children the periosteum is only attached at the metaphysis, while in adults a firm attachment is made at the metaphysis and diaphysis. Histologically, two layers are evident—an outer fibrous and an inner cambium layer. The fibrous layer functions to provide the mechanical means of attachment of itself, tendons, and ligaments by way of Sharpey's fibers. The inner cambium layer is metabolically labile, containing osteoblastic and osteoclastic potential. This inner zone may therefore produce or resorb bone, in response to a

pulling away from the underlying bone by pus, blood, or tumors, and is an important indicator of bone disease.

Endosteum

All trabeculae and inner cortical margins are covered with a single layer that has both osteoclastic and osteoblastic properties. At the cortex a balance between the outer periosteum and inner endosteum maintains cortical thickness.

BONE METABOLISM

Bone metabolism is a complex and dynamic process. Many factors are responsible in promoting or reducing bone activity. The discussion to follow focuses on the effects of minerals and hormones active in normal and abnormal conditions.

Bone Minerals

The major bone minerals are calcium and phosphorus, which usually exist in bone at a ratio of 2 to 1.

Calcium.   Calcium plays numerous roles in body metabolism, including muscle and nerve function. Within bone, calcium forms many different complexes, especially with phosphorus. The main calcium-phosphorus complex is that of crystaline hydroxyapatite—$Ca_{10}(PO_4)_6(OH)_2$. Less than one percent of bone calcium is readily available for turnover at any particular time. The most active sites are at the Haversian canal linings and resorption cavities. The major factors controlling calcium deposition include mechanical stress, vitamin D, parathormone, trace minerals, and alkaline phosphatase.

Phosphorus.   Serum levels of phosphorus are inversely related to calcium. The role of phosphorus is to allow precipitation of calcium at the bone crystal surface.

Hormones

Parathormone (PTH).   Produced by the parathyroid gland, PTH functions to increase serum calcium by promoting bone, kidney, and gut resorption of calcium. In bone this is accomplished by increasing osteoclastic activity. In addition, phosphorus levels are decreased.

Calcitonin.   Its origin is uncertain, though the thyroid and parathyroid glands are likely sites. It is directly antagonistic to PTH by acting to decrease serum calcium levels by reversed effects on the skeleton, kidney, and gut.

Estrogen.   Produced by the ovarian follicle, its presence stimulates bone production by inducing protein anabolic activity. It closely controls longitudinal growth and maturity.

Androgen.   This is the male conterpart of estrogen. It is produced in the testes and adrenal cortex and controls longitudinal growth and maturity.

Growth Hormone (GH).   Arising from the acidophilic cells of the anterior pituitary, GH controls the chondrocyte proliferation and hypertrophy at the growth plate. An absence of GH in the growing period produces dwarfism; an excess of GH produces giantism. If an excess is present in an adult, acromegaly results, with increased membranous ossification in the skull and mandible, and subperiostally in long bones. Additionally, joint cartilage proliferates and degenerates prematurely.

Glucocorticoids. The most important glucocorticoid with effects on bone is hydrocortisone. It induces protein catabolism and phosphorus excretion and therefore encourages osteoclasis. Strong gluconeogenic influences also have the potential to produce diabetes.

The Categorical Approach to Bone Disease

A general etiological classification which aids in arriving at differential and definitive diagnoses is encompassed in seven categories—congenital, trauma, arthritis, tumor, infection, hematologic, and nutritional, metabolic, and endocrine. (Table 7.2) An attempt to approach a given abnormality by using this framework will greatly simplify the process of including and excluding different entities.

CONGENITAL

This includes localized and generalized skeletal anomalies, such as spinal block vertebrae, hip dysplasia, achondroplasia, and cleidocranial dysplasia.

TRAUMA

Traumatic injuries include fractures, subluxations, dislocations, and soft tissue abnormalities such as myositis ossificans.

ARTHRITIS

Joint afflictions as manifested by alterations in alignment, articular contour, and joint space are readily identifiable. By identifying specific features a diagnosis can usually be made.

TUMOR

Neoplastic conditions, whether benign or malignant, can be recognized by their destructive and productive features. The recognition that a lesion has neoplastic characteristics excludes other categories as being possible considerations except in isolated instances.

INFECTION

Disorders of infective processes in bone (osteomyelitis) and joints (septic arthritis) may be difficult to differentiate from tumors but usually can be suggested, given pertinent clinical features, and recognized by key radiological signs.

HEMATOLOGIC

This category encompasses those abnormalities which are characterized by their origins within the bone marrow, such as the various hemolytic anemias or an absence of blood supply typified by epiphyseal avascular necrosis.

NUTRITIONAL, METABOLIC, ENDOCRINE

This is a broad category which contains a number of entities such as nutritional osteopenias (scurvy, rickets, etc.), parathyroid, and hormonal diseases.

Radiological Predictor Variables

A number of methodologies in the assessment of skeletal abnormalities have been suggested. (14,15) A computer-assisted approach based on standard criteria has also been developed. (16,17) A systematic step-by-step analysis is the most optimum method to arrive at an appropriate diagnosis. (Table 7.3) One of the most important decisions based on the accumulated data is to differentiate between slow and aggressive lesions. (Table 7.4)

PRELIMINARY ANALYSIS

Clinical Data

Age. Many disorders exhibit peak ages and age ranges of occurrence. For example, bone tumors such as osteosarcoma, Ewing's sarcoma, and aneurysmal bone cyst are most common under the age of 20 years. Over 50 years, disorders such as Paget's disease, metastasis, and multiple myeloma become more common. Knowledge of these age predilections greatly assists in forming diagnostic possibilities.

Sex. Similarly, some disorders exhibit a gender predominance. Examples of male prevalences include Paget's disease, gout, ankylosing spondylitis, Reiter's syndrome, (9) and hemophilia. Female-dominated disorders include

Table 7.2.
The Seven Categories of Bone Disease

Congenital
Trauma
Arthritis
Tumor
Infection
Hematologic
Nutritional, Metabolic, Endocrine

Table 7.3.
Radiological Predictor Variables

PRELIMINARY ANALYSIS
  Clinical data: age, sex, race, history
  Number of lesions
  Symmetry of lesions
  Systems involved
ANALYSIS OF THE LESION
  Skeletal location
  Position within bone
  Site of origin
  Shape
  Size
  Margination
  Cortical integrity
  Behavior of the lesion
  Matrix
  Periosteal response
  Soft tissue changes
  Joint changes
SUPPLEMENTARY ANALYSIS
  Other radiologic procedures
  Laboratory examination
  Biopsy

Table 7.4.
Radiological Criteria of Benign and Aggressive Lesions

	Benign	Aggressive Primary	Aggressive Secondary
Age (Decades)	123	1234567	4567
Size:			
0–6 cm	+++	+	+
6+ cm	+	+++	+++
Monostotic	+++	+++	++
Polyostotic	+	+	+++
Cortical destruction	−	+++	+++
Periosteal reaction			
Solid	+++	+	−
Laminated	++	++	−
Spiculated	−	+++	+
Codman's	++	++	+
Destruction			
Geographic	+++	+	−
Motheaten	−	+++	+++
Permeative	−	+++	+++
Margins			
Sharp	+++	+	+
Imperceptible	−	+++	+++
Matrix	+++	++	−
Soft tissue mass	−	+++	+
Joint space	−	−	−

    − Absent
    + Occasionally
   ++ Common
  +++ Very common

Table 7.5.
Monostotic Versus Polyostotic Bone Disease

	Monostotic	Polyostotic
CONGENITAL	Block vertebra Polydactyly	Bone dysplasia Achondroplasia
TRAUMATIC	Localized injury	Battered child Severe injury
ARTHRITIS	Degenerative joint disease	Rheumatoid arthritis
TUMOR	Osteoid osteoma Osteosarcoma	Multiple myeloma Metastasis
INFECTION	Staphylococcal	Salmonella
HEMATOLOGIC	Perthes disease	Sickle cell anemia
NUTRITIONAL, METABOLIC, ENDOCRINE	None	Hyperparathyroidism Rickets, scurvy

osteoporosis, systemic lupus erythematosus, osteitis condensans ilii and rheumatoid arthritis.

Race. Certain racial populations are predisposed to some skeletal diseases. Sickle cell anemia in Blacks and thalassemia, in Italian and other Mediterranean populations are classic examples.

History. An accurate, current history is vital to radiological interpretation. Specific information such as the history of trauma, previous diagnosis and associated conditions, and pain and swelling often dictates the followup procedures necessary to confirm or disprove the suspected diagnosis.

Number of Lesions

Numerous disorders may be polyostotic (multiple bones) or monostotic (single bone). (Table 7.5) Polyostotic bone disease includes congenital dysplasias, fibrous dysplasia, Paget's disease, metastatic disease, multiple myeloma, and histiocytoses. (Fig. 7.18) Solitary sites of involvement are usually indicative of a bone tumor or infection. This is an important feature to demonstrate, since the differential possibilities change greatly according to the number of sites affected.

Symmetry of Lesions

Symmetrical and equally distributed skeletal lesions are usually due to disseminated diseases which interfere with bone function and metabolism, such as hyperparathyroidism, osteomalacia, osteoporosis, and leukemia. Asymmetric, haphazardly arranged lesions suggest chance seeding of lesions, such as in metastasis and Paget's disease.

Determination of Systems Involved

If only bone involvement is present, then numerous disorders can be excluded, such as hyperparathyroidism and metastasis. Singular involvement of bone is distinctive of benign bone tumors, occasionally Paget's disease, and selected congenital disorders.

ANALYSIS OF THE LESION

Careful scrutiny of a lesion according to the following criteria will aid in arriving at a diagnosis and will provide clinical insight into its present and possible future behavior.

Skeletal Location

Statistical evaluations of bone lesions, especially tumors, reveal a frequent site predilection. (Table 7.6) For example, most cases of chordoma selectively involve the sacrum and skull base, while osteosarcoma is predominantly encountered around the knee. Knowledge of these common sites of occurrence greatly aid in making a diagnosis.

Position Within Bone

Specific lesions are found in the various anatomic divisions of bone. (Table 7.7) (Fig. 7.19) In the epiphysis congenital dysplasia, ischemic necrosis, and neoplasms such as chondroblastoma and giant cell tumor occur. Metaphyseal lesions are the most common due to the high metabolic rate and high vascularity of the region. Diaphyseal disorders usually are related to marrow disease such as multiple myeloma, Ewing's, and non-Hodgkin's lymphoma ("round cell" tumors).

Site of Origin

By attempting to designate the tissue site of origin within the bone important clues to the diagnosis can be obtained. (Fig. 7.20)

Medullary. These lesions are mostly centric in location. There may be evidence of scalloping and thinning of the cortex from the endosteal surface, a sign which is often found associated with fibrous and cartilagenous lesions. (Fig. 7.20A)

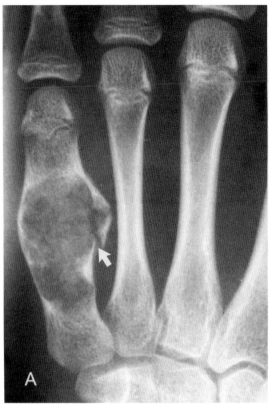
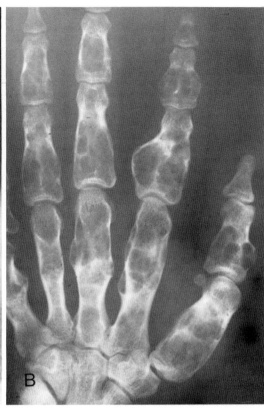

Figure 7.18. MONOSTOTIC AND POLYOSTOTIC BONE DISEASE. A. Monostotic Lesion. A solitary osteolytic lesion is present in the fifth metacarpal. Observe the pathological fracture in this enchondroma (arrow). **B. Polyostotic Lesions.** Multiple expansile osteolytic lesions are seen throughout all metacarpals and phalanges. Similar changes were present in the opposite hand, feet, and long bones in this patient with multiple enchondromatosis (Ollier's disease).

Table 7.6.
Most Common Locations of Bone Tumors

	Tumor	Skeletal Sites
MALIGNANT	Adamantinoma	Mandible, tibia
	Chondrosarcoma	Pelvis, scapula, sternum, femur, humerus
	Chordoma	Sacrococcygeal, skull base
	Ewing's sarcoma	Pelvis, femur, humerus
	Fibrosarcoma	Femur, tibia
	Multiple myeloma	Pelvis, spine, sternum, femur, humerus
	Osteosarcoma	Femur, tibia, humerus
	Parosteal sarcoma	Femur
	Non-Hodgkin's lymphoma	Femur, humerus, pelvis, spine
QUASIMALIGNANT	Giant cell tumor	Femur, tibia, radius
BENIGN	Aneurysmal bone cyst	Femur, tibia, humerus, neural arch
	Bone island	Pelvis, femur
	Chondroblastoma	Humerus, femur
	Chondromyxoid fibroma	Tibia, rib, ulna
	Enchondroma	Metacarpal, phalanges, metatarsals, femur
	Fibrous cortical defect	Femur, tibia
	Hemangioma	Spine, skull
	Nonossifying fibroma	Femur, tibia
	Osteoblastoma	Femur, humerus, neural arch
	Osteochondroma	Femur, tibia, humerus
	Osteoid osteoma	Femur, tibia, neural arch
	Osteoma	Sinuses, skull
	Simple bone cyst	Humerus, femur, calcaneus

Table 7.7.
Tumor Positions in Bone

	Benign	Malignant
EPIPHYSEAL	Chondroblastoma Giant cell tumor	Giant cell tumor
EPIPHYSEAL—METAPHYSEAL	Aneurysmal bone cyst Giant cell tumor	Giant cell tumor Metastasis
METAPHYSEAL	Bone island Enchondroma Fibrous cortical defect Nonossifying fibroma Osteoid osteoma Osteochondroma Simple bone cyst	Chondrosarcoma Fibrosarcoma Metastasis Osteosarcoma
METAPHYSEAL—DIAPHYSEAL	Chondromyxoid fibroma Nonossifying fibroma Osteoid osteoma	Chondrosarcoma Metastasis Multiple myeloma Osteosarcoma
DIAPHYSEAL	Osteoid osteoma	Adamantinoma Ewing's sarcoma Metastasis Multiple myeloma Non-Hodgkin's lymphoma

Cortical. The most distinctive feature is the frequent eccentric position in at least one projection of the lesion. (Fig. 7.20B) Notably, there is usually destruction, distortion, or expansion of the cortical bone. These lesions commonly provoke an overlying periosteal response. Cortical lesions are more readily identifiable than medullary lesions. (Fig. 7.21)

Periosteal. These are typified by their close apposition but definite separation from the majority of the underlying bone. There is usually a notable lesion in the soft tissues but very little actual bony abnormality. (Fig. 7.20C)

Extraosseous. The abnormality is conspicuous by its distant location from the bone or adjacent cleft which separates the mass from the cortical surface. (Fig. 7.20D) Sites of origin include muscle, nerves, arteries, and synovium. A large extraosseous mass may produce an extrinsic pressure atrophy of bone conspicuous by the presence of a sclerotic rim.

Shape

Benign slow-growing lesions are usually elongated along the axis of the bone ("long lesion in a long bone"). (Fig. 7.22) Typical examples include fibrous dysplasia, nonossifying fibroma, and unicameral bone cyst. Rapidly growing lesions can be pleomorphic and do not exhibit definitive morphologic shapes. Shapes of lesions must not be considered as a reliable differential sign between slow- and fast-developing abnormalities.

Size

Size of a lesion can be useful. Most benign tumors are under 6 cm in size at the time of discovery, while aggressive lesions tend to be larger. Exceptions to this rule include benign conditions such as aneurysmal bone cyst, unicameral bone cyst, giant cell tumor, and fibrous dysplasia, all of which may be very large at the initial examination.

Margination

The peripheral margins of a lesion closely reflect its growth rate. Two terms are used to describe this zone of transition into normal bone—imperceptible and sharp. (Fig. 7.23)

Imperceptible Margination. Other terms which are commonly used include poor, hazy, and ill-defined margins, or a wide zone of transition. The gradation between the lesion and normal bone occurs gradually, with no distinct demarcating line or change in density. (Fig. 7.23A and B) This type of boundary is indicative of aggressive bone destruction such as seen in infections and malignant tumors.

Sharp Margins. Synonyms include definite and sclerotic margins or a narrow zone of transition. The interface between the lesion and normal bone is clearly identified and may be outlined by a sclerotic line. (Fig. 7.23C and D) The inference in this type of bone abnormality is usually slow growing, such as in fibrous dysplasia and unicameral bone cyst.

Cortical Integrity

A key factor in assessing the growth rate of a bone lesion is the integrity of the cortex. A number of appearances may occur—thinning, thickening, expansion, destruction, and fracture. (Fig. 7.24)

Cortical Thinning. Normally, the cortex gradually

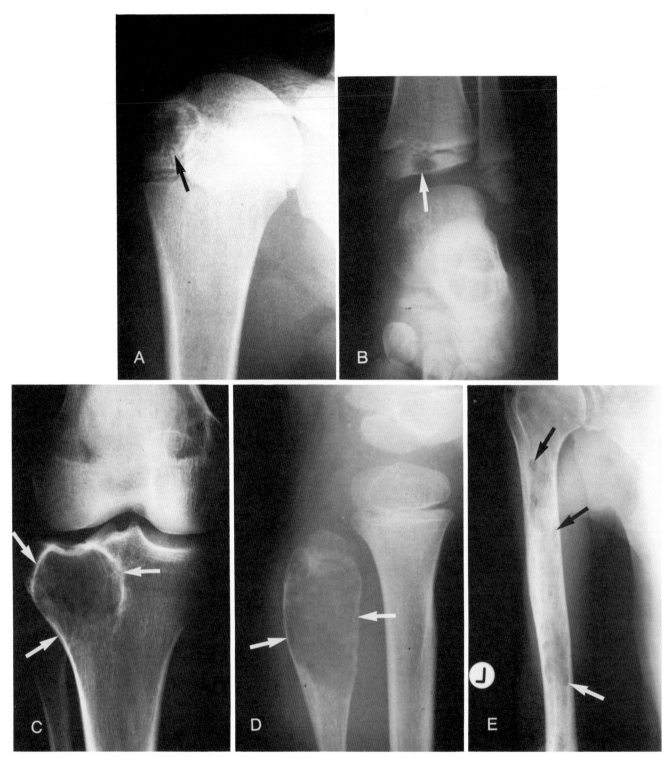

Figure 7.19. LOCATIONS OF LESIONS WITHIN BONE. A. Apophysis. An apophysis is analogous to an epiphysis and is therefore prone to developing similar lesions. Observe the osteolytic lesion in the greater tuberosity of this 10-year-old patient, a chondroblastoma (arrow). **B. Epiphysis.** A well-defined osteolytic lesion is evident within the distal tibial epiphysis of this 7-year-old patient, also a chondroblastoma (arrow). **C. Epiphyseal-Metaphyseal.** Within the lateral tibial epiphysis and metaphysis a sharply circumscribed abnormality is present, a giant cell tumor (arrows).

D. Metaphysis. An expansile, osteolytic, aneurysmal bone cyst occupies the fibular metaphysis (arrows). Note that the epiphysis is unaffected. **E. Diaphysis.** Multiple, sharply demarcated, osteolytic lesions are present throughout the humeral diaphysis. Note the inner cortical destruction (endosteal scalloping), indicating the medullary origins of the tumor (arrows); in this case, multiple myeloma. **Comment:** Knowledge of locational predispositions greatly enhances the observer's diagnostic accuracy.

thins toward the metaphysis and remains uniform into the epiphysis. (Fig. 7.24A) Osteoporosis generally thins all cortices (pencil thin). Localized thinning is seen in lesions such as tumors. When the inside surface of the cortex is eroded and undulated, it is referred to as endosteal scalloping and is frequently seen in medullary tumors

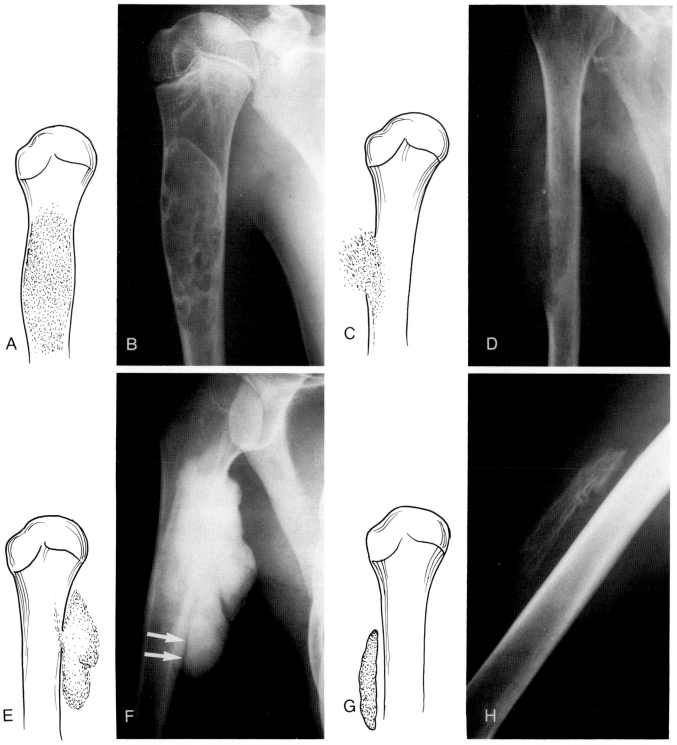

Figure 7.20. SITES OF ORIGIN.   A and B. Medullary. Note the central location, slight expansion, thin but intact cortex, and scalloped endosteal margin. Diagnosis: Simple bone cyst (unicameral bone cyst).   **C and D. Cortical.** Note the eccentric location, cortical destruction, and periosteal new bone formation. Diagnosis: Ewing's sarcoma.   **E and F. Periosteal.** A dense soft tissue mass is the dominant feature, with no evidence of bone destruction. Observe the thin, separating, radiolucent cleft between the mass and cortex (arrows) indicating its extracortical origin. Diagnosis: Periosteal osteosarcoma. (Courtesy of Friedrich H. W. Heuck, MD, Stuttgart, West Germany).   **G and H. Extraosseous.** A well-demarcated soft tissue lesion is visible which demonstrates cortical and trabecular bone. Diagnosis: Traumatic myositis ossificans of the anterior thigh.

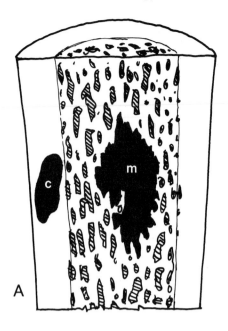

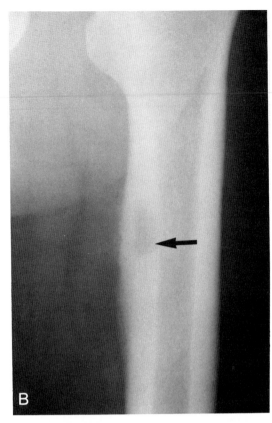

Figure 7.21. VISIBILITY OF LESIONS. **A.** Cortical lesions (c) are more readily identified than medullary lesions (m) because of the surrounding compact bone.

B. A localized cortical lesion in the femur is easily recognized (arrow). Diagnosis: Brodie's abscess. (Courtesy of Steven P. Brownstein, MD, Springfield, New Jersey)

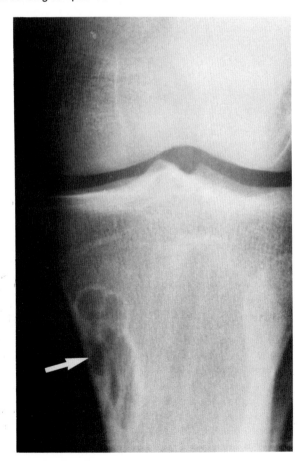

Figure 7.22. LONG LESION IN A LONG BONE. This eccentrically placed, well-defined radiolucent lesion displays typical features of a slowly developing neoplasm which is distorted with long bone growth (arrow). Note that the length far exceeds its width. Diagnosis: Nonossifying fibroma.

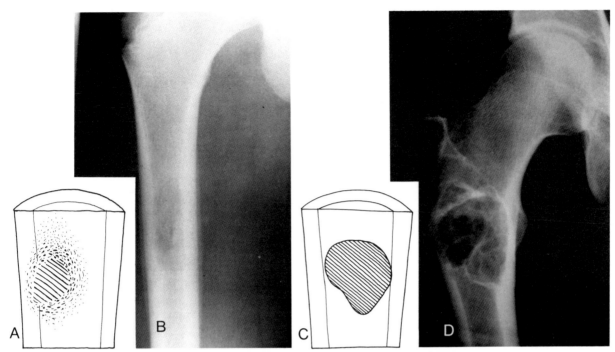

Figure 7.23. MARGINATION.   A. Diagram.   B. Radiograph: Imperceptible Margination. A motheaten osteolytic lesion is present in the medullary cavity, with some adjacent endosteal destruction. It is difficult to perceive where the lesion begins and ends, which is typical of an aggressive abnormality (Ewing's sarcoma).

C. Diagram.   D. Radiograph: Sharp Margination. Conversely, this geographic lesion exhibits a conspicuous zone of transition accentuated by the sclerotic margin. This appearance usually denotes a contained, slowly growing lesion which, in this case, was fibrous dysplasia.

such as enchondroma and multiple myeloma. Thinning without loss of integrity usually denotes slow growth of the abnormality.

Cortical Thickening.   This may occur either locally or generally within a bone. (Fig. 7.24B) Localized causes include osteoid osteoma and stress fracture due to periosteal and endosteal appositional new bone. The most classic disorder to thicken cortices generally is Paget's disease, due to disordered bone remodeling.

Cortical Expansion.   Bulging of an intact cortex outward is a sign of slow but continued growth. (Fig. 7.24C) The outer cortex represents a balance between continuous erosion from within and periosteal new bone on the outside. Generally, this is a sign of a benign lesion but can be seen in slow-growing malignant tumors.

Cortical Destruction.   Disruption of the cortical bone is a strong indicator of aggressive bone disease. (Fig. 7.24D) This is usually easier to identify than destruction within the medullary cavity. Manifestations of cortical destruction include loss of definition and identifying permeative or motheaten lesions.

Fracture.   A sharp, irregular radiolucent line is visible, creating discontinuity of the cortical surface. (Fig. 7.24E)

BEHAVIOR OF LESION

Bone lesions are of three types—osteolytic, osteoblastic, or mixed. (Table 7.8)

Osteolytic Lesions

These are typified by their loss of localized bone structure and density. It is the subtle loss of bone density which is the most difficult to perceive of all patterns of bone disease. Neoplastic bone destruction is due to pressure or hyperemic-generated osteoclastic resorption, not direct tumor lysis. (18) As a result, these lesions are radiolucent on radiological examination. Three patterns of bone destruction are identified—geographic, motheaten, and permeative—which may occur separately but usually in varying degrees of combination. (16,18) (Fig. 7.25)

Geographic Lesions.   Another term used is circumscribed and uniformly lytic lesion. (Fig. 7.25A and B) The morphologic criteria of geographic lesions is that it is usually solitary, is greater than 1 cm, and has a sharp margin. Occasionally, multiple geographic lesions may occur. Internal septations (trabeculation) may isolate separate chambers, giving a "soap bubble" type appearance. (Fig. 7.26) In general, geographic lesions are slower-growing abnormalities.

Motheaten Lesions.   Multiple, poorly marginated, small, or moderately sized (2–5 cm) lucencies are characteristic of this pattern. (Fig. 7.25C and D) Frequently, the margins of each lesion are ragged and irregular. Confluence with adjacent lesions is common. This type of destruction reflects an aggressive abnormality such as lytic metastatic bone disease or osteomyelitis.

Permeative Lesions.   Numerous tiny, pinhole-sized lucencies (less than 1 mm) constitute the permeative pattern. (Fig. 7.25E and F) A wide zone of transition is evident. These lesions are frequently overlooked, because of their size, and with progression may enlarge enough to become motheaten in character. They are usually seen in the most rapidly aggressive malignant bone tumors.

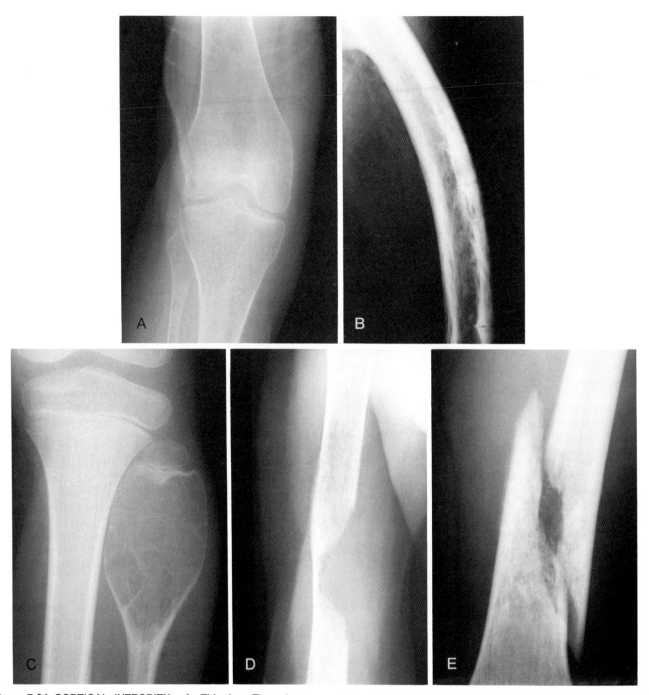

Figure 7.24. CORTICAL INTEGRITY. A. Thinning. There is extreme thinning of all visible cortices ("pencil thin") and generalized demineralization of all bones in this patient with osteoporosis. **B. Thickening.** The two cortices are grossly thickened, with compromise of the adjacent medullary space. Additionally, the bone is deformed and has transverse lucencies on its convex surface (pseudofractures), all consistent with the diagnosis of Paget's dis-

ease. **C. Expansion.** Note the thin bulging but intact cortex of the proximal fibula. This represents continued endosteal erosion and periosteal deposition, with continued growth of the lesion. Diagnosis: Aneurysmal bone cyst. **D. Destruction.** Disruption of the cortex is indicative of an aggressive bone lesion; in this case, from metastatic carcinoma. **E. Fracture.** An oblique fracture line and disruption of the cortex is readily identified through a malignant lesion.

Osteoblastic Lesions

These show increased density due to an overproduction of bone or calcium laden tissue. (Fig. 7.27) These may be diffuse ivory-like or localized ("snowball"). Examples include blastic metastasis, osteosarcoma, and Paget's disease.

Mixed Lesions

Both lytic and blastic patterns are evident. (Fig. 7.28) The most common cause is mixed metastasis.

MATRIX

The dominant internal extracellular substance of a

Table 7.8.
Radiological Features of Lesion Behavior

OSTEOLYTIC BEHAVIOR
   Geographic Lesion
      Solitary
      Greater than 1 cm
      Sharp margin
   Motheaten lesion
      Multiple
      2–5 mm
      Ragged margins and coalescence
      Imperceptible transition
   Permeative Lesion
      Multiple
      Less than 1 mm
      Imperceptible transition
OSTEOBLASTIC BEHAVIOR
   Diffuse Lesion
      Homogenously sclerotic ("ivory")
      Obliterated corticomedullary junction
   Localized Lesion
      Single or multiple
      Irregular, hazy border
      Asymmetrical
MIXED BEHAVIOR
   Both osteolytic and osteoblastic features

lesion is termed the matrix. Radiologically, the matrix can be determined based on its appearance. (19,20) (Table 7.9)

Fat. Intraosseous fat matrix (lipoma) as a rule cannot be suggested on plain films but occasionally may have central calcification. (Fig. 7.29) Soft tissue lipomas, however, can be identified due to the relatively low contrast with surrounding muscle. CT scanning will be definitive in both instances in identifying the low-density fat.

Cartilage. Cartilaginous matrix frequently calcifies in distinct patterns which are readily identifiable. (20) (Fig. 7.30)

Stippled Calcification. Small, discrete, spotty densities typify this variety. (Fig. 7.30A) It represents localized dense mineralization of hyaline cartilage. This type is best identified in enchondroma.

Flocculent Calcification. Larger but still spotty densities represent confluence of stippled regions. (Fig. 7.30B) As a result, floccules and stipples may be seen together.

Arc and Ring Calcification. Thin, eggshell-like curvilinear calcifications occur at the periphery of mature cartilage lobules. (Fig. 7.30C) This is usually seen in chondrosarcoma.

Osseous. Bone production by tumors shows varying degrees of density from diffuse to hazy or very dense (ivory-like). (Fig. 7.31) The most characteristic bone-producing tumor is osteosarcoma.

Fibrous. Fibrous matrix lesions are difficult to identify, since the internal density changes may be subtle. (Fig. 7.32) The most definitive feature is the "smokey" or hazy internal density. Some have referred to it as the "ground glass" appearance. (21) This type of matrix is usually identified in fibrous dysplasia.

PERIOSTEAL RESPONSE

The recognition of periosteal new bone is an important radiological feature seen in many abnormalities, especially infection and tumor. Generally, a "radiographic latent period" following the initial stimulus of between 10–21 days is necessary before it can be identified on the radiograph. (22) The stimulus to produce periosteal new bone may be due to subperiosteal extensions of blood, pus, or tumor. These migrate beneath the periosteum by way of the Haversian canals, which freely intercommunicate throughout the cortex and into the medullary cavity. Additional bone-forming irritants include hyperemia, inflammation, and edema. The mechanisms active in these factors inducing periosteal new bone formation by the inner cambium layer are complex. Proposed mechanisms include the physical elevation of the periosteum away from the cortical bone, compensation to underlying destruction, tumor containment, hyperemia, and tumor-secreted osteogenic substances. (22) Whatever the stimulus, three basic periosteal patterns of new bone formation are encountered—solid, laminated, and spiculated. (Table 7.10) (Fig. 7.33)

Solid Response

A solid periosteal response is defined as a continuous layer of new bone which attaches to the outer cortical surface. (Fig. 7.33A and B) Variations of this pattern focus on its shape and external contour. For example, a localized reaction may render the external contour eliptical in shape. In some instances the surface may be undulating. Despite these deviations a solid pattern is readily identified and typically is related to a very slow form of irritation. Disorders associated include osteoid osteoma, stress fracture, venous stasis, and hypertrophic osteoarthropathy.

Laminated Response

Alternative terms include lamellated, layered, and "onion-skin." The most conspicuous feature is the alternating layers of lucent and opaque densities on the external bone surface. (Fig. 7.33C and D) At times only a single lamination will be visible. Recognition of this pattern can be interpreted as a cyclical variation in growth of the underlying lesion. Histopathological studies show the radiolucent zones to be filled with prominent dilated blood vessels in loose connective tissue which have not ossified. (22,23) With time, a laminated response may transform to a solid form as the opaque bony layers thicken and infringe on the adjacent connective tissue. The significance of the laminated response is varied, since it can be seen in slow and aggressive tumors as well as with infections. The most classic associated disorder is Ewing's sarcoma.

Spiculated Response

Additional terms include perpendicular, brushed whiskers, and hair-on-end. (Fig. 7.33E and F) The term "sunburst" has been used to describe radiating spicules of bone from a point source. (Fig. 7.34) The most conspicuous finding is the fine, linear spiculations of new bone orientated perpendicularly away from the cortex. Each spicule

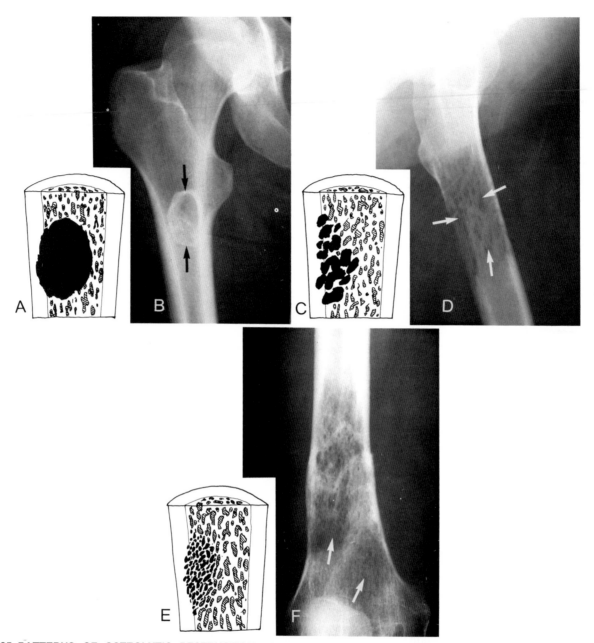

Figure 7.25. PATTERNS OF OSTEOLYTIC DESTRUCTION. A. Diagram. B. Radiograph: Geographic. A solitary, well-demarcated lesion is seen in the proximal femur (arrows). Diagnosis: Fibrous dysplasia. **C. Diagram.   D. Radiograph: Motheaten.** Multiple, poorly outlined radiolucencies are visible (arrows). Note the wide zone of transition. Diagnosis: Metastatic carcinoma. (Courtesy of Lawrence A. Cooperstein, MD, Pittsburgh, Pennsylvania). **E. Diagram.   F. Radiograph: Permeative.** Numerous, tiny, pinhole-sized lesions can be seen (arrows). Diagnosis: Non-Hodgkin's Lymphoma.

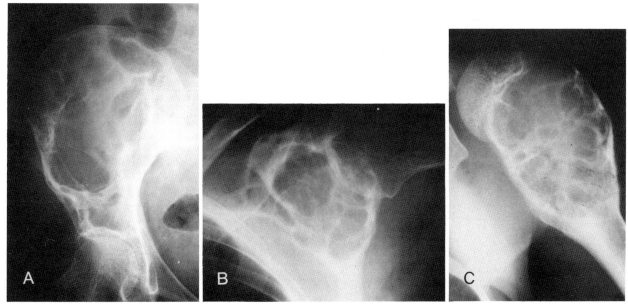

Figure 7.26. TRABECULATION ("SOAPBUBBLE"). A. Plasmacytoma. Observe the expansile, lightly septated appearance of this lesion in the ilium. **B. Chondrosarcoma.** A similarly appearing lesion involves the subglenoid region of the scapula.

C. Aneurysmal Bone Cyst. Note the metaphyseal expansile, septated lesion in the proximal humerus. ***Comment:*** A trabeculated lesion may be benign or malignant and is found in various bone neoplasms.

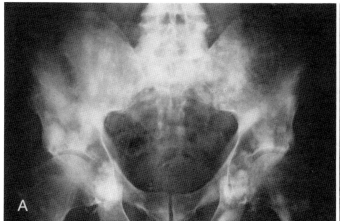
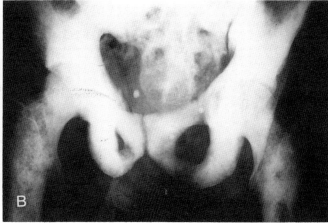

Figure 7.27. OSTEOBLASTIC METASTATIC PATTERNS. A. Localized. Multiple osteoblastic lesions are seen throughout the pelvis ("snowball").

B. Diffuse. All bones demonstrate a generalized increase in bone density ("ivory-like").

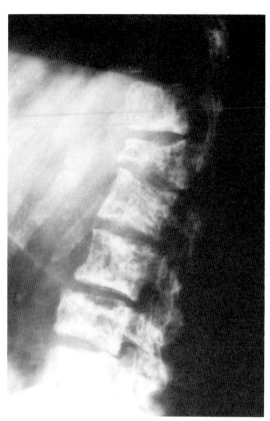

Figure 7.28. MIXED OSTEOBLASTIC AND OSTEOLYTIC LE-SIONS. Multiple lytic and blastic changes are seen disseminated throughout the lumbar spine. Diagnosis: Mixed metastatic carcinoma. (Reprinted with permission: Yochum TR, et al: A radiographic anthology of vertebral names. *J Manip Physiol Ther* 8:87, June 1985)

Table 7.9.
Radiological Features of Lesion Matrix

Matrix	Lesion
Fat	Lipoma
Lucent	
Calcification	
Cartilage	Enchondroma, chondrosarcoma
Lucent	
Calcification	
(stippled, floccules,	
arcs and rings)	
Osseous	Osteosarcoma, osteoma
Dense	
Fibrous	Fibrous dysplasia
Hazy (ground glass)	

is separated from the other by an interposed radiolucent region. (22,24) Frequently, the length of the spicules decreases peripherally away from the midpoint of the lesion. This pattern of new bone formation is indicative of a very aggressive bone tumor, usually osteosarcoma.

Codman's Triangle

Other synonyms include Codman's angle, periosteal cuff, and periosteal buttress. First described by Ribbert in 1914, Codman associated the triangle of periosteal new bone at the peripheral lesion-cortex junction as due to subperiosteal extension of the lesion. (25) (Fig. 7.35) This had long been interpreted as a pathognomonic sign of a primary malignant bone tumor but is now known also to be seen accompanying benign tumors, infections, and many other disorders.

SOFT TISSUE CHANGES

Many diagnostic clues can be found in soft tissue changes. Signs of soft tissue abnormality include displaced overlying skin lines, displaced or obliterated myofascial planes, increased density, calcification, and air. (Fig. 7.36) When an adjacent cortex is disrupted in the presence of a soft tissue mass the diagnosis of an aggressive primary bone tumor is almost certain. Notably, infectious lesions which extend into the soft tissue usually

obliterate fascial fat lines due to edema, while tumors displace them.

JOINT CHANGES

Careful scrutiny of adjacent articulations when a bone lesion is found frequently renders helpful information. Generally speaking, tumors do not break the articular cortex, spread into the joint, or involve the opposing articular cortex. This is in direct contrast to infections which, when in close proximity to a joint, destroy the opposing articular cortices and intervening joint cartilage. (Fig. 7.37, 7.38) This rule applies to all articulations, including the sacroiliac and intervertebral discs.

Essentially, two forms of joint space loss occur—nonuniform and uniform. (Fig. 7.39) A nonuniform decrease in joint space is defined as only part of a single joint cavity demonstrating a loss in width. This type of localized joint compromise is distinctive for degenerative joint disease. A uniform loss of joint space conversely shows diminution throughout the entire articulation and is suggestive of an inflammatory arthropathy such as rheumatoid arthritis.

Also, certain arthritic disorders have associated bone lesions which may be misinterpreted as tumors. A good example is the subarticular degenerative cyst (geode) which simulates an epiphyseal neoplasm. (Fig. 7.40) The recognition of coexistent articular changes characteristic of degenerative joint disease, however, makes this misdiagnosis less likely. Other arthritic conditions which may have confusing, coexistent bone lesions include rheumatoid arthritis, gout, and pigmented villonodular synovitis.

SUPPLEMENTARY ANALYSIS

Imaging

The combination of additional, more sophisticated forms of imaging with the plain film information will frequently allow a diagnosis to be established. These are discussed earlier in this chapter. Additionally, treatment procedures may be appropriately directed.

Laboratory Examination

Numerous laboratory parameters can be assessed in the evaluation of various bone and joint disorders. An absolute minimum skeletal profile should include a com-

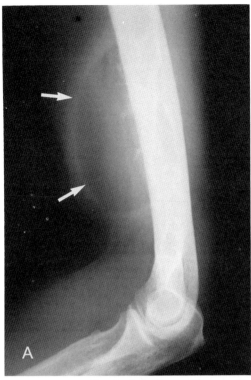

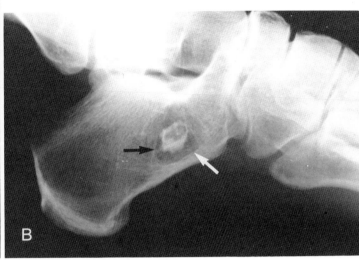

Figure 7.29. FAT MATRIX.   A. Soft Tissue Lipoma. Observe the radiolucent soft tissue lesion on the anterior arm (arrows). **B. Intraosseous Lipoma.** Note the radiolucent lesion (arrows) with central target calcification in the calcaneus. (Courtesy of Steven P. Brownstein, MD, Springfield, New Jersey)

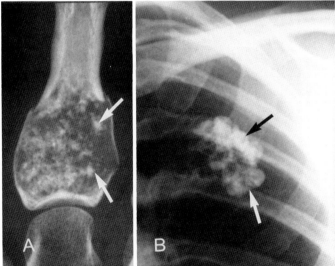

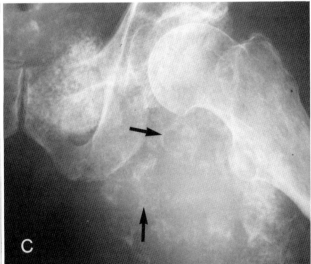

Figure 7.30. CARTILAGE MATRIX.   A. Stippled Calcification. The small, discrete opacities can be identified (arrows). Diagnosis: Enchondroma with pathological fracture.   **B. Flocculent Calcification.** Larger, more confluent densities are present at the anterior second rib (arrows). Diagnosis: Osteochondroma.   **C. Arc and Ring Calcification.** Thin, curvilinear densities typify this type of calcification (arrows). Diagnosis: Chondrosarcoma.

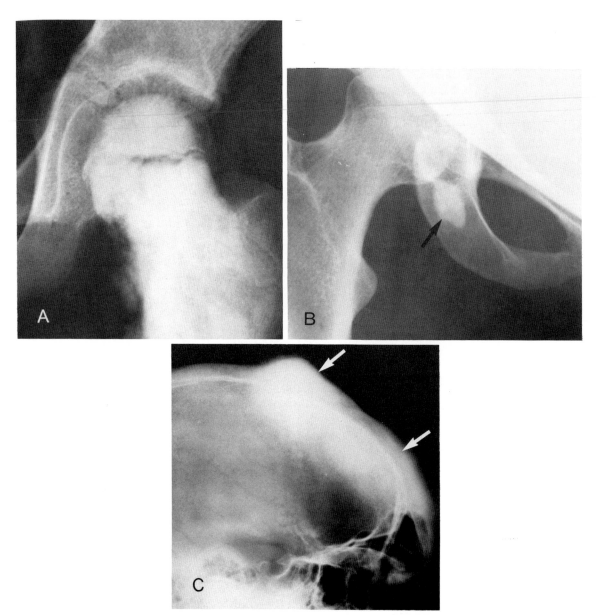

Figure 7.31. BONE MATRIX. A. Osteosarcoma. Dense, wavy-like new bone formation is evident in the proximal femoral metaphysis and epiphysis. **B. Bone Island.** A well-circumscribed, homogenous, opaque lesion is present in the ischium (arrow). The radiopaque density overlying the pelvic basin represents an ovarian shield. (Courtesy of Gary M. Guebert, DC, DACBR, St Louis, Missouri). **C. Osteoma.** A smooth, dense, and wavy-like calvarial overgrowth typifies this lesion of intramembranous bone (arrows).

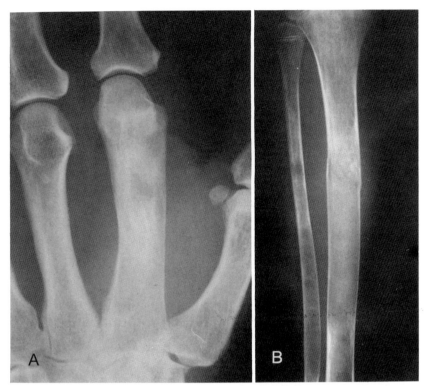

Figure 7.32. FIBROUS MATRIX. A. Note the blurred trabecular markings and the overall "smokey" appearance to the medullary portion of the diaphysis of the second metacarpal. **B.** Observe the cortical thinning and hazy trabecular pattern of the mid-diaphysis of the tibia and fibula. Note the pathological fracture of the tibia. The diagnosis in A and B was fibrous dysplasia.

Table 7.10.
Radiological Features of Periosteal Response

Pattern	Lesion
Solid	Osteoid osteoma
Homogenous, single at-tached layer	
Laminated	Ewing's sarcoma
Alternating layers of lucency and opacity	
Spiculated	Osteosarcoma
Radiating spicules	
Codman's Triangle	Any
Solid or laminated	

plete blood count, erythrocyte sedimentation rate, serum calcium and phosphorus, serum alkaline and acid phosphatase, and total serum proteins. More specialized procedures are applied when a particular diagnostic entity is suspected or to be excluded. Standard values, while not universally uniform, provide the baseline for comparisons. (26) (Table 7.11)

Complete Blood Count (CBC). A cell differential, hematocrit, hemoglobin, red cell count, and other cellular features are evaluated.

Erythrocyte Sedimentation Rate (ESR). An increased tendency of red blood cells to sediment is noted in many disease states. As such, it represents a nonspecific index of disease, particularly those of an inflammatory nature.

C-Reactive Protein (CRP). In normal individuals no C-reactive protein will be present. Any inflammatory change or tissue necrosis will elevate the release of this substance. It usually precedes changes in the ESR; however, like the ESR, it is not a specific sign for any particular disorder but remains as a general index of pathologic activity.

Serum Calcium. Serum calcium is normally kept within very strict limits. In disorders of bone destruction or increased parathormone activity serum calcium will be elevated.

Serum Phosphorus. This is also an indicator of bone destruction and an important index of bone activity. It usually will show an inverse relationship to calcium levels.

Alkaline Phosphatase. This is a group of isoenzymes which are found in strong concentrations in bone, liver, spleen, kidney, intestine, and placenta. They are designated as "alkaline" because they exhibit optimal activity at a pH of 9. Their main clinical application is in the detection of liver or bone disease. In bone abnormalities such as Paget's or metastatic disease an increased alkaline phosphatase level is a direct reflection of increased osteoblastic activity.

Acid Phosphatase. Within the prostate, red blood cells and platelet isoenzymes of acid phosphatase are found. They are grouped together as "acid" since their optimal activity is at a pH of 5. The major disorders which demonstrate abnormal levels of the enzyme are in metastasis from prostatic carcinoma and Gaucher's disease. In prostate cancer it is usual for the prostate capsule to be

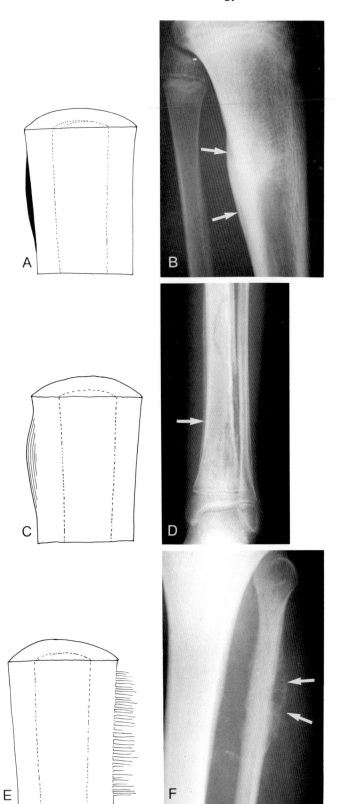

Figure 7.33. PATTERNS OF PERIOSTEAL RESPONSE. **A. Diagram.** **B. Radiograph: Solid Response.** An elliptical, homogenous layer of bone is evident (arrows) adjacent to this stress fracture. **C. Diagram.** **D. Radiograph: Laminated Response.** Alternating lucent and opaque laminations are seen adjacent to a focus of osteomyelitis (arrow). **E. Diagram.** **F. Radiograph: Spiculated Response.** Radiating spicules of bone (arrows) characterize this aggressive osteosarcoma.

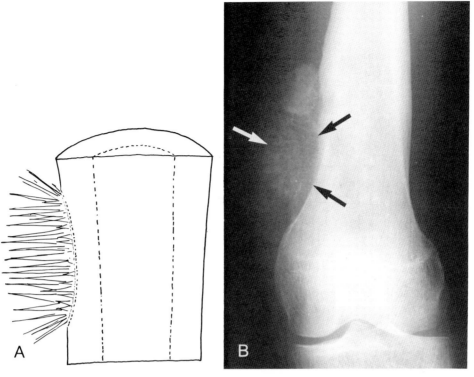

Figure 7.34. "SUNBURST" PERIOSTEAL RESPONSE. A. Diagram. B. Radiograph. The periosteal spicules appear to radiate away from a point source (arrows). Diagnosis: Osteosarcoma.

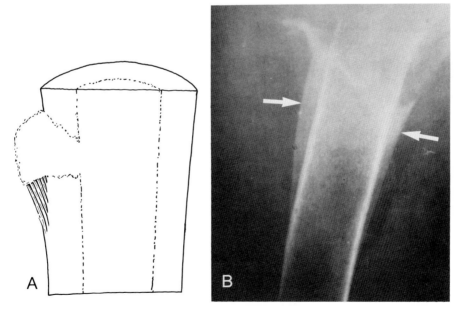

Figure 7.35. CODMAN'S TRIANGLE. A. Diagram. B. Radiograph. A triangular-shaped periosteal new bone formation typifies this named response (arrows) and is a significant but nonspecific finding in many disorders, including infection, neoplasm, and trauma.

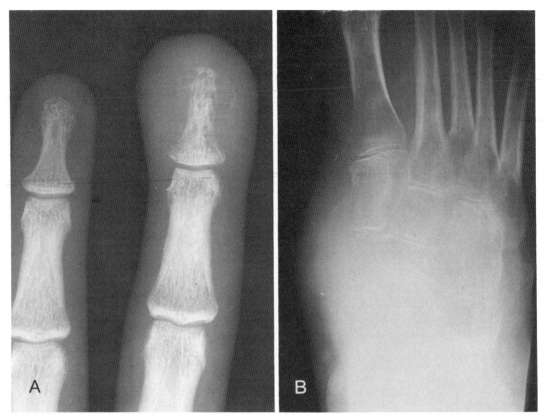

Figure 7.36. SOFT TISSUE CHANGES.   A. Ewing's Sarcoma. Observe the combination of motheaten bone destruction and soft tissue mass in this digit.   **B. Malignant Synovioma.** Note the severe bone destruction and large soft tissue mass in the foot.   ***Comment:*** The combination of bone destruction and soft tissue mass makes the diagnosis of primary malignant tumor or infection likely.

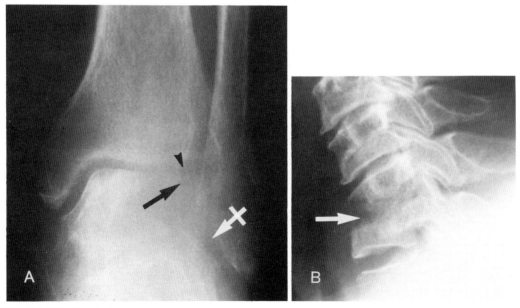

Figure 7.37. JOINT INFECTION.   A. Ankle. Note the destruction of the cortical outlines of the lateral talus (arrow), plafond of the tibia (arrowhead), and distal medial fibula (crossed arrow).   **B. Cervical Spine.** Loss of the intervertebral disc height and contiguous vertebral end plates are evident at C6/C7 (arrow).   ***Comment:*** Joint infections distinctively tend to involve both opposing articular cortices ("crossing the joint").

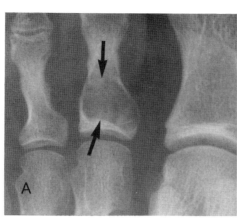

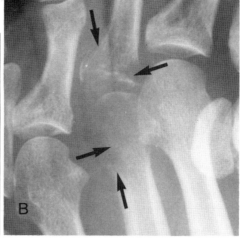

Figure 7.38. TUMOR VERSUS INFECTION OF THE JOINT. A. Enchondroma. Note the loss of bone density extending to but not beyond the articular cortex (arrows). (Courtesy of David M. Walker, DPM, Melbourne, Australia)   **B. Infection.** Observe the lytic destruc-tion of the opposing metatarsal head and proximal phalanx (arrows). *Comment:* This demonstrates the tendency for neoplasms to respect the joint surfaces, while infections readily infiltrate and involve all joint components.

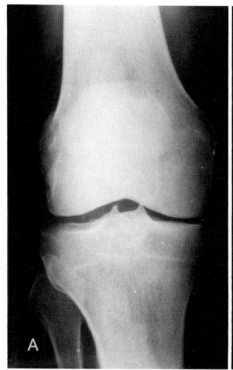

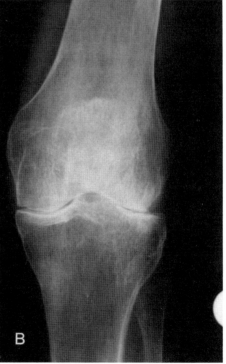

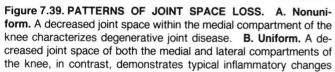

Figure 7.39. PATTERNS OF JOINT SPACE LOSS. A. Nonuniform. A decreased joint space within the medial compartment of the knee characterizes degenerative joint disease.   **B. Uniform.** A decreased joint space of both the medial and lateral compartments of the knee, in contrast, demonstrates typical inflammatory changes such as seen in rheumatoid arthritis. Also, observe the diffuse osteoporosis. *Comment:* No matter where the site of involvement is, the pattern of joint space loss frequently provides the clue to arriving at a definitive diagnosis.

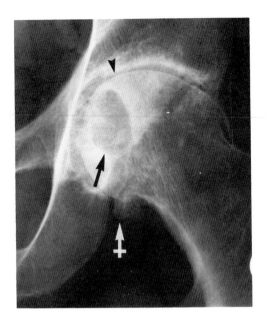

Figure 7.40. SUBCHONDRAL CYST MIMICKING NEOPLASM. The large geographic radiolucency within the femoral head has the appearance of a destructive neoplasm (arrow); however, close scrutiny of the adjacent narrowed joint space (arrowhead) and associated osteophytes (crossed arrow) makes the diagnosis of a degenerative subchondral cyst most likely. (Courtesy of Mahinder Lall, MSc, DC, Melbourne, Australia) *Comment:* This case demonstrates the importance of evaluating the joint in bone disease.

Table 7.11
Normal Laboratory Values*

	Adult Values		Indication
	Male	Female	
Acid phosphatase	0.5–2 (Bodansky)		Prostate metastasis
Alkaline phosphatase	2–4.5 (Bodansky)		Liver, bone disease
Calcium	8.5–10.5 mg/100 ml		Tumor, destruction
Complete blood count (CBC)			Anemia, tumor, infection
Hematocrit	42–52 ml/100 ml	37–47 ml/100 ml	
Hemoglobin	14–18 gm/100 ml	12–16 gm/100 ml	
Red blood cell (total)	4.6–6.2 mill/mm^3	4.2–5.4 mill/mm^3	
White blood cell (total)	4500–11000 mm^3		
C-reactive protein (CRP)	Absent		Inflammation, tumor
Erythrocyte sedimentation rate (ESR)	0–15 mm/hr	0–20 mm/hr	Inflammation, tumor
Phosphorus	2–4.5 mg/100 ml		Tumor, destruction
Protein	6–8 gm/100 ml		Tumor
Total			
Fractions			
Albumin	3.5–5.5 gm/100 ml		
Globulin	1.5–3.0 gm/100 ml		Multiple myeloma
Special antigens			
HLA B27	6–8% of population		Seronegative arthritis
RA factor	3% of population		Rheumatoid arthritis
Uric acid	3–6 mg/100 ml		Gout

* Adapted from: Wallach J: *Interpretation of Diagnostic Tests. A Handbook Synopsis of Laboratory Medicine*, ed 2, Boston, Little, Brown & Co., 1974.

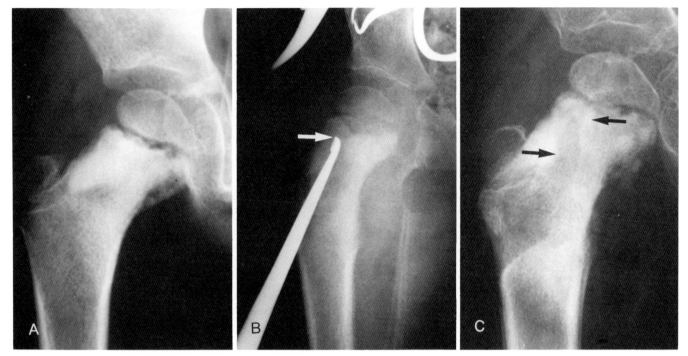

Figure 7.41. BIOPSY PROCEDURE.   A. Initial Film. Based on the osteoblastic nature of the lesion, its location, and the age of the patient, a presumptive diagnosis of osteosarcoma was made.   **B. Biopsy Film.** Note the position of the biopsy tool within the matrix of the tumor (arrow).   **C. Postbiopsy Film.** With the procedure completed, a residual linear lucency remains at the biopsy site (arrows). Final biopsy confirmed the diagnosis of osteosarcoma.

disrupted before the serum acid phosphatase will be found in abnormal concentrations. It appears that the abnormal amounts of the enzyme are liberated by the bone and soft tissue metastatic lesions. As such, a patient may have carcinoma of the prostate yet still show normal acid phosphatase levels as long as the capsule remains intact.

Total Protein.   Protein levels are frequently altered in certain bone disorders, especially malignancy. A raised total serum protein often indicates metastatic disease or multiple myeloma. More specific examination of the various protein fractions will reveal a more definitive diagnosis. In multiple myeloma, for example, there is an overproduction of a specific immunoglobulin (monoclonal gammopathy) which reverses the normal albumin-globulin ratio (A:G ratio) and on electrophoresis shows as an IgG or IgA spike. In the urine the presence of Bence-Jones proteins may be found in almost 40 percent of those with multiple myeloma.

Additional Studies.   When indicated, certain labora-

tory examinations will provide additional data in the evaluation of a skeletal or rheumatologic disorder. Uric acid levels are of assistance in the evaluation of gout, chromosomal studies for dysplasias, and the special antigens such as HLA-B27 in seronegative arthritis and rheumatoid factor in inflammatory arthritis. More sophisticated studies include electrophoresis, calcium balance studies, renal function, synovial fluid and blood studies, and bioassay.

Biopsy

The definitive diagnosis frequently rests on the histologic evaluation of biopsy material. This can be obtained by numerous methods, including incisional and needle aspiration. (27) Frequently, the radiograph determines the site for biopsy and further follow-up procedures. (Fig. 7.41) In bone marrow evaluations the most common sites for obtaining specimens include the sternum and iliac crest.

CAPSULE SUMMARY. Principles of Radiological Interpretation

TECHNICAL CONSIDERATIONS

Plain Film: Most common employed method. Based on differential absorption of x-rays by body tissues. Five densities—air, fat, water, bone, and metal. Minimum of two views, perpendicular to each other. Need 30–50 percent destruction to be visible on film.

Tomography: Increased detail at fulcrum between moving tube and cassette.

Xeroradiography: Enhanced sharpness but high dose. Used mainly in mammography.

Contrast Studies: Arthrogram—joints; angiogram—vessels; lymphangiogram—lymph channels; myelogram—spinal subarachnoid space.

Radionuclide Imaging: Technetium-99m taken up selectively by osteoblasts. Only 3–5 percent destruction needed to be visible. Abnormal uptake regions referred to as "hot spots." Quantitative imaging only.

Computerized Tomography: Computer formulated cross-sectional images.

Magnetic Resonance Imaging: Uses magnetic fields to create sectional images.

SKELETAL ANATOMY AND PHYSIOLOGY

Intramembranous Ossification: Bone formation from a fibroblastic membrane.

Enchondral Ossification: Bone formation from a cartilaginous model.

Parts of a Bone: Epiphysis, physis, metaphysis, diaphysis, apophysis, cortex, medulla, and periosteum. Epiphysis vulnerable to dysplasia and ischemia.

Physis: Responsible for longitudinal growth (enchondral) and periosteum for bone width (intramembranous).

Metaphysis: Most active part of a bone and is prone to tumors and infections.

Periosteum: Has an inner, metabolically active layer which can lay down or take away cortical bone.

Calcium and phosphorus are the most important bone minerals; usually in the form of hydroxyapatite (Ca10 (PO4)6 (OH)2).

Hormones most active in bone metabolism are parathormone, calcitonin, estrogen, androgen, growth hormone, and glucocorticoids.

CATEGORICAL APPROACH TO BONE DISEASE

Seven categories—congenital, trauma, arthritis, tumor, infection, hematologic, and nutritional, metabolic, and endocrine.

RADIOLOGICAL PREDICTOR VARIABLES

The evaluation of certain features of a lesion leads to the correct diagnosis or differential diagnosis:

Clinical data—age, sex, race, history

Number of lesions—polyostotic, monostotic

Symmetry of lesions

Systems involved

Skeletal location

Position within bone—predilection to a bone site an important diagnostic clue. *Epiphysis:* giant cell tumor, chondroblastoma. *Diaphysis:* round cell tumors.

Site of origin

Shape—elongated lesions frequently due to slow growth and development during bone growth.

Size

Margination: imperceptible (aggressive), sharp (benign).

Cortical integrity: thin, thick, expansion, destruction, and fracture.

Behavior of lesion: lytic, blastic, or mixed. Lytic lesions will be either geographic (slow), motheaten or permeative (rapid). *Geographic:* single, greater than 1 cm, sharp margins, and may be septated ("soap bubble"). *Motheaten:* multiple, 2–5 mm, imperceptible margins, and confluent. *Permeative:* multiple, less than 1 mm, and imperceptible margins. Blastic lesions: diffuse (ivory) or localized (snowball).

Matrix: fat, cartilage, bone, fibrous.

Periosteal response: solid, laminated, spiculated.

Codman's triangle: takes 10–21 days to appear.

Soft tissue changes: displaced skin and muscle planes, increased density, calcification or air. When combined with broken cortex, primary malignant bone tumor is the most likely cause.

Joint changes: arthritis, infection—rarely, tumors.

Supplementary procedures: other imaging modalities, laboratory and biopsy. Most standard lab tests for bone include CRP, CBC, ESR, calcium, phosphorus, alkaline and acid phosphatase, and serum proteins.

REFERENCES

1. Ardran GM: Bone destruction not demonstrable by radiography. *Br J Radiol* 24:107, 1951.
2. Borak J: Relationship between the clinical and roentgenological findings in bone metastases. *Surg Gynecol Obstet* 75:599, 1942.
3. Lachman E: Osteoporosis: The potentialities and limitations of its roentgenologic diagnosis. *AJR* 74:712, 1955.
4. Dupuis PR, Yong-Hing K, Cassidy JD, et al: Radiologic diagnosis of degenerative lumbar spinal instability. *Spine* 10 (3):287, 1985.
5. Bassett LW, Gold RH, Webber MM: Radionuclide bone imaging. *Radiol Clin North Am* 19: (4) 645, 1981.
6. Porter RW, Ottowell E, Wicks M: Use of diagnostic ultrasound for spinal canal measurements. *J Bone Joint Surg (Br)* 59 (2):249, 1977.
7. Howe JW: Observations from cineroentgenographic studies of the spinal column. *J Am Chiropractic Assn* 7 (10):65, 1970.
8. Pennal GF, Garson SC, McDonald G, et al: Motion studies of the lumbar spine. A preliminary report. *J Bone Joint Surg (Br)* 54 (3):442, 1972.
9. Hounsfield GN: Computerized transverse axial scanning (tomography) Part I: Description of system. *Br J Radiol* 46:1016, 1973.
10. Genant HK, Cann CE, Chapetz NI, et al: Advances in computed tomography of the musculoskeletal system. *Radiol Clin North Am* 19 (4):645, 1981.
11. McCullough EC, Payne JT: Patient dosage in computed tomography. *Radiology* 129:457, 1978.
12. Kramer DM: Basic principles of magnetic resonance imaging. *Radiol Clin North Am* 22 (4):765, 1984.
13. Han JS, Benson JE, Yoon YS: Magnetic resonance imaging in the spinal column and craniovertebral junction. *Radiol Clin North Am* 22 (4):805, 1984.
14. Sherman RS: General principles of the radiologic diagnosis of bone disorders. *Radiol Clin North Am* 8:173, 1970A.
15. Sherman RS: The nature of radiologic diagnosis in diseases of bone. *Radiol Clin North Am* 8:227, 1970B.
16. Lodwick GS: Solitary malignant tumors of bone: The application of predictor variables in diagnosis. *Semin Roentgenol* 1:293, 1966.
17. Lodwick GS: *Atlas of Tumor Radiology. The Bones and Joints*, Chicago, Year Book Medical Publishers, 1971.
18. Madewell JE, Ragsdale BD, Sweet DE: Radiologic and pathologic analysis of solitary bone lesions. Part I: Internal margins. *Radiol Clin North Am* 19 (4):715, 1981.
19. Edeiken J, Hodes PJ, Caplan LH: New bone production and periosteal reaction. *AJR* 97:708, 1966.
20. Sweet DE, Madewell JE, Ragsdale BD: Radiologic and pathologic analysis of solitary bone lesions. Part III: Matrix patterns. *Radiol Clin North Am* 19 (4):785, 1981.
21. Greenfield GB: *Radiology of Bone Diseases*, ed 3, Philadelphia, JB Lippincott, 1980.
22. Ragsdale BD, Madewell JE, Sweet DE: Radiologic and pathologic analysis of solitary bone lesions. Part II: Periosteal reactions. *Radiol Clin North Am* 19 (4):749, 1981.
23. Volberg FM Jr, Whalen JP, Krook L, et al: Lamellated periosteal reactions: A radiologic and histologic investigation. *AJR* 128:85, 1977.
24. Brunschwig A, Harman PH: Studies in bone sarcoma. Part III: An experimental and pathological study of the role of the periosteum in formation of bone in various primary bone tumors. *Surg Gynecol Obstet* 60:30, 1935.
25. Codman EA: Registry of bone sarcoma. *Surg Gynecol Obstet* 42:105, 1925.
26. Wallach J: *Interpretation of Diagnostic Tests. A Handbook Synopsis of Laboratory Medicine*, ed 2, Boston, Little, Brown & Co., 1974.
27. Hajdu SI, Melamed MR: Needle biopsy of primary malignant bone tumors. *Surg Gynecol Obstet* 133:829, 1971.

Skeletal Dysplasias

MARGARET A. SERON
TERRY R. YOCHUM
LINDSAY J. ROWE

Introduction

The skeletal dysplasias are a vast and often confusing group of disorders. They have been the subject of much curiosity and speculation over the years. Recently, with the advent of sophisticated genetic and laboratory studies the various causes of skeletal dysplasias have been better understood. However, they still remain a heterogeneous group, with considerable variation noted even within specific entities.

By definition, skeletal dysplasias are the result of faulty development. Many are known to be the result of specific genetic mutations and are inherited. Many are congenital; fewer develop in adolescence or early adulthood.

This chapter addresses only the more commonly encountered skeletal dysplasias. Some are important to correctly diagnose in order to rule out more serious conditions such as malignancy or toxicity. Other dysplasias require proper diagnosis in order to adequately recognize and sometimes prevent serious sequelae of the entity itself. Major examples include the life-threatening dissecting aneurysm of Marfan's syndrome and the frequent development of paralysis in achondroplasia due to congenital spinal stenosis.

Although this chapter is primarily in alphabetical order, similar or related entities have been grouped together for ease of understanding.

Achondroplasia

GENERAL CONSIDERATIONS

Achondroplasia, the most common form of dwarfism, is a hereditary, autosomal dominant disturbance in epiphyseal chondroblastic growth and maturation. The name "achondroplasia" was first used in 1878 by Parrot. (1) Other synonyms that have been used include chondrodystrophia fetalis, (2) chondrodystrophic dwarfism, and micromelia. A congenital abnormality, the etiology of achondroplasia is unknown.

The phenotypic appearance is remarkably similar in all cases and is the result of a single mutant gene. The parents of achondroplastic dwarfs are normal in 90 percent of cases; it is thought that sporadic mutations account for 80 percent of achondroplastic births. (3) The offspring of the rare mating of two achondroplastics often manifest a severe form (homozygous) which is usually lethal within the first weeks of life.

CLINICAL FEATURES

Achondroplasia is one of the oldest growth disorders known to man. In ancient times these individuals were kept as advisors to emperors and entertainers to the wealthy. It is only since the 19th Century that these people have been known to be normal except for their physical appearance. (4) The average height is approximately 50 inches.

The characteristics of this dwarfing dysplasia are recognizable at birth. The long bones are markedly shortened, especially the more proximal ones (rhizomelia). The upper extremity is more affected than the lower. The cranium is large, with a prominent forehead and depressed nasal bridge. Associated hydrocephalus may be obstructive or nonobstructive. (5) The length of the spinal column is relatively normal, thus the dwarfism is due primarily to limb shortening. The abdomen is protuberant, and the buttocks are prominent. Thoracolumbar kyphosis often develops. A characteristic rolling gait is caused by the posterior tilt of the pelvis and posterior angulation of the hip joints. (6)

Additional clinical features include elbow deformities with limitation of supination and extension, (7) flexion contractures of the hips, and genu varum. The characteristic "trident hand" is due to a separation of the third and fourth digits (8) and the inability to approximate them in extension.

Achondroplastics may die at birth due to a difficult delivery, a small foramen magnum, or a constricted thorax. (6) However, the majority survive and enjoy a normal life span. The most significant complication in adulthood is congenital spinal stenosis, often leading to paraplegia. Mental and sexual development are normal.

PATHOLOGICAL FEATURES

In the past it was thought that achondroplasia was due to an endocrine abnormality, but exhaustive studies have found no functional disturbances. The major abnormality is failure of normal enchondral cartilage growth at the physis. Periosteal and membranous ossification are normal. Some enchondral ossification centers are affected more than others, particularly those at the base of the skull and at the ends of long bones.

RADIOLOGICAL FEATURES

The most characteristic radiographic features are found in the skull, spine, pelvis, and limbs. (9) The base of the skull (which is formed by enchondral ossification) is small, often with a stenotic foramen magnum. Basilar impression is frequent. The cranium is large, though short in its anterior-posterior dimension (brachycephaly). The frontal bones are prominent, and the nasal bones are small. The mandible forms normally and thus gives the impression of prognathism.

There is symmetrical shortening of all long bones, with the proximal portions being most affected. (Fig. 8.1) The

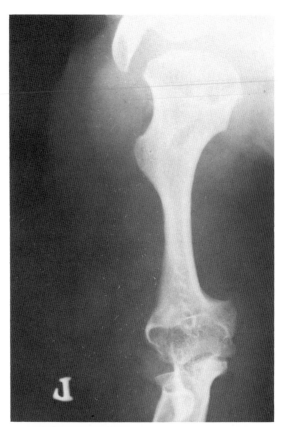

Figure 8.1. ACHONDROPLASIA: HUMERUS.   Note the shortening of the humerus. This shortening is most apparent in the proximal portions of the limbs.   *Comment*: Achondroplasia is the most common form of dwarfism; the average height is 50 inches.

bone ends are often splayed, with metaphyseal cupping. (Fig. 8.2) Because periosteal ossification proceeds normally, there is relative widening of the shafts. The ulna and tibia are often shorter than the radius and fibula. The tubular bones of the hands and feet are short and thick. (Fig. 8.3) The fingers are all the same length, with separation of the middle and ring fingers (trident hand). (Fig. 8.4) The ribs are quite short and often do not extend around the thorax. The scapulae may be squared inferiorly, (10) with shallow glenoids. The entire pelvis is small. The ilium is shortened caudally, and flattened, with small sciatic notches. The acetabulae are horizontally oriented, and there is excessive thickening of the "Y" cartilage. (Fig. 8.5) The length of the spinal column is generally normal at birth, though mild platyspondyly may be seen. The amount of cartilage is increased, causing the height of the discs to equal that of the vertebral bodies. Posterior scalloping of the bodies is common. The interpedicular spaces decrease caudally in the lumbar region, whereas they increase from L1 to L5 in the normal individual. The pedicles are short and thick. (Fig. 8.6) The lumbar lordosis is often exaggerated, complicated by a horizontally oriented sacrum. An angular kyphosis often develops at the thoracolumbar junction, resulting from anteriorly wedged or "bullet-nosed" vertebra. (11) (Fig. 8.7)

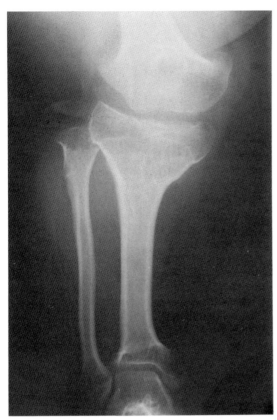

Figure 8.2. ACHONDROPLASIA: LOWER LIMB. Observe the splayed and cupped metaphyses, as well as the shortening of the leg.

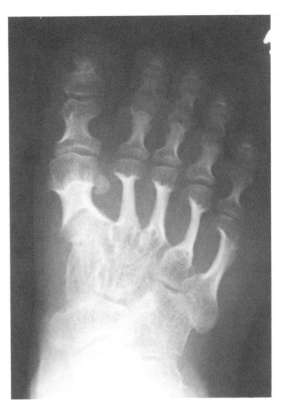

Figure 8.3. ACHONDROPLASIA: FEET. Note the short, thick tubular bones. (Courtesy of David P. Thomas, MD, Melbourne, Australia)

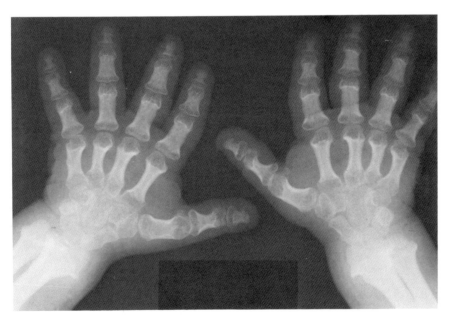

Figure 8.4. ACHONDROPLASIA: "TRIDENT" HANDS. Observe the characteristic "trident" hand, with separation of the third and fourth digits. Also note that the fingers are all the same length. (Courtesy of Bryan Hartley, MD, Melbourne, Australia)

NEUROLOGICAL COMPLICATIONS

Neurological manifestations are seen at all ages. In the infant the small foramen magnum and hydrocephalus can lead to cord compression. Spinal stenosis is a frequent neurological complication. In fact, Holder et al (4) consider achondroplasia to be the archetype of congenital spinal stenosis. Although the entire spine is involved, cord compression and resultant paraplegia more commonly de-

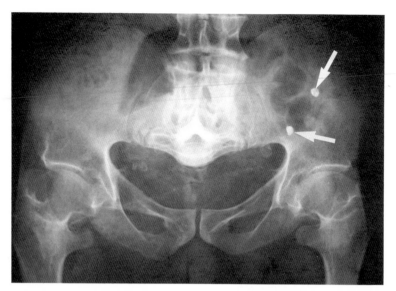

Figure 8.5. ACHONDROPLASIA: PELVIS. Observe the characteristic "champagne glass" pelvis. The ilii are short and flat. Also observe that the acetabulae are horizontally oriented. Of incidental notation is retention of barium in two colonic diverticuli (arrows).

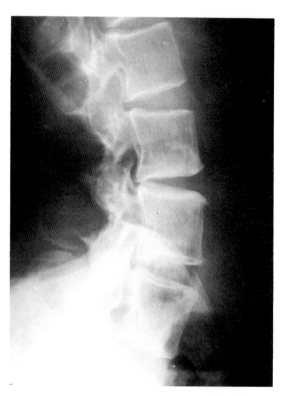

Figure 8.6. ACHONDROPLASIA: LUMBAR SPINE. Note the posterior scalloping of the vertebral bodies. The pedicles are short and thick and contribute to the development of lumbar spinal stenosis. *Comment:* These individuals are usually hyperlordotic.

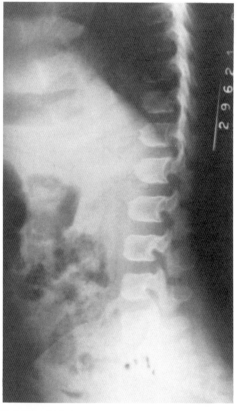

Figure 8.7. ACHONDROPLASIA: SPINAL COLUMN. Note the increased disc height and "bullet-nosed" vertebrae. (Courtesy of Paul E. Siebert, MD, Denver, Colorado)

velop in the adult at the thoracolumbar and lumbar regions.

Several anatomical factors contribute to the development of spinal stenosis in achondroplastics. These include decreased interpedicular distance, thick and short pedicles and facets, decreased AP diameter of the canal (which may be decreased by as much as 50 percent at L5) (6), decreased transverse diameter of the spinal canal, and stenosis of the nerve root canal. Surgical decompression comprising laminectomies from T11 to L5 is a frequent treatment. (4) (Fig. 8.8)

Four clinical syndromes have been described: (12)

(1) Nerve root compression caused by disc herniation and osteophyte formation;

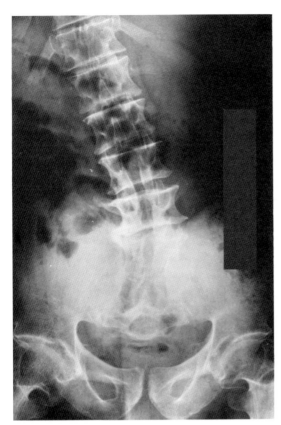

Figure 8.8. ACHONDROPLASIA, LUMBAR SPINE: SURGICAL DE-COMPRESSION. This patient has had laminectomies from L3 to L5 as treatment for the common complication of achondroplasia, spinal stenosis. (Courtesy of Douglas B. Hart, DC, Carina, Queensland, Australia)

(2) Transverse myelopathy developing over several years and associated with severe kyphosis;

(3) Acute transverse myelopathy, with sudden paraplegia following trauma; and

(4) Intermittent claudication of the cauda equina, possibly due to ischemia. Patients have symptoms suggesting vascular disease of the lower extremities associated with activity.

Achondroplasia has been confused with other dwarfing dysplasias. These include the mucopolysaccharidoses, trisomy, and spondyloepiphyseal dysplasia. However, careful biochemical and radiographic evaluation of these individuals should readily reveal the proper diagnosis.

Cleidocranial Dysplasia

GENERAL CONSIDERATIONS

Cleidocranial dysplasia is an uncommon autosomal dominant disorder which affects ossification of mainly intramembranous bones and is characterized by skull and clavicular anomalies and midline defects. According to Soule, (1) the first case was described by Cutter in 1870. (2) In 1898 the condition was recognized as an entity by Marie and Sainton and given the name cleidocranial

dysostosis. (3) The condition is congenital and has an extremely varied presentation. Infrequently, cases are seen which do not have clavicular or cranial findings, and Rhinehart has suggested the name "mutational dysostosis." (4) In more recent times the term "dysostosis" has been replaced by the term "dysplasia" when used in the context of cleidocranial abnormalities.

CLINICAL FEATURES

The typical individual presents with a large head, small face, and drooping shoulders. While small stature is common, dwarfism is not a usual feature. The chest is frequently narrowed or cone-shaped. The patient's mental status is normal. Gait disturbances due to deformities of the hips and femurs and abnormal dentition with severe caries and periodontitis are the most common complaints. Hearing loss has been reported, apparently secondary to structural abnormalities of the ossicles. (5) Clavicular hypoplasia or agenesis produces extreme mobility of the shoulders. Often, the patient can touch the two acromial regions together under the chin. (Fig. 8.9) Laboratory findings are consistently normal.

RADIOLOGICAL FEATURES

The radiographic signs are characteristic and leave little room for difficulty in diagnosis.

Skull

Early in infancy there is delayed or absent ossification of the calvarium. With time, multiple Wormian bones are formed in the sutures and often the metopic suture persists. Widening of the principal sutures (sagittal and coronal) gives a "hot cross-bun" appearance. (6) (Fig. 8.10A and B) There is marked brachycephaly with a widened interparietal diameter. The supraorbital region, temporal squama, and occipital bone are frequently thickened. The foramen magnum is deformed and enlarged, and there may be platybasia. (7)

The small face is the result of underdeveloped facial bones. Frequently, the nasal bones fail to ossify and the paranasal sinuses are hypoplastic. While the maxilla is small, the mandible is large, and the mandibular suture closes late. A high arched or cleft palate is not uncommon. Delayed and defective dentition is a prominent and often symptomatic finding. (8)

Thorax

Anomalous clavicular development is a nearly constant finding. Since the clavicle is formed from three separate ossification centers (sternal, middle, and acromial) and any one or even all can be affected, there is considerable variation in the clavicular involvement. (Fig. 8.11A–C) In 10 percent of cases the clavicle is completely absent. A pseudarthrosis may develop when the middle portion is missing. The scapulae are often small, winged, or even elevated. The shoulder girdle deformities allow great mobility of the shoulders. While the ribs are usually normal, the chest is narrow and cone-shaped.

Pelvis

The bones of the pelvis are small and underdeveloped, forming a small pelvic bowl. Commonly, there is a midline

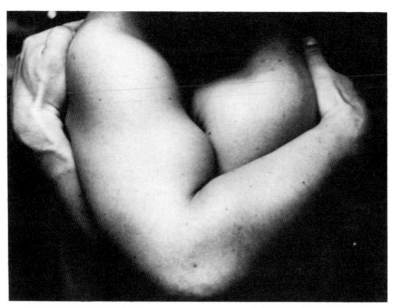

Figure 8.9. CLEIDOCRANIAL DYSPLASIA: HYPERMOBILE SHOULDERS. Extreme hypermobility of the shoulders is secondary to agenesis or hypoplasia of the clavicles. This patient can approximate his shoulders under the chin. (Courtesy of Kenneth E. Yochum, DC, St. Louis, Missouri)

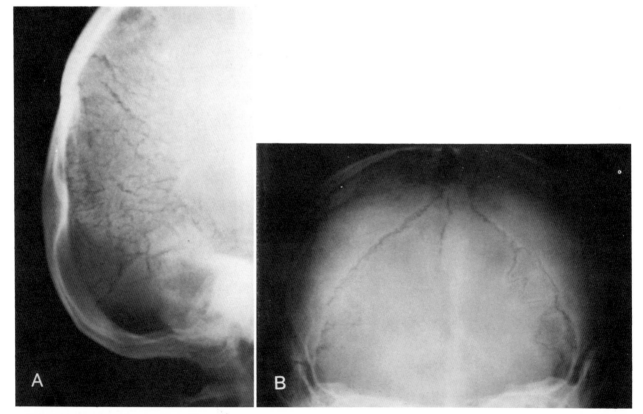

Figure 8.10. CLEIDOCRANIAL DYSPLASIA: SKULL INVOLVEMENT. **A. Lateral Occiput: Wormian Bones.** Note the numerous Wormian bones throughout the occipital region. These sutural bones are fairly common in cleidocranial dysplasia but are not pathognomonic, as they are found in other disorders as well. (Courtesy of Bruce Farkas, DO, Chicago, Illinois). **B. Sutural Widening.** As in this patient, widening of the sutures and persistence of the fetal sutures are common findings.

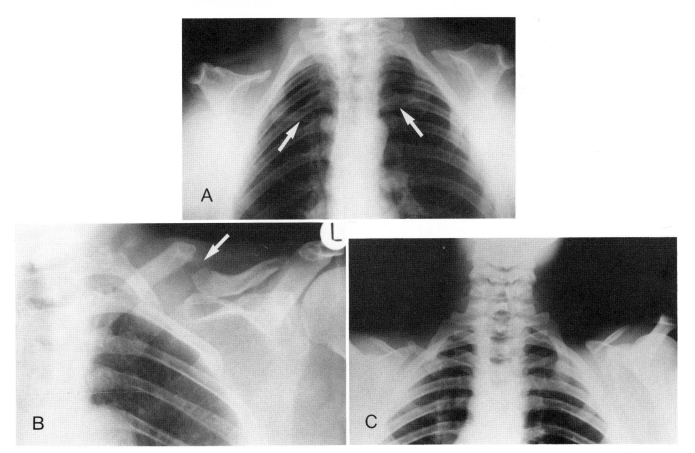

Figure 8.11. CLEIDOCRANIAL DYSPLASIA: CLAVICULAR INVOLVEMENT. **A.** There is agenesis of the middle and lateral portions of the clavicle, with only the medial portion present (arrows). **B.** Note the agenesis of the middle ossification center of the clavicle, with a pseudarthrosis (arrow). **C.** All three ossification centers are present but are hypoplastic, with resultant pseudarthroses. ***Comment***: In 10 percent of individuals with cleidocranial dysplasia the clavicles are completely absent.

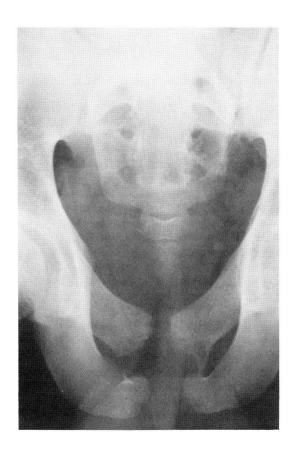

Figure 8.12. CLEIDOCRANIAL DYSPLASIA: PUBIC SYMPHYSIS. Note the midline diastasis of the pubic symphysis. (Courtesy of Bruce Farkas, DO, Chicago, Illinois)

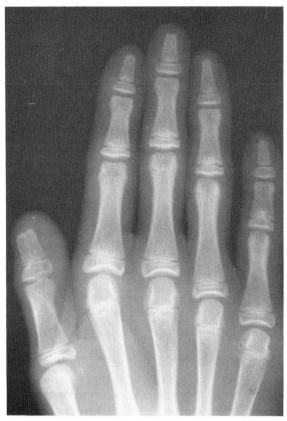

Figure 8.13. CLEIDOCRANIAL DYSPLASIA: HANDS. The distal phalanges are hypoplastic and flattened. (Courtesy of Bruce Farkas, DO, Chicago, Illinois)

defect at the pubic symphysis, where the rami fail to approximate anteriorly. (Fig. 8.12) Valgus and varus deformities of the femoral neck are frequent. Lateral notching of the capital femoral epiphysis has been reported. (9)

Spine

Hyperlordosis, excessive kyphosis, and scoliosis are found secondary to neural arch defects and hemivertebrae.

Extremities

The most marked changes are found in the hands, where an accessory epiphysis for the base of the second metacarpal occurs, creating an elongated digit. The distal phalanges are hypoplastic and often pointed. (10) (Fig. 8.13) Similar changes may be found in the feet but are less common. The long tubular bones are less frequently involved but, occasionally, shortening of the radius with an abnormal wrist articulation is seen.

COMPLICATIONS

Hearing loss, severe dental problems, dislocations of the shoulders and hips, and scoliosis are troublesome but do not lead to a shortened life span.

The Epiphyseal Dysplasias

The epiphyseal dysplasias are a diverse and overlapping group of entities. Often, differentiation between the

various types is not easily made. For academic and teaching purposes, they will be described here in their more classic presentations. But it is important for the reader to realize that the clinical and radiographic features of any one case may not be clear-cut. The epiphyseal dysplasias covered in this text include chondrodysplasia punctata, dysplasia epiphysealis hemimelica (Trevor's disease), epiphyseal dysplasia multiplex, and spondyloepiphyseal dysplasia.

Chondrodysplasia Punctata

GENERAL CONSIDERATIONS

Chondrodysplasia punctata is a type of epiphyseal dysplasia characterized by punctate or stippled calcification of multiple epiphyseal centers during the first year of life. The entity is rare and has been classified into two types: 1) an autosomal dominant form (Conradi-Hunermann syndrome) with a normal life expectancy; and 2) a recessive form which is rhizomelic (proximal limb) and is frequently fatal in the first years of life. (1) Synonyms include stippled epiphyses, dysplasia epiphysialis punctata, (2) chondrodystrophia fetalis calcificans, and chondrodystrophia calcificans congenita. (3)

CLINICAL FEATURES

The lethal rhizomelic form features symmetric proximal limb shortening, joint contractures, mental retardation, cataracts, optic atrophy, and skin changes. Most infants die in the first year of life, often as a result of respiratory failure (4) or recurrent infection. Less frequently, tracheal stenosis (5) or spinal cord compression is the cause of death. (6) A female predominance has been noted. (7)

The dominant form, Conradi-Hunermann syndrome, has asymmetric features, with less limb shortening and deformity. The intelligence is normal, but there are prominent spinal changes. There is speculation that this form is actually composed of several different genetic disorders, ranging from a mild nondeforming type to a lethal type found in males, carried on the X chromosome. (8,9) Recently, there have been reports of Conradi-Hunermann syndrome in children born to women who received Coumadin and Warfarin medication during pregnancy. (10,11)

PATHOLOGICAL FEATURES

The epiphyseal centers undergo mucoid degeneration, and hypervascularity is prominent. This leads to fragmentation of the epiphysis. Calcific and ossific punctate deposits are scattered through the fragments. These calcifications may eventually disappear and ossification will proceed, though often in an abnormal fashion, resulting in deformity.

RADIOLOGICAL FEATURES

The roentgen findings in the two forms differ.

Lethal Recessive Type

The epiphyseal stippling is noted primarily in the hips, shoulders, knees, and wrists. There is symmetric shortening of the limbs, particularly proximally, and more frequently in the upper extremities. The metaphyses are often flared, and the long bones are bowed. (Fig. 8.14) In most cases there are coronal clefts of the vertebrae, but stippling of the spine is usually absent.

Conradi-Hunermann Syndrome

The stippling may be mild to severe, with asymmetric limb shortening occasionally seen. The metaphyses and diaphyses are normal. (Fig. 8.15A and B) The vertebral end plates and sometimes the centra are stippled, leading to abnormally shaped vertebrae and a resultant kyphoscoliosis. Stippling may also affect the ends of the ribs, the hyoid, the thyroid cartilage, and the base of the skull. Laryngeal and tracheal calcifications may occur.

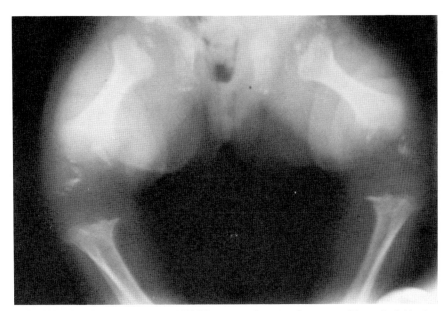

Figure 8.14. CHONDRODYSPLASIA PUNCTATA, LETHAL RECESSIVE FORM: EPIPHYSEAL STIPPLING. Along with epiphyseal stippling, there is symmetrical limb shortening and the metaphyses are flared. *Comment:* These individuals usually die within the first year of life.

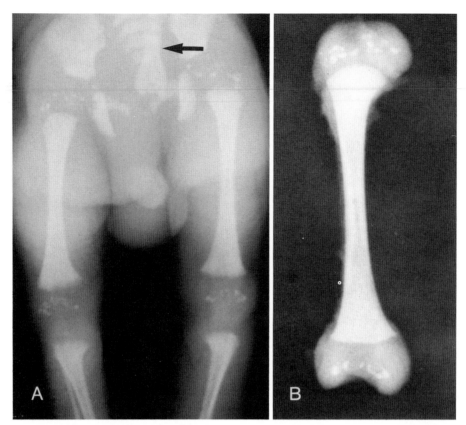

Figure 8.15. CHONDRODYSPLASIA PUNCTATA: CONRADI-HU-NERMANN SYNDROME (DOMINANT FORM). A. Pelvis and Legs. Limb shortening is less commonly encountered, and stippling may be mild to severe. The artifact is a clamp for the newborn's umbilicus (arrow). **B. Autopsy Specimen.** Note that in this dominant form the metaphysis and diaphysis are normal. *Comment:* In this dominant form life expectancy is normal. This disorder may be associated with the use of Coumadin and Warfarin during pregnancy.

Dysplasia Epiphysealis Hemimelica

GENERAL CONSIDERATIONS

This rare bone dysplasia involving the epiphyses was first defined by Trevor in 1950 and given the name "tarso-epiphyseal aclasis." (1) While still referred to as Trevor's disease, it was Fairbank who suggested the name dysplasia epiphysealis hemimelica, as he felt that this entity was not a true aclasis, and there were cases where bones other than the tarsals were involved. (2) Aegerter and Kirkpatrick have suggested that it be called epiphyseal hyperplasia. (3) Resnick refers to the lesions found in this peculiar entity as articular chondromas. (4)

Dysplasia epiphysealis hemimelica may be hereditary and familial and occurs as a solitary finding or is found in conjunction with other benign cartilaginous lesions of bone. Within one family some members displayed solitary dysplasia epiphysealis hemimelica, while others were found to have associated extraskeletal osteochondromas, typical osteochondromas, and intracapsular chondromas. (5)

CLINICAL FEATURES

Presenting in males during the first decade of life, dysplasia epiphysealis hemimelica becomes symptomatic when the asymmetrical epiphyseal overgrowth interferes with normal joint range of motion. It is found predominantly in the lower extremity and is usually monomelic (one limb). (Fig. 8.16) The most commonly involved bones are the distal femur, distal tibia, and talus. (Fig. 8.17) The small bones of the hands and feet may be affected, displaying premature appearance of the ossification centers which are enlarged. (2,6,7) Involvement of the ulna has been reported. (8) (Fig. 8.18) Functional impairment of the joint may be seen, along with varus and valgus deformities. Hard, bony swellings are noted clinically in the region of involvement, but pain is infrequent. Painful "locking" of the knee, regional muscular atrophy, and clumsy gait have been reported. (9) Shortening or lengthening of the limb may also be associated.

RADIOLOGICAL FEATURES

Focal overgrowth of one-half of an epiphysis in the lower extremity is the characteristic feature. The overgrowth is a bony mass covered with epiphyseal cartilage which is attached to the remainder of the epiphysis. The lesion is sometimes composed of multiple centers and may be separated from the epiphysis. Histologically, the lesions are identical to osteochondromas. With skeletal maturity, these osteocartilagenous masses fuse with the remainder of the epiphysis or, less frequently, remain as separate bodies. The distribution and roentgen appearance of this entity generally present no diagnostic dilemma.

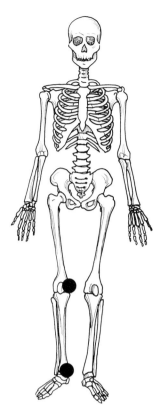

Figure 8.16. SKELETAL DISTRIBUTION OF DYSPLASIA EPIPHYSEALIS HEMIMELICA.

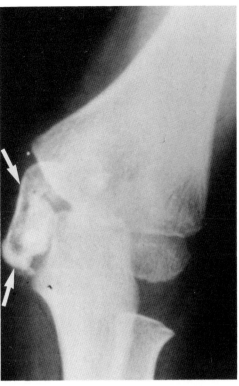

Figure 8.18. DYSPLASIA EPIPHYSEALIS HEMIMELICA: PROXIMAL ULNA. Note the less commonly encountered involvement of the proximal ulna (arrows). (Courtesy of Gary M. Guebert, DC, DACBR, St. Louis, Missouri)

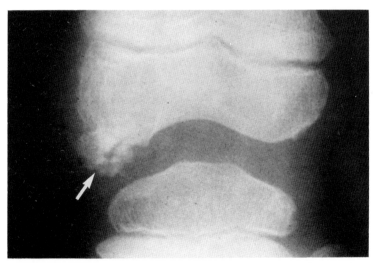

Figure 8.17. DYSPLASIA EPIPHYSEALIS HEMIMELICA: DISTAL FEMUR. Note the focal overgrowth of the medial femoral condyle (arrow). **Comment:** These overgrowths become symptomatic when there is interference with normal joint movement; varus and valgus deformities may develop in affected joints. (Courtesy of Gary M. Guebert, DC, DACBR, St. Louis, Missouri)

Epiphyseal Dysplasia Multiplex

GENERAL CONSIDERATIONS

Epiphyseal dysplasia multiplex is a disorder with epiphyseal abnormalities that are generally manifested in childhood and lead to severe degenerative changes. Most cases appear to be of autosomal dominant transmission, but varied severity is noted within families. Ribbing described the disorder in 1937, and Fairbank coined the term dysplasia epiphysealis multiplex in 1947. (1,2) Rubin believes epiphyseal dysplasia multiplex to be a tarda form of chondrodysplasia punctata. (3) Synonyms include multiple epiphyseal dysplasia, Fairbank-Ribbing disease, and dysplasia polyepiphysaire.

CLINICAL FEATURES

Generally, the disorder is first noticed when the child begins to walk, with common complaints of a waddling gait and difficulty running. Milder cases may not become apparent until early adulthood, when premature joint degeneration occurs. Both sexes are equally affected. Mental status is normal. Most individuals are of short stature, but dwarfism is not a prominent feature. The hands and feet are short and stubby. Other findings include flexion deformities, genu valgum or varus and, occasionally, coxa vara. Approximately 50 percent of cases reveal a tibiotalar slant produced by deformity of the lateral portion of the distal tibial epiphysis. (4) This sign is not pathognomic, however, since it can also be seen in hemophilia and juvenile rheumatoid arthritis. The most frequent sites of epiphyseal involvement are the hips, knees, and ankles, with the shoulders and wrists being less commonly affected.

PATHOLOGICAL FEATURES

Epiphyseal dysplasia multiplex appears to be caused by an abnormality of the epiphyseal chondrocytes. (5–7) The number of chondrocytes is decreased and their arrangement is abnormal, leading to delayed and disorderly ossification of the epiphyses.

RADIOLOGICAL FEATURES

Mottled and irregular mineralization is noted in the epiphyses usually during the second or third year of life. The involvement is bilateral and symmetric, with the hips, knees, and ankles most commonly involved. While growth is abnormal and delayed, maturation and fusion are usually within norms. Frequently, the epiphyses will develop from multiple centers. Occasionally, the metaphyses are flared, most likely due to the abnormal epiphyses. The carpal and tarsal bones are hypoplastic, and the long tubular bones of the hands (and sometimes the feet) are short and thick. (Fig. 8.19)

With maturation, the epiphyses have irregular articular surfaces. The femoral heads and condyles are flattened. (Fig. 8.20) Slipped femoral epiphyses complicate coxa vara deformities. (8) Approximately two-thirds of patients have spinal changes. (9,10) These are similar to Scheuermann's disease or, more rarely, platyspondyly. Also associated is anterior wedging and scoliosis. The irregular epiphyses lead to premature and often severe degenerative changes, especially in the hip and knee joints.

Several entities, including Legg-Calve-Perthes' disease, Morquio's disease, and cretinism, may offer similar roentgen findings. However, the symmetrical nature and characteristic joints of involvement should provide sufficient evidence to adequately diagnose epiphyseal dysplasia multiplex.

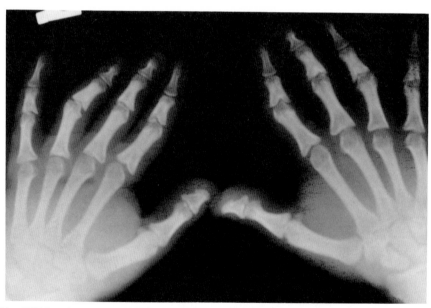

Figure 8.19. EPIPHYSEAL DYSPLASIA MULTIPLEX: HANDS. Note the symmetrically short and thick tubular bones. There is irregularity of the phalangeal articular surfaces. The hands and feet are short and stubby.

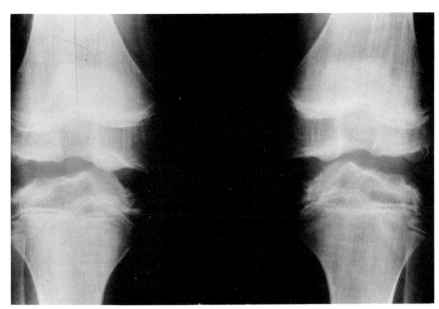

Figure 8.20. EPIPHYSEAL DYSPLASIA MULTIPLEX: KNEES. There is symmetrical flattening of the femoral condyles and irregularity of the tibial plateaus. *Comment:* The irregular epiphyses often lead to premature and severe degenerative changes. (Courtesy of Jack Edeiken, MD, Houston, Texas)

Spondyloepiphyseal Dysplasia

GENERAL CONSIDERATIONS

Spondyloepiphyseal dysplasia is a group of inheritable bone dysplasias with a wide range of expression. It is generally divided into congenital and tarda forms. Spondyloepiphyseal dysplasia congenita is recognized at birth and is transmitted by an autosomal dominant trait. (1) The tarda type is manifested only in males, usually in late childhood, and is transmitted in an "X" linked recessive mode. (2)

Spondyloepiphyseal Dysplasia Congenita

Clinical Features. At birth affected infants have short limbs, their faces are flat, and the eyes are widely spaced. (1) Other clinical features include a cleft palate, hearing loss, myopia, and retinal detachment. (3,4) The neck and spine are short, and often exaggerated kyphoses, lordoses, and scolioses develop. Pectus carinatum occurs. Muscle tone is poorly developed, with genu valgum or varum and hip contractures. (5,6) The height attained ranges from 37 to 52 inches. (1) The hands and feet are normal.

Radiological Features. The most prominent features are found in the spine and pelvis. Ossification is delayed, and in the newborn there may be lack of ossification of the pubic bone, distal femur, proximal tibia, calcaneus, and talus. Ossification of the femoral head is greatly retarded throughout childhood, and marked coxa vara is common. The acetabular roofs are horizontal, and the iliac wings are short. In the spine the vertebral bodies have an anterior bulbous appearance ("pear-shaped" vertebrae) which then flattens into platyspondyly and persists into adulthood. (7) The platyspondyly, along with thin discs, results in extreme shortening of the trunk. Often, several vertebral bodies at the thoracolumbar junction are hypoplastic. (8) Scolioses and severe kyphoses and lordoses develop, and odontoid hypoplasia is common. The proximal long bones are often shortened (rhizomelia), with flared metaphyses. The articular surfaces are irregular, and carpal and tarsal maturation may be retarded.

The major entity which must be differentiated from spondyloepiphyseal dysplasia congenita is Morquio's syndrome. Morquio-type mucopolysaccharidosis is autosomal recessive and has keratosulfaturia and corneal opacities, unlike spondyloepiphyseal dysplasia. In the spine, the shape of the vertebral bodies is different, and Morquio discs are of normal height.

Spondyloepiphyseal Dysplasia Tarda

Clinical Features. Spondyloepiphyseal dysplasia tarda usually manifests between the ages of 5 and 10 and is found only in males. There is mild loss of stature, with the adult height varying from 52 to 62 inches. (9,10) Back pain is a frequent complaint, and premature osteoarthritis begins shortly after puberty.

Radiological Features. Loss of stature is due primarily to the platyspondyly, which is most marked in the thoracic region. A characteristic configuration of the vertebral body is noted in which there is hyperostotic bone deposited on the posterior two-thirds of the end plates. This is referred to as a "hump-shaped" or "heaping-up" vertebra. (11) (Fig. 8.21) The ring epiphyses do not ossify, and the disc spaces are thin. Mild kyphosis, scoliosis, and early degenerative changes are frequent, and early and marked osteoarthritis of the hips is the most prominent clinical complaint. Loss of joint space, spurring, and cyst formation result in deformity of the femoral head and neck, and the pelvis is often small. There may be a broad thorax with sternal prominence, and degenerative changes are occasionally seen in the shoulders and less frequently in the knees and ankles.

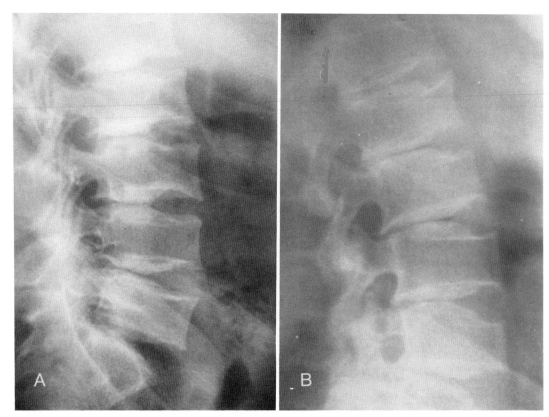

Figure 8.21. SPONDYLOEPIPHYSEAL DYSPLASIA: TARDA FORM. A. Lumbar Spine. Hyperostotic bone is deposited on the posterior two-thirds of the vertebra, referred to as "hump-shaped" or "heaping-up" vertebra. (Courtesy of John R. Nolan, DC, Wanganui, New Zealand). **B. Lumbar Spine.** This patient also demonstrates a "heaping-up" configuration. **Comment:** Note the thinness of the disc. The changes in spondyloepiphyseal dysplasia lead to back pain and premature osteoarthritis.

Fibrodysplasia Ossificans Progressiva

GENERAL CONSIDERATIONS

Fibrodysplasia ossificans progressiva (1) is a rare, disabling hereditary mesodermal disorder which leads to progressive ossification of striated muscles, tendons, ligaments, fascia, and aponeuroses. McKusick believes it to be of autosomal dominant transmission with a wide range of expression. (2) Patin first described a case in 1692 of a young woman who "turned to wood." (2) Munchmeyer reported the first series of cases, and the disorder is sometimes referred to as Munchmeyer's disease. (3) Other synonyms include fibrogenesis ossificans progressiva, myositis ossificans progressiva, and fibrositis ossificans progressiva. The etiology is unknown.

CLINICAL FEATURES

The disease is usually seen in the first years of life. There is no sex predominance. The most common presenting symptom is torticollis, with painful, hot, edematous masses in the sternocleidomastoid muscle. Involvement then progresses to the soft tissues of the remainder of the neck, shoulders, spine, and upper arms. Later in the course of the disease the lower extremities may be affected. Occasionally, these masses follow trivial trauma. Fever may accompany this acute phase. As the acute tenderness of the masses subsides, the lesions become smaller and harden, as ossification occurs. The extensive ossification leads to severely disabling restriction of joint movement, and involvement of the intercostal musculature interferes with respiration. Wasting follows ossification of the muscles of mastication. The smooth muscles of the tongue, larynx, diaphragm, heart, and sphincters are not involved. (1) An abnormal electrocardiogram has been reported. (4)

Seventy-five percent of patients with fibrodysplasia ossificans progressiva have bilateral microdactyly of the first toes, with synostosis of the phalanges. A smaller percentage have similar anomalies of the thumbs. These congenital digital anomalies are present in 5 percent of the family members of fibrodysplasia ossificans progressiva patients, thus supporting the hereditary but varied presentation theory of this disease. (5–7) Two sets of homozygous twins have been reported with fibrodysplasia ossificans progressiva. (8,9)

LABORATORY FEATURES

Chemistry findings are generally noncontributory, with blood chemistry, serum alkaline phosphatase, renal function, and parathormone levels all within normal limits. (4)

PATHOLOGICAL FEATURES

Early, the soft tissue masses are composed of edema and inflammatory exudate, forming a mass of collagen. Calcium salts then are deposited within the collagenous mass, which eventually develops into irregular masses of lamellar and woven bone. McKusick suggests that fibrodysplasia ossificans progressiva affects the interstitial tissues primarily, and that muscle involvement is secondary to pressure atrophy. (1) It has been suggested that the calcium salts are deposited due to lack of a circulating inhibitor, (4) or due to a primary defect in the collagen. (1) Still other reports reveal abnormalities suggestive of a myopathy. (10,11)

RADIOLOGICAL FEATURES

The radiographic findings can be divided into two categories—digital anomalies and ectopic ossification.

Digital Anomalies

The digital abnormalities are present at birth and precede the ectopic ossification. As previously stated, microdactyly of the first toe is present in 75 percent of individuals with fibrodysplasia ossificans progressiva and in 5 percent of unaffected family members. (Fig. 8.22) Another common finding is microdactyly of the thumbs. (Fig. 8.23) The microdactyly results from phalangeal shortening, synostosis or, rarely, absence. Short metacarpals may be found in the hand, especially the first and the fifth. Hallux valgus is nearly always present. (10) Other associated congenital anomalies include brachydactyly, clinodactyly, large epiphyses, and broad femoral necks. (Fig. 8.24)

Ectopic Ossification

During the acute inflammatory stage the lesions appear radiographically as soft tissue masses. As the collagen organizes and collects calcium salts, then progresses to ossification, linear and spheroid deposits of bone are seen. (Fig. 8.25) Eventually, columns of bone replace tendons, fascia, and ligaments and are seen in the muscles. (Fig. 8.26) Ossification of tendon and ligament insertions gives the appearance of exostoses. Sesamoid bones may fuse to the digits. Joint ankylosis results from involvement of the surrounding soft tissues. Spinal changes add to the severe lack of mobility and include fusion of the apophyseal articulations and vertebral bodies, reminiscent of ankylosing spondylitis. Early ossification of the neck soft tissue structures results in premature fusion of the cervical spine growth centers with hypoplastic ankylosed vertebral bodies. (Fig. 8.27) The diagnosis is usually readily made when congenital digital anomalies are present in association with widespread soft tissue ossification.

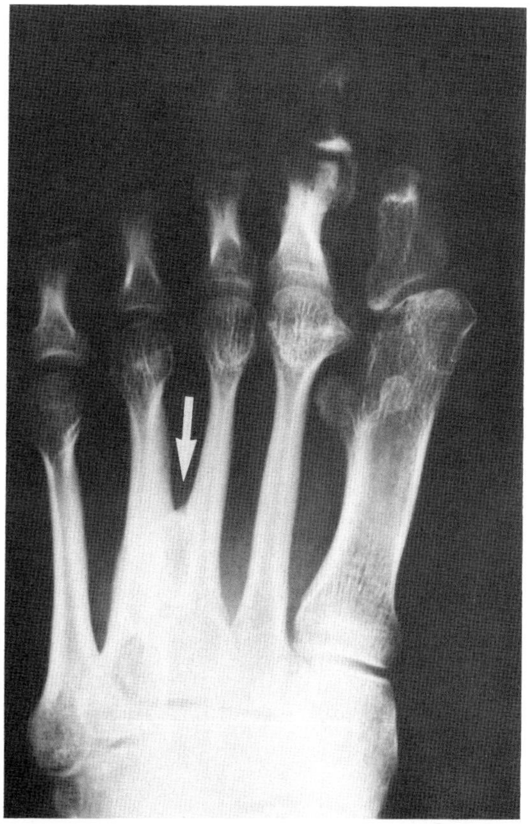

Figure 8.22. FIBRODYSPLASIA OSSIFICANS PROGRESSIVA: MICRODACTYLY OF THE GREAT TOE. Microdactyly of the great toe is present in 75 percent of individuals with fibrodysplasia ossificans progressiva and in 5 percent of unaffected family members. Also note the hallux valgus and the synostosis of the third and fourth metatarsal bases (arrow).

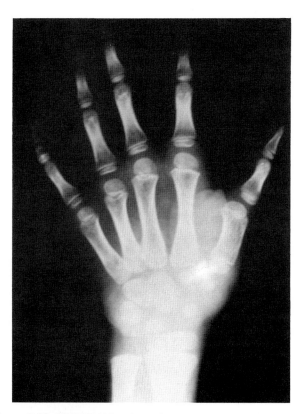

Figure 8.23. FIBRODYSPLASIA OSSIFICANS PROGRESSIVA: MICRODACTYLY OF THE THUMB. The microdactyly results either from phalangeal shortening or synostosis. In this case the first metacarpal is short as well.

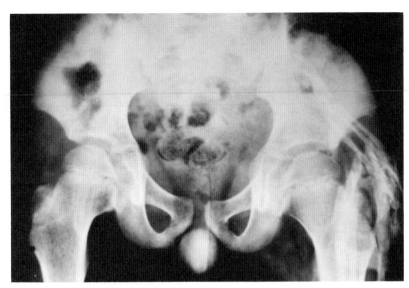

Figure 8.24. FIBRODYSPLASIA OSSIFICANS PROGRESSIVA, PELVIS: BROAD FEMORAL NECKS. Broad femoral necks are often associated with fibrodysplasia ossificans progressiva. Note the extensive ossification around the hip joint.

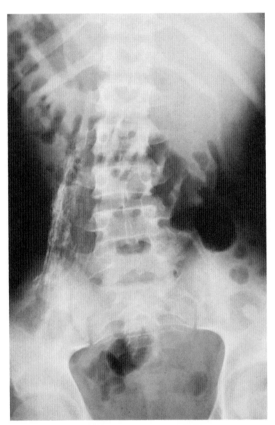

Figure 8.25. FIBRODYSPLASIA OSSIFICANS PROGRESSIVA: PSOAS MUSCLE OSSIFICATION. There is unilateral ossification of the psoas muscle. Eventually, columns of bone replace tendons, fascia, ligaments, and muscle, leading to severe disability.

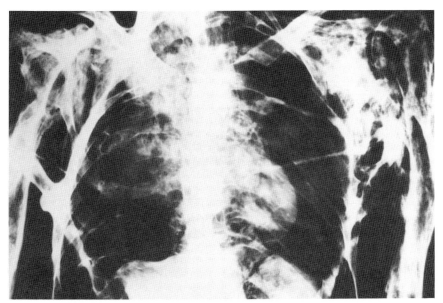

Figure 8.26. FIBRODYSPLASIA OSSIFICANS PROGRESSIVA: THORACIC AND AXILLARY INVOLVEMENT. Columns of bone traverse the axillary regions and extend around the chest. Involve-ment of the intercostal muscles interferes with respiration. Respira-tory failure and cor pulmonale are severe complications.

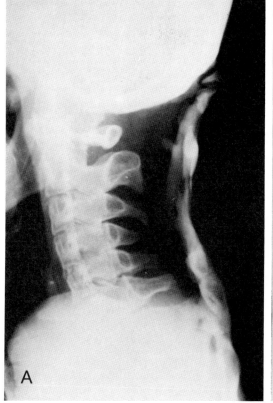

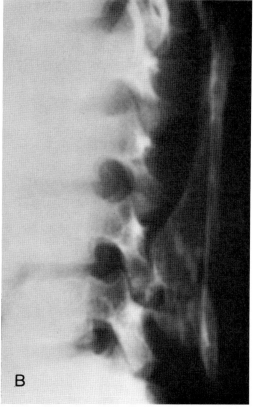

Figure 8.27. FIBRODYSPLASIA OSSIFICANS PROGRESSIVA: SPINE.   A. Cervical Spine. Note the ossification extending caudally from the occiput along the spine. Also note the hypoplastic fused vertebral bodies.   **B. Lumbar Spine.** The ossification extends into the lumbar region.   *Comment:* The most common presenting symp-tom is torticollis. The muscles of the neck are inflamed and become progressively ossified. Premature fusion of the cervical spine growth centers leads to hypoplastic, ankylosed vertebral bodies. Involve-ment then progresses to the shoulders and upper arms.

Infantile Cortical Hyperostosis

GENERAL CONSIDERATIONS

Infantile cortical hyperostosis is an uncommon and puzzling disease of infants, nearly always presenting before the age of five months. It was first described by Caffey and Silverman in 1945 and is sometimes referred to as Caffey's disease or Caffey's syndrome. (1) Sexual distribution is equal, and cases have been found throughout the world with no racial predilection. Familial involvement over several generations has been noted, (2) but most cases are sporadic.

CLINICAL FEATURES

Patients usually manifest a clinical triad of hyperirritability, swellings of the soft tissues, and palpable, hard masses over affected bones. Fever is nearly always present, along with an increased erythrocyte sedimentation rate and elevated serum phosphatase levels. More than half of Caffey's patients showed reduced hemoglobin and red blood cell levels. (3) Anemia and a moderate leukocytosis may be present. Serologic and culture tests for viral and bacterial agents have all been unrewarding. Pseudoparalysis, pleuritis, and pallor are additional clinical features, and remissions and exacerbations are common. Some cases have shown improvement with corticosteroid medication. The soft tissue swellings and hard masses are extremely tender to palpation but lack warmth and discoloration. Swelling is most marked over the mandible. (4) The average age at onset is nine weeks, but it has been present at birth and has even been recognized in utero. (5,6)

The severity and course of the disease are extremely variable. Most cases resolve within a few weeks to several months, but there have been cases persisting into adolescence. (7) Mild cases may go without clinical notice, while severe involvement can produce deformities that persist into adulthood. (8)

PATHOLOGICAL FEATURES

Pathological features show initial involvement in the periosteum, which swells, then loses its distinct margins and blends with the adjacent soft tissues. During this inflammatory stage the cortex undergoes resorption. With progression, connective tissue and trabeculae are laid down, sometimes enlarging the bone to profound proportions. With healing, remodeling takes place; however, bony deformities may persist.

The etiology of infantile cortical hyperostosis is still unknown. Most of the clinical and pathological features suggest an infectious agent, most likely a virus. Similar findings in hamsters and cats have been reported. (3) Further viral implication is supported by the lack of response to antibiotic and sulfonamide therapy. The importance of genetic and inheritable conditions is suggested by familial incidence in several generations.

RADIOLOGICAL FEATURES

Periosteal new bone formation takes place within the soft tissue swelling adjacent to the cortex. This new bone may be very dense and may increase to the extent that the bone doubles its original size. The hyperostosis usually persists for some time after evidence of soft tissue swelling has subsided. During the healing phase, the new bone formation may have a "laminated" appearance, but this is not noted during the acute stage.

The most commonly involved bones are the mandible, clavicle, and ribs, where involvement is frequently symmetrical. (4) (Fig. 8.28, 8.29) The ulna is the most frequently involved of the long bones, often without concomitant involvement of the radius. (Fig. 8.30) All bones of the skeleton have been implicated, with the exception of the vertebral column, phalanges, and round bones (carpals and tarsals). (3) In the past it was believed that infantile cortical hyperostosis never manifested without involvement in the mandible, but Wilson has reported one such case. (9) The cortical hyperostosis is most prominent in the lateral ribs, and there may be associated pleural effusions and diaphragmatic eventration. The epiphyses are spared when long bone involvement occurs. (Fig. 8.31) In the skull various presentations may occur. Thickening of the calvarium or destructive lesions may simulate histiocytosis or metastatic neuroblastoma. Involvement around the anterior fontanelle yields an appearance not unlike bulging due to increased intracranial pressure. Scapular lesions have been mistaken for malignant tumors. Several cases with shoulder girdle involvement have presented with Erb's palsy. (10)

Severe and chronic cases often have residual changes such as medullary expansion and long bone undertubulation, bowing deformities, length growth disturbances, and facial asymmetry. (11) Extremely large hyperostotic areas may lead to death of adjacent periosteum due to pressure, causing local fusion of cortical walls and interosseous bridging. This is most frequently encountered in the ribs and between the ulna and radius or the tibia and fibula. Radioulnar synostosis can lead to radial head dislocation. (12)

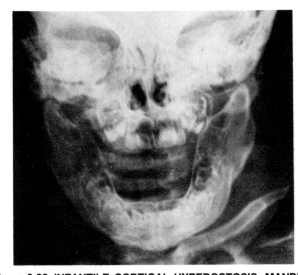

Figure 8.28. INFANTILE CORTICAL HYPEROSTOSIS: MANDIBULAR INVOLVEMENT. Note the bilateral mandibular hyperostosis, with soft tissue swelling. *Comment:* The most commonly involved bones are the mandible, clavicle, and ribs. (Reprinted with permission: Edeiken J: *Roentgen Diagnosis of Diseases of Bone*, ed 3, Baltimore, Williams & Wilkins, p 818, 1981)

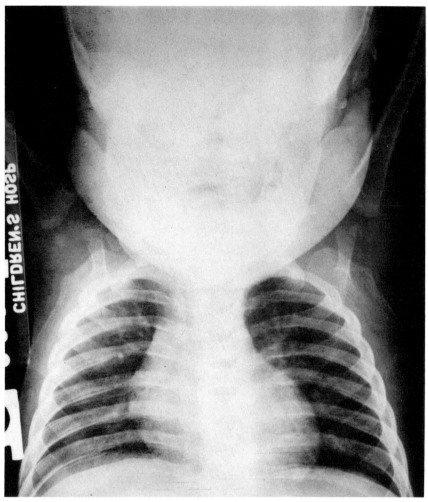

Figure 8.29. INFANTILE CORTICAL HYPEROSTOSIS: RIB AND MANDIBULAR INVOLVEMENT. There is symmetrical hyperostosis of ribs and mandible. (Reprinted with permission: Edeiken J: *Roentgen Diagnosis of Diseases of Bone*, ed 3, Baltimore, Williams & Wilkins, p 822, 1981)

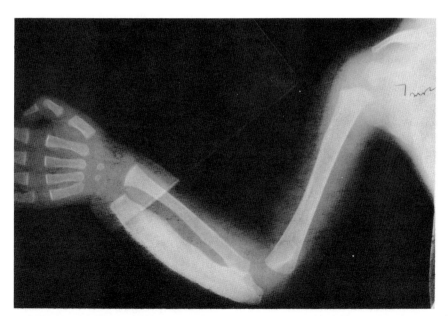

Figure 8.30. INFANTILE CORTICAL HYPEROSTOSIS: ULNAR INVOLVEMENT. Note involvement of the ulna, with sparing of the radius and humerus. The ulna is the most frequently involved long bone in infantile cortical hyperostosis.

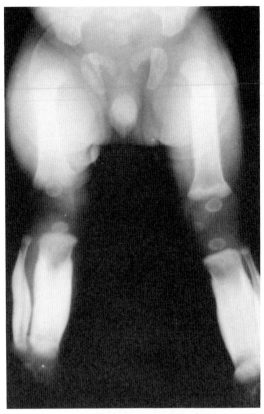

Figure 8.31. INFANTILE CORTICAL HYPEROSTOSIS: LOWER EX-TREMITIES. Note the symmetrical involvement in the lower extremities, with sparing of the epiphyses.

Marfan's Syndrome

GENERAL CONSIDERATIONS

Marfan's syndrome is an autosomal dominant entity consisting of long, slender tubular bones, ocular abnormalities, and aneurysm of the aorta. First described in 1896 by Marfan, (1) it is now thought that his patient had congenital contractural arachnodactyly, a similar disorder. (2) Synonyms for Marfan's syndrome include arachnodactyly and dolichostenomelia. (3) Marfan's syndrome is not rare, and the majority of patients will have familial incidence, though some cases are sporadic.

CLINICAL FEATURES

No sexual or racial predominance has been established. The severity of involvement varies greatly, but most individuals can be diagnosed clinically. The extremities are markedly elongated, with very sparse soft tissue, owing to muscular hypoplasia and a scarcity of subcutaneous fat. The elongation of the tubular bones (the trunk is spared) is most marked in the distal portion of the extremities, especially the phalanges, metacarpals, and metatarsals. The lower extremity exhibits greater overgrowth than the upper. Underdevelopment and hypotonicity of the muscular system contributes to joint laxity and dislocation. Associated findings include hip dislocations, genu recurvatum, patellar dislocations, and pes planus. Persist-

ent bilateral perilunate dislocations have been reported. (4) Generally, affected individuals are taller than six feet. Scoliosis is found in approximately 45 percent of patients with Marfan's syndrome. (5)

Classically, the skull reveals dolichocephaly. The face is elongated, with a high, arched palate and prominent jaw. Mental capacity is generally normal. Poor dentition is frequent, often with two rows of misplaced, long teeth. Approximately 50 percent of cases of Marfan's syndrome have dislocation of the ocular lens; this is the most common ocular abnormality. (6–8) Also frequently encountered are myopia and contracted pupils, which are secondary to absence of the dilator muscle of the pupil. There may also be strabismus and retinal detachments. In adulthood cataracts may form secondary to lens detachment.

Some form of congenital heart disease is present in about one-third of affected individuals, and cardiac abnormalities contribute to the shortened life span of Marfanoid individuals. Atrial septal defect is the most frequent congenital heart lesion. (8) Abnormal tunica media and cystic medial necrosis predispose to dissection and rupture of the aorta and pulmonary artery. Dilatation of the ascending aorta, along with abnormalities of the valves, leads to valvular incompetence and left-sided insufficiency referred to as the "floppy valve" syndrome. (2,9)

To allow proper diagnosis in less classical cases, clinical and radiographic tests have been described. Steinberg suggests the "thumb sign," which refers to the protrusion of the flexed thumb beyond the confines of a clenched fist. (10) Radiographically, the metacarpal index (the ratio of the length to the width of the second through fifth metacarpal bones) is increased in Marfan patients. (11)

Pathologically, Marfan's syndrome is a connective tissue disorder, with a failure to produce normal collagen. It appears to be the poor quality rather than an insufficient quantity of collagen which leads to the vast array of changes. The etiology is still unknown, and there are no consistently abnormal laboratory findings.

RADIOLOGICAL FINDINGS

Elongation of the extremities without an increase in width is classic. There is no osteoporosis. The tubular bones of the hands and feet are particularly long, slender, and gracile; hence, the name arachnodactyly or "spider-like" fingers. (Fig. 8.32) The cortices are generally thinned, and the trabecular pattern is often delicate.

In the spine the findings include tall vertebrae (12) and often a severe scoliosis or kyphoscoliosis. The spinal canal is frequently widened, and there may be posterior scalloping of the vertebral bodies which is thought to be due to dural ectasia. (13)

A pectus excavatum deformity with elongated ribs is often encountered, and McKusick suggests that this finding is indicative of hereditary Marfan's syndrome. (8) Similar roentgen findings are seen in homocystinuria, an inheritable methionine metabolism disorder. However, osteoporosis is present, along with vertebral body flattening and mental retardation, to aid in differentiating the two entities.

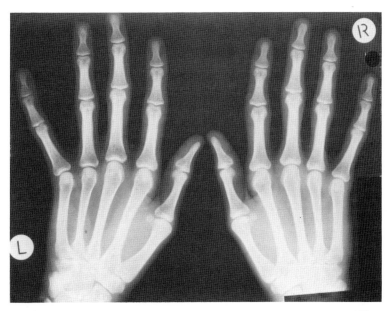

Figure 8.32. MARFAN'S SYNDROME: HANDS. The tubular bones of the hands and feet are long, slender, and gracile; hence, the name "arachnodactyly" or "spider-like" fingers. **Comment:** Fifty percent of cases have ocular lens dislocations and cardiac abnormalities which contribute to shortened lifespans. Also encountered are dissecting aortic aneurysms. (Courtesy of Bryan Hartley, MD, Melbourne, Australia)

Metaphyseal Dysplasia

GENERAL CONSIDERATIONS

First described by Pyle in 1931, metaphyseal dysplasia is a rare autosomal recessive disorder characterized by splaying or flaring of the ends of long bones. (1) Familial incidence has been reported. (2,3) Synonyms include Pyle's disease and familial metaphyseal dysplasia.

CLINICAL FEATURES

The disorder manifests at variable ages, most commonly in late childhood. Many patients are taller than normal, presenting with bulbous enlargements of the lower extremity joints and often with genu valgum. There are few clinical symptoms; occasionally, patients complain of joint pain and muscular weakness. The process is apparently due to failure of subperiosteal remodeling in the metaphyses; the cause of this is thought to be chronic hyperemia of the perichondrial ring of osteoblasts. The hyperemia may be due to congenital hyperplasia of the perichondrial ring arteries. (4)

RADIOLOGICAL FEATURES

While clinical manifestations are not seen until late childhood, the skeleton of a newborn with Pyle's disease may be overly radiopaque, simulating osteopetrosis. (5) With growth, most bones assume a normal density, but there is failure of metaphyseal modeling, producing splaying or an "Erlenmeyer flask" deformity. The cortex in the involved area is thinner and is predisposed to fracture. The lower extremity is more markedly affected than the upper. The most commonly involved bones are the distal femur, tibia (proximal and distal), and proximal fibula. In the upper extremity involvement of the distal radius and ulna and proximal humerus is most frequent. Occasionally, the hands and feet show metaphyseal flaring in the small tubular bones. There may be involvement of the sternal ends of the clavicles and ribs (3) or the rami of the ischium and pubis. Involvement in the skull manifests as hypoplasia of the sinuses (2) and hyperostosis of the calvarium and mandible, with ocular hypertelorism. (6) Vertebra plana or platyspondyly with increased density of the central bodies is also associated. (5)

Mucopolysaccharidoses

The mucopolysaccharidoses are a group of inherited metabolic disorders which result in widespread skeletal, visceral, and mental abnormalities. A defect in metabolic degradation leads to the storage of mucopolysaccharide macromolecules in the nervous system and other body tissues. There is also excessive urinary excretion of mucopolysaccharides, which are components of connective tissue.

Brante was the first to use the term mucopolysaccharidosis in 1952 in describing a patient with gargoylism. (1) Further investigation has shown that the absence of certain enzymes causes the clinical and radiological disorders which characterize the mucopolysaccharidoses. McKusick has classified these entities into six distinct syndromes: (2)

MPS-I: Hurler
MPS-II: Hunter
MPS-III: Sanfilippo
MPS-IV: Morquio
MPS-V: Scheie
MPS-VI: Maroteaux-Lamy

This text will describe only two of these entities, MPS-

I: Hurler's syndrome, and MPS-IV: Morquio's syndrome, which are more commonly encountered and rather characteristic clinically and radiographically.

MPS-I: Hurler's Syndrome

GENERAL CONSIDERATIONS

Hurler's syndrome is a rare autosomal recessive (3) disorder of mucopolysaccharide metabolism which leads to excessive lipoid accumulation in the central nervous system (4) and other viscera. (5) It occurs in approximately 1 in 10,000 births. (6) The excessive mucopolysaccharides excreted in the urine are dermatan sulfate and heparin sulfate. Synonyms include lipochondrodystrophy, gargoylism, osteochondrodystrophy, and dysostosis multiplex.

CLINICAL FEATURES

Patients are usually normal at birth and remain so until after the first year of life. Facial features then begin to coarsen, with the development of a large head, widely set eyes (hypertelorism), a sunken nose, large lips, and a protruding tongue. Corneal opacities develop and the teeth are short and malformed. Mental deterioration ensues and loss of hearing develops. Hepatosplenomegaly produces a protuberant abdomen, and umbilical and inguinal hernias are common. As physical development ceases in the early years of life, affected individuals become dwarfed. A severe dorsolumbar kyphosis develops, along with multiple flexion contractures. The hands are "trident" and sometimes "clawed." At about the same time, cardiomegaly and heart murmurs become evident. Death usually occurs in the second decade, often following pneumonia or cardiac failure.

RADIOLOGICAL FEATURES

Changes seen in the skull include frontal bossing, calvarial thickening, and premature closure of the sagittal and lambdoidal sutures. Hydrocephalus is common. The sella turcica is enlarged and "J" shaped. (Fig. 8.33A) Often, the facial bones are small and the mandibular angle is widened. Spinal changes are fairly typical. A dorsolumbar kyphosis develops secondary to vertebral body hypoplasia. (Fig. 8.33B) The lower thoracic and upper lumbar bodies are small in their anterior-superior aspect and may be beaked inferiorly. The remaining vertebral centra may be oval due to convexity of the upper and lower surfaces. The pedicles are often long and slender. The ribs are overly wide, with tapered ends, producing a "paddle" or "spatulated" appearance. (Fig. 8.33C) The ilia are flared, with obliquely-directed acetabular roofs. Coxa valga or vara is common. The varus deformity of the humerus is characteristic. The tubular bones have widened diaphyses; this is more obvious in the upper extremities than in the lower. Often, the metacarpals and phalanges are short and wide, producing the "trident" hand, and osteoporosis is frequent. (Fig. 8.33D)

Differential diagnosis from Morquio's syndrome is easily accomplished by observing the spinal differences, as well as the lack of hepatosplenomegaly in Morquio-type patients. While some resemblance to achondroplasia exists, the Hurler patient is normal at birth and achondroplasia is easily discerned in the infant.

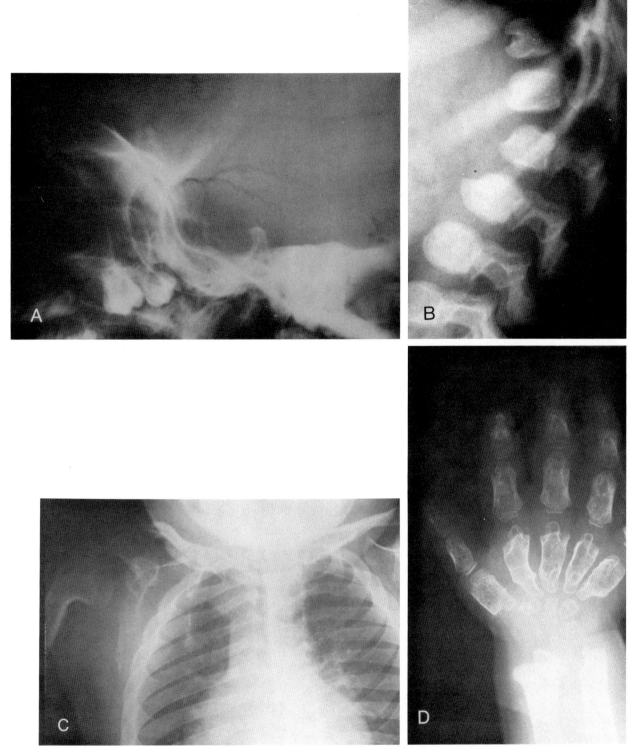

Figure 8.33. HURLER'S SYNDROME.   A. "J" Shaped Tur-cica. A characteristic feature is an enlarged and "J" shaped sella.   **B. Dorsolumbar Kyphosis.** The lower thoracic and upper lumbar vertebral bodies are small and are beaked inferiorly, resulting in a thoracolumbar kyphosis.   **C. Paddle Ribs.** The ribs are overly wide, producing a "paddled" or "spatulated" appearance. Note the characteristic varus deformity of the humerus.   **D. Hands.** The metacarpals and phalanges are short and wide. Note also the osteoporosis. (Courtesy of Bryan Hartley, MD, Melbourne, Australia)

MPS-IV: Morquio's Syndrome

GENERAL CONSIDERATIONS

Morquio's syndrome is an autosomal recessive disorder occurring in 1 in 40,000 births. (7) A mucopolysaccharide metabolism error leads to keratosulfaturia which is present at birth and establishes the diagnosis. Morquio (8) and Brailsford (9) independently described the syndrome in 1929. Synonyms include chondrodystrophy, familial osteodystrophy, eccentro-osteochondrodysplasia, Morquio-Ullrich syndrome, and Morquio-Brailsford syndrome (10).

CLINICAL FEATURES

Patients often appear normal at birth, with the manifestation of skeletal changes becoming apparent only upon weightbearing. During early childhood individuals develop marked dwarfism, dorsal kyphosis, weakness, and muscular hypotonia. Adult height rarely exceeds four feet. The sternum is usually horizontal and protuberant (pectus carinatum), the neck is short, and the head appears sunken into the chest. The nose is short, with a depressed bridge, and the eyes are wide-set. The maxillae are wide, with deformed, poorly spaced teeth. Fine corneal opacities develop around the age of 10. (11) Mental capacity is generally normal, but deafness often develops.

Genu valgum and flexion contractures of the extremities are common. Enlarged wrists and deformed hands are noted. Atlantoaxial dislocations occur due to odontoid hypoplasia and may result in paraplegia and respiratory paralysis. Most patients survive into the third and fourth decades.

RADIOLOGICAL FEATURES

By age two or three the spinal changes are characteristic. Universal platyspondyly with central beaking is nearly pathognomonic. (Fig. 8.34A–C, 8.35) Often, the first or second lumbar vertebra is posteriorly displaced and hypoplastic. The disc spaces are normal or increased. Atlantoaxial instability results from a hypoplastic or absent odontoid. (Fig. 8.36) Hip dislocations occur due to poorly formed acetabulae and femoral heads. (Fig. 8.37) The femoral necks are wide (Fig. 8.38), and coxa valga or vara is common. The long tubular bones are short and thick, especially in the upper extremity. The hands and feet are deformed secondary to carpal, tarsal, and phalangeal growth disturbances.

The major entity which must be differentiated from Morquio's syndrome or MPS-IV is spondyloepiphyseal dysplasia. On close inspection the spinal changes are characteristic in each disorder, and the biochemical findings which are present in Morquio's syndrome are absent in spondyloepiphyseal dysplasia.

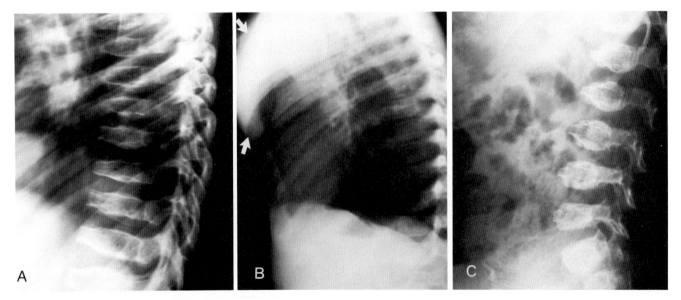

Figure 8.34. MORQUIO'S SYNDROME: PLATYSPONDYLY WITH CENTRAL BEAKING AND PECTUS CARINATUM. A. Thoracic Spine. Note the flat vertebral bodies and central beaking. **B. Pectus Carinatum.** The sternum is horizontally oriented and protuberant (pectus carinatum) (arrows). **C. Lumbar Spine.** Note the characteristic central beaking in the lumbar spine. Also note that the disc heights are normal. (Courtesy of Leonard R. Levine, MD, Melbourne, Australia)

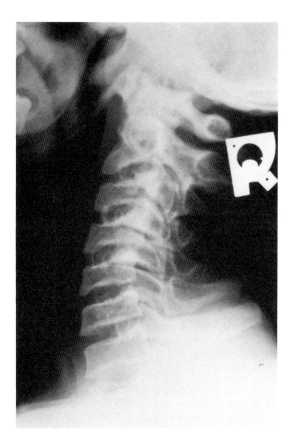

Figure 8.35. MORQUIO'S SYNDROME: UNIVERSAL PLATYSPON-DYLY OF THE CERVICAL SPINE. All cervical vertebrae are flat, but the discs are normal. (Courtesy of Andrew H. Jackson, Jr., DC, DACBR, Belleville, Illinois)

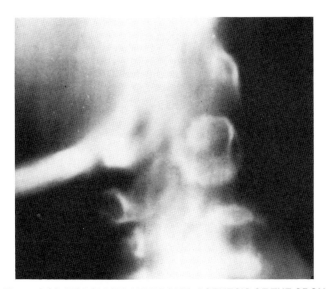

Figure 8.36. MORQUIO'S SYNDROME: AGENESIS OF THE ODON-TOID. This tomogram of the upper cervical spine demonstrates odontoid agenesis. *Comment*: Atlantoaxial instability results from hypoplasia or agenesis of the odontoid. (Courtesy of Andrew H. Jackson, Jr., DC, DACBR, Belleville, Illinois)

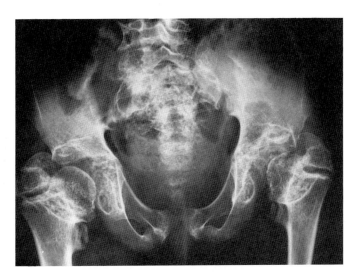

Figure 8.37. MORQUIO'S SYNDROME: PELVIS. Note the poorly formed acetabulae and femoral heads. Hip dislocations are frequently encountered. (Courtesy of Leonard R. Levine, MD, Melbourne, Australia)

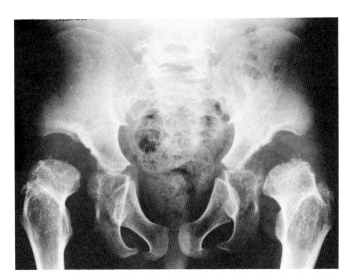

Figure 8.38. MORQUIO'S SYNDROME, PELVIS: WIDENED FEM-ORAL NECKS. The femoral necks are widened. Also note the flared ilii. (Courtesy of Leonard R. Levine, MD, Melbourne, Australia)

Nail-Patella Syndrome

GENERAL CONSIDERATIONS

The presence of bilateral posterior iliac horns as an isolated finding is referred to as Fong's disease (1) and was described in 1946 by Fong. (2) Iliac horns may also occur in an autosomal dominant syndrome, hereditary onycho-osteodysplasia, in association with abnormalities of the nails, skeletal deformities involving the elbows, knees, and pelvis, and numerous soft tissue abnormalities including renal dysplasia. (3–5) This syndrome is also referred to as the HOOD or nail-patella syndrome.

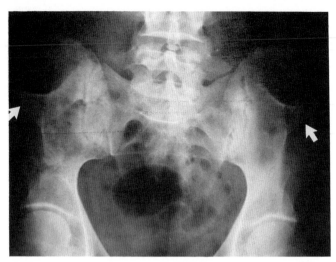

Figure 8.39. NAIL-PATELLA SYNDROME: ILIAC HORNS. Observe the bilateral central posterior iliac horns, which are characteristic of this syndrome (arrows). **Comment:** An isolated finding of iliac horns, without nail and patellar findings, is referred to as Fong's disease.

CLINICAL FEATURES

Agenesis or hypoplasia of the nails is most commonly seen on the thumbs and index fingers. Clinodactyly and short fifth metacarpals may also be found. Soft tissue abnormalities manifest as joint contractures, web formations, and muscular hypoplasia. Found in conjunction with renal dysplasia, there may be proteinuria, hypertension, and other forms of renal impairment. (6)

RADIOLOGICAL FEATURES

A pair of central posterior iliac horns formed by separate ossification centers is the characteristic radiographic sign. (7) (Fig. 8.39, 8.40) While these outgrowths resemble osteochondromas, they may actually be analogous to the acromion processes of the scapulae. (8) The ilia may also be shortened and flared. The patellae may be absent or small, frequently with lateral subluxations. Hypoplasia of the head of the radius allows the elbow to dislocate quite readily. Occasionally seen is hyperplasia of the medial condyles of the humerus and femur, which produces valgus deformities. The presence of a unilateral posterior iliac horn has been reported and is not associated with nail-patella syndrome. (9)

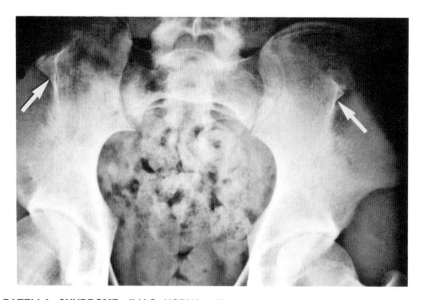

Figure 8.40. NAIL-PATELLA SYNDROME: ILIAC HORNS. This patient demonstrates small posterior iliac horns (arrows).

Osteogenesis Imperfecta

GENERAL CONSIDERATIONS

Osteogenesis imperfecta is a generalized inheritable disorder of connective tissue with widespread abnormalities. The most serious involvement is in the skeleton, but changes in ligaments, skin, sclera, the inner ear, and dentition are also noted. The disease is thought to have an autosomal dominant transmission. Many synonyms have been used in the literature, including osteopsathy-rosis idiopathica, (1) mollities ossium, (2) fragilitas ossium, (3) and Lobstein's disease.

There are three major clinical criteria for diagnosis: 1) osteoporosis with abnormal fragility of the skeleton (Fig. 8.41); 2) blue sclerae; and 3) abnormal dentition (dentinogenesis imperfecta). (4) Only two of these need be present to confirm the diagnosis. Other findings include premature otosclerosis with resultant hearing loss, generalized ligamentous laxity, episodic diaphoresis (sweating) with abnormal temperature regulation, easy bruising, hyperplastic scars, and premature vascular calcification.

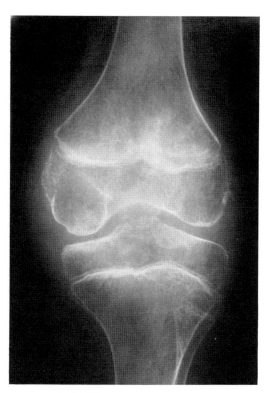

Figure 8.41. OSTEOGENESIS IMPERFECTA: SEVERE OSTEO-POROSIS OF THE KNEE. Observe not only the severe osteoporosis but also the extreme thinness of the cortices, both of which contribute to the skeletal fragility of osteogenesis imperfecta. (Courtesy of David P. Thomas, MD, Melbourne, Australia)

Osteogenesis imperfecta has been subdivided into two forms: the congenita form, with a high rate of stillborns and infant mortality; and the tarda form, often with a normal life expectancy. Initially, this subdivision was based on the age at the time of first fracture, (5) but recently investigators use the designation of congenita and tarda to refer to the presence or absence of osseous deformities at birth. (5,6) The presence or absence of bowing deformities of the long bones is useful as a guide to the severity of the disease. The tarda form is further subdivided into Type I, with acquired bowing, and Type II, with no bowing deformities. (4) These divisions of osteogenesis imperfecta are purely descriptive and are not based on the genetic patterns of inheritance.

CLINICAL FEATURES

The sexual predominance of osteogenesis imperfecta is stated to be equal (7) or slightly increased in females. (6,8) It is found in all races. The severe congenita form is characterized by osseous fractures and deformities which often are observable in utero. (9) The skull is paper thin and soft. Death occurs in utero, during the birthing process or shortly thereafter, usually following intracranial hemorrhage.

Osteogenesis imperfecta tarda is less severe and has a widely varied presentation. Fractures following trivial trauma occur during childhood, after puberty and, more rarely, later in adulthood. (Fig. 8.42) Blue sclerae are found in the majority of individuals with osteogenesis

imperfecta (over 90 percent) (5,6) and result from the appearance of the brown choroid when seen through the abnormal collagen in the thin sclera. (7) A white ring of normally colored sclera called "Saturn's ring" often surrounds the cornea. (4) Many patients have bluish-gray to yellowish-brown opalescent teeth, referred to as dentinogenesis imperfecta. While the enamel is normal, the dentin is malformed and defective, leading to easy chipping and severe caries. The otosclerosis, aside from early onset, is similar to idiopathic conduction deafness. The abnormal temperature regulation may be related to a disturbance in cellular ATPase. (10) A defect in platelet aggregation results in bleeding tendencies.

Most patients show some evidence of growth retardation. Severely affected individuals are dwarfed due to both the abnormal growth patterns and the severe fractures and deformities. (Fig. 8.43A and B) The lower extremities are more affected than the upper. Kyphoscoliosis and bowing of the limbs contribute to the shortening. Bone fragility appears to decrease with increasing age. Females may especially show remission following puberty. Estrogen therapy has shown some benefit.

PATHOLOGICAL FEATURES

Osteogenesis imperfecta is characterized by abnormal maturation of collagen affecting both intramembranous and enchondral bone formation. Primitive fetal collagen and bone are not replaced with mature lamellar and woven bone. An enzyme deficiency (ATPase) may be the cause of the abnormal connective tissue proteins. (5,7,10,11) The numerous fractures heal within a normal period of time but produce an exuberant callus which yields only a poor cellular matrix.

RADIOLOGICAL FEATURES

The cardinal roentgen features of osteogenesis imperfecta are a diffuse decrease in bone density, pencil-thin cortices, and multiple fractures. Fairbank (12) has subdivided osteogenesis imperfecta into three groups based on radiographic findings: 1) thin and gracile bones (Fig. 8.44); 2) short, thick bones (Fig. 8.45A and B); and 3) cystic bones. (Fig. 8.46A and B) The thin and gracile type is most frequent and these are generally osteogenesis imperfecta tarda patients. Patients with the congenita form often have the "thick bone" radiographic appearance. This description, however, is a misnomer because, although the bone is wider than normal owing to fracture deformity, the cortices are paper thin and the overall density is diminished. The cystic type is rare. The metaphyseal regions are flared and radiolucent. This flared, cystic appearance may extend into the diaphyses. The radiographic subtypes are purely descriptive, and patients may be seen to change from one type to another.

Multiple fractures, often transverse and in the lower extremities, are the hallmarks of osteogenesis imperfecta. Subsequent healing with tumoral callus leads to shortening (the result of telescoping), bowing deformities, and pseudarthroses. The excessive callus formation (called "pseudotumors") has been mistaken for osteosarcoma. (13)

Skull radiographs reveal persistent Wormian bones

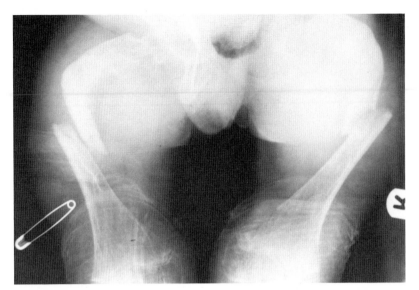

Figure 8.42. OSTEOGENESIS IMPERFECTA: MULTIPLE FRAC-TURES OF THE LOWER EXTREMITIES. Observe the bilateral midshaft fractures and the bowing deformity of the proximal fem-ora. **Comment:** Fractures are more commonly encountered in the lower extremities in osteogenesis imperfecta. (Courtesy of Tyrone Wei, DC, DACBR, Portland, Oregon)

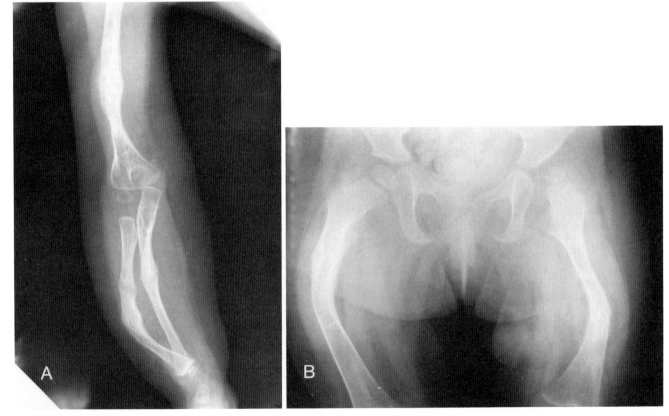

Figure 8.43. OSTEOGENESIS IMPERFECTA: BOWING DEFORMI-TIES. A. Upper Extremity. Multiple fractures have contributed to bowing deformities. **B. Femora.** Note the bilateral bowing deform-ities of the femora, occurring secondary to the fractures.

(Fig. 8.47) and enlarged sinuses. The calvarium is lucent and thin. Platybasia is a frequent finding and may be accompanied by basilar impression. Kyphoscoliosis is common, resulting from ligamentous laxity, osteoporosis, and fracture deformity. The vertebral bodies may be anteriorly wedged and often appear evenly flattened or biconcave (creating the "biconcave lens vertebra"). (14) (Fig. 8.48) Protrusio actabuli may occur, and a shepherd's crook deformity of the proximal femur has been noted. (Fig. 8.49) Premature degenerative joint disease results from multiple fractures of the articular surfaces as well as the ligamentous laxity.

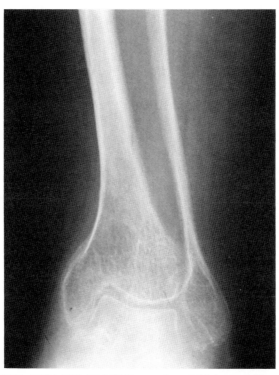

Figure 8.44. OSTEOGENESIS IMPERFECTA, THIN AND GRACILE TYPE: TIBIA AND FIBULA. Observe the thin and gracile configu-ration of the bones of lower extremity. **Comment:** Thin and gracile bones are the most common type found in osteogenesis imperfecta.

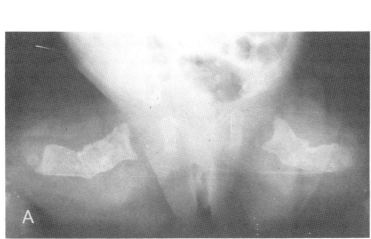

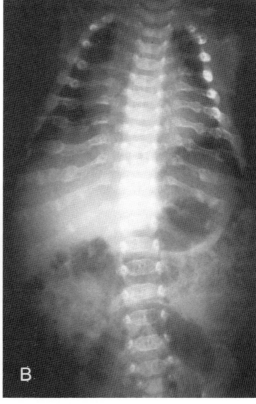

Figure 8.45. OSTEOGENESIS IMPERFECTA: SHORT, THICK BONES. A. Femora. Note the short, thick appearance of the femora. **B. Ribs.** Multiple fractures also contribute to the thick appearance of the ribs. (Courtesy of Alf Turner, MIR, BAppSc (Chiro), Sydney, Australia)

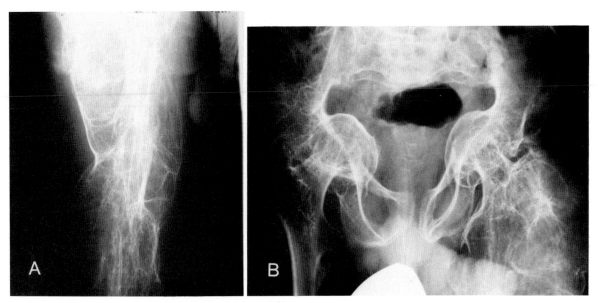

Figure 8.46. OSTEOGENESIS IMPERFECTA: CYSTIC BONES. A. Femur. Note the expanded cystic nature of the femur. **B. Pelvis.** Observe, also, the bilateral protrusio acetabuli. **Comment:** Intraosseous hemorrhage is believed to be the mechanism leading to the cystic appearance of bone in osteogenesis imperfecta.

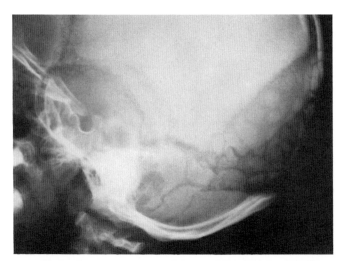

Figure 8.47. OSTEOGENESIS IMPERFECTA, SKULL: WORMIAN BONES. Numerous small Wormian bones are found in the occipital region in this patient. **Comment:** Wormian bones are not pathognomonic of osteogenesis imperfecta and are found in several of the dysplasias. (Courtesy of C. H. Quay, MD, Melbourne, Australia)

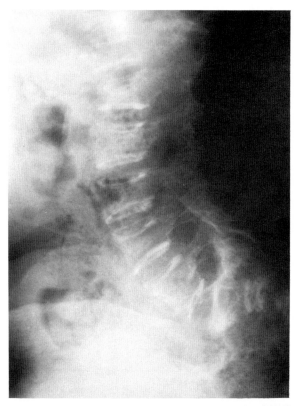

Figure 8.48. OSTEOGENESIS IMPERFECTA, LUMBAR SPINE: BICONCAVE LENS VERTEBRA. Note the severe osteoporosis of the spine and the biconcave appearance of the vertebral bodies. (Courtesy of Tyrone Wei, DC, DACBR, Portland, Oregon)

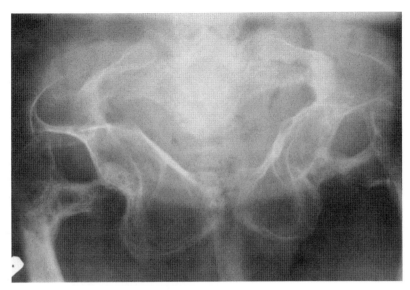

Figure 8.49. OSTEOGENESIS IMPERFECTA: PROTRUSIO ACE-TABULI. This patient has bilateral protrusio acetabuli and coxa vara. (Courtesy of Tyrone Wei, DC, DACBR, Portland, Oregon)

The Sclerosing Dysplasias

This section is devoted to those skeletal dysplasias that cause an increase in bony density or sclerosis. Some demonstrate overall increase in bone density, while others have a peculiar and often pathognomonic pattern of sclerosis.

Several of the entities in this section are thought to be intimately related; these are osteopoikilosis, osteopathia striata, and melorheostosis. Patients have been reported who exhibit signs of all three of these disorders. The remaining entities show no relationship to the others but are grouped here because of their sclerotic presentation.

Melorheostosis

GENERAL CONSIDERATIONS

Melorheostosis is a rare, sclerosing bone dysplasia which was first described in 1922 by Leri and Joanny. (1) Synonyms include Leri type of osteopetrosis, osteosi eberneizzante monomelica, (2) and flowing hyperostosis. The name melorheostosis is of Greek derivation, meaning limb, flow, and bone, and aptly describes the hyperostotic appearance which has been likened to "wax flowing down a lighted candle." (3)

CLINICAL FEATURES

The etiology is unknown, and there is no sex predilection. While most authors agree that melorheostosis is a congenital entity, most individuals do not manifest any symptoms until late childhood or early adolescence. The most common presenting symptom is pain, though some cases are found incidentally. (4) Joint swelling and limitation of motion are seen and are usually more marked in adults than in children. (5) Joint contractures and deformities may ensue, with reported cases of genu varus and valgum, valgus deformities of the feet, and dislocation of the patella. Severe involvement in children may lead to premature epiphyseal closure, with resultant limb shortening.

Soft tissue changes are frequently present and include anomalous pigmentation, scleroderma-like atrophy of the skin, and muscular wasting. Pressure on adjacent vessels may contribute to lymphedema. The soft tissue changes may precede the osseous findings and have been demonstrated on thermography. (6) An association with arteriovenous malformations has been reported. (7) This disorder is most frequently monomelic and usually involves the lower limb. (8) (Fig. 8.50A–C) Often, the innominate or scapula corresponding to the involved limb is affected. The process appears to begin proximally and progress distally. Other sites of involvement include the vertebrae, ribs, skull, and facial bones.

The histological findings are nonspecific, with hyperostotic sclerotic bone and thickened trabeculae. The marrow space may contain fibrotic tissue. While many hypotheses have been offered, especially vascular insufficiency, the best explanation has been proposed by Murray and McCredie, who suggest that the lesions follow sclerotomes and myotomes which are supplied by an individual spinal sensory nerve. (9) Disease of a sensory nerve could result in the segmental distribution of this bone dysplasia and its associated soft tissue abnormalities. Laboratory findings are classically normal.

RADIOLOGICAL FINDINGS

Cortical thickening in a streaked or wavy pattern is the most marked roentgen feature. (Fig. 8.51) The hyperostotic bone protrudes under the periosteum and usually follows along one side of a long bone. (Fig. 8.52A and B, 8.53A and B) Endosteal involvement may encroach upon the medullary space. Bony masses resembling osteochondromas extend into adjacent articulations. Involvement of the carpal and tarsal bones resembles the multiple bone islands which are seen in osteopoikilosis. In the pelvis

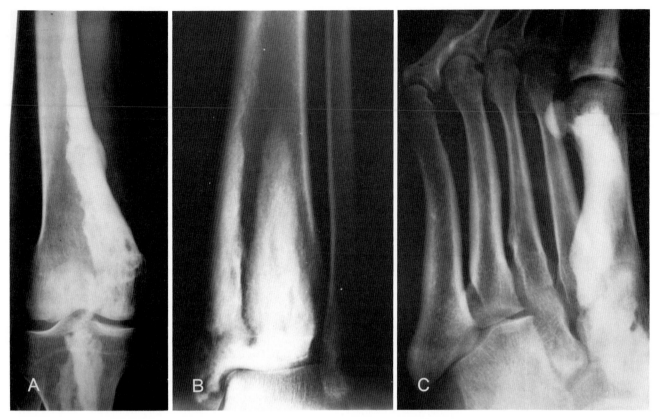

Figure 8.50. MELORHEOSTOSIS: LOWER LIMB INVOLVE-MENT. A. Femur. Note the flowing, dense, cortical bone along the medial aspect of the femur. **B. Tibia.** Observe that the dense bone formation appears to flow distally down the tibia. **C. Foot.** The bone formation continues down the lower extremity into the foot, where it is found along the medial aspect of the tarsals and metatarsals. ***Comment:*** Melorheostosis is usually monomelic and is found in the lower limbs. (Courtesy of Steven P. Brownstein, MD, Springfield, New Jersey)

and scapulae (flat bones) the sclerotic bone may be in the form of dense radiations from the joint. Heterotopic bone formation and soft tissue calcification is encountered and may lead to joint ankylosis. (10)

A number of other disorders have been found in association with melorheostosis. These include linear scleroderma, osteopoikilosis, osteopathia striata, neurofibromatosis, tuberous sclerosis, and hemangiomas. (7, 11–15)

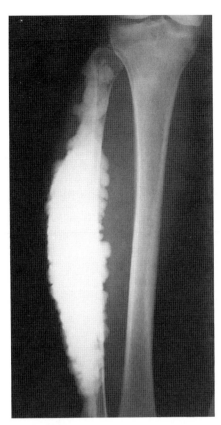

Figure 8.51. MELORHEOSTOSIS, FIBULA: WAVY NEW BONE FORMATION.   A wavy, undulating, cortical bone formation appears to surround the fibula. This appearance has been referred as "wax flowing down a lighted candle." (Courtesy of Gilbert M. Meal, DC, Christchurch, Great Britain)

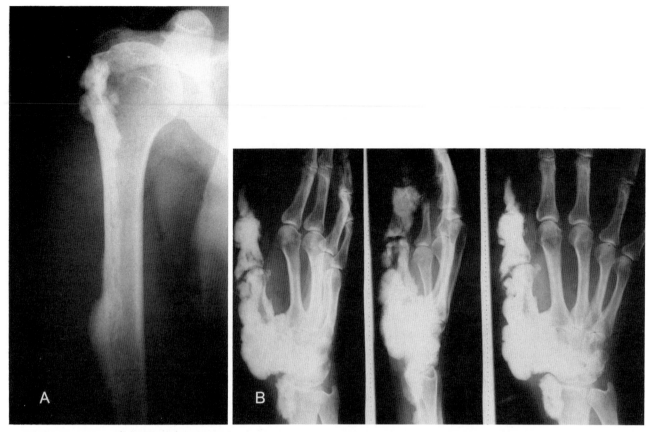

Figure 8.52. MELORHEOSTOSIS: DISTRIBUTION ALONG ONE SIDE OF THE BONE. A. Humerus. The hyperostotic bone flows along one side of the humerus. **B. Hand.** Extensive involvement is seen along the lateral aspect of the hand. (Reprinted with permission: Yochum TR, et al: Melorheostosis—A report of two patients. *ACA Council Roent, Roentgen Brief*, April 1981)

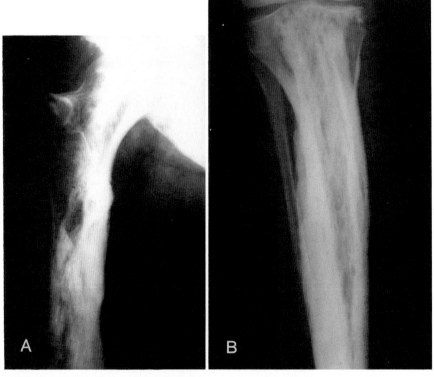

Figure 8.53. MELORHEOSTOSIS: ENDOSTEAL INVOLVEMENT. A. Femur. Endosteal involvement of the femur encroaches on the medullary space. **B. Tibia.** Note that the medullary canal appears compromised due to endosteal bone formation. (Courtesy of Paul D. Sykes, DC, Adelaide, Australia)

Osteopathia Striata

GENERAL CONSIDERATIONS

Osteopathia striata is a rare and unusual entity first described in 1924 by Voorhoeve as a variant of osteopoikilosis. (1) Fairbank in 1950 applied the name osteopathia striata, (2) but the disease still bears the synonym Voorhoeve's disease. Characteristic findings are linear bands of dense bone involving the metaphyses and diaphyses of long bones. While the etiology is unknown, a genetic transmission may be involved, especially in light of its suspected variance from osteopoikilosis, a disease of autosomal dominance. (3) Curiously, patients with osteopathia striata often show evidence of other conditions causing increased bone density, such as melorheostosis and osteopetrosis. (4,5) A limited study of individuals with focal dermal hypoplasia (Goltz syndrome) has revealed a high incidence of concomitant osteopathia striata. (6,7)

CLINICAL FEATURES

The majority of patients are asymptomatic, with osteopathia striata found incidentally on x-ray examination. Some individuals present with vague joint pains. (2) Laboratory findings are normal, and no age or sex predilection has been demonstrated.

RADIOLOGICAL FINDINGS

The majority of involvement is in the major long bones of the body. Usually bilateral in distribution, (8,9) vertical radiopaque lines in the metaphyses extend for some distance into the diaphyses. More rarely, striations are seen crossing the epiphyseal line to involve the epiphysis. The length of these densities appears to be related to the growth rate of the bone; the long bone with the greatest growth potential (the femur) consistently demonstrates the longest striations. (10)

A fan-like pattern radiating from the acetabulum to the iliac crest is characteristic of involvement in the ilium and has been referred to as the "sunburst effect." (11) (Fig. 8.54) Occasionally, densities are encountered in the small tubular bones of the hands and feet or the spine. Thickening and sclerosis of the base of the skull has been reported.

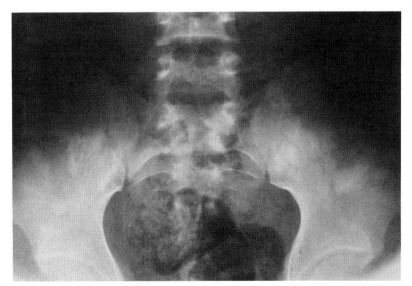

Figure 8.54. OSTEOPATHIA STRIATA, PELVIS: "SUNBURST" EFFECT. The dense bone formation is seen in a fan-like pattern radiating from the acetabulum toward the iliac crest. This has been referred to as the "sunburst" effect of osteopathia striata. (Courtesy of Bryan Hartley, MD, Melbourne, Australia)

Osteopetrosis

GENERAL CONSIDERATIONS

Osteopetrosis is a rare hereditary and familial bone abnormality characterized by lack of resorption of normal primitive osteochondroid tissue. This persistence of osteochondroid inhibits the formation of a normal mature adult bone with a medullary canal containing marrow tissue. (1) There appear to be two forms: 1) a benign form which is autosomal dominant; and 2) a severe malignant form that is autosomal recessive. (2) Consanguinity apparently plays a role in the severe malignant form. (3) Synonyms include Albers-Schönberg's disease, osteosclerosis, osteopetrosis generalisata, osteosclerosis generalisata, marble bones, and chalk bones.

CLINICAL FEATURES

The severe form of osteopetrosis is recognized in infancy; (4) often, the patient dies within the second year of life. Florid cases are inevitably stillborn. The clinical picture is one of severe anemia, hepatosplenomegaly, lymphadenopathy, thrombocytopenia, and failure to thrive. The dense but extremely brittle bones fracture easily. Involvement of the cranium may lead to optic nerve atrophy, with blindness or other cranial nerve defects. The most frequent cause of death is massive hemorrhage and recurrent infection. Leukemia and sarcoma are known sequelae.

Fifty percent of benign cases are asymptomatic (5) and are discovered incidentally on radiographic examination, or the individuals present with fractures. Others reveal anemia, facial palsies, deafness, and hepatosplenomegaly. Defective dentition with severe caries may lead to osteomyelitis of the maxilla or mandible. (6)

LABORATORY FINDINGS

Anemia is invariably present and does not correlate well with the degree of sclerosis. Some individuals with marked increased density have mild anemia, while those with little change in bony density may have severe anemia. Myelophthisic, aplastic, and hypoplastic types of anemia are encountered. Often, thrombocytopenia is severe and leads to hemorrhage. The serum calcium levels may be elevated.

PATHOLOGICAL FEATURES

Failure of the normal resorptive mechanism which replaces calcified cartilage with mature bone accounts for the bone changes. The osteoclasts may be unresponsive to parathyroid hormone and unable to resorb bone and cartilage. (7) The primitive calcified cartilage persists in abundance, and a medullary space is never allowed to form. This leads to anemia and extramedullary hematopoiesis, causing hepatosplenomegaly. Failure of remodeling also produces flared metaphyses (Erlenmeyer flask deformity). (Fig. 8.55)

While the bone is very radiopaque in appearance and hard to the touch, it is actually very brittle and subject to pathological fracture. (Fig. 8.56) These are characteristically transverse, healing quickly but producing a callus of defective, osteopetrotic bone. Frequently, there are vertical or horizontal striations of normal bone interspersed with the more abundant primitive tissue, suggesting that the disease may have an intermittent nature.

RADIOLOGICAL FEATURES

There is generalized sclerosis of the skeleton, and there may be a homogenous appearance of increased density, without trabeculation, and little or no differentiation between cortical and medullary regions. (Fig. 8.57) Frequently, however, there are striations producing a "bone within a bone" appearance. (Fig. 8.58A–C) One case has been reported which presented with alternating dense and radiolucent metaphyseal transverse lines as the only evidence of the disease. (8) The long bones have flared and elongated metaphyses (Fig. 8.59A and B); occasionally, the shafts may be widened. Involvement of the hands and feet parallel changes in the long bones, and tuftal erosion has been reported. (9) Characteristically, the ilium demonstrates multiple, dense curved lines paralleling the iliac crest. (Fig. 8.60A and B) In the spine a number of presentations are seen. The vertebrae may be uniformly dense or, more commonly, there are dense bands adjacent to the endplates, with a more normal appearing midbody—the "sandwich vertebra." (9) (Fig. 8.61A and B) The "bone within a bone" appearance is also commonly seen in the vertebral bodies. (10) (Fig. 8.62A–D) Skull changes include calvarial and basilar thickening and sclerosis, with poor sinus development. (Fig. 8.63A and B) These changes may produce macro-

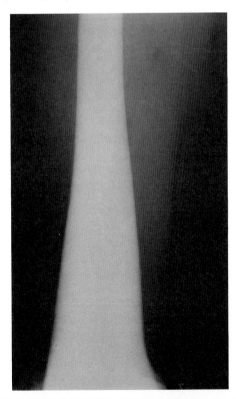

Figure 8.55. OSTEOPETROSIS, DISTAL FEMUR: FLARED METAPHYSIS (ERLENMEYER FLASK DEFORMITY). Note the uniformly dense appearance of the femur. Failure of remodeling produces flared metaphyses.

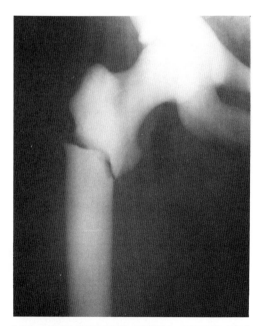

Figure 8.56. OSTEOPETROSIS, FEMUR: PATHOLOGICAL FRACTURE. Observe the pathological fracture through the subtrochanteric region of the femur. *Comment:* While the bone is very radiopaque in appearance, it is actually very brittle.

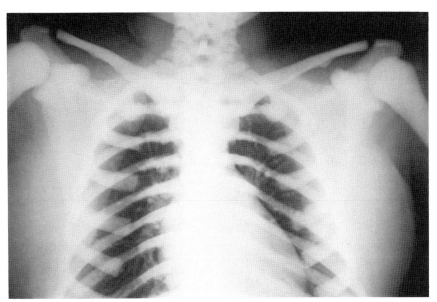

Figure 8.57. OSTEOPETROSIS, THORAX: HOMOGENEOUS IN-CREASED DENSITY. Note the homogeneous increased density without trabeculation or differentiation between cortical and medullary regions throughout the ribs.

cephaly. Involvement of the mandible may result in prognathism. Complications include pathological fractures (especially of the femur), hemorrhage, infection, blindness, and deafness. Leukemia and sarcoma are also known sequelae. Differential diagnosis includes idiopathic hypercalcemia and heavy metal poisoning.

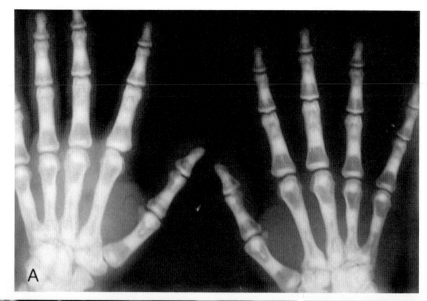

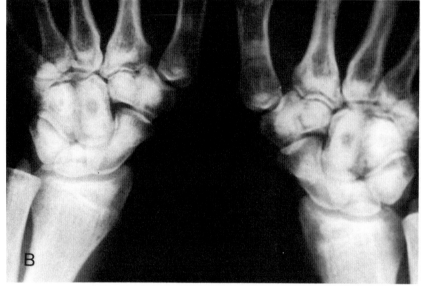

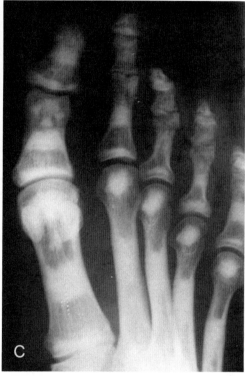

Figure 8.58. OSTEOPETROSIS: "BONE WITHIN A BONE" APPEARANCE. A. Hands. Note the increased densities within the metacarpals and phalanges, producing a "bone within a bone" effect. **B. Wrists.** Note the areas of increased density within the carpal bones. **C. Foot.** The "bone within a bone" appearance here is similar to that seen in the small bones of the hand.

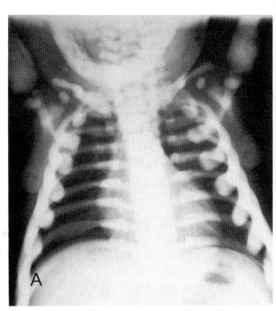

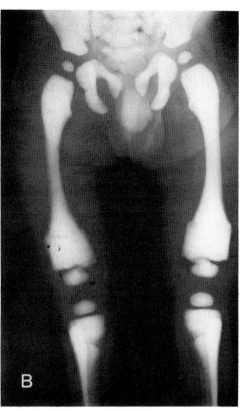

Figure 8.59. OSTEOPETROSIS: FLARED METAPHYSIS. A. Thorax. Note the flared metaphyses of the ribs and proximal humeri. **B. Lower Extremities.** There is a uniform increase in density and flared metaphyses in the distal femora. *Comment:* Anemia is invariably present in osteopetrosis but does not correlate well with the degree of sclerosis.

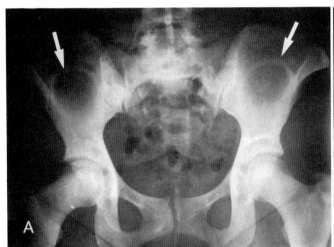

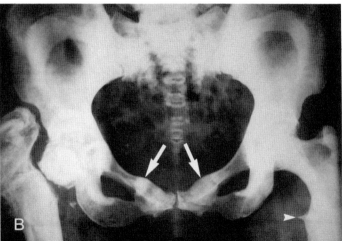

Figure 8.60. OSTEOPETROSIS: CURVED LINE PARALLELING THE ILIAC CREST. A. Pelvis. Note the single curved line paralleling each iliac crest, with a "bone within a bone" appearance (arrows). A similar appearance is visualized in the femoral heads and supra-acetabular regions bilaterally. (Courtesy of Brian V. Lonsdale, DC, Geelong, Victoria, Australia). **B. Pelvis: Pathological Fracture of the Femur.** Note the thick, dense bands paralleling the iliac crests and the pathological subcapital fracture of the femur. Thickening of the pubic rami bilaterally is secondary to previous fractures (arrows). Of incidental note is a musculotendinous exostosis at the lesser trochanter (arrowhead).

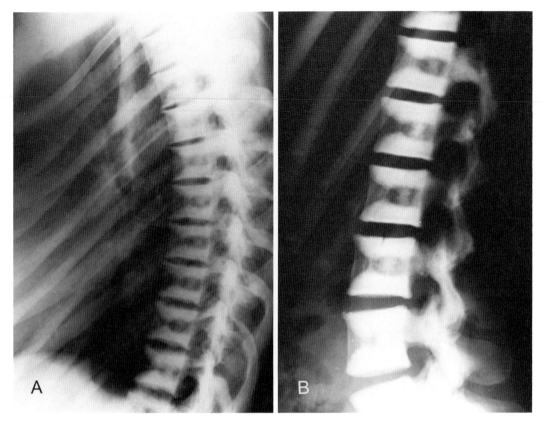

Figure 8.61. OSTEOPETROSIS: "SANDWICH" VERTEBRA. A. Thoracic Spine. Note the dense bands along the superior and inferior end plates, referred to as the "sandwich" vertebra.

B. Lumbar Spine. Another patient with "sandwich" vertebrae of the lumbar spine. (Courtesy of Bryan Hartley, MD, Melbourne, Australia)

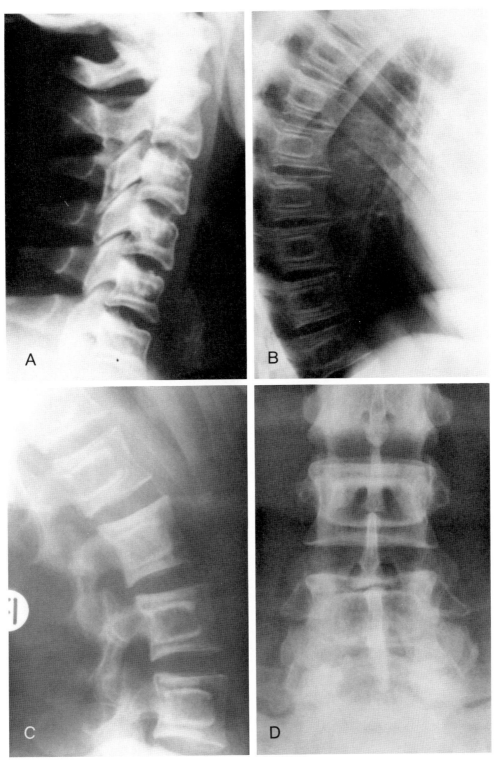

Figure 8.62. OSTEOPETROSIS: "BONE WITHIN A BONE" AP-PEARANCE. A. Cervical Spine. Note the sclerotic lines paralleling the cervical spine end plates. (Courtesy of Robin R. Canterbury, DC, DACBR, Davenport, Iowa). **B. Thoracic Spine.** Note the appearance of tiny vertebrae within larger vertebral bodies.

C. Lateral Lumbar Spine. Note the "bone within a bone" effect, similar to the cervical and thoracic vertebral bodies. **D. AP Lumbar Spine.** Observe the "bone within a bone" appearance as viewed frontally. (B–D, courtesy of Brian V. Lonsdale, DC, Geelong, Victoria, Australia)

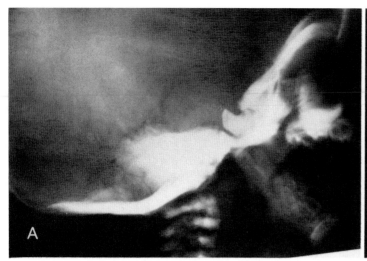
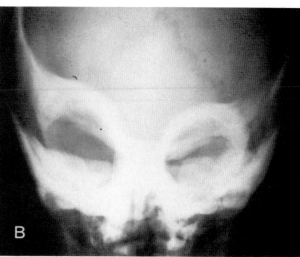

Figure 8.63. OSTEOPETROSIS: SKULL INVOLVEMENT. A. Lateral Skull. Observe the basilar thickening and sclerosis. Also note involvement of the facial bones. **B. AP Skull.** Observe the involvement of the facial bones and basilar region, as viewed frontally.

Osteopoikilosis

GENERAL CONSIDERATIONS

This uncommon but interesting bone disorder was first described by Albers-Schönberg (1) and Ledoux-Lebard and Chabaneux (2) in the early 1900's. Osteopoikilosis is characterized by small round or ovoid radiopacities appearing in the juxta-articular regions of bone. It would appear to be autosomal dominant in transmission and has been found to become more prominent in succeeding generations in some cases. (3–6) Synonyms include osteopathia condensans disseminata and spotted bones.

CLINICAL FEATURES

The majority of cases are asymptomatic and found on radiographic studies taken for other reasons. It can be detected at any age but is rarely seen below age three. (7) In approximately 25 percent of cases cutaneous abnormalities are present, including dermatofibrosis lenticularis disseminata, (8,9) a predisposition to keloid formation, (10,11) and scleroderma-like lesions. (12) In 15–20 percent of cases there may be mild joint pain, with or without joint effusion. (13) Laboratory findings are normal.

PATHOLOGICAL FEATURES

While the etiology of this disorder is still unknown, the lesions appear to reflect spongy bone remodeling related to mechanical stress but unrelated to healing secondary to microfractures. (14) It has been suggested that osteopoikilosis, because of its diffuse nature, hereditary mode of transmission, and association with cutaneous abnormalities, may be a manifestation of a metabolic disorder of connective tissue. (14)

The lesions are foci of compact lamellar bone containing haversian systems. Histologically, osteopoikilotic bone closely resembles the solitary bone island. However, while bone islands are sometimes found to be active on bone scans, this is not a regular feature of osteopoikilosis.

RADIOLOGICAL FEATURES

Multiple small radiopacities found scattered in epiphyseal and metaphyseal regions are generally pathognomonic. (Fig. 8.64A and B) The lesions are symmetric, with a predilection for the long tubular bones, carpals, and tarsals. (Fig. 8.65A and B) In the pelvis and scapula the densities are found adjacent to the acetabulum and glenoid. (Fig. 8.66A and B) Rarely, lesions are found in the skull, spine, ribs, and clavicles. (Fig. 8.67A–C) Occasionally, their size may change, with reports of disappearance and reappearance in children and, more rarely, in adults. (15) Generally, the size ranges from 1–10 mm in diameter. Rarely, larger lesions are found. Most commonly, they are uniformly dense but occasionally exhibit lucent centers. Infrequently, the sclerotic areas in osteopoikilosis become more radiopaque with age. (16)

Osteopoikilosis has been found in association with both osteopathia striata and melorheostosis, and there is a suggestion that these are related conditions. (17) It is of interest that a patient has been described who had both osteopoikilosis and osteosarcoma, since osteosarcoma may be related to active osteogenesis, and perhaps the chronic remodeling of osteopoikilosis transformed into the malignant osteogenic tumor. (18–20)

The considerations for differential diagnosis include blastic metastasis, tuberous sclerosis, and mastocytosis. However, a radiographic skeletal survey will demonstrate the symmetric juxta-articular distribution and uniform size so characteristic of osteopoikilosis to aid in the definitive diagnosis.

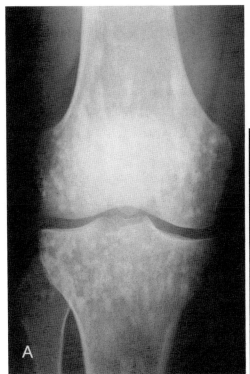

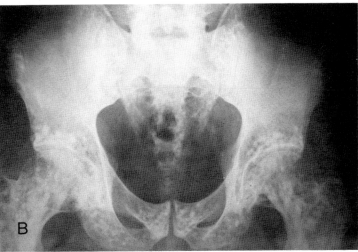

Figure 8.64. OSTEOPOIKILOSIS: METAPHYSEAL AND EPIPHY-SEAL RADIOPACITIES. A. Knee. Note the clustering of small opacities in the metaphyseal and epiphyseal regions.

B. Pelvis. Also note the small roundish densities that are found surrounding the acetabulae and proximal femora. (Courtesy of Brian V. Lonsdale, DC, Geelong, Victoria, Australia)

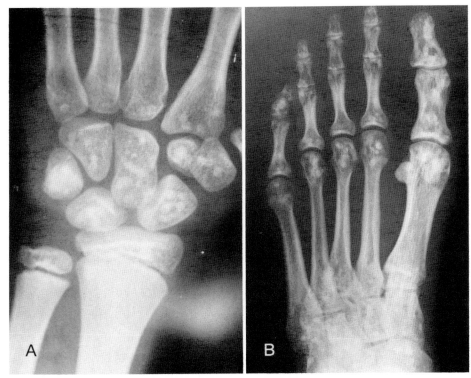

Figure 8.65. OSTEOPOIKILOSIS: INVOLVEMENT OF THE HANDS AND FEET. A. Wrist. Small roundish radiopacities resembling bone islands are seen in the carpal bones and proximal metacarpals in

this patient. **B. Foot.** All of the visualized bones of the foot show roundish radiopacities. (Courtesy of Bryan Hartley, MD, Melbourne, Australia)

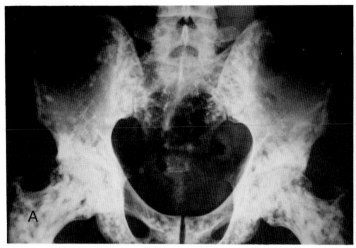

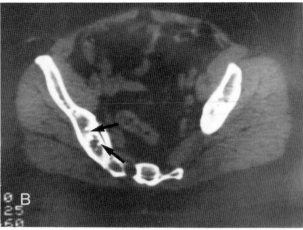

Figure 8.66. OSTEOPOIKILOSIS: PELVIC INVOLVEMENT. A. AP Pelvis: Plain Film. Note the diffuse involvement of osteopoikilosis, with radiopacities scattered throughout the pelvis and proximal femora. **B. CT Scan: Midpelvis.** Also note the small densities located in the medullary portion of the innominates (arrows). (Courtesy of Bryan Hartley, MD, Melbourne, Australia)

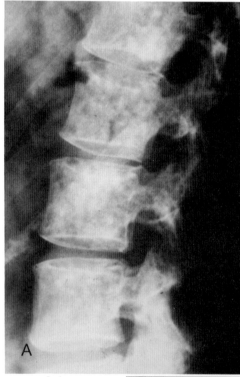

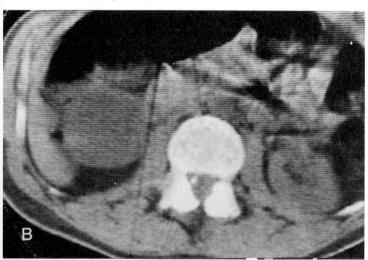

Figure 8.67. OSTEOPOIKILOSIS: SPINAL INVOLVEMENT. A. Lateral Lumbar Spine. Note the diffuse involvement of the lumbar vertebrae. **B. CT Scan: Lumbar Segment.** A CT scan of the same patient reveals the presence of these radiopacities in the spongy bone of the vertebral body. **C. Shoulder.** Also observe in this patient clustering of densities within the glenoid and proximal humerus. **Comment:** Osteopoikilosis rarely involves the skull, spine, ribs, and clavicles. (Courtesy of Bryan Hartley, MD, Melbourne, Australia)

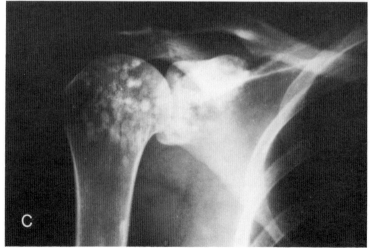

Progressive Diaphyseal Dysplasia

GENERAL CONSIDERATIONS

Progressive diaphyseal dysplasia is a rare congenital, familial, and hereditary disorder characterized by cortical thickening and sclerosis of mainly the long tubular bones. Camurati in 1922 (1) and Engelmann in 1929 (2) were the first to describe this disorder, and it is frequently referred to as Engelmann-Camurati or Engelmann's disease. It is now considered an autosomal dominant entity, but the expression is extremely variable.

CLINICAL FEATURES

Progressive diaphyseal dysplasia is usually manifest in the first decade. Males are more frequently affected than females. (3) Often, the patient presents clinically with a waddling gait and poor muscular development. There is profound weakness of mainly the lower extremities, and malnutrition. Tenderness over the involved long bones may be found. (4) Occasionally, the serum alkaline phosphatase level (5) and erythrocye sedimentation rate are elevated. Anemia is not a regular feature. The clinical signs of weakness and malnutrition often resolve following adolescence and the radiographic features are the most marked findings.

Pathologically, the classic features include greatly increased osteoblastic activity, with cancellous bone laid down at the periosteal and endosteal surfaces of the cortex. A sparse vascular supply to the region of involve-

ment has been suggested as the stimulus for the marked new bone formation. (6,7)

RADIOLOGICAL FEATURES

Neuhauser and associates present an excellent description of the roentgen features. (8) The skeleton is involved in a symmetric distribution with fusiform widening of the diaphyseal portions of long bones. (Fig. 8.68) The metaphyses and epiphyses are spared. (Fig. 8.69) New radiopaque bone is produced by the cortex, widening the diameter of the diaphysis, while encroaching on the medullary canal. There may be relative elongation of the bone as well. (Fig. 8.70) The new bone formation begins in the midshaft, progressing proximally and distally but ending abruptly, without involving the metaphysis.

The most commonly involved bones are the femur, tibia, radius, ulna, and humerus. While all long bones may be affected, the tubular bones of the hands and feet are frequently spared. (Fig. 8.71) The skull may show basilar sclerosis and, less commonly, calvarial hyperostosis. The ribs, clavicles, pelvis, and spine occasionally display similar changes in bone density. Complications may occur and include increased intracranial pressure and encroachment on cranial nerves. The distribution and radiographic features of progressive diaphyseal dysplasia do not generally offer a diagnostic dilemma.

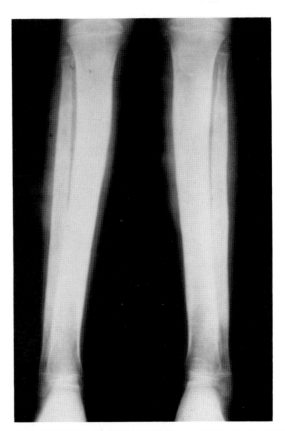

Figure 8.69. PROGRESSIVE DIAPHYSEAL DYSPLASIA, LOWER LEGS: SPARING OF THE METAPHYSES AND EPIPHYSES. There is symmetrical widening and sclerosis of the tibial and fibular diaphyses, with sparing of the metaphyses and epiphyses.

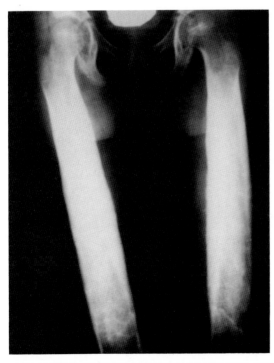

Figure 8.68. PROGRESSIVE DIAPHYSEAL DYSPLASIA, FEMORA: SYMMETRICAL DIAPHYSEAL INVOLVEMENT. Note the symmetrical fusiform widening of the femoral diaphyses.

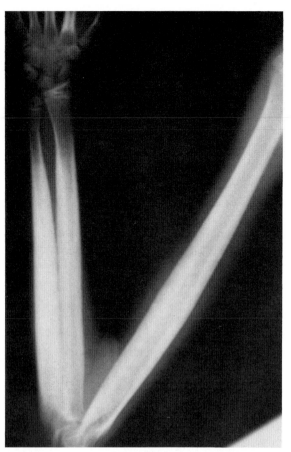

Figure 8.70. PROGRESSIVE DIAPHYSEAL DYSPLASIA, UPPER EXTREMITY: RELATIVE ELONGATION OF THE LONG BONES. Along with widening and increased density of the diaphyses, there is a relative elongation of the long bones. Also note the poor muscular development.

Pyknodysostosis

GENERAL CONSIDERATIONS

Defined in 1962 by Maroteaux and Lamy, (1) pyknodysostosis is the dysplasia which afflicted the French painter, Toulouse-Lautrec. (2) The condition is transmitted by an autosomal recessive trait (3) and is characterized by increased bone density, dwarfism, and skeletal fragility. Though considered a distinct entity by most, similarities with osteopetrosis and cleidocranial dysplasia do exist.

CLINICAL FEATURES

Individuals manifest disproportionate short stature in early childhood and rarely exceed five feet in height as adults. Additional loss of stature may be due to multiple fractures occurring during the patient's lifetime. (4) The facial appearance is characteristic, with a beaked nose, prognathic jaw, small face, and a prominent forehead. Failure of closure of the cranial sutures produces an enlarged head. Dentition is anomalous, and the palate is high and arched. Lowered intelligence has been noted in approximately 10 percent of cases. (5) The hands and feet are stubby, with spoon-shaped nails (koilonychia) and finger clubbing. Laboratory findings are consistently normal; there is no anemia (as found in osteopetrosis) (6) or thrombocytopenia, and no splenomegaly.

RADIOLOGICAL FEATURES

A generalized increase in bone density is seen, with preservation of the medullary canal. This osteosclerosis is most prominent in the long bones, which are subject to transverse pathological fractures. Stress fractures of

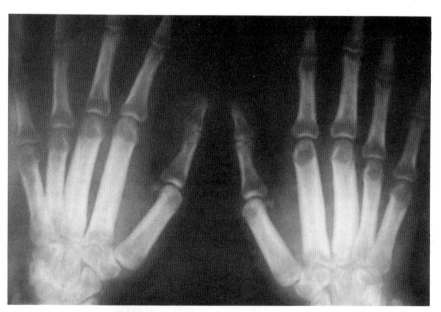

Figure 8.71. PROGRESSIVE DIAPHYSEAL DYSPLASIA: BILATERAL HAND INVOLVEMENT. Note the widening and increased density of the metacarpals bilaterally. **Comment:** The hands and feet are frequently spared in progressive diaphyseal dysplasia.

weightbearing bones as well as fractures of the clavicle and mandible are not infrequent. (5) Numerous abnormalities are found in the skull. The cranial sutures remain open, with a wide anterior fontanelle; the facial bones and sinuses are hypoplastic, and numerous Wormian bones are present. Mandibular hypoplasia with an obtuse angle results in a receding jaw. (7) (Fig. 8.72) Retention of the decidous teeth is often present, with unerupted or malformed permanent teeth. Platybasia is frequent. Hypoplasia or absence of the lateral ends of the clavicles and terminal tufts of the fingers and toes (acro-osteolysis) is a consistent finding. (Fig. 8.73) In the pelvis there may be shallow and obliquely roofed acetabulae and coxa valga. Bowing and overgrowth of the radius or Madelung's deformity contribute to abnormal radioulnar articulations. Spinal abnormalities include block vertebrae, especially at the craniovertebral, and the lumbosacral region. (8) "Spool-shaped" vertebrae (5) and persistence of anterior infantile notching are frequently present. The lack of anemia and the preservation of the medullary canal help to distinguish pyknodyostosis from osteopetrosis. The short stature and dense bones of pyknodsyostosis are absent in cleidocranial dyostosis.

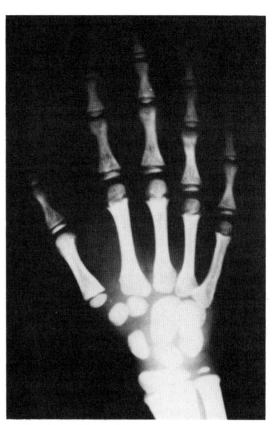

Figure 8.73. PYKNODYSOSTOSIS, HAND: TERMINAL TUFT HYPOPLASIA. Note the acro-osteolysis, which is a consistent finding in pyknodysostosis. There is also a generalized increase in bone density.

Tuberous Sclerosis

GENERAL CONSIDERATIONS

Tuberous sclerosis is a rare autosomal dominant multisystem disorder of neuroectodermal origin. First described in 1880 by Bourneville, (1) the disease has an extremely wide variation in both clinical and radiographic presentation. The classic clinical triad consists of mental retardation, epileptic seizures, and skin lesions, but one or more of these characteristics may be lacking. Synonyms include Bourneville's disease and epiloia (meaning "mindless epileptic"). (1)

CLINICAL FEATURES

Diagnosis of tuberous sclerosis is most often made during adolescence or early adulthood but may be delayed until autopsy because of the paucity of symptoms. The most common clinical presentation is mental deficiency with epilepsy. (2) The seizures usually manifest in the first decade of life but are nonspecific. The skin lesions are considered to be hamartomas and may involve many

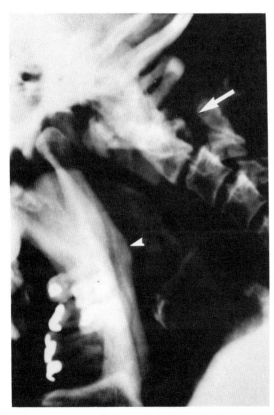

Figure 8.72. PYKNODYSOSTOSIS, LATERAL MANDIBLE: RECEDING JAW. Hypoplasia of the mandible with an obtuse angle (arrowhead) produces a receding jaw. Abnormal dentition and nonunion of a hangman's fracture (arrow) are also noted.

noncutaneous sites as well, including eyes, lungs, kidneys, liver, spleen, brain, heart, and bones.

Cutaneous Manifestations

The most widely recognized skin change is adenoma sebaceum, which is present in 80–90 percent of cases. This is frequently evident in childhood but may not manifest until puberty or pregnancy. (3,4) The earliest skin manifestations are thought to be hypopigmented macules which occur on the legs and trunk. (5–8) These are oval or leaf-shaped, with irregular margins, and may be evident at birth. Other cutaneous lesions include café au lait spots, shagreen, or peau-chagrin patches (20–50% of cases), gingival and periungual fibromas, and skin tags. Retinal phacomas (white patches) often appear.

Cranial Abnormalities

Intracerebral calcifications are found on x-ray examination in 50–80 percent of cases. (9) (Fig. 8.74A and B) The most common locations are in the basal ganglia and paraventricularly. The incidence increases with the patient's age. Cortical tubers and subependymal nodules (hamartomas) are common near the ventricles and may calcify. The calcifications may be multiple or singular and appear as discrete nodules or, occasionally, as linear conglomerates. Cerebellar calcifications are found in 10–15 percent of patients. (10,11)

Visceral Abnormalities

Hamartomas are found in many organs and, depending on the predominant tissue, are classified as myolipomas, angiomyomas, angiofibromas, adenomas, or rhabdomy-

omas. These lesions are rarely present at birth, but their incidence increases with age and they may grow slowly.

Renal hamartomas (angiomyolipomas) occur in 40–80 percent of patients (12) and may cause them to present with flank pain and hematuria. The majority of renal hamartomas in tuberous sclerosis are bilateral, and 50 percent of individuals with renal angiomyolipomas may have no other manifestations of the disease. (9) Renal artery tortuosity and aneurysms are not infrequent.

The rare cardiac involvement is usually with rhabdomyoma, and then it is commonly multiple. Colonic adenomas are infrequently seen. Fewer than one percent of patients with tuberous sclerosis have pulmonary lesions. When present, they occur late and develop into a uniform and diffuse or basilar interstitial infiltrative process. (13,14) Tuberous sclerosis is a rare cause of "honeycomb" lung. (Fig. 8.75)

Endocrine and metabolic dysfunctions are common in these patients and may be evidenced as abnormal pituitary or adrenal function and thyroid disorders. Abnormal glucose tolerance tests and high levels of serum alkaline phosphatase have also been reported. (15)

RADIOLOGICAL FEATURES

Skeletal lesions occur in approximately 50 percent of cases and have a varied presentation. (16) In addition to the intracranial calcifications, generalized thickening and hyperostosis of the cranial vault is noted.

The tubular bones of the hands and feet frequently have cortical manifestations. (Fig. 8.76) Irregular subperiosteal new bone formation and nodules are common.

Figure 8.74. TUBEROUS SCLEROSIS: INTRACRANIAL CALCIFICATION. A. Lateral Skull. Note the numerous calcifications scattered throughout the skull. **B. PA Skull.** A frontal view of this patient's skull aids in localizing the calcifications primarily in the basal ganglia and paraventricularly. (Courtesy of Bryan Hartley, MD, Melbourne, Australia)

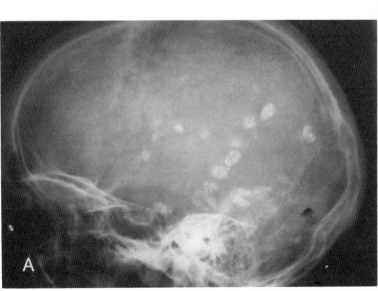

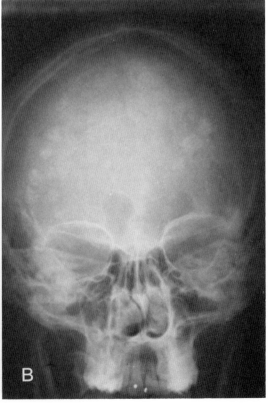

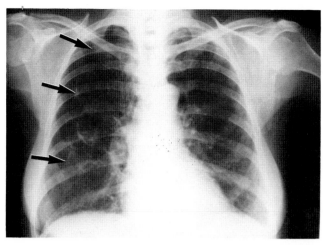

Figure 8.75. TUBEROUS SCLEROSIS: PULMONARY INVOLVE-MENT. Note the diffuse interstitial infiltrate. Tuberous sclerosis is one of the rare causes of "honeycomb" lung. Also note the right spontaneous pneumothorax (arrows). (Courtesy of Bryan Hartley, MD, Melbourne, Australia)

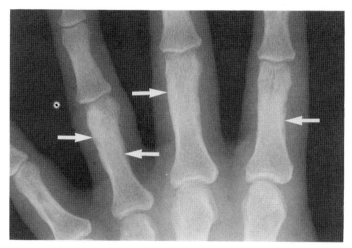

Figure 8.76. TUBEROUS SCLEROSIS, PROXIMAL PHALANGES: SMALL TUBULAR BONE INVOLVEMENT. Note the irregular subperiosteal new bone and nodules along the proximal phalangeal shafts (arrows).

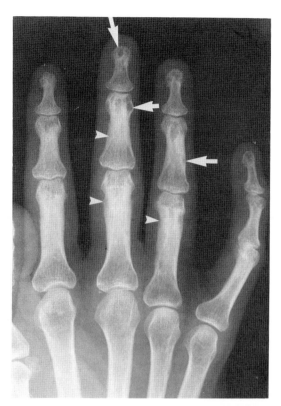

Figure 8.77. TUBEROUS SCLEROSIS, HAND: PHALANGEAL CYSTS. Observe the small, well-defined cysts in the distal and middle phalanges (arrows). There is also subperiosteal new bone formation in the middle and proximal phalangeal shafts (arrowheads).

Small, well-defined cysts are seen in the phalanges, particularly distally. (Fig. 8.77) The trabecular pattern may be coarsened.

The spine and innominate bones are often involved, with osteoblastic deposits of varied size and contour. (17) (Fig. 8.78A and B) The reactive new bone may be in response to osseous hamartomas. (16) The areas of increased density may be diffuse or seen as discrete islands and are most common in the vertebral bodies, pedicles, and pelvic brim. (11) Cortical excrescences affecting the tibia in tuberous sclerosis patients have been referred to as "periosteal warts." (18) Enlargement and sclerosis of a rib has been reported in association with tuberous sclerosis. (19)

The fatty component of most renal hamartomas may allow for their detection on plain radiographs, accompanied by kidney enlargement and contour irregularities. When present, the interstitial fibrotic changes that occur in the lungs are apparent radiographically.

Complications of tuberous sclerosis include urinary tract infection, pulmonary disease (e.g., pneumothorax, hemoptysis, dyspnea, aspiration pneumonia), cor pulmonale, and neoplastic degeneration of the hamartomatous lesions.

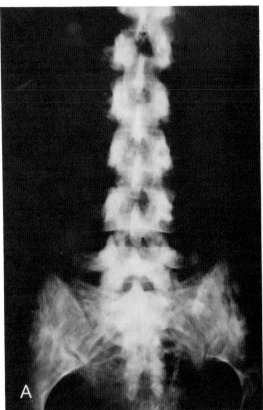

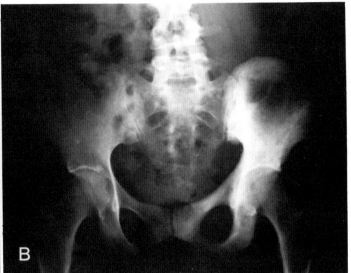

Figure 8.78. TUBEROUS SCLEROSIS: SPINAL AND PELVIC IN-VOLVEMENT.   A. Lumbar Spine. Note the diffuse increased bone density and bright sclerotic pedicles.   **B. AP Pelvis.** There is unilateral innominate sclerosis. (Courtesy of Bryan Hartley, MD, Melbourne, Australia)

Table 8.1.
The Skeletal Dysplasias: Major Clinical Features

Entity	Transmission	Major Clinical Features	Lifespan	Complications
Achondroplasia	Autosomal dominant	Rhizomelic dwarf Waddling gait Increased lumbar lordosis Large head, prominent forehead, depressed nasal bridge Spinal column normal length "Trident" hand	Normal	Back pain Spinal stenosis
Cleidocranial Dysplasia	Autosomal dominant	Large head, small face, drooping, hypermobile shoulders Abnormal gait Severe dental caries	Normal	Deafness Severe dental caries Hip and shoulder dislocations Scoliosis
Chondrodysplasia Punctata	Mild form: Autosomal dominant Lethal form: Autosomal recessive; increased in females	Mild dwarfing Normal mental status Rhizomelic dwarf Mental retardation Joint contractures	Normal Death in first years of life	Thoracic kyphoscoliosis Respiratory failure Recurrent infection
Dysplasia Epiphyseal Hemimelica	Thought to be hereditary	Monomelic limb deformity Functional impairment Valgus and varus deformity	Normal	Functional impairment of involved limb Rarely, limb shortening or elongation
Epiphyseal Dysplasia Multiplex	Autosomal dominant	Waddling gait Stubby hands and feet Flexion deformities Valgum and varus deformities	Normal	Premature degenerative joint disease, especially of the hips and knees

Table 8.1. *Continued*

Entity	Transmission	Major Clinical Features	Lifespan	Complications
Spondyloepiphyseal Dysplasia	Congenita form: Autosomal dominant	Short limbs, flat face, wideset eyes (hypertelorism) Increased thoracic kyphosis, lumbar lordosis, scoliosis, pectus carinatum, dwarfing	Normal	Scoliosis, increased lumbar lordosis, increased thoracic kyphosis
	Tarda form: Males only X-linked recessive	Mild loss of stature, back pain	Normal	Premature DJD
Fibrodysplasia Ossificans Progressiva	Autosomal dominant	Progressive ossification of striated muscles, with loss of motion and wasting	Death in 2nd–3rd decade	Respiratory failure Severe wasting Short thumbs and great toes
Infantile Cortical Hyperostosis	Unknown May be viral	Hyperirritability; painful swellings Fever Exacerbations and remissions Increased ESR	Normal	Usually resolves without complications
Marfan's Syndrome	Autosomal dominant	Tall, slender individual with muscular hypoplasia; many have scoliosis Joint laxity and dislocations Lens dislocations, cataracts	Life is shortened when complications occur	Dissecting aneurysms Lens dislocations
Metaphyseal Dysplasia	Autosomal dominant	Tall individuals with bulbous enlargement of lower extremity joints	Normal	Rarely, fractures through thin cortices
Hurler's Syndrome	Autosomal recessive	Large head, hypertension, corneal opacities Mental deterioration, hepatosplenomegaly Severe dwarfing, dorsal kyphosis, flexion contractures Hydrocephalus	Death in 2nd decade	Cardiac failure, pneumonia
Morquio's Syndrome	Autosomal recessive	Marked dwarfism, dorsal kyphosis, muscular hypotonia Horizontal sternum, short neck Deafness, genu valgum, flexion contractures C1/C2 dislocations	Death in 3rd–4th decade	Paraplegia, respiratory failure Atlantoaxial subluxation
Nail-Patella Syndrome	Autosomal dominant	Hypoplasia of nails, thumb, and index fingers Joint contractures, muscular hypoplasia Renal dysplasia	Normal	Occasionally, renal impairment Patellar and radial head dislocations
Osteogenesis Imperfecta	Autosomal dominant	Osteoporosis with skeletal fragility Blue sclera, abnormal dentition } triad	Congenital form: stillborn or early death	Multiple fractures with severe deformity Hearing loss Pneumonia
Melorheostosis	Congenital	Pain over involved bone Joint contractures, restricted motion Skin abnormalities (scleroderma-like)	Normal	Rarely, premature epiphyseal closure with limb shortening
Osteopathia Striata	Congenital Probably genetic	Usually asymptomatic	Normal	None
Osteopetrosis	Benign form: Autosomal dominant	Often asymptomatic, defective dentition Rare, anemia, deafness	Usually normal	Pathological fracture, hemorrhage, mandibular osteomyelitis
	Severe form: Autosomal recessive	Severe anemia, hepatosplenomegaly, failure to thrive Blindness	Death within 2 years of life	Massive hemorrhage, recurrent infections, anemia Rarely, leukemia and sarcoma

Table 8.1. *Continued*

Entity	Transmission	Major Clinical Features	Lifespan	Complications
Osteopoikilosis	Autosomal dominant	Usually asymptomatic	Normal	None
Progressive Diaphyseal Dysplasia	Autosomal dominant in males	Waddling gait, poor muscular development Weakness of lower extremity	Normal	Increased intracranial pressure Encroachment on neural canals
Pyknodysostosis	Autosomal recessive	Dwarfism Skeletal fragility Block vertebrae Characteristic facies: enlarged head, receding jaw Stubby hands and feet Anomalous dentition	Normal	Pathological fractures
Tuberous Sclerosis	Autosomal dominant	Mental retardation, epileptic seizures } triad Skin lesions	Normal or shortened from complications	Urinary tract infection, pulmonary disease Cor pulmonale Hamartomas, renal angiomyolipomas

Table 8.2.
The Skeletal Dysplasias: Major Roentgen Features

Entity	Major Roentgen Features	Major Sites of Involvement	Bone Density
Achondroplasia	Symmetric limb shortening, especially proximal Relative widening of shafts, "champagne glass" pelvis, narrow thorax Posterior scalloping of vertebral bodies Narrowed interpedicular distance "Trident" hand	Skull, spine, pelvis, limbs Proximal long bones—rhizomelia Congenital spinal stenosis, especially lumbar	Normal
Cleidocranial Dysplasia	Persistent sutures, Wormian bones, agenetic or hypoplastic clavicles Hypoplastic facial bones Midline defects of pelvis, small pelvis Neural arch defects	Skull, clavicles, pelvis, spine	Normal
Chondrodysplasia Punctata	Mild form: Fragmented epiphyses, normal metaphyses and diaphyses Vertebral stippling	Spine, limbs	Normal
	Lethal form: symmetric rhizomelic shortening due to fragmented epiphyses, flared metaphyses Rarely, spinal involvement	Hips, shoulders, knees, wrists	Normal
Dysplasia Epiphysealis Hemimelica	Focal overgrowth of one half of the epiphysis	Lower extremity predominates	Normal
Epiphyseal Dysplasia Multiplex	Bilateral symmetric epiphyseal irregularity End plate irregularity Hypoplastic carpals and tarsals Flattened femoral heads and condyles	Hips, knees, and ankles	Normal
Spondyloepiphyseal Dysplasia	Congenita: Delayed ossification Rhizomelic dwarfing Platyspondyly (short spine) Irregular articular surfaces	Spine, pelvis	Normal
	Tarda: "Heaping-up" vertebrae Narrowed discs	Spine, pelvis	Normal

Table 8.2. *Continued*

Entity	Major Roentgen Features	Major Sites of Involvement	Bone Density
Fibrodysplasia Ossificans Progressiva	Ossification of striated muscle Short thumbs and great toes	Neck, trunk, pelvis, upper extremity	Normal or decreased
Infantile Cortical Hyperostosis	Periosteal new bone formation	Mandible, clavicle, ribs	Normal or increased when acute
Marfan's Syndrome	Long, slender bones Thin cortices	Most marked in distal extremities but involves the entire skeleton	Normal
Metaphyseal Dysplasia	Failure of metaphyseal remodeling with splaying or "Erlenmeyer flask" deformity	Distal femur, proximal and distal tibia, proximal fibula	Normal
Hurler's Syndrome	Frontal bossing, calvarial thickening, large, "J" shaped sella, dorsolumbar kyphosis Paddle ribs Flared ilia Coxa valga and vara	Entire skeleton	Osteoporosis
Morquio's Syndrome	Universal platyspondyly, hypoplastic or agenetic odontoid Short, thick tubular bones	Entire skeleton	Normal
Nail-Patella Syndrome	Bilateral, central posterior iliac horns Patella is small or absent	Ilium, patella, nails Kidney	Normal
Osteogenesis Imperfecta	Severe osteoporosis with pencil-thin cortices Multiple fractures, especially lower extremities "Biconcave lens" vertebrae	Entire skeleton	Decreased
Melorheostosis	Streaked or wavy periosteal new bone "Wax flowing down a lighted candle" appearance	Lower extremity (usually monomelic) Often, with innominate also involved	Increased
Osteopathia Striata	Vertical metaphyseal striations of increased density	Long bones	Increased
Osteopetrosis	Benign and Severe Form: Generalized osseous sclerosis or "bone within a bone" "Sandwich" vertebrae	Entire skeleton	Increased
Osteopoikilosis	Multiple small radiopacities in metaphyseal and epiphyseal regions Usually symmetric	Long tubular bones, carpals, tarsals, pelvis, scapula	Increased
Progressive Diaphyseal Dysplasia	Symmetric fusiform widening of the diaphyses	Femur, tibia, radius, ulna, humerus	Increased
Pyknodysostosis	Generalized increase in bone density with preservation of medullary canals	Most prominent in long bones	Increased
Tuberous Sclerosis	Intracranial calcifications Hyperostosis of cranium Periosteal new bone (warts) in tubular bones, coarsened trabeculae Osteoblastic deposits in spine and pelvis	Skin, viscera, skeleton	Increased

Table 8.3.
Synonyms of Skeletal Dysplasias

Entity	Synonyms	Entity	Synonyms
Achondroplasia	Chondrodystrophia fetalis Chondrodystrophic dwarfism Micromelia	Morquio's Syndrome	Chondrodystrophy Familial osteodystrophy Eccentro osteochondrodysplasia Morquio-Ullrich syndrome Morquio-Brailsford's syndrome
Cleidocranial Dysplasia	Mutational dysostosis Cleidocranial dysostosis	Nail-Patella Syndrome	Hereditary onycho osteodysplasia HOOD syndrome Fong's syndrome
Chondrodysplasia Punctata	Conradi-Hunermann syndrome Stippled epiphyses Dysplasia epiphysialis punctata Chondrodystrophia fetalis calcificans Chondrodystrophia calcificans congenita	Osteogenesis Imperfecta	Osteopsathyrosis idiopathica Mollities ossium Fragilitas ossium Lobstein's disease
Dysplasia Epiphysealis Hemimelica	Tarsoepiphyseal aclasis Trevor's disease Epiphyseal hyperplasia Articular chondromas	Melorheostosis	Flowing hyperostosis Leri-type osteopetrosis Osteosi eberneizzante monomelica
Epiphyseal Dysplasia Multiplex	Multiple epiphyseal dysplasia Fairbank-Ribbing disease Dysplasia polyepiphysaire	Osteopathia Striata	Voorhoeve's disease
Spondyloepiphyseal Dysplasia	None	Osteopetrosis	Albers-Schönberg's disease Osteosclerosis Osteopetrosis generalisata Osteosclerosis generalisata Marble bones Chalk bones
Fibrodysplasia Ossificans Progressiva	Munchmeyer's disease Fibrogenesis ossificans progressiva Fibrositis ossificans progressiva	Osteopoikilosis	Osteopathia condensans disseminata Spotted bones
Infantile Cortical Hyperostosis	Caffey's disease Caffey's syndrome	Progressive Diaphyseal Dysplasia	Engelmann's disease Engelmann-Camurati disease
Marfan's Syndrome	Arachnodactyly Dolichostenomelia	Pyknodysostosis	None
Metaphyseal Dysplasia	Pyle's disease Familial metaphyseal dysplasia	Tuberous Sclerosis	Bourneville's disease Epiloia
Hurler's Syndrome	Lipochondrodystrophy Gargoylism Osteochondrodystrophy Dysostosis multiplex		

REFERENCES

Achondroplasia

1. Parrot MJ: Sur la malformation achondroplasique et le dieu Ptah. *Bull Soc Anthropol Paris* 1 (3rd ser):296, 1878.
2. Kaufmann E: *Untersuchungen über die sogenannte foetale Rachitis (Chondrodystrophy Foetalis)*, Berlin, Georg Reimer, 1892.
3. Caffey J: *Pediatric X-Ray Diagnosis*, ed 7, Chicago, Year Book Medical Publishers, 1978.
4. Holder JC, FitzRandolph RL, Flanigan S: The spectrum of spinal stenosis. *Curr Prob Diag Radiol* 15:16, 1985.
5. Wise BL, Sondheimer F, Kaufman S: Achondroplasia and hydrocephalus. *Neuropaediatrie* 3:106, 1971.
6. Edeiken J: *Roentgen Diagnosis of Diseases of Bone*, ed 3, Baltimore, Williams & Wilkins, 1981.
7. Bailey JA II: Elbow and other upper limb deformities in achondroplasia. *Clin Orthop* 80:75, 1971.
8. Marie P: L'achondroplasie dans l'adolescence et l'age adult. *Presse Med* 8:17, 1900.
9. Saldino RM: Radiographic diagnosis of neonatal short-limbed dwarfism. *Med Radiogr Photogr* 49:61, 1973.
10. Fairbank T: *An Atlas of General Affections of the Skeleton*, Baltimore, Williams & Wilkins, 1951.
11. Murray RO, Jacobson HG: *The Radiology of Skeletal Disorders*, ed 2, New York, Churchill Livingston, 1977.
12. Galanski M, Herrmann R, Knoche V: Neurological complications and myelographic features of achondroplasia. *Neuroradiology* 17:59, 1978.

Cleidocranial Dysplasia

1. Soule AB Jr: Mutational dysostosis (cleidocranial dysostosis). *J Bone Joint Surg (Am)* 28:81, 1946.
2. Cutter E: *Descriptive Catalogue of the Warren Anatomical Museum*, (JBS Jackson) 21, No. 217, Boston, 1870.
3. Marie P, Sainton P: Sur la dysostose cleidocranienne hereditaire. *Rev Neurol* 6:835, 1898.
4. Rhinehart BA: Cleidocranial dysostosis (mutational dysostosis), with a case report. *Radiology* 26:741, 1936.
5. Hawkins HB, Shapiro R, Petrillo CJ: The association of cleidocranial dysostosis with hearing loss. *AJR* 125:944, 1975.
6. Aegerter E, Kirkpatrick JA: *Orthopedic Diseases*, ed 4, Philadelphia, WB Saunders, 1975.
7. Keats TE: Cleidocranial dysostosis. Some atypical roentgen manifestations. *AJR* 100:71, 1967.
8. Anspach WE, Huepel RC: Familial cleidocranial dysostosis (cleidal dysostosis). *Am J Dis Child* 58:786, 1936.
9. Jarvis JL, Keats TE: Cleidocranial dysostosis. A review of 40 new cases. *AJR* 121:5, 1974.
10. Caffey J: *Pediatric X-Ray Diagnosis*, ed 7, Chicago, Year Book Medical Publishers, 1978.

Chondrodysplasia Punctata

1. Spranger J: The epiphyseal dysplasias. *Clin Orthop Rel Res* 114:46, 1976.
2. Bateman D: Two cases, and specimens from a third case, of punctate epiphyseal dysplasia. *Proc R Soc Med* 29:745, 1936.

3. Hunermann C: Chondrodystrophia calcificans congenital als abortive form der chondrodystrophie. *Z Kinderheilkd* 51:1, 1931.
4. Cremin BJ, Beighton P: Dwarfism in the newborn: The nomenclature and genetic significance. *Br J Radiol* 47:77, 1974.
5. Kaufmann HJ, Mahoubi S, Sprackman TJ, et al: Tracheal stenosis as a complication of chondrodysplasia punctata. *Ann Radiol* 1:203, 1976.
6. Afshani E, Girdany BR: Atlanto-axial dislocation in chondrodysplasia punctata. Report of the findings in two brothers. *Radiology* 102:399, 1972.
7. Fairbank T: *An Atlas of General Affectations of the Skeleton*, Baltimore, Williams & Wilkins, 1951.
8. Sheffield LJ, Danks DM, Mayne V, et al: Chondrodysplasia punctata—23 cases of a mild and relatively common variety. *J Pediatr* 86:916, 1976.
9. Happle R, Matthias HH, Macher E: Sex linked chondrodysplasia punctata? *Clin Genet* 11:73, 1977.
10. Jacobson HG: Dense bone—Too much bone: Radiological considerations and differential diagnosis. *Skel Radiol* 13:1, 1985.
11. Shaw WL, Emery J, Hall JG: Chondrodysplasia punctata and maternal warfarin use during pregnancy. *Am J Dis Child* 129:360, 1975.

Dysplasia Epiphysealis Hemimelica

1. Trevor D: Tarso-epiphyseal aclasis: Congenital error of epiphyseal development. *J Bone Joint Surg (Br)* 32:204, 1950.
2. Fairbank TJ: Dysplasia epiphysealis hemimelica (tarso epiphyseal aclasis). *J Bone Joint Surg (Br)* 38:237, 1956.
3. Aegerter E, Kirkpatrick JA: *Orthopedic Diseases*, ed 4, Philadelphia, WB Saunders, 1975.
4. Resnick D, Niwayama G: *Diagnosis of Bone and Joint Disorders*, Philadelphia, WB Saunders, 1981.
5. Hensinger RN, Cowell HR, Ramsey PL, et al: Familial dysplasia epiphysealis hemimelica, associated with chondromas and osteochondromas. Report of a kindred with variable presentations. *J Bone Joint Surg (Am)* 56:1513, 1974.
6. Keats TE: Dysplasia epiphysealis hemimelica (tarso epiphyseal aclasis). *Radiology* 68:558, 1957.
7. D'Angio GJ, Ritvo M, Ulin R: Clinical and roentgen manifestations of tarso-epiphyseal aclasis; review of the manifestations of tarso-epiphyseal aclasis; review of the literature and report of an additional case. *AJR* 74:1068, 1955.
8. Buckwalter JA, El-Khoury GY, Flatt AE: Dysplasia epiphysealis hemimelica of the ulna. *Clin Orthop Rel Res* 135:36, 1978.
9. Caffey J: *Pediatric X-Ray Diagnosis*, ed 7, Chicago, Year Book Medical Publishers, 1978.

Epiphyseal Dysplasia Multiplex

1. Ribbing S: Studien über hereditare, multiple epiphysenstörungen. *Acta Radiol Suppl* 34:1, 1937.
2. Fairbank T: Dysplasia epiphysialis multiplex. *Br J Surg* 34:225, 1947.
3. Rubin P: *Dynamic Classification of Bone Dysplasias*, Chicago, Year Book Publishers, 1964.
4. Leeds NE: Epiphyseal dysplasia multiplex. *AJR* 84:506, 1960.
5. Maroteaux P: *Birth Defects Compendium*, New York, National Foundation, March of Dimes, Alan R Liss, 1979.
6. Berg PK: Dysplasia epiphysialis multiplex. *AJR* 97:31, 1966.
7. Hoefnagel D, Sycamore LK, Russel SW, et al: Hereditary multiple epiphyseal dysplasia. *Ann Hum Genet* 30:201, 1967.
8. Resnick D, Niwayama G: *Diagnosis of Bone and Joint Disorders*, Philadelphia, WB Saunders, 1981.
9. Hulvey JT, Keats T: Multiple epiphyseal dysplasia. A contribution to the problem of spinal involvement. *AJR* 106:170, 1969.
10. Hunt DD, Ponseti IV, Pedrine-Mille A, et al: Multiple epiphyseal dysplasia in two siblings. *J Bone Joint Surg (Am)* 49:1611, 1967.

Spondyloepiphyseal Dysplasia

1. Spranger JW, Langer LO Jr: Spondyloepiphyseal dysplasia congenita. *Radiology* 94:313, 1970.
2. Maroteaux P, Lamy M, Bernard J: La dysplasie spondyloepiphysaire tardive; description clinique et radiologigue. *Presse Med* 65:1205, 1957.
3. Kozlowski K, Bittel D, Budzinska A: Spondylepiphyseal dysplasia congenita. *Ann Radiol* 11:367, 1968.
4. Roaf R, Longmore JB, Forrester RM: A childhood syndrome of bone dysplasia, retinal detachment and deafness. *Dev Med Child Neurol* 9:464, 1967.
5. Spranger JW, Langer LO Jr, Wiedemann HR: *Bone Dysplasias. An Atlas of Constitutional Disorders of Skeletal Development*, Philadelphia, WB Saunders, 1974.
6. Saldino RM: Radiographic diagnosis of neonatal short-limbed dwarfism. *Med Radiogr Photogr* 49:61, 1973.
7. Murray RO, Jacobson HG: *The Radiology of Skeletal Disorders*, ed 2, New York, Churchill Livingston, 1977.
8. Edeiken J: *Roentgen Diagnosis of Diseases of Bone*, ed 3, Baltimore, Williams & Wilkins, 1981.
9. Langer LO Jr: Spondyloepiphyseal dysplasia tarda. *Radiology* 82:833, 1964.
10. Poker N, Finby N, Archibald R: Spondyloepiphyseal dysplasia tarda. *Radiology* 85:474, 1965.
11. Aegerter E, Kirkpatrick JA: *Orthopedic Diseases*, Philadelphia, WB Saunders, 1975.

Fibrodysplasia Ossificans Progressiva

1. Young JWR, Haney PJ: Case Report 314. *Skel Radiol* 13:318, 1985.

2. McKusick VA: *Heritable Disorders of Connective Tissue*, ed 4, St. Louis, CV Mosby, 1972.
3. Resnick D, Niwayama G: *Diagnosis of Bone and Joint Disorders*, Philadelphia, WB Saunders, 1981.
4. Lutwak L: Myositis ossificans progressiva; mineral, metabolic and radioactive calcium studies of the effects of hormones. *Am J Med* 37:269, 1964.
5. Koontz AR: Myositis ossificans progressiva. *Am J Med Sci* 174:406, 1927.
6. VanCreveld S, Soeters JM: Myositis ossificans progressiva. *Am J Dis Child* 62:1000, 1941.
7. Riley HD Jr, Christie A: Myositis ossificans progressiva. *Pediatrics* 8:753, 1951.
8. Letts RM: Myositis ossificans progressiva. A report of two cases with chromosome studies. *Can Med Assoc J* 99:856, 1976.
9. Eaton WL, Conkling WS, Daeschner CW: Early myositis ossificans progressiva occurring in homozygotic twins; a clinical and pathological study. *J Pediatr* 50:591, 1957.
10. Fletcher E, Moss MS: Myositis ossificans progressiva. *Ann Rheum Dis* 24:267, 1965.
11. Smith DM, Zerman W, Johnston CC, et al: Myositis ossificans progressiva. Case report with metabolic and histochemical studies. *Metabolism* 15:521, 1966.

Infantile Cortical Hyperostosis

1. Caffey J, Silverman WA: Infantile cortical hyperostoses; preliminary report on a new syndrome. *AJR* 54:1, 1945.
2. Clemett AR, Williams JG: The familial occurrence of infantile cortical hyperostosis. *Radiology* 80:409, 1963.
3. Caffey J: *Pediatric X-Ray Diagnosis*, ed 7, Chicago, Year Book Medical Publishers, 1978.
4. Resnick D, Niwayama G: *Diagnosis of Bone and Joint Disorders*, Philadelphia, WB Saunders, 1981.
5. Bennett HS, Nelson TR: Prenatal cortical hyperostosis. *Br J Radiol* 26:47, 1953.
6. Barba WP II, Freriks DJ: The familial occurrence of infantile cortical hyperostosis in utero. *AJR* 42:141, 1953.
7. Taj-Eldin S, Al-Jawak J: Cortical hyperostosis: Infantile and juvenile manifestations in a boy. *Arch Dis Child* 46:564, 1971.
8. Blank E: Recurrent Caffey's cortical hyperostosis and persistent deformity. *Pediatrics* 55:856, 1975.
9. Wilson AK: Infantile cortical hyperostosis: A review of the literature and report of a case without mandibular involvement. *Clin Orthop* 62:209, 1969.
10. Holtzman D: Infantile cortical hyperostosis of the scapula presenting as an ipsilateral Erb's palsy. *J Pediatr* 81:785, 1972.
11. Milton LR, Elliott JH: Ocular manifestations of infantile cortical hyperostosis. *Am J Ophthalmol* 64:902, 1967.
12. Scott EP: Infantile cortical hyperostosis: Report of an unusual complication. *J Pediatr* 62:782, 1963.

Marfan's Syndrome

1. Marfan AB: Un cas de deformation congenitale des quatre membres, tres prononcee aux extremities caracterisee par l'allongement des os avec un certain degre d'amincissement. *Bull Mem Soc Med Hop Paris*, 3rd series, 13:220, 1896.
2. Resnick D, Niwayama G: *Diagnosis of Bone and Joint Disorders*, Philadelphia, WB Saunders, 1981.
3. Achard C, Grenet H: Persistance de la lymphocytose arachnoidienne, et des douleurs dans un cas de zona. *Bull Mem Soc Med Hop Paris* 19:1069, 1902.
4. Pennes DR, Braunstein EM, Shirazi KK: Carpal ligamentous laxity with bilateral perilunate dislocation in Marfan syndrome. *Skel Radiol* 13:62, 1985.
5. Robins PR, Moe JH, Winter RB: Scoliosis in Marfan's syndrome. Its characteristics and results of treatment in thirty-five patients. *J Bone Joint Surg (Am)* 57:358, 1975.
6. Burch FE: Association of ectopia lentis with arachnodactyly. *Arch Ophthalmol* 15:645, 1936.
7. Etter L, Glover LP: Arachnodactyly complicated by dislocation of lens and death from rupture of dissecting aneurysm of aorta. *JAMA* 123:88, 1943.
8. McKusick VA: *Heritable Disorders of Connective Tissue*, St. Louis, CV Mosby, 1966.
9. Edeiken J: *Roentgen Diagnosis of Diseases of Bone*, ed 3, Baltimore, Williams & Wilkins, 1981.
10. Steinberg I: A simple screening test for the Marfan syndrome. *AJR* 97:118, 1966.
11. Parrish JG: Heritable disorders of connective tissue. *Proc R Soc Med* 53:515, 1960.
12. Greenfield GB: *Radiology of Bone Diseases*, ed 3, Philadelphia, JB Lippincott, 1975.
13. Nelson JD: The Marfan syndrome, with special reference to congenital enlargement of the spinal canal. *Br J Radiol* 31:561, 1958.

Metaphyseal Dysplasia

1. Pyle E: A case of unusual bone development. *J Bone Joint Surg (Am)* 13:874, 1931.
2. Hermel MB, Gershon-Cohen J, Jones DT: Familial metaphyseal dysplasia. *AJR* 70:413, 1953.
3. Bakwin H, Krida R: Familial metaphyseal dysplasia. *Am J Dis Child* 53:1521, 1937.
4. Caffey J: *Pediatric X-ray Diagnosis*, ed 7, Chicago, Year Book Medical Publishers, 1978.

5. Jacobson HG: Dense bone—Too much bone: Radiological considerations and differential diagnosis. *Skel Radiol* 13:1, 1985.
6. Mori PA, Holt JF: Cranial manifestations of familial metaphyseal dysplasia. *Radiology* 66:335, 1956.

Mucopolysaccharidoses

1. Brante G: Gargoylism: A mucopolysaccharidosis. *Scan J Clin Lab Invest* 4:43, 1952.
2. McKusick VA: *Heritable Disorders of Connective Tissue*, ed 3, St. Louis, CV Mosby, 1966.
3. Lamy M, Maroteaux P, Bader JP: Etude genetique du gargoylisme. *J Genet Hum* 6:156, 1957.
4. Tuthill CR: Juvenile amaurotic idiocy; marked adventitial growth associated with skeletal malformations and tuberculomas. *Arch Neurol Psychiatr* 32:198, 1934.
5. Kressler RJ, Aegerter EE: Hurler's syndrome (gargoylism); summary of literature and report of case with autopsy findings. *J Pediatr* 12:579, 1938.
6. McKusick VA, Milch RA: The clinical behavior of genetic disease; selected aspects. *Clin Orthop* 33:22, 1964.
7. McKusick VA, et al: The genetic mucopolysaccharidoses. *Medicine* 44:445, 1965.
8. Morquio L: Sur une forme de dystrophie osseuse familiale. *Bull Soc Pediatr Paris* 27:145, 1929.
9. Brailsford JE: Chondro-osteo-dystrophy; roentgenographic and clinical features of a child with dislocation of vertebra. *Am J Surg* 7:404, 1929.
10. Zellweger H, Pnsetti IV, Pedrini V, et al: Morquio-Ullrich's disease. *J Pediatr* 59:549, 1961.
11. Fairbank T: *An Atlas of General Affections of the Skeleton*, Baltimore, Williams & Wilkins, 1951.

Nail-Patella Syndrome

1. Greenfield GB: *Radiology of Bone Diseases*, ed 3, Philadelphia, JB Lippincott, 1980.
2. Fong EE: "Iliac horns" (symmetrical bilateral central posterior iliac processes); a case report. *Radiology* 47:517, 1946.
3. Hawkins CF, Smith DE: Renal dysplasia in a family with multiple hereditary abnormalities including iliac horns. *Lancet* 1:803, 1950.
4. Thompson EA, Walker ET, Weens HS: Iliac horns (an osseous manifestation of hereditary arthrodysplasia associated with dystrophy of the fingernails). *Radiology* 53:88, 1949.
5. Darlington D, Hawkins CF: Nail-patella syndrome with iliac horns and hereditary nephropathy. *J Bone Joint Surg (Br)* 49:164, 1967.
6. Eisenberg KS, Potter DE, Bovill EG: Osteoonychodystrophy with nephropathy and renal osteodystrophy. A case report. *J Bone Joint Surg (Am)* 54:1301, 1972.
7. Edeiken J: *Roentgen Diagnosis of Diseases of Bone*, ed 3, Baltimore, Williams & Wilkins, 1981.
8. Murray RO, Jacobson HG: *Radiology of Skeletal Disorders*, ed 2, New York, Churchill Livingstone, 1977.
9. Wasserman D: Unilateral iliac horn (central posterior iliac process). Case report. *Radiology* 120:562, 1976.

Osteogenesis Imperfecta

1. Lobstein JGCFM: *Lehrbuch der Pathologischen Anatomie* Bd II, Stuttgart, 1835.
2. Ormerod EL: An account of a case of mollities ossium. *Br Med J* 2:735, 1859.
3. Gurlt E: *Handbuch der Lehre von den Knochenbrüchen*, Bd 1, Berlin, 1862–1865.
4. Resnick D, Niwayama G: *Diagnosis of Bone and Joint Disorders*, Philadelphia, WB Saunders, 1981.
5. Falvo KA, Root L, Bullough PG: Osteogenesis imperfecta: Clinical evaluation and management. *J Bone Joint Surg (Am)* 56:783, 1974.
6. Bauze RJ, Smith R, Francis MJO: A new look at osteogenesis imperfecta. *J Bone Joint Surg (Br)* 57:2, 1975.
7. McKusick VA: *Heritable Disorders of Connective Tissue*, ed 4, St. Louis, CV Mosby, 1972.
8. Ibsen KH: Distinct varieties of osteogenesis imperfecta. *Clin Orthop Rel Res* 50:279, 1967.
9. Danelius G: Osteogenesis imperfecta intrauterin diagnostiziert. *Arch Gynaekol* 154:160, 1933.
10. Solomons CC, Miller EA: Osteogenesis imperfecta—New perspectives. *Clin Orthop Rel Res* 96:229, 1973.
11. Giordano A: Hereditary disease of the osteocartilagenous system; comparative morphological basis. *Acta Genet* 7:155, 1957.
12. Fairbank T: *An Atlas of General Affections of the Skeleton*, Baltimore, Williams & Wilkins, 1951.
13. Jacobson HG: Dense bone—Too much bone: Radiological considerations and differential diagnosis. *Skel Radiol* 13:1, 1985.
14. Meschan I: *Analysis of Roentgen Signs in General Radiology*, vol 1, Philadelphia, WB Saunders, 1973.

Melorheostosis

1. Leri A, Joanny J: Une affection non decrite des os. Hyperostose "en coulee" sur toute la longueur d'un membre ou "melorheostose." *Bull Mem Sco Hop Paris* 46:1141, 1922.
2. Putti V: L'osteosi eberneizzante monomelica (una nuova sindrome osteopatica). *Chir Organi Mov* 11:335, 1927.
3. Yochum TR, et al: Melorheostosis—A report of two patients. *ACA Council Roentgenol, Roentgen Brief*, April 1981.
4. Franklin EL, Matheson I: Melorheostosis; report on case with review of literature. *Br J Radiol* 15:185, 1942.
5. Younge D, Drummond D, Herring J, et al: Melorheostosis in children. Clinical features and natural history. *J Bone Joint Surg (Br)* 61:415, 1979.
6. Bied JC, Malsh C, Meunier P: La melorheostose chez l'adulte. A propos de deux cas dont l'un traite par un diphosphonate. *Rev Rhum Mal Osteoartic* 43:193, 1976.
7. Patrick JH: Melorheostosis associated with arteriovenous aneurysm of the left arm and trunk. *Skel Radiol* 51:126, 1969.
8. Jacobson HG: Dense bone—Too much bone: Radiological considerations and differential diagnosis. *Skel Radiol* 13:1, 1985.
9. Murray RO, McCredie J: Melorheostosis and the sclerotomes: A radiological correlation. *Skel Radiol* 4:57, 1979.
10. Dissing I, Zafirovski G: Para-articular ossifications associated with melorheostosis Leri. *Acta Orthop Scand* 50:717, 1979.
11. Soffa DJ, Sire DJ, Dodson JH: Melorheostosis with linear sclerodermatous skin changes. *Radiology* 114:577, 1975.
12. Green A, Ellswood WH, Collins JR: Melorheostosis and osteopoikilosis—with a review of the literature. *AJR* 87:1096, 1962.
13. Abrahamson MN: Disseminated asymptomatic osteosclerosis with features resembling melorheostosis, osteopoikilosis, and osteopathia striata. Case report. *J Bone Joint Surg (Am)* 59:991, 1968.
14. McCarroll HR: Clinical manifestations of congenital neurofibromatosis. *J Bone Joint Surg (Am)* 32:601, 1950.
15. Hall GS: A contribution to the study of melorheostosis: Unusual bone changes associated with tuberous sclerosis. *Q J Med* 12:77, 1943.

Osteopathia Striata

1. Voorhoeve N: L'image radiologique non encore decrite de'une anomalie due squelette. *Acta Radiol* 3:407, 1924.
2. Fairbank HAT: Osteopathia striata. *J Bone Joint Surg (Br)* 32:117, 1950.
3. Jacobson HG: Dense bone—too much bone: Radiological considerations and differential diagnosis. *Skel Radiol* 13:1, 1985.
4. Abrahamson MN: Disseminated asymptomatic osteosclerosis with features resembling melorheostosis, osteopoikilosis, and osteopathia striata. Case report. *J Bone Joint Surg (Am)* 50:991, 1968.
5. Hurt RL: Osteopathia striata—Voorhoeve's disease. Report of a case presenting the features of osteopathia striata and osteopetrosis. *J Bone Joint Surg (Br)* 35:89, 1953.
6. Knockaert D, Dequecker J: Osteopathia striata and focal dermal hypoplasia. *Skel Radiol* 4:223, 1979.
7. Larreque M, Maroteaux P, Michey Y, et al: L'osteopathie striee, symptome radiologique de l'hypoplasia dermique en aives. *Ann Radiol* 15:287, 1972.
8. Carlson DH: Osteopathia striata revisited. *J Can Assoc Radiol* 28:190, 1977.
9. Fairbank HAT: A case of unilateral affection of the skeleton of unknown origin. *Br J Surg* 12:594, 1925.
10. Gehweiler JA, Bland WR, Carden TS Jr, et al: Osteopathia striata—Voorhoeve's disease. Review of the roentgen manifestations. *AJR* 118:450, 1973.
11. Aegerter E, Kirkpatrick JA: *Orthopedic Diseases*, ed 4, Philadelphia, WB Saunders, 1975.

Osteopetrosis

1. Zawisch C: Marble bone disease; a study of osteogenesis. *Arch Pathol* 43:55, 1947.
2. Lamy ME: *The Delineation of Birth Defects, IV: Skeletal Dysplasias*, Baltimore, Williams & Wilkins, 1969.
3. Nussey AM: Osteopetrosis. *Arch Dis Child* 13:161, 1938.
4. Beighton PH, Horan FT, Hamersma H: A review of the osteopetroses. *Postgrad Med J* 53:507, 1977.
5. Greenfield GB: *Radiology of Bone Diseases*, ed 3, Philadelphia, JB Lippincott, 1980.
6. Murray RO, Jacobson HG: *The Radiology of Skeletal Disorders*, ed 2, New York, Churchill Livingstone, 1977.
7. Shapiro F, Glimcher MJ, Holtrop ME, et al: Human osteopetrosis. *J Bone Joint Surg (Am)* 62:384, 1980.
8. Sear HR: A case of Albers-Schönberg's disease. *Br J Surg* 14:657, 1927.
9. Moss AA, Minzer F: Osteopetrosis: An unusual cause of terminal tuft erosion. *Radiology* 97:631, 1970.
10. Jacobson HG: Dense bone—too much bone: Radiological considerations and differential diagnosis. *Skel Radiol* 13:1, 1985.

Osteopoikilosis

1. Albers-Schönberg H: Eine seltene, bisher nicht bekannte strukturanomalie des skelettes. *Fortschr Geb Roentgenstr Nuklear Med* 23:174, 1915–1916.
2. Ledoux-Lebard R, Chabaneix D: L'osteopoecilie forme nouvelle d'osteite condensante generalisee sans symptomes cliniques. *J Radiol Electrol Med Nucl* 2:133, 1916–1917.
3. Szabo AD: Osteopoikilosis in a twin. *Clin Orthop Rel Res* 79:156, 1971.
4. Wilcox LF: Osteopoikilosis. *AJR* 30:615, 1933.
5. Risseeuw J: Familiäre osteopoikilie. *Ned Tijdschr Geneeskd* 80:3827, 1936.
6. Melnick JC: Osteopathia condensans disseminata (osteopoikilosis). Study of a family of four generations. *AJR* 82:229, 1959.
7. Busch KFB: Familial disseminated osteosclerosis. *Acta Radiol* 18:693, 1937.
8. Sutherland CG: Osteopoikilosis. *Radiology* 25:470, 1935.

9. Windholz F: Über familiäre osteopoikilie und dermatofibrosis lenticularis disseminata. *Fortschr Geb Roentgenstru Nuklear Med* 45:566, 1932.
10. Buschke A, Ollendorff H: Ein fall von dermatofibrosis lenticularis disseminata und osteopathia condensans disseminata. *Dermatol Wochenschr* 86:257, 1928.
11. Raskin MM: Osteopoikilosis. Possible association with dystocia and keloid. *South Med J* 68:270, 1975.
12. Weissmann G: Scleroderma associated with osteopoikilosis. *Arch Intern Med* 101:108, 1958.
13. Bethge JFJ, Ridderbusch KE: Über osteopoikilie und das neue krankheitsbild hyperostose bei osteopoikilie. *Ergeb Chir Orthop* 49:138, 1967.
14. Lagier R, Mbakop A, Bigler A: Osteopoikilosis: A radiological and pathological study. *Skel Radiol* 11:161, 1984.
15. Holly LE: Osteopoikilosis: 5-year study. *AJR* 36:512, 1936.
16. Blank N, Lieber A: The significance of growing bone islands. *Radiology* 85:508, 1965.
17. Abrahamson MN: Disseminated asymptomatic osteosclerosis with features resembling melorheostosis, osteopoikilosis, and osteopathia striata. Case report. *J Bone Joint Surg (Am)* 50:991, 1968.
18. Mindell ER, Northup CS, Douglass HO Jr: Osteosarcoma associated with osteopoikilosis. Case report. *J Bone Joint Surg (Am)* 60:406, 1978.
19. Dahlin DC: Pathology of osteosarcoma. *Clin Orthop Rel Res* 111:23, 1975.
20. Resnick D, Niwayama G: *Diagnosis of Bone and Joint Disorders*, Philadelphia, WB Saunders, 1981.

Progressive Diaphyseal Dysplasia
1. Camurati M: Di un rara case di osteite simmetrica creditaria delgi arti inferiori. *Chir Organi Mov* 6:662, 1922.
2. Engelmann G: Ein fall von osteopathia hyperostotica (sclerotisans) multiplex infantilis. *Fortschr Geb Roentgenstru Nuklear Med* 39:1101, 1929.
3. Jacobson HG: Dense bone—too much bone: Radiological considerations and differential diagnosis. *Skel Radiol* 13:1, 1985.
4. Sear HR: Engelmann's disease. *Br J Radiol* 21:236, 1948.
5. Bingold AC: Engelmann's disease: osteopathia hyperostotica (sclerotisans) multiplex infantilis; progressive metaphyseal dysplasia. *Br J Surg* 37:266, 1950.
6. Singleton EB: Progressive diaphyseal dysplasia (Engelmann's disease). *Radiology* 67:233, 1956.
7. Aegerter E, Kirkpatrick JA: *Orthopedic Diseases*, ed 4, Philadelphia, WB Saunders, 1975.
8. Neuhauser EBD: Progressive diaphyseal dysplasia. *Radiology* 51:11, 1948.

Pyknodysostosis
1. Maroteaux P, Lamy M: La pycnodysostosis. *Presse Med* 70:999, 1962.
2. Maroteaux P, Lamy M: The malady of Toulouse-Lautrec. *JAMA* 191:715, 1965.
3. Elmore S, Nance W, McGee B, et al: Pycknodysostosis with a familial chromosome anomaly. *Am J Med* 40:273, 1966.
4. Aegerter E, Kirkpatrick J: *Orthopedic Diseases*, ed 4, Philadelphia, WB Saunders, 1975.

5. Murray RO, Jacobson HG: *The Radiology of Skeletal Disorders*, ed 2, New York, Churchill Livingstone, 1977.
6. Emami-Ahari Z, Zarabi M, Javid B: Pycknodysostosis. *J Bone Joint Surg (Br)* 51:307, 1969.
7. Dusenberry JF Jr, Kane JJ: Pycknodysostosis: Report of three new cases. *AJR* 99:717, 1967.
8. Elmore SM: Pycknodysostosis: A review. *J Bone Joint Surg (Am)* 49:153, 1967.

Tuberous Sclerosis
1. Bourneville DM: Contribution a l'etude de l'idiotie. *Arch Neurol* 1:69, 1880.
2. Edeiken J: *Roentgen Diagnosis of Diseases of Bone*, ed 3, Baltimore, Williams & Wilkins, 1981.
3. Lagos JC, Holman CB, Gomez MR: Tuberous sclerosis: Neuroentgenologic observations. *AJR* 104:171, 1968.
4. Medley BE, McLeod RA, Houser OW: Tuberous sclerosis. *Semin Roentgenol* 11:35, 1976.
5. Bunde S: The significance of a white macule on the skin of a child. *Dev Med Child Neurol* 12:805, 1970.
6. Fitzpatrick TB, Sxabo G, Hori Y, et al: White leaf-shaped macules: Earliest visible signs of tuberous sclerosis. *Arch Dermatol* 98:1, 1968.
7. Gold AP, Freeman JM: Depigmented nevi: The earliest sign of tuberous sclerosis. *Pediatrics* 35:1003, 1965.
8. Hurwitz S, Braverman IM: White spots in tuberous sclerosis. *J Pediatr* 77:587, 1970.
9. Resnick D, Niwayama G: *Diagnosis of Bone and Joint Disorders*, Philadelphia, WB Saunders, 1981.
10. Ross AT, Dickerson WW: Tuberous sclerosis. *Arch Neurol Psychiatr* 50:233, 1943.
11. Green GJ: The radiology of tuberous sclerosis. *Clin Radiol* 10:135, 1968.
12. Crosett AD Jr: Roentgenographic findings in the renal lesion of tuberous sclerosis. *AJR* 98:739, 1966.
13. Dwyer JM, Hickie JB, Gravan J: Pulmonary tuberous sclerosis: Report of three patients and a review of the literature. *Q J Med* 40:115, 1971.
14. Malik SK, Pardee N, Martin CJ: Involvement of the lungs in tuberous sclerosis. *Chest* 58:538, 1970.
15. Sareen CK, Ruvalcaba RHA, Scotvold MJ, et al: Tuberous sclerosis. Clinical, endocrine, and metabolic studies. *Am J Dis Child* 123:34, 1972.
16. Jacobson HG: Dense bone—too much bone: Radiological considerations and differential diagnosis. *Skel Radiol* 13:1, 1985.
17. Komar NN, Gabrielsen TD, Holt JF: Roentgenographic appearance of lumbosacral spine and pelvis in tuberous sclerosis. *Radiology* 89:701, 1967.
18. From *The Learning File*, Skeletal Section, SK-2617, with permission of the Center for Devices and Radiological Health, FDA, and the American College of Radiology, 1978.
19. Nathanson N, Anvet NL: An unusual x-ray finding in tuberous sclerosis. *Brit J Radiol* 39:786, 1966.

Trauma

TERRY R. YOCHUM
LINDSAY J. ROWE

Introduction

Traumatic lesions of the skeleton are common occurrences in everyday living and at all ages. The presence of a fracture upon clinical examination may or may not be obvious, thus leaving the radiological investigation as a focal point for definitive diagnosis. With today's sophisticated imaging systems which render a minimal dosage of radiation to the patient, whenever there is any doubt concerning the presence of a fracture, radiographs should be performed. There may be severe medicolegal ramifications when fractures have been overlooked due to the lack of appropriate radiographs being taken or the oversight of the observer. When a fracture or dislocation is identified, key features must be evaluated. (Table 9.1, 9.2)

Successful treatment of fractures starts with accurate diagnosis, which requires a well-performed and accurately interpreted radiographic examination. The minimum examination is considered to be two radiographs at 90 degrees to each other; anything less is considered an incomplete examination. The standard recommended series for each body part is clearly outlined in the positioning component of Chapter 1.

The purpose of this chapter is to familiarize the reader with the most common types of fractures and dislocations. The chapter is presented in a regional manner, with a preliminary presentation of descriptive terminology, definitions, and a review of fracture repair.

Types of Fractures

TERMINOLOGY

Open Fracture

An open fracture is one which penetrates the skin over the fracture site. (Fig. 9.1A) The older term for this type of fracture was "compound," which is a confusing term.

Closed Fracture

A closed fracture does not break the skin or communicate with the outside environment. (Fig. 9.1B) The older term used for this type of fracture was "simple."

Table 9.1.
Key Features to Identifying and Classifying a Fracture

Fracture Type
    Skin penetration
    Comminution
    Mechanism (avulsion, impaction, etc.)
    Complete/incomplete
    Pathological
    Stress
Fracture Orientation
    Oblique
    Transverse
    Spiral
Spatial Relationships
    Alignment
    Apposition
    Rotation
Soft Tissue Involvement

Table 9.2.
Key Features to Identifying and Classifying Dislocations

Position
    Relative to proximal bone
Type
    Subluxation
    Dislocation
    Diastasis
Associated Fractures

Comminuted Fracture

A comminuted fracture is a fracture from which two or more bony fragments have separated. (Fig. 9.2A and B) If a triangular cortical fragment is isolated, this is called a "butterfly" fragment.

Noncomminuted Fracture

A noncomminuted fracture is one which penetrates completely through the bone, separating into two fragments. (Fig. 9.2C and D)

Avulsion Fracture

An avulsion fracture consists of a tearing away of a portion of the bone by a forceful muscular or ligamentous pulling. (Fig. 9.3) Frequent sites are the tuberosities of tubular bones and the lower cervical spinous processes.

Impaction Fracture

An impaction fracture occurs when a portion of bone is driven into its adjacent segment. Because of the compressive forces, the radiolucent fracture line is seldom visualized; instead, a subtle radiopaque white line is seen in the region of impaction. (Fig. 9.4) The two subtypes of impaction fractures are

Depressed Fracture. (1) This type of fracture represents an inward bulging of the outer bone surface. Two characteristic sites for depressed fractures are the tibial plateau and frontal bone.

Compression Fracture. (1) This fracture demonstrates decreased size of the involved bone due to trabecular telescoping and occurs primarily in the spine following a

forceful hyperflexion injury. The vertebral end plates are driven towards each other, creating compression of the intervening spongy bone.

The mechanism of injury in impaction and compression fractures is similar, with the term "compression fracture" used for fractures of the vertebrae and "impaction fracture" primarily for those bones of the appendicular skeleton, the most common of which is the femoral neck. (Fig. 9.5A and B)

Incomplete Fracture

Incomplete fractures are broken on only one side of the bone, leaving a buckling or bending of the bone as the only sign of fracture (1). Angular deformity is common; however, no displacement is expected. The following represent various types of incomplete fracture.

Greenstick (hickory stick) Fracture. (1) This occurs primarily in infants and children under the age of 10 because of the relatively greater component of pliable woven bone. The bone is permitted to bend, thus demonstrating a disruption of the cortex on only one side. (Fig. 9.6A) The affected bone bends like a green twig does upon trying to break it. (1) Greenstick fractures heal without any complication in most instances.

Torus (Buckling) Fracture. Those injuries which insufficiently disrupt the continuity of a bone may result in a buckling of the cortex through forces applied to the long axis of the bone (1). Most occur in the metaphysis and are very painful. The term "torus" is derived from the

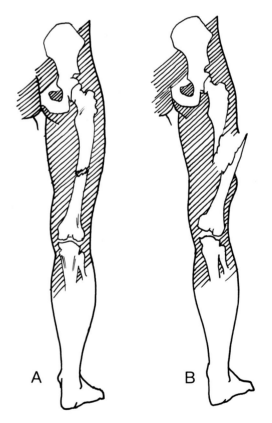

Figure 9.1. FRACTURE AND SKIN RELATIONSHIPS. A. Closed Fracture. B. Open Fracture.

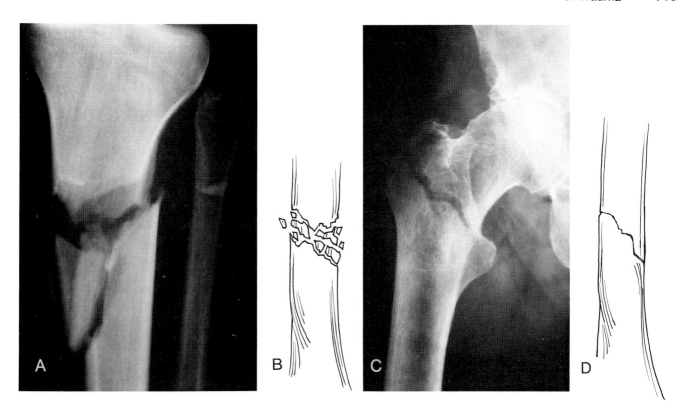

**Figure 9.2. COMMINUTED VERSUS NONCOMMINUTED FRAC-
TURE.   A. AP Tibia and Fibula.** Observe the comminuted fracture
of the proximal tibia. There is associated diastasis of the proximal
tibiofibular articulation.   **B. Diagram: Comminuted Fracture.**

C. AP Femur. Observe the singular radiolucency present between
the intertrochanteric space of the proximal femur without fragmentation. **D. Diagram: Noncomminuted Fracture.**

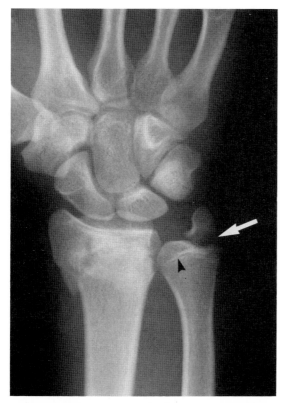

Figure 9.3. AVULSION FRACTURE: WRIST.   Observe the avulsion
fracture of the distal ulnar styloid process (arrow). The growth plate
of the distal ulna should not be confused with a fracture (arrowhead).

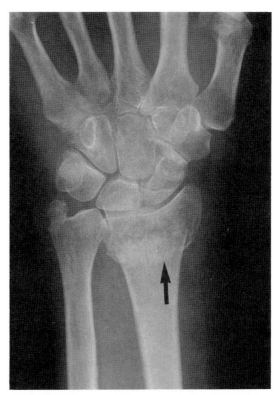

Figure 9.4. IMPACTION FRACTURE: WRIST.   There is an area of
increased bone density (arrow) associated with this impaction fracture of the distal radius.

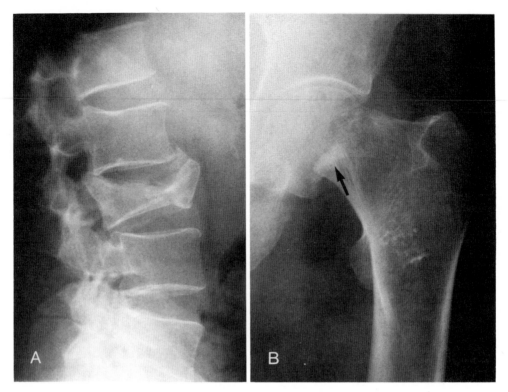

Figure 9.5. COMPRESSION OR IMPACTION FRACTURE. A. Lateral Lumbar Spine. Observe the significant loss in height of the L3 vertebral body. This is an old compression fracture.

B. AP Hip. Note the linear band of radiopacity, representing the area of impaction in this subcapital fracture (arrow).

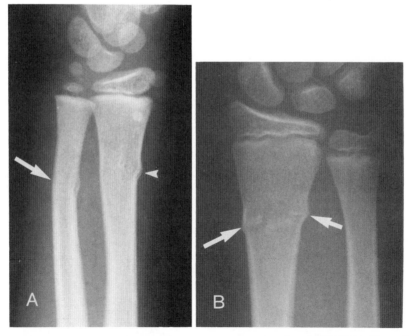

Figure 9.6. GREENSTICK FRACTURE: FOREARM. A. PA Forearm. Observe the altered angulation of the distal ulna, representing a greenstick fracture (arrow). A torus fracture of the radius is also seen (arrowhead). **B. PA Wrist: Torus Fracture.** Note the bulging of the cortex of the distal radius consistent with a torus fracture (arrows).

Latin root meaning "to bulge." (Fig. 9.6B) This has been likened to the lip or bulge at the base of a Greek column or pillar.

Infraction

This type of fracture is actually a form of impaction fracture which is only moderately severe in nature (1). It is used to explain a minor localized break in the cortex, leaving minimal bone deformity. This term is vague, and its use should be discouraged (1).

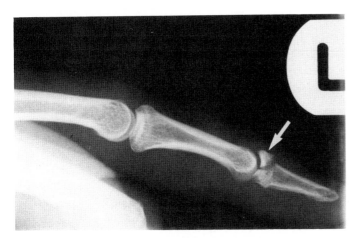

Figure 9.7. CHIP FRACTURE: LATERAL FINGER.   There is a chip fracture present at the base of the distal phalanx (arrow).

Chip (Corner) Fracture

This represents a form of avulsion fracture which is usually limited, demonstrating the separation of a small chip of bone from the corner of a phalanx or other short or long tubular bone. (1) (Fig. 9.7)

Pathological Fracture

A pathological fracture is a fracture through a bone which is weakened by a localized or systemic disease process. The orientation of pathological fractures are usually *transverse* and often appear quite smooth. (1) (Fig. 9.8A and B)

Stress (Fatigue) Fracture

A stress fracture is caused by repetitive stress, causing gradual formation of microfractures and, eventually, an interruption in the bone structure at a greater rate than can be offset by the reparative process. (Fig. 9.9) It represents an actual fatigue failure of the bone. A stress fracture through a diseased bone is called an "insufficiency" fracture. (1,2)

Occult Fracture

An occult fracture represents a special presentation whereby the fracture gives clinical signs of its presence without any radiological evidence. Often, followup radiological examination, usually within 7 to 10 days, reveals resorption of bone at the fracture site or frank displacement. The most common *occult* fracture site involves the

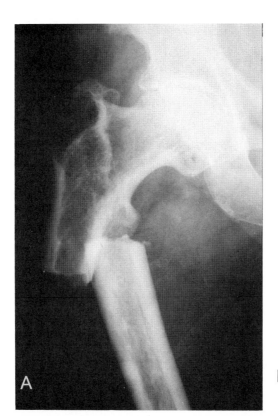
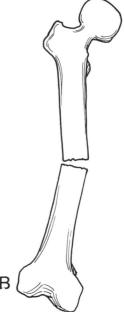

Figure 9.8. PATHOLOGICAL FRACTURE: FEMUR.   A. AP Femur. There is a transverse fracture noted through the proximal diaphysis of the femur. Observe the cortical thickening and accentuated tra-becular patterns consistent with Paget's disease.   **B. Diagram: Pathological Fracture.**

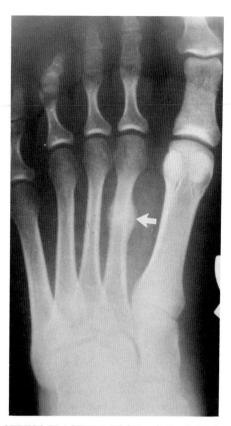

Figure 9.9. STRESS FRACTURE: FOOT. Callus formation is noted surrounding the mid-diaphysis of the second metatarsal (arrow). A subtle transverse fracture line can be identified through the overlying callus formation. **Comment:** This is one of the most common sites for stress fractures and is most frequently found in increased physical activities related to walking, running, and jumping.

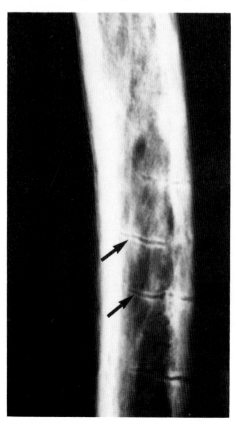

carpal navicular (scaphoid), with the ribs being the second most common. Occult fractures in the spine are very rare.

Pseudofracture

A pseudofracture is not a true fracture. It is thought that it actually represents an insufficiency fracture or is due to vascular pulsations. (3) Histologically, pseudofractures are discrete regions of uncalcified osteoid. Radiographically, they appear as linear lucencies on the convex surface of the bone which are orientated at 90 degrees to the long axis of the bone. (Fig. 9.10) They are often multiple in occurrence and are found in association with bone softening diseases such as Paget's disease, rickets, osteomalacia, and fibrous dysplasia. Various synonyms are applied to pseudofractures, including "Looser's lines," "Milkman's syndrome," "increment fractures," and "umbau zonen."

Fracture Orientation

MODE OF PRESENTATION

Oblique Fracture

The oblique fracture runs in a course of approximately 45 degrees to the long axis of the bone. This occurs commonly in the shaft of a long tubular bone. (2)

Spiral Fracture

A spiral fracture is created by torsional forces, along with axial compression and angulation. The ends of a spiral fracture are pointed like a pen, which is contrasted to the blunt edge of an oblique fracture. (2)

Transverse Fracture

A transverse fracture runs at a right angle to the long axis of a bone. It is uncommon through healthy bone but is frequently seen in diseased bone (pathological fracture). An example of this type of fracture is the "banana" transverse pathological fracture found associated with Paget's disease of bone. (2) (Fig. 9.8A and B)

Spatial Relationships of Fractures

POSITION OF THE FRAGMENT

Alignment

The alignment of a fracture is described as the position of the distal fragment in relation to the proximal fragment. Fractures are in "good" alignment when there is no perceptible angulation in frontal and side views. The relationship of fracture fragments must be accurately described in the x-ray report, especially when reduction is anticipated. (1)

Apposition

The appositional state of the fracture site concerns the closeness of the bony contact at the fracture site. *Good apposition* means near complete surface contact of the

Figure 9.10. PSEUDOFRACTURE: FEMUR. Pseudofractures are present on the convex contour of this pagetoid femur (arrows).

fractured area. *Partial apposition* refers to partial bony contact. If the fractured ends are pulled apart by muscle force or therapeutic traction, it is referred to as *distraction*. (1)

Rotation

Twisting forces on a fractured bone along its longitudinal axis produce rotational deformity. Inclusion of the proximal and distal joints on the film is necessary in determining rotation malposition. (1)

Traumatic Articular Lesions

DISPLACEMENT

Subluxation

Subluxation occurs when there is a partial loss of contact between the usual articular surface components of a joint. (Fig. 9.11B) The joint surfaces are incongruous, but a significant portion remains apposed. (2)

Dislocation (Luxation)

Dislocation refers to a complete loss of contact between the usual articular components of a joint. (Fig. 9.11C) When found associated with a fracture, it is referred to as a fracture dislocation. In the extremities a dislocated bone is always described in relation to the proximal bone. In the spine the dislocated segment is described relative to the segment below. (1)

Diastasis

Diastasis represents displacement or frank separation of a slightly movable joint (syndesmoses). (1) The most common locations for this to occur are the pubic symphysis, sutures of the skull, or the distal tibiofibular syndesmosis. (Fig. 9.12) A separated suture is a *diastatic fracture*. (2)

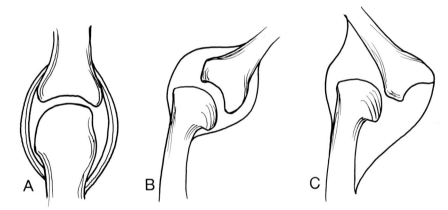

Figure 9.11. TRAUMATIC ARTICULAR LESIONS.   A. Normal Articular Alignment.   B. Subluxation. There is partial displacement of the articular components.   **C. Dislocation.** There is total disrelationship of the articular components.

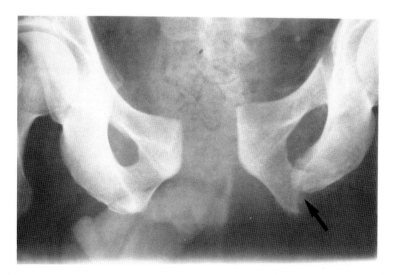

Figure 9.12. DIASTATIC FRACTURE: SYMPHYSIS PUBIS. Widening of the symphysis pubis is present. Additionally noted is a fracture through the ischium and pubic rami (arrow).

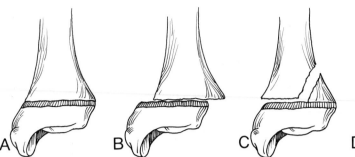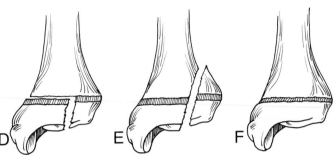

Figure 9.13. SALTER-HARRIS CLASSIFICATION OF EPIPHYSEAL INJURIES.   A. Normal.   B. Type I.   C. Type II.   D. Type III.   **E. Type IV.   F. Type V.**

Epiphyseal Fractures

SALTER-HARRIS CLASSIFICATION

A classification system of growth plate injuries based on the radiological findings was proposed by Salter and Harris in 1963. (4) This system has gained widespread acceptance and is a standard in the description of these injuries which allows for certain prognostic predictions to be made. Essentially, the components involved in the fracture determine its classification type. (Fig. 9.13) (Table 9.3)

Salter-Harris Type I

This represents pure and simple fracture through the growth plate. (Fig. 9.14A) Usually, the radiograph appears normal, with the diagnosis being made clinically because of tenderness over the epiphyseal plate and soft tissue swelling. This type of fracture often complicates scurvy, rickets, osteomyelitis, and hormone imbalance, presenting, for example, as a slipped capital femoral epiphysis.

Salter-Harris Type II

This is a fracture through the displaced growth plate which carries with it a corner of the metaphysis. (Fig. 9.14B) The metaphyseal fragment has been called the "Thurston-Holland sign." (5) This is the most common epiphyseal injury, comprising approximately 75 percent of cases. (6) The most common sites are the distal radius (50 percent), as well as the distal tibia, fibula, femur, and ulna. (6) The epiphyseal separation is usually easily reduced, and the prognosis generally favorable. (6)

Salter-Harris Type III

This fracture is directed along the growth plate and

Table 9.3.
Salter-Harris Classification of Epiphyseal Injuries

Type	Growth Plate	Metaphysis	Epiphysis
I	*		
II	*	*	
III	*		*
IV	*	*	*
V	Compression		

Fracture Site (spanning Growth Plate, Metaphysis, Epiphysis)

then turns toward the epiphysis. (Fig. 9.14C) It results in intra-articular fracture which may require open reduction treatment. The most frequent site is the distal tibia. (6)

Salter-Harris Type IV

This is an obliquely oriented, vertical fracture which passes through the epiphysis, growth plate, and metaphysis. (Fig. 9.14D) The fracture fragment consists of a portion each of the metaphysis, growth plate, and epiphysis. The most common sites are the lateral condyle of the distal humerus in patients under 10 years of age, and the distal tibia in those over the age of 10. Prognosis is poor without expedient open reduction and internal fixation and may result in permanent deformity. (4)

Salter-Harris Type V

This injury is the least common of all the Salter-Harris epiphyseal lesions, resulting in a compressive deformity of the growth plate. Initially, the radiographs are normal, until cessation of growth creates bone shortening or partial arrest which leads to progressive angular deformity. (1) These children should be monitored for at least two years following injury to ensure that the normal growth of bone is occurring at the growth plate. The most common sites are the distal tibial and distal femoral epiphyseal centers. (6)

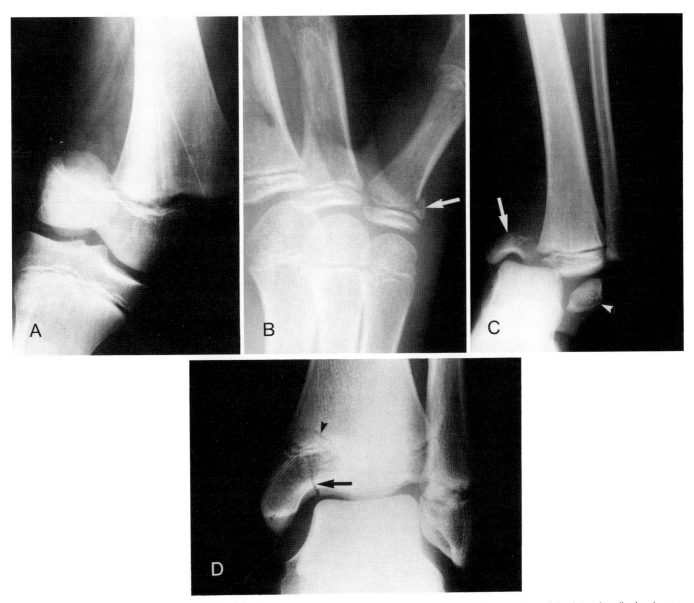

Figure 9.14. SALTER-HARRIS CLASSIFICATION OF EPIPHYSEAL INJURIES: RADIOLOGICAL FEATURES. A. AP Knee: Type I. Epiphyseal separation at the distal femur. **B. Fifth Digit of the Hand: Type II.** Epiphyseal separation with an additional metaphyseal fragment (Thurston-Holland fragment) (arrow). **C. AP Ankle: Type III.** Separation of the medial distal epiphysis (arrow) of the distal tibia, with an associated Type I separation of the lateral malleolus (arrowhead). **D. AP Ankle: Type IV.** Fracture lines extend through the medial aspect of the tibial epiphysis (arrow), with extension into the adjacent metaphysis (arrowhead). A Type I epiphyseal separation is present affecting the distal fibula.

Fracture Repair

THREE PHASES OF HEALING

Circulatory or Inflammatory Phase

The initial circulatory or inflammatory phase is conveniently subdivided into three distinct phases—cellular (with hematoma), vascular, and primary callus—each phase lasting approximately 10 days. (7)

Cellular Phase. Trauma sufficient to cause fracture in bone also damages the overlying muscle, tendon, periosteum, numerous blood vessels, and marrow tissue, resulting in hematoma or clot formation. (8) The injured cells as well as the hematoma incite a cellular inflammatory response which is particularly prominent during the first 5 days of the fracture. Surviving cells in the area of injury and new cells brought in by the granulation tissue create a blastema of undifferentiated mesenchymal cells. This granulation tissue invades and replaces the hematoma. These cells are ultimately capable of modulating into the mature components of callus.

Vascular Phase. The cellular phase is promptly followed by the vascular phase. A specialized circulatory network develops around the fracture. This network consists of dilated tributaries of major vessels that form around the periphery of the injured area and a central swamp-like area of wide-open capillaries and result in formation of a vascular spindle. Following injury, the blood flow of the entire limb is augmented, with active hyperemia at the edges of the injured area. The vigorous blood flow in the arteries and arterioles is slowed when it reaches the vascular "swamp," and passive hyperemia or congestion occurs. This passive hyperemia establishes the milieu for the active secretion of osteoid matrix by the mesenchymal cells that have migrated into the area.

The active hyperemia on the periphery of the vascular spindle, by reason of its high-speed, well-oxygenated blood flow, induces osteoclastic activity in the cortex surrounding the fracture which is easily demonstrable on sequential radiographs. It also activates the vascular bed of the old growth plate and subchondral plate, producing radiographically identifiable subchondral and submetaphyseal resorption bands. Augmented circulation to the entire limb also produces hypertrichosis due to stimulation of hair follicles and tanning of the skin from stimulation of the melanocytes.

Trauma in the muscle and stripping of the periosteum add to the initial fracture hematoma. Periosteal cells adjacent to the fracture become activated, reproduce, and secrete a matrix about themselves which, in effect, "elevates" the periosteum. Simultaneously, changes take place in the injured muscle tissue outside the periosteum, with granulation tissue replacing muscle cells. These cells then give rise to mature callus. As the process continues, a new periosteum forms at the line of demarcation between the normal muscle and callus. This makes moot the argument of whether to put plates beneath or outside the injured periosteum, since the eventually healed periosteum is a newly formed structure. In actuality, the periosteum is not "elevated"; the old is destroyed and a new membrane is formed. "Elevated" periosteal callus, when mineralized, may produce a Codman's triangle on radiographs.

Primary Callus Phase. Callus is the plastic exudate and tissue that develops around the ends of and ultimately unites the fracture fragments. (2) The term is derived from the Latin word "callum," meaning "hard" or "thickened."

Once the vascular phase is well established, more and more "raw material" becomes available. Cellular elements arise from injured bone, connective tissue, marrow, and muscle to form undifferentiated mesenchymal cells. Whether these cells are modulated rhabdomyoblasts, fibroblasts, or osteoblasts or are new cells arising out of the necrotic tissue has not been resolved; nevertheless, muscle, connective tissue, and bone marrow are all essential in producing a blastema that accounts for approximately 70 percent of the callus in a femur shaft fracture. High-speed deposition of osteoid occurs in the form of coarsely woven bone, deposited in a more or less haphazard fashion in the area of the fracture. This osteoid becomes mineralized and earliest radiographic visualization occurs after 14 days. Depending on the degree of motion and vascularization, cartilage is formed within the callus at the same time.

The development of this primitive material in the blas-

temal zone represents the formation of the primary callus. The first stage of fracture healing can be summarized as 1) necrosis, hematoma (approximately 10 days); 2) vascular spindle formation (approximately 10 days); and 3) primary callus.

Reparative or Metabolic Phase

This is the second phase of fracture healing and is characterized by a more orderly secretion of callus and the removal and replacement of coarsely woven osteoid by a more mature form of bone. The process is one of remodeling, mimicking the generalized remodeling processes that occur during normal growth and development. The callus can be divided into separate entities, separated more by nomenclature than by function, and are identifiable as sealing, buttressing, bridging, and uniting callus. Buttressing callus is adjacent to the outer surface of the cortex and is formed by the periosteum as well as surrounding skeletal musculature. Sealing callus fills the medullary cavity and arises from the marrow to "seal" it from the fracture site. Bridging callus unites the gap between the two buttress ends, and uniting callus joins the cortical portions of the fractured bone. Clinical union is achieved when the callus is sufficiently developed to allow weightbearing or similar stress.

Remodeling or Mechanical Phase

The final phase in fracture repair is the remodeling or mechanical phase, which involves realignment and remodeling of bone and callus along lines of stress. Extra bone is deposited in stress lines and removed in areas in which stress is not applied (Wolff's law). The final stage of fracture healing is restoration of the medullary cavity and bone marrow.

The sequence of events in the healing of a fracture, as described previously, have definite practical consequences in the management of the patient.

Although a hematoma is not essential to the healing of a fracture, the hematoma plays a role in inducing granulation tissue response. The greater the response, the more cellular the granulation tissue and the better the ultimate callus. Therefore, the less disturbance of the hematoma, the better.

Large necrotic bone fragments will have to be removed by phagocytic processes and may impede callus formation. Sequestered bone fragments may require removal to help the healing process. Injury induces increased vascularity, which promotes callus. Injured soft tissue should, therefore, be left alone. Muscle contributes extensively to formation of callus and is richly vascularized; it should be minimally disturbed, despite injury. Poor fracture healing usually occurs in bones with little or no adjacent musculature.

Clinical healing will precede anatomic reconstitution. Extensive remodeling will proceed for years after the fracture; therefore, realignment of fracture fragments should emphasize maintained viable bone and all fragments within the field of the vascular spindle. Anatomic reconstitution will usually occur as a consequence of extensive remodeling and does not require exact replacement of fracture fragments.

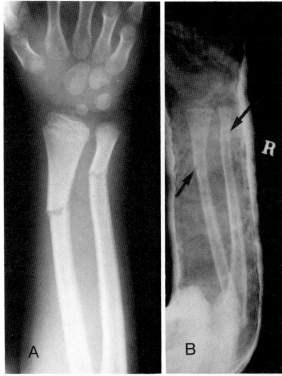

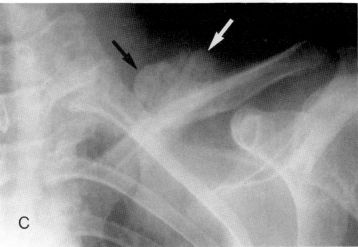

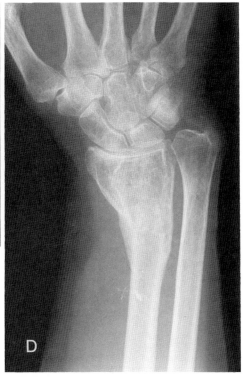

Figure 9.15. RADIOLOGICAL FEATURES OF FRACTURE HEALING.   A. PA Forearm. There are complete fractures present in the distal diaphysis of the radius and ulna, with associated angular deformity.   **B. Postreduction Film Through Cast.** Observe the realignment at the fracture sites (arrows). There is no evidence of callus formation at the fracture site, distinctive of the early phase of fracture repair.   **C. AP Clavicle: Healing Fracture.** Observe the exuberant callus formation secondary to a healing fracture in the midclavicle (arrows).   **D. PA Wrist: Healed Fracture.** There is complete absence of the fracture line in the distal metaphysis of the radius, with residual deformity noted. Of incidental notation is an old avulsion fracture of the distal ulnar styloid process.

RADIOLOGICAL FEATURES OF FRACTURE HEALING

Within the first 5 days following fracture resorption of the fracture line occurs, creating an increase in width of the actual fracture line. (Fig. 9.15A and B) In the following 10–30 days a "veil" of new bone formation occurs adjacent to the fracture site (callus). (Fig. 9.15C) Gradually, the callus formation is remodeled, filling in the previous site of cortical disruption. (Fig. 9.15D) This entire healing process takes 4–6 weeks in the young patient and 6–12 weeks in the geriatric patient.

Complications of Fracture

Complications include nonunion, osteomyelitis, reflex sympathetic dystrophy syndrome, and premature joint disease. (Table 9.4)

NONUNION

"Nonunion" is defined as a failure to complete osseous fusion across the fracture site. Contributing factors of nonunion include distraction, inadequate immobilization, infection, or impaired circulation. The most common sites for nonunion are the midclavicle, ulna, and tibia.

The radiographic signs of nonunion take a number of months to develop. These signs include fracture rounding, lack of callus, sclerosis, and pseudarthrosis. (Fig. 9.16A and B) (Table 9.5)

Rounding of the Fracture Margins

Fractures which are not going to unite often become smooth at their margins, losing the roughened and irreg-ular appearance. Later, the fractured end becomes rounded off and sclerotic.

Lack of Calcified Callus

Failure to demonstrate callus formation across the frac-ture site is a sure sign of nonunion.

Sclerosis of the Fracture Fragment Margins

The fragment ends of the fracture may undergo in-creasing sclerosis when bony union fails to occur.

Pseudarthrosis

If the fracture is not adequately immobilized, motion between the fractured bony ends persists and small ves-sels that grow into the fracture site are constantly sheared. The callus is thus poorly vascularized and tends to pro-duce cartilage instead of bone. Continued motion results in myxoid degeneration and liquefaction of the cartilage, with the formation of a pseudo joint space. This pseud-arthrosis, once established, can be healed only by refrac-ture, removal of the cartilaginous component, and the re-

Table 9.4.
Complications of Fractures

Nonunion
Osteomyelitis
Premature Degenerative Joint Disease
Reflex Sympathetic Dystrophy Syndrome

Table 9.5.
Radiographic Signs of Fracture Nonunion

Rounding of the Fracture Margin
Lack of Callus Formation
Sclerosis of Fracture Margins
Pseudarthrosis

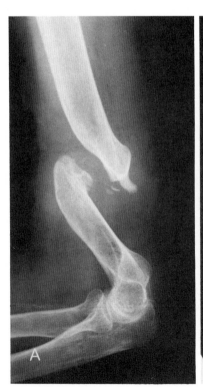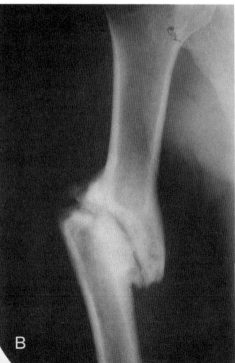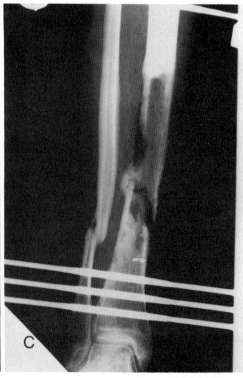

Figure 9.16. FRACTURE COMPLICATIONS.   A. Nonunion: Lateral Humerus. A failure of union of the fracture sites is evidenced by rounding and sclerosis of the adjacent fracture margins.   **B. Non-union with Pseudarthrosis: Humerus.** A pseudarthrosis has formed as the result of failure of union of this fracture. Observe the exuberant sclerosis at the fracture margins.   **C. Osteomyelitis: Tibia and Fibula.** Following removal of a tibial fixation plate, an extensive osteomyelitis has formed, as evidenced by a "motheaten" pattern of bone destruction and cortical disruption.

establishment of a vascular spindle with new callus formation.

OSTEOMYELITIS

Those fractures which become complicated with osteomyelitis are usually open or compound in nature or are those which have required surgical reduction. The incidence of osteomyelitis in fracture of this type is 15 percent. (9) The most common organism is *Staphylococcus aureus*, occurring in 60–70 percent of cases. (9) Most cases manifest within a month of the occurrence of open fracture or open surgical reduction. (2) The dominant symptom is pain, and the radiological features are destructive "moth-eaten" lesions, sequestra formation, and periosteal response near the fracture site. (Fig. 9.16C)

REFLEX SYMPATHETIC DYSTROPHY SYNDROME (SUDECK'S ATROPHY)

Severe and painful regional osteoporosis following rather trivial trauma is referred to as reflex sympathetic dystrophy syndrome (RSDS) or Sudeck's atrophy. This is a relatively rare complication of trauma to a limb.

A more detailed discussion of this entity is found in Chapter 14.

PREMATURE JOINT DISEASE

If a fracture is intra-articular, damage to the articular cartilage often occurs. This is seen most commonly in weightbearing joints such as the hip, knee, or ankle. The arthritic changes represent secondary degenerative joint disease (post-traumatic arthritis).

Fractures of the Skull and Facial Bones

SKULL FRACTURES

General Comments

Because of the complexity of anatomical structures and the difficulty in interpretation of skull radiographs the overall incidence in detection of skull fractures is less than 10 percent on plain film radiographs. (1) Many of the skull series are performed for medicolegal reasons only. Intracranial soft tissue lesions such as intracerebral or subdural hematomas are found without the presence of fracture in 15 percent of cases. (2) (Fig. 9.17) The minimum routine radiographic study of the skull includes the PA Caldwell and AP Towne, with right and left laterals. More specialized projections such as the tangential or submentovertex views may be helpful, along with tomography and computed tomograms, as clinically indicated.

Linear Fracture

Linear fractures represent 80 percent of all skull fractures. (3) They are seen radiographically as sharp, radiolucent, irregular lines without a rim of sclerosis surrounding them. (Fig. 9.18A and B) They are usually several centimeters long and, often, their entire length cannot be determined. Since its course may be straight, angular, or

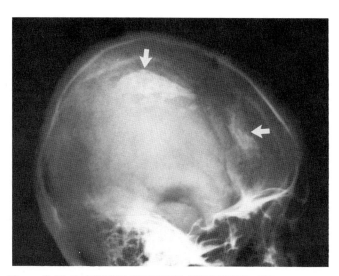

Figure 9.17. CALCIFIED SUBDURAL HEMATOMA: SKULL. A thin plaque-like calcification is seen adjacent to the parietal bones (arrows).

curvilinear, the linear fracture must be differentiated from a vascular groove or suture. The fracture line is more radiolucent than a vascular groove, since it involves both the inner and outer table of the skull, whereas, the vascular groove only represents an impression of varying depth on either the inner or outer table, rendering it less sharp in appearance. Fractures will cross a suture, while a vascular groove will not. The presence of a serrated edge around a radiolucent line usually represents a sutural line rather than fracture. The most common bones involved are the temporal or parietal area, but all skull bones are subject to linear fracture.

Depressed Fracture

Depressed fractures occur as a result of impact by a small mass at high velocity, such as a direct blow with a small object, and are nearly always located within the cranial vault. (3) (Fig. 9.19, 9.20) They represent 15 percent of all skull fractures. (3) The depression usually affects several fragments of bone which are usually angulated inward.

This type of fracture may appear *stellate*, due to the radiating pattern of the multiple fragments, and will appear very radiopaque when viewed *en face* due to the overlap of the fractured fragments.

Depressed fractures must be seen in profile to determine the depth of displacement of the fracture fragments. Approximately one-third of depressed fragments are associated with dural tears that require surgical repair. (3) Displacement of 5 mm or more of depression beyond the inner table suggests a high probability of dural tear.

Ping Pong Fracture. This fracture represents a variation of the depressed fracture and is seen most often in the young child whose skull is very soft and pliable. (3) The skull sustains a deep and broad depression without an associated overt fracture, much like the indentation produced by one's fingers being pushed into a ping pong ball. (4) They are best seen on frontal radiographs, since most lesions occur on the lateral surface of the skull.

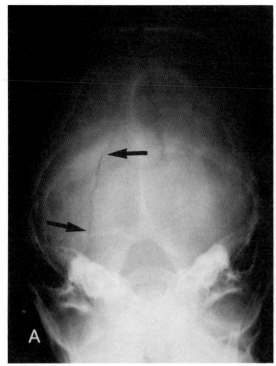

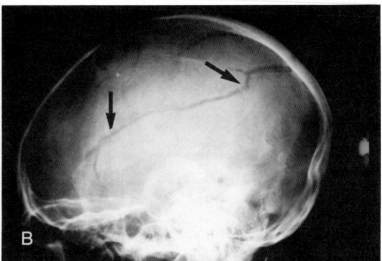

Figure 9.18. LINEAR SKULL FRACTURES.   A. Occipital Bone. A linear fracture line extends through the occipital bone (arrows).   **B. Parietal Bone.** A linear fracture extends from the posterior aspect of the cranial fault anteriorly (arrows).

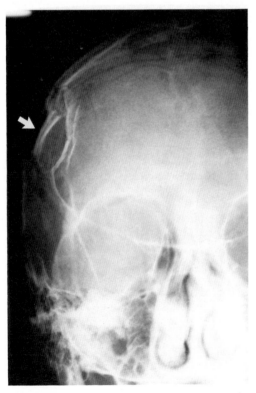

Figure 9.19. DEPRESSED SKULL FRACTURE.   Multiple fracture fragments are seen displaced inward (arrow).

Basal Skull Fracture

One of the most difficult areas to radiographically demonstrate a fracture of the skull is in the area of the skull base. (5) The most reliable index of the presence of a basal skull fracture is an air/fluid (hemorrhage) level or complete opacification of the sphenoid sinus. (6) This sign is seen in up to three-fourths of patients with basal skull fractures. (6) Horizontal-beam lateral radiographs of the skull are required in order to demonstrate an air/fluid level in the sphenoid sinus. (6)

Diastatic Fracture

Diastatic fracture represents a traumatic sutural separation which is usually unilateral and seen most commonly in children. (Fig. 9.21A and B) They account for 5 percent of all cranial fractures. (7) The lambdoidal and sagittal sutures are the most common areas of diastasis. (7) Unilateral separation of a suture greater than 2 mm is considered a sufficient roentgen sign to make the diagnosis of a *diastatic* fracture.

Complications of Skull Fractures

Leptomeningeal Cyst.   Dural tears may occur beneath an area of fracture and may become adherent to the bone adjacent to the margins of the fracture. (8) The accumulation of cerebrospinal fluid forms a cyst within this relative space. The pulsation within the cyst erodes bone, increasing the size of the bony and dural defect, which increases the size of the fracture ("growing" fracture). (3) Therefore, any widening of a fracture line within the skull suggests the possibility of development of a *leptomeningeal cyst.* The importance of this lesion is the pressure on the subadjacent cerebral cortex, leading to focal neurologic deficit, not bone erosion.

Pneumocephalus.   When a fracture extends through the bony wall of a paranasal sinus or mastoid air cell, air may dissect its way through to the subarachnoid space, reaching the ventricular system. Less than 3 percent of all skull fractures are associated with pneumocephalus, with

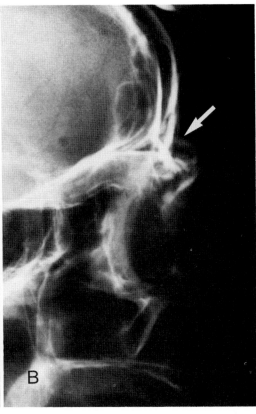

Figure 9.20. DEPRESSED FRACTURE: FRONTAL BONE. A. PA Skull. The loss of aeration throughout the inferior portions of both frontal sinuses represents accumulated hemorrhage (arrows) associated with a comminuted fracture of the frontal bone. **B. Lateral Skull.** Observe the depressed contour of the frontal bone adjacent to the frontal sinus (arrow). (Courtesy of Richard T. Coade, MIR, DC, Kempsey, New South Wales, Australia)

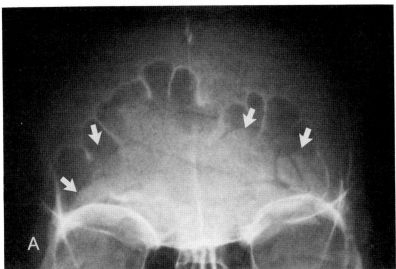

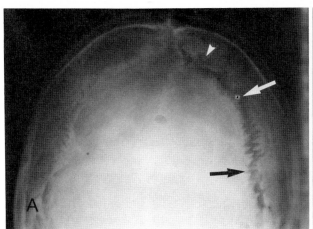

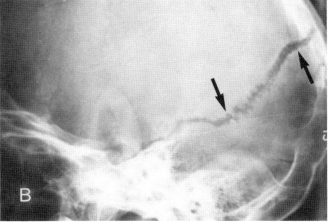

Figure 9.21. DIASTATIC FRACTURES. A. AP Towne's View. A widening of the lambdoidal suture is evident (arrows). A communi- cating linear fracture extends into the adjacent parietal bone (arrowhead). **B. Lateral Skull.** The lambdoidal suture is widened (arrows).

8 percent of fractures of the paranasal sinuses resulting in pneumocephalus. (9)

Subdural and Epidural Hematoma.   Patients do not need to have a fracture of the skull to develop a serious hematoma. (Fig. 9.17) Today's diagnostic imaging devices, the computed tomogram (CT) and magnetic resonance (MR), are the most accurate and least invasive examinations to demonstrate hematoma formation.

FACIAL BONE FRACTURES

General Considerations

More than 70 percent of victims of auto accidents sustain facial injury, the majority of which are soft tissue in nature. (3) The standard radiographic evaluation of facial trauma includes four projections—a PA Water's, PA Caldwell, lateral, and submentovertex. These views should include the entire mandible.

Nasal Bones

Nasal fractures are sustained by high-velocity forces directly impacting in the region of the nasion. They may occur as isolated entities or may be associated with more complex fractures. (10) Most nasal fractures are transverse and tend to depress the distal portion of the nasal bones; however, longitudinal fractures do occur. (3) The nasal

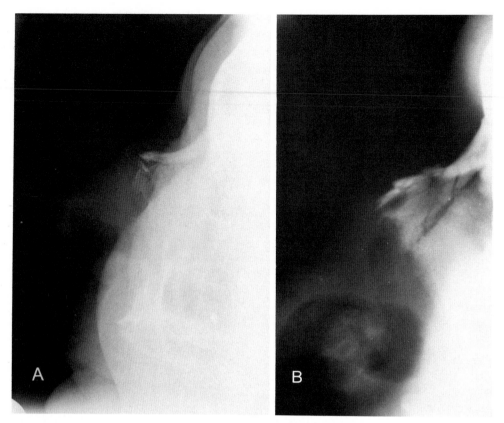

Figure 9.22. NASAL FRACTURES. A. Lateral View. A simple fracture is evident through the nasal bone, with adjacent soft tissue swelling. **B. Lateral Nose**. A comminuted fracture of the nasal bone is observed.

bone fractures are best seen on the lateral projection, which may be underexposed somewhat in order to enhance the visualization of the fracture site. (Fig. 9.22A and B)

Orbital Blowout Fracture

The mechanism of injury in the *blowout* fracture was first described by Smith and Regan in 1957. (11) It is defined as a fracture which disrupts the infraorbital plate of the maxillary bone. The orbital rim may remain intact. Orbital blowout fractures usually occur as a result of a blow by a fist or a ball directly over the globe of the eye or just caudal to it. Additional occular damage occurs in 30 percent of cases. (12) The patient often complains of diplopia.

The radiographic presentation of a blowout fracture is dense opacification of the maxillary sinus, with an inverted dome-like or polypoid mass (usually representing the inferior rectus muscle) hanging from the roof of the maxillary sinus. (3) Intraorbital emphysema (air) may also be found, if the fracture involves an aerated sinus. These findings are best seen on the Water's projection. (3) The opacification of the maxillary sinus is due to hemorrhage or herniated orbital contents, periorbital fat, and the inferior rectus muscle. (12) The inferior orbital rim is usually intact but may be displaced. A thin spicule of bone is often seen caudal to the orbit, representing the depressed portion of the orbital floor.

Tripod Fracture

The tripod fracture is the most common fracture of the facial bones. (3) The mechanism of injury represents a blow over the malar eminence and primarily involves the zygoma. (3) The patient complains of restricted jaw movement due to trapping of the coronoid process of the mandible by the zygoma. The focal points of the fracture affect the three distinct limbs of the zygomatic bone—the zygomatic arch, the orbital process, and the maxillary process surrounding the superior and lateral margins of the maxillary sinus. (Fig. 9.23) Because of the three components of this fracture, it was named "tripod" fracture.

LeFort Fracture

This fracture classification was named for the french investigator Rene LeFort, whose original studies were upon cadavers. (13) By a series of experiments where he varied the direction and strength of forces upon the face, three consistent patterns of fracture lines emerged.

LeFort 1.   This type represents a fracture through the midportion of the maxilla and the pterygoid plates. (13)

LeFort 2.   This type occurs as a result of a blow to the nasofrontal area. The fracture line extends across the ethmoidal bone obliquely, across the medial maxillary surface of the orbit, and shears obliquely through the lateral maxilla between the inferior orbital fissure and the lateral maxillary wall. (13)

LeFort 3.   The fracture line completely separates the

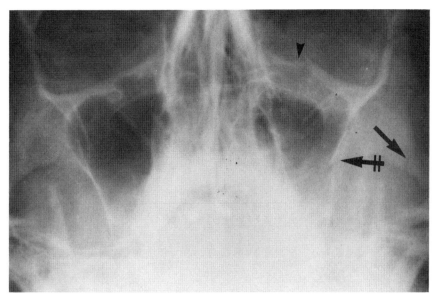

Figure 9.23. TRIPOD FRACTURE: WATER'S VIEW. Three fracture sites are visible, involving the zygomatic arch (arrow), orbital process (arrowhead), and maxillary process (crossed arrow). Adjacent clouding of the maxillary antrum due to hemorrhage is also apparent.

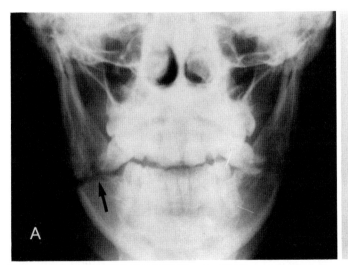

Figure 9.24. MANDIBLE FRACTURE.   A. AP View. A fracture line is seen to extend through the body of the mandible (arrow).

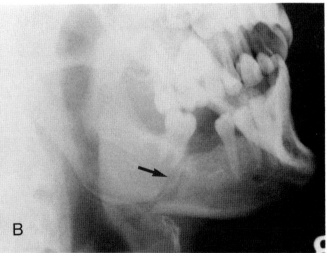

B. Oblique View. The fracture line is clearly seen (arrow).

facial skeleton from the skull. The actual fracture line extends from the nasofrontal area across the ethmoid, posteriorly, to the inferior orbital fissures and pterygoid process, then laterally through the lateral wall of the orbit and the zygomatic arches. (13) This is best seen on the Caldwell and Water's projections and is poorly seen on the lateral. Occasionally, tomography may be needed to demonstrate any of the three types of LeFort fractures.

Fractures of the Mandible

Most mandibular fractures occur in automobile accidents or fist fights, accounting for approximately 80 percent of all mandibular fractures. (14) The most common site for fracture of the mandible is the body, occurring in 30–40 percent of cases. (15) (Fig. 9.24A and B) Other sites include the mandibular angle, condyle, symphysis, ramus, coronoid process, and those limited to the alveolar process. (14,15) Fractures of the mandibular condyle are best seen on overpenetrated Towne views. Notably, the mandible is the slowest healing bone in the body. (14,15)

Fractures and Dislocations of the Spine

INTRODUCTION

Fractures of the spinal column are found most commonly in the cervical spine and the lower thoracic/upper lumbar spine. There has been a significant rise in spinal fractures and spinal cord injuries which appears to be attributable to an increase in automobile accidents and sports activities. (1) Approximately 20 percent of spinal fractures are associated with fractures elsewhere. (2) Spinal cord injuries occur in 10–14 percent of spinal fractures and dislocations. (3) Fractures of the cervical spine produce neurological damage in approximately 40 percent of cases, whereas, the incidence in fractures of the thoracolumbar junction is 4 percent, and in the thoracic spine it is approximately 10 percent. (4) The incidence of neurological deficit is much higher when the fractures affect the neural arch as well as the vertebral body. (4) In 10 percent of the spinal cord injuries there are no associated fractures. (3,4)

Flexion is the most common line of force in spinal injuries, with extension, rotation, shearing, compression, and distraction occurring less frequently. In order to demonstrate the presence of any fracture or dislocation the radiographic examination must be comprehensive and of good diagnostic quality. Therefore, a complete series in each region of the spine should be performed, and, occasionally, pillar views, tomograms, bone scans, or computed tomograms (CT) may be necessary in order to demonstrate the presence or absence of a fracture.

FRACTURES AND DISLOCATIONS OF THE CERVICAL SPINE

Fractures of the Atlas

Jefferson's Fracture ("Bursting" Fracture of the Atlas). A bursting fracture of the ring of the atlas, with fractures through the anterior and posterior arches, was first described by Sir Geoffrey Jefferson, a British neurosurgeon, in 1920. (5) (Fig. 9.25A–D) In 1970 only 191 cases had been reported in the world literature. (6) Jefferson's fracture is created by a forceful blow upon the skull vertex which is transmitted through the occipital condyles to the lateral masses of the atlas. Most of these fractures occur from automobile accidents or diving injuries, usually into too shallow water. The force displaces the lateral masses laterally, classically producing the fractures on each side of the anterior and posterior arches of the atlas. Computed tomography (CT) has since demonstrated variations in this fracture pattern. The lateral masses are subsequently spread apart, creating increased lateral paraodontoid spaces bilaterally and offset of the lateral edge of the atlas lateral masses and the axis superior articular processes. This is best seen on the AP open-mouth radiograph, which may be supplemented with tomography. Often, the transverse ligament will be ruptured as well.

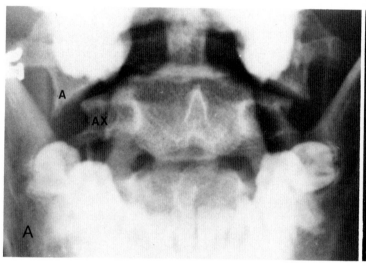

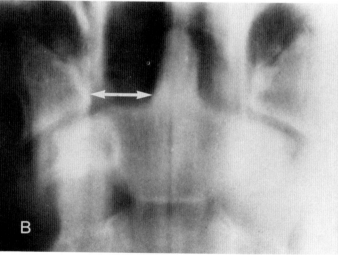

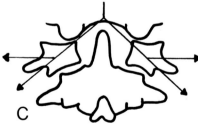

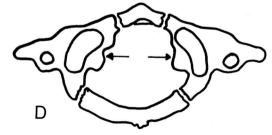

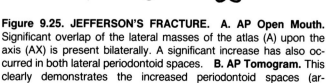

Figure 9.25. JEFFERSON'S FRACTURE. A. AP Open Mouth. Significant overlap of the lateral masses of the atlas (A) upon the axis (AX) is present bilaterally. A significant increase has also occurred in both lateral periodontoid spaces. **B. AP Tomogram.** This clearly demonstrates the increased periodontoid spaces (arrows). **C. Mechanism of Jefferson's Fracture.** A compression force applied through the skull results in lateral displacement of the lateral masses of the atlas. **D. Schematic Diagram.** Observe the bilateral fractures through the anterior and posterior arches of the atlas.

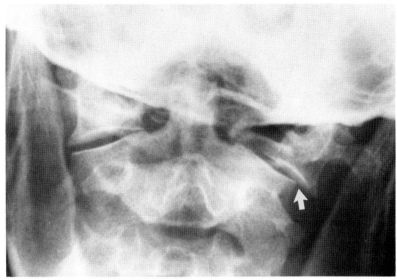

Figure 9.26. UNILATERAL JEFFERSON'S FRACTURE. Significant overlap of the lateral mass of the atlas has occurred unilaterally (arrow).

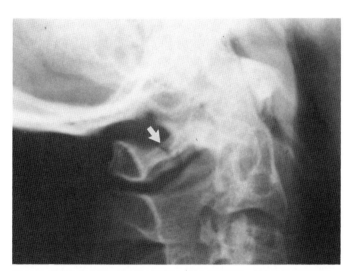

Figure 9.27. POSTERIOR ARCH FRACTURE: ATLAS. Bilateral fracture lines are seen at the junction of the posterior arch with the lateral masses (arrow). Observe the close proximity of the fracture lines to the course of the vertebral artery, which may be injured in this fracture.

Most lesions are bilateral, except when the causative force is eccentrically applied to the skull and is transmitted in greater magnitude to one lateral mass. Unilateral Jefferson's fracture is not as common as the bilateral type. (Fig. 9.26)

Posterior Arch Fracture of the Atlas. The most common fracture of the atlas is a bilateral vertical fracture through the neural arch, usually through or close to the junction of the arch to the posterior surfaces of the lateral masses. (6) This fracture occurs as a result of the posterior arch of the atlas being compressed between the occiput and the large posterior arch of the axis during severe hyperextension. (7) It is best seen on the lateral projection

(Fig. 9.27) and usually carries no serious complications for the patient, as the spinal canal is decompressed. However, because of the close anatomical proximity of the vertebral artery to the fracture site, a serious vascular injury may occur.

Rupture of the Transverse Ligament. Isolated post-traumatic disruption of the transverse ligament is infrequent. The ligament is strong, with the odontoid usually breaking before the ligament is completely compromised. Rupture of the ligament is common in association with Jefferson's fracture, inflammatory arthritis (e.g., rheumatoid arthritis, psoriasis, ankylosing spondylitis, and Reiter's syndrome.) (8) Additionally, 20 percent of Down's syndrome patients exhibit laxity or agenesis of this ligament.

The key radiological features of a ruptured transverse ligament consist of an abnormal atlantodental interspace (ADI) (more than 3 mm in adults and 5 mm in children), especially apparent in a flexion study. (Fig. 9.28A and B) The posterior cervical line will also be disrupted. Cord compression may not be clinically apparent until considerable anterior displacement of the atlas (up to 10 mm) has occurred due to the protective effect of the surrounding tissues of the cord which make up approximately one-third of the diameter of the atlas ring. The division of the atlas into thirds—one-third cord, one-third space, and one-third odontoid—is an important anatomical factor in determining the amount of atlas displacement required to produce cord compression (Steele's Rule of Thirds). (Fig. 9.28C and D)

Fractures of the Axis

Hangman's Fracture (Traumatic Spondylolisthesis). Fractures of the neural arch of the axis are one of the most common injuries of the cervical spine. It is usually the result of an automobile accident in which there is abrupt deceleration from a high speed, but the

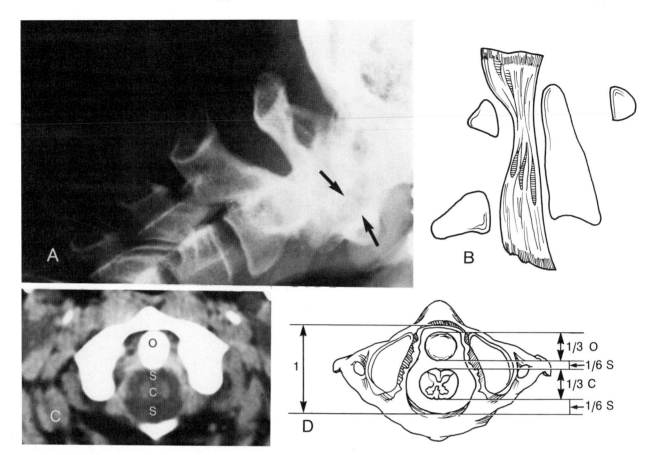

Figure 9.28. RUPTURE OF THE TRANSVERSE LIGAMENT. A. Lateral Cervical With Flexion. An increase in the atlantodental interspace is seen during flexion which measures approximately 7 mm (arrows). This is a radiological sign of transverse ligament instability. **B. Diagrammatic Representation.** Anterior displacement of the atlas upon the axis due to rupture of the transverse ligament may result in significant cord compression with entrapment between the posterior tubercle and odontoid process (guillotine mechanism). **C. Computerized Tomogram Through the C1/C2 Articulation.** The relationship of the odontoid (O), spinal cord (C), and soft tissues surrounding the cord (S) is clearly depicted. **D. Diagrammatic Representation of the C1/C2 Articulation.** Approximately one-third of the atlas ring is occupied by the odontoid (O), one-third by the spinal cord (C), and the remaining one-third by the space surrounding the cord (S). This anatomical division explains why patients with anterior atlas displacement may be relatively asymptomatic until a large degree of translation has occurred (Steele's Rule of Thirds).

fracture occurs during hyperextension. The close similarity of the pathological skeletal characteristics of this injury to that caused by judicial hanging has prompted the term "hangman's fracture." (9) This fracture is actually misnamed, since the hangman is not the recipient of this act. It should more accurately be called the *"hangee's fracture."*

This fracture occurs as a bilateral disruption through the pedicles of the axis and is usually associated with anterior displacement of C2 upon C3. (Fig. 9.29A–C) This displacement is usually persistent following osseous union, a sign of previous injury which should be recognized. The lateral view best demonstrates the fracture, with the frontal radiograph revealing little information.

This injury is usually accompanied by prevertebral hemorrhage, which increases the retropharyngeal interspace (RPI) and, if large enough, may compromise the adjacent airway. There is a surprising lack of neurological findings in fractures of the neural arch of the axis due to the large spinal canal at this level. (10)

Teardrop Fracture. This fracture is an avulsion of a triangular-shaped fragment from the anteroinferior corner of the axis body. (Fig. 9.30A and B) Although teardrop fractures can occur at any cervical body, the lesion is most common at the axis. (11) At this level an acute hyperextension is the usual mechanism of injury, which explains its common occurrence in combination with a hangman's fracture.

Odontoid Process Fracture. Fractures of the odontoid process are common traumatic injuries of the cervical spine. The fracture types were initially described by Anderson and D'Alonzo on the basis of their location. (12) (Fig. 9.31A–C) (Table 9.6) They divided them into three types:

Type I. This type is an avulsion of the tip of the odontoid process as a result of apical or alar ligament stress. It is an uncommon injury which is rarely complicated by nonunion.

Type 2. This is a fracture at the junction of the odontoid process and the body of the axis. This is the most common type of odontoid process fracture and the

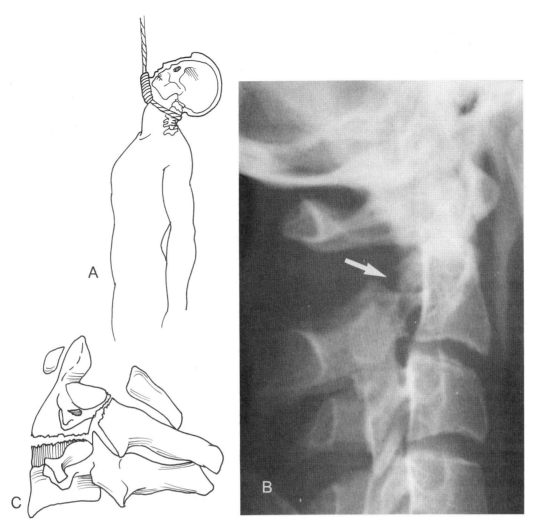

Figure 9.29. HANGMAN'S FRACTURE. A. Mechanism of Injury. During judicial hangings, a hyperextension and rotatory force to the neck directs the impact to the pedicle regions of the C2 segment, resulting in fracture. **B. Radiological Manifestations.** An irregular fracture line (arrow) is seen to extend through the pedicle of the axis. Minimal anterior displacement of the C2 segment upon C3 is also apparent. **C. Diagrammatic Representation.** In addition to the fracture through the pedicle region, disruption at the discovertebral junction may result in vertebral displacement.

most frequent type to not heal. (13) It is often mimicked by the Mach effect, which occurs at the junction of the base of the odontoid process and the body of the axis. (Fig. 9.32A) This Mach effect is caused by superimposition of the anterior and posterior arch of the atlas, which frequently resembles a fracture line and is seen on an AP open-mouth radiograph. The Mach effect is not associated with prevertebral soft tissue swelling and changes with the alteration of the head position, which will often remove its appearance. (3)

Type 3.   This fracture is found deep within the vertebral body, below the base of attachment of the odontoid process to the body. This type heals readily, without incident.

The odontoid process fracture is best seen on AP open-mouth radiographs as an irregular radiolucent line. Occasionally, a side tilt of the odontoid process indicates an underlying fracture. (Fig. 9.32C) The lateral radiograph reveals displacement of the odontoid in either the anterior or posterior position in most cases. This displacement creates an offset of the posterior cervical line (PCL) of the atlas as it relates to the normally positioned axis. Some spinal cord pressure occurs with anterior displacement of the odontoid and the atlas. Greater spinal cord pressure occurs in an isolated rupture of the transverse ligament with an intact odontoid process, creating a "guillotine" or "pincers" effect upon the cord. (Fig. 9.33A–C) Occasionally, an apparent vertical cleft within the odontoid process occurs from the space between the frontal incisors which will simulate a fracture. (Fig. 9.32B) Vertical cleft fractures of the odontoid are virtually impossible to create, and none have been reported. (14)

An additional entity which must be differentiated from an odontoid fracture is an os odontoideum. (Fig. 9.34A and B, 9.35) (Table 9.7) Os odontoideum represents a failure of union of the odontoid peg to the body of the odontoid. Since this entity occurs as a developmental anomaly around the age of 12–14 years, its presence in

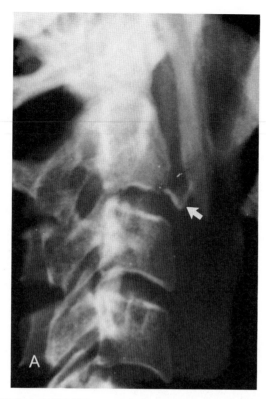

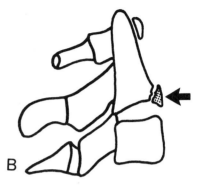

Figure 9.30. TEARDROP FRACTURE. A. C2. Observe the anteroinferior corner of C2, which has been avulsed, creating a free triangular fragment (teardrop) (arrow). **B. Diagrammatic Representation** (arrow).

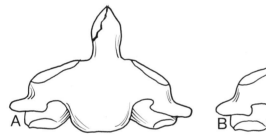
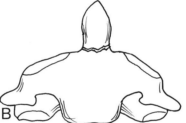
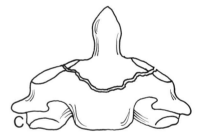

Figure 9.31. CLASSIFICATION OF ODONTOID FRACTURES. A. Type I. B. Type II. C. Type III.

the adult patient may confuse the observer into believing it is a fracture. Radiographically, os odontoideum shows a large radiolucent gap between the peg and the body of the axis which is far too wide to be a fracture. The margins at the base of the os odontoideum are usually smooth and exhibit a sclerotic appearance, whereas odontoid fractures have a serrated or jagged, nonsclerotic margin. Both odontoid fracture and os odontoideum may allow atlantoaxial subluxation (AAS) to occur. In equivocal cases or for medicolegal purposes a bone scan may provide a definitive means of differentiating fracture from congenital anomaly. Odontoid fractures will be positive on a bone scan, with a negative scan being found with os odontoideum.

An additional roentgen sign which is frequently overlooked is enlargement of the anterior tubercle of the atlas in association with os odontoideum. This occurs as a result of hypertrophy secondary to an abnormal amount of

Table 9.6.
Classification of Odontoid Fractures

Type	Location	Stability
I	Odontoid tip	Stable (union)
II	Odontoid base	Unstable (nonunion)
III	Extension into body	Stable (union)

biomechanical stress being placed upon the anterior tubercle of the atlas from the underlying instability of the os odontoideum. The presence of this roentgen sign lends supportive evidence of an anomaly rather than fracture. This sign must be used as an aid to the differential diagnosis, not as the definitive means of diagnosis. This roentgen sign may also be found in association with other upper cervical anomalies such as agenesis or hypoplasia of the posterior arch of the atlas, agenesis or hypoplasia of the odontoid process, and spina bifida of the atlas or

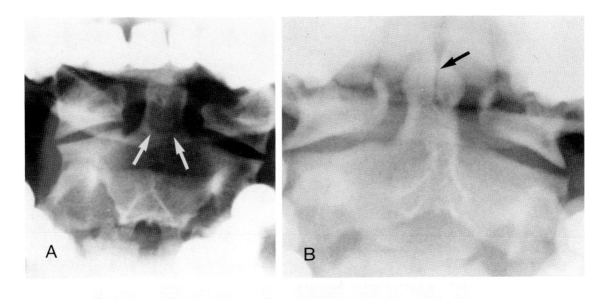

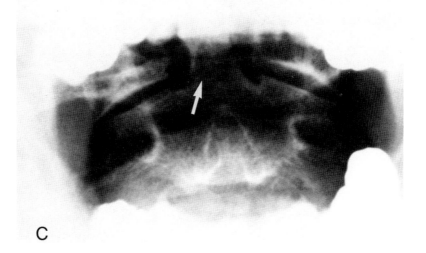

Figure 9.32. UPPER CERVICAL ABNORMALITIES SIMULATING ODONTOID FRACTURE. A. Mach Band Effect: APOM. Observe the simulation of a radiolucent fracture line present at the base of the odontoid process (arrows) as a result of the mach band effect. This pseudoradiolucent line is due to the superimposition of the arch of the atlas near the base of the odontoid process. **B. Pseudocleft of the Odontoid: APOM.** There is a radiolucent pseudocleft (arrow) in the odontoid processes noted as a result of superimposition of the space between the upper incisors. **C. True Odontoid Fracture: APOM.** Observe the jagged radiolucent line at the base of the odontoid, representing a true fracture (arrow). Tilting of the odontoid process is an additional roentgen sign of odontoid fracture.

axis. Close scrutiny of the posterior surface of the anterior tubercle will show it to be straight in odontoid fractures and occasionally angular in os odontoideum, the angle having its apex adjacent to the separating odontoid cleft.

Vertebral Body Compression Fractures

Wedge Fracture. The wedge fracture occurs as a result of mechanical compression of the involved vertebra between the adjacent vertebral bodies. Forceful hyperflexion is the usual mechanism. Two thirds of wedge fractures occur at the fifth, sixth, and seventh cervical segments. (15) This is a stable fracture, because the intervertebral disc, anterior longitudinal ligament, and posterior ligamentous structures are intact.

The lateral radiograph is diagnostic, demonstrating a sharp, triangular, anterior wedging of the superior verte-

bral end plate. (Fig. 9.36) If the anterior height of a vertebral body measures 3 or more millimeters less than the posterior height, a fracture of the vertebral body can be assumed. (14) An increase in the retropharyngeal interspace (RPI) above the normal limit of 20 mm can occur as the result of prevertebral hemorrhage. Displacement of the prevertebral fat stripe may also occur secondary to hemorrhage and edema. Occasionally, a fragment of bone may occur near the anterior surface of the vertebral end plate as a remnant of the traumatic incident. The frontal radiograph is usually of little help in evaluation of the fracture. The absence of a vertical fracture line in the vertebral body in a wedge fracture helps distinguish the wedge fracture from the burst fracture on the frontal film.

Burst Fracture. The burst fracture occurs as a result of vertical compression to the head which usually occurs

**Figure 9.33. GUILLOTINE EFFECT OF ANTERIOR ATLAS DIS-
PLACEMENT. A. Schematic Diagram.** Transverse ligament rupture creates a potential for cord compression between the approximated posterior arch and odontoid process. **B. Schematic Diagram.** Odontoid process fractures result in less compression of the
spinal cord, since the odontoid process and atlas move as a unit. **C.
Lateral Cervical.** A Type III odontoid process fracture (arrows) is
present, with anterior translation of the atlas (arrowheads). **Comment:** The incidence of isolated transverse ligament
rupture following trauma is much less than odontoid process fractures, since the transverse ligament is stronger than the odontoid
attachment. Transverse ligament ruptures, however, represent a
more life-threatening situation as a result of the guillotine effect.

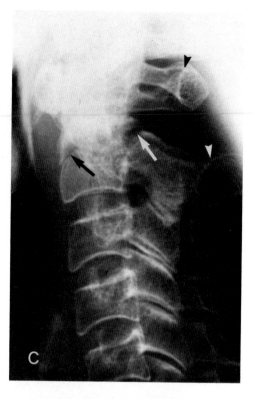

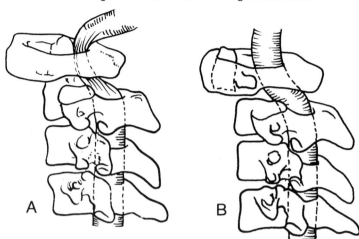

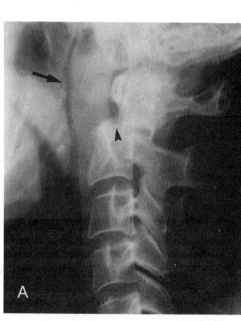

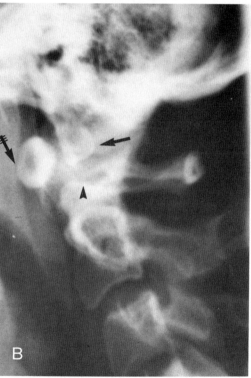

**Figure 9.34. DIFFERENTIATION OF ODONTOID FRACTURES AND
OS ODONTOIDEUM. A. Lateral Cervical: Odontoid Fracture.** A
Type II fracture of the odontoid process with posterior displacement
of the atlas has occurred. An increase in the prevertebral soft tissue
space (arrow) secondary to hemorrhage in association with an
irregular fracture line (arrowhead) at the base of the odontoid process
is seen. Observe the normal size and shape of the anterior tubercle
of C1. **B. Lateral Cervical: Os Odontoideum.** A small bony ossicle
represents the separated odontoid ossicle (arrow). The radiolucent

space between the odontoid ossicle and base of the axis, and the
smooth and sclerotic margins (arrowhead), are distinctive. Significant
enlargement and increased density of the anterior tubercle (crossed
arrow) is also a frequent finding in os odontoideum. The enlargement
of the anterior tubercle with an increase in density is a stress
response secondary to chronic upper cervical instability. This radiographic sign is found in chronic instability and is not seen in acute
fractures. Close observation of the posterior surface of the anterior
tubercle reveals an angular surface with its apex directed posteriorly.

in the mid to lower cervical vertebral bodies. The burst fracture occurs when the nucleus pulposus is propelled through the end plate into the vertebral body at the moment of impact. This force fractures the vertebra vertically, causing a literal explosion of the vertebral body, leading to communition. (Fig. 9.37A and B) The explosion of the vertebral body leads to posteriorly displaced fragments of bone, which may create extrinsic pressure on the ventral surface of the cord. This is best seen with transaxial images created by computed tomography (CT scan). A burst fracture may lead to neurological deficit or paralysis.

The lateral radiograph reveals a comminuted vertebral body which is usually flattened centrally. The frontal radiograph demonstrates a vertical fracture line of the vertebral body in the burst fracture, a sign not seen with the simple wedge fracture.

Teardrop Fracture. "Teardrop fracture" is the term used to describe the triangular-shaped bone that has been separated from the anteroinferior corner of a vertebral body. These may occur from a hyperextension injury as an avulsive process (extension teardrop fracture) or from

a hyperflexion force which compresses the anterior body corners and shears off a significant anteroinferior fragment (flexion teardrop fracture). (Fig. 9.38A and B, 9.39)

These fractures produce severe and unstable injuries of the cervical spine. Forward dislocation of the involved vertebra occurs frequently, because of complete tearing of the anterior longitudinal ligament and partial tearing of the disc and its attachment to the vertebral end plates. Occasionally, rupture of the posterior ligaments allows unilateral or bilateral facet dislocation to occur. These

Table 9.7.
Differential Features Between Os Odontoideum and Odontoid Fracture

	Os Odontoideum	Fracture
Zone of separation	Wide	Narrow
Marginal details	Round, smooth, sclerotic	Irregular
Odontoid orientation	Vertical	Often tilted
Posterior cervical line	Interrupted	Interrupted
Anterior tubercle size/ density	Increased	Normal
Anterior tubercle posterior shape	Angular	Straight

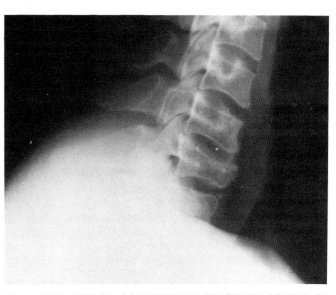

Figure 9.36. WEDGE COMPRESSION FRACTURE OF THE C7 VERTEBRAL BODY. A characteristic wedge-type deformity with loss of intervertebral height and preservation of the posterior vertebral margins secondary to a hyperflexion injury. **Comment:** The lower cervical spine in the C5 through C7 area is the most common location for these fractures.

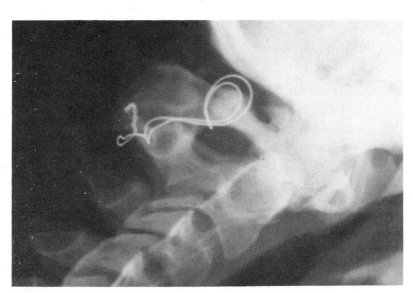

Figure 9.35. SURGICAL STABILIZATION FOR ODONTOID FRACTURE. A combination of osseous and wire arthrodesis has been performed, fixing the posterior arch of the atlas to the spinous process of the axis. Note the residual anterior displacement of the atlas.

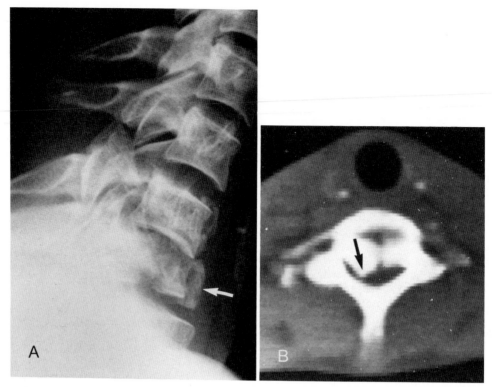

Figure 9.37. BURST FRACTURE OF THE VERTEBRAL BODY. A. Lateral Cervical. There are multiple fracture fragments of the C7 vertebral body (arrow) which have been displaced in various directions. **B. Computed Tomogram: C7.** The displaced fracture frag- ments are seen to extend posteriorly, which has resulted in significant spinal stenosis (arrow). This demonstrates the clinical value of computed tomography in vertebral body fractures.

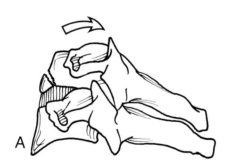
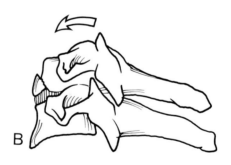

Figure 9.38. MECHANISMS OF THE DEVELOPMENT OF TEAR- DROP FRACTURE. A. Extension Teardrop Fracture. This is an avulsion fracture following a hyperextension injury, which pulls off a small triangular fragment from the anteroinferior corner of the ver- tebral body. **B. Flexion Teardrop Fracture.** Compression of the anterior vertebral body corners creates a shearing effect which disrupts the triangular fragment from the anteroinferior aspect of the vertebral body following a hyperflexion cervical injury.

dislocations should be carefully looked for when a tear- drop avulsion fracture is seen.

If the injury is totally unstable, it may be associated with the *acute anterior cervical cord syndrome.* (12) This is defined as immediate, complete motor paralysis and loss of the anterior column sensations of pain and tempera- ture. The posterior column sensations of position, vibra- tion, and motion are maintained. Involvement of the upper extremities is greater than the lower extremities, due to the neuroanatomy of the cord.

Articular Pillar Fractures

The articular pillar fracture is one of the most fre- quently missed fractures of the cervical spine, (16) partly because the pillars are not well seen on standard views. The articular pillar is formed by the superior and inferior articular processes, which fuse to form a rhomboidal- shaped structure. These articular pillars, C3 through C7, are best demonstrated by pillar views (AP projection obtained with a 20–30-degree caudal tube tilt) of the

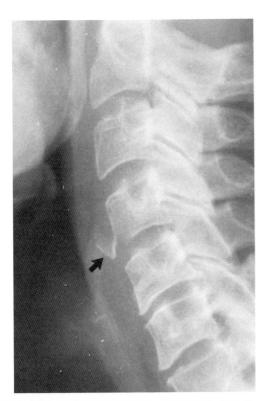

Figure 9.39. TEARDROP FRACTURE: CERVICAL SPINE. There is a teardrop avulsion fracture noted at the anteroinferior aspect of the C4 vertebral body (arrow). **Comment:** Teardrop fractures are often unstable and may be associated with facet dislocation and an acute anterior cervical cord syndrome. (Courtesy of Margaret A. Seron, DC, DACBR, Denver, Colorado)

cervical spine, thus allowing a better profile visualization of these structures.

Pillar fractures most commonly occur at C4 through C7, with C6 representing the site of approximately 40 percent of cases. (15) The most common form of pillar fracture is the compression type, with compression distraction and displacement and avulsion also occurring. Most articular pillar fractures are caused by automobile accidents, and the mechanism of injury is severe compressive hyperextension of the cervical spine, with a lateral flexion component.

Articular pillar fractures have a variable appearance. There may be a horizontal or vertical fracture line, compression with wedging or flattening of the articular pillar, or they may even present as elliptical lucencies within the pillar itself. (Fig. 9.40) Therefore, asymmetry in the height of the articular pillars may occur as a result of unilateral compression, and a fracture line or separation is usually seen with such pillar fractures. It is important to note that congenital developmental asymmetry of the articular pillars is common, and variations from the normal pillar height do occur. Thus, pillar height asymmetry should not be used as the definitive criteria to diagnose fracture, as a diligent search for a fracture line will usually reveal such. (17)

Clay-Shoveler's Fracture

Clay-shoveler's fracture (coal-miner's fracture) is an avulsive injury of the spinous process. The injury derives its name from its common occurrence in clay miners in Australia during the 1930's. (18) The injury usually occurs following an abrupt flexion of the head, such as is found in automobile accidents, diving, or wrestling injuries, or from repeated stress caused by the pull of the trapezius and rhomboid muscles on the spinous process. The spinous avulsion most commonly occurs at C7, with C6 and T1 also frequently involved. (19) This is a stable fracture, since it involves the spinous process only, without neurological deficit. It is best seen on the lateral projection as an oblique radiolucent fracture line through the base of the spinous process or distal tip. (Fig. 9.41A and B) Its margins are rough and serrated, a helpful roentgen sign which enables the observer to differentiate a nonunion of the secondary growth center for the spinous process from a clay shoveler's fracture. The distal portion of the spinous process which is fractured often is displaced caudally a sign not seen with nonunion.

The frontal radiograph demonstrates the apparent presence of two spinous processes for one vertebra which is called the "double spinous process" sign of clay shoveler's fracture. (20) (Fig. 9.42) This roentgen sign may be helpful for patients in whom the cervicothoracic junction is hard to visualize on lateral radiographs. Realignment of the avulsed fragment with the remaining spinous process seldom occurs with healing.

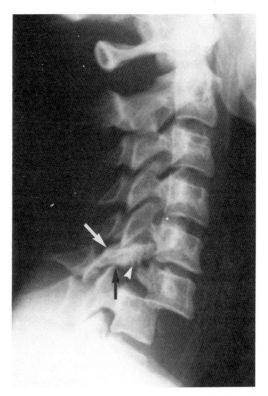

Figure 9.40. PILLAR FRACTURE ASSOCIATED WITH DISLOCATION. Significant decrease in the vertical height of the articular pillar of C6, along with an increase in density of the compressed articular pillar, is characteristic of a pillar fracture (arrows). Additionally, a fracture of the pedicle (arrowhead) and complete dislocation of the C6 vertebral body has occurred.

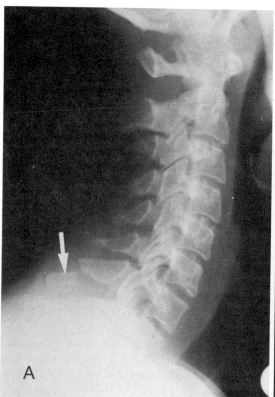

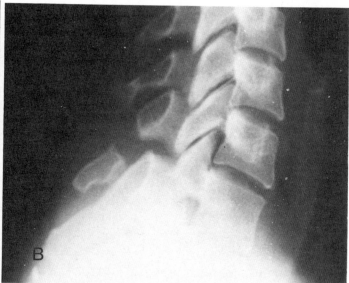

Figure 9.41. CLAY SHOVELER'S FRACTURE. A. Acute Clay Shoveler's Fracture: Lateral Cervical. An avulsion fracture of the spinous process of C7 with inferior displacement of the distal fragment is noted (arrow). Observe the fracture line, which is irregular and exhibits no sclerosis. **B. Old Clay Shoveler's Fracture.** The presence of smooth and sclerotic opposing margins indicates an old clay shoveler's fracture. (Courtesy of Peter Christensson, DC, Rome, Italy)

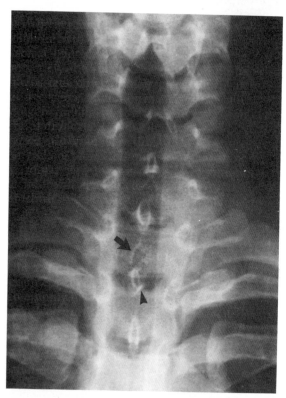

Figure 9.42. DOUBLE SPINOUS PROCESS SIGN: CLAY SHOVELER'S FRACTURE. Two spinous process shadows are seen at the T1 segment, the first of which shows the intact base of the spinous process (arrow). The second shadow is the caudally displaced distal fragment (arrowhead). (Courtesy of Lawrence C. Pyzik, DC, DACBR, Chicago, Illinois)

Lamina and Transverse Process Fractures

Laminar fractures occur in the mid to lower cervical spine, with C5 and C6 being the most common sites. (21) They present as radiolucent vertical or oblique fracture lines through the lamina and are best seen on lateral films. Standard tomography is often necessary in order to demonstrate the fracture line. (Fig. 9.43A and B)

Transverse process fractures of the cervical spine are uncommon. The most frequent location is C7, since the transverse processes are the largest at this level. These fractures are thought to be produced by forced lateral bending of the cervical spine, which results in avulsion of the transverse process by the pull of attached muscles and ligaments. They are usually unilateral lesions, tend to be obliquely or vertically oriented, and occur most commonly at the junction of the mid and distal two-thirds. (Fig. 9.44) Transverse process fractures of the lower cervical spine are associated with severe trauma, and a diligent search for other fractures is prudent. Differential diagnosis should include nonunion of the secondary growth center for the transverse process. The margins adjacent to this nonunion are invariably smooth and exhibit a sclerotic border, while the fracture site is usually jagged.

Whiplash Syndrome

The whiplash syndrome occurs following a deceleration hyperflexion/hyperextension movement of the head and neck which is usually associated with an automobile accident. The term "whiplash" has been popularized by the legal profession and the lay press.

Whiplash injury usually results in soft tissue damage

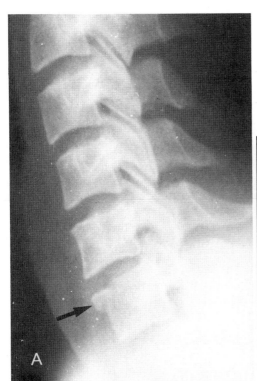

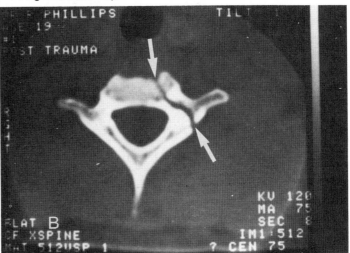

Figure 9.43. VERTEBRAL BODY AND ASSOCIATED NEURAL ARCH FRACTURE.   A. C7 Body Fracture. An anterior compression fracture with a "step defect" is present at the anterosuperior corner of the body of C7 (arrow). **B. Computed Tomogram: C7.** The fracture line is seen to extend through the vertebral body, pedicle, and base of the transverse process (arrows). The extension into the posterior arch could not be appreciated on the plain film radiographs. (Courtesy of Reed B. Phillips, DC, DACBR, MSCM, Ph.D, Los Angeles, California)

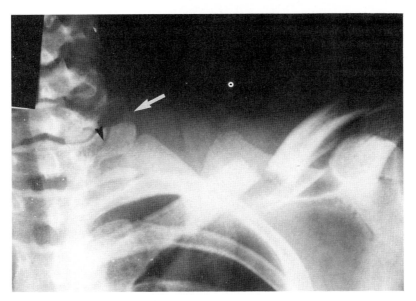

Figure 9.44. TRANSVERSE PROCESS FRACTURES OF C7 AND T1. There is a small avulsion fracture noted at the tip of the C7 transverse process (arrow), along with an oblique transverse process fracture of T1 (arrowhead). Additionally noted is a fracture with malalignment of the mid one-third of the clavicle.   *Comment:* Transverse process fractures in the cervical spine are infrequent and, when present, signify severe injury.

rather than fractures and/or dislocations. These soft tissue changes are often subtle and require careful observation and specific radiological evaluations. (Table 9.8) An integral part of the radiological examination is performing a complete seven view series of the cervical spine (Davis series), (22) which allows evaluations to be made on both osseous and ligamentous structures. These views consist of an anteroposterior open mouth, anteroposterior lower cervical, neutral lateral, right and left obliques, and, most importantly, flexion and extension laterals. Additional pillar views may be taken to assess the integrity of these articular structures, when indicated.

Changes in the cervical curve may provide information on the presence of soft tissue injuries. Straightening, reversal, and acute angulation may all be manifestations of varying degrees of soft tissue damage. A complete kyphotic reversal of the curve (arcual kyphosis) is identified by the spinous processes being spread apart, and this has been referred to as "fanning" of the spinous processes. (Fig. 9.45A and B) These generalized alterations in the cervical curve are usually secondary to protective intrinsic muscular spasm; (14) however, the same curvature configuration can be produced in a nonwhiplash patient by slightly depressing the chin at the time of the radiographic exposure. (23)

Localized changes in the curvature may also be present and usually represent isolated intersegmental damage to

Table 9.8.
Radiological Features in Whiplash Injuries

Alignment Abnormalities
  Alordosis
  Arcual kyphosis
  Segmental flexion/extension
  Anterolisthesis
  Apophyseal joint space widening
  Widened interspinous spacing (fanning)
Soft Tissue Abnormalities
  Increased prevertebral space
  Acute loss of disc height
  Displaced prevertebral fat stripe
  Vacuum cleft sign (extension)

the posterior ligamentous complex. A key sign of this injury is a sudden angular change in the direction of the curvature (acute kyphosis sign), as signified by a flexed vertebral body and widening of the interspinous space (divergent spinous process sign). (24) These localized ligamentous injuries are optimally demonstrated (following resolution of muscle spasm) on flexion/extension films, where additional signs of anterolisthesis, widening of the joint space, and increased superior movement of the pillar may become visible. (22) (Fig. 9.46A–C)

Following trauma, a prevertebral hemorrhage may be precipitated. (Fig. 9.47) This is appreciated on the lateral radiograph by measuring the retropharyngeal interspace (RPI), which should not be greater than 7 mm at the C2 level, or the retrotracheal interspace (RTI), which should not exceed 20 mm at the C6 vertebral level. This prevertebral hemorrhage may also anteriorly displace the prevertebral fat stripe.

An additional soft tissue sign which has not been given sufficient recognition is the "lucent cleft" sign. (25) This sign is created when there is partial disc avulsion from the anterior corner of the cartilaginous end plate. It is best seen on lateral extension radiographs, appearing as a radiolucent "vacuum cleft" lying parallel to the anterior aspect of the inferior end plate. (Fig. 9.48A and B) Often,

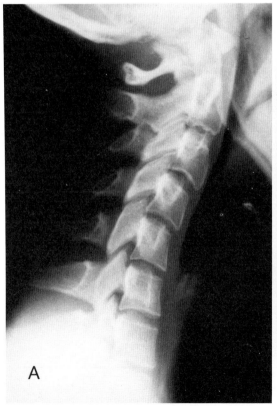

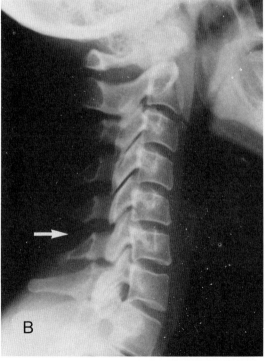

Figure 9.45. ALTERATIONS OF THE CERVICAL LORDOSIS. A. Arcual Kyphosis: Lateral Cervical. There is a reversal of the cervical lordosis, creating an arc-like kyphotic configuration. **B. Acute Angular Kyphosis: Lateral Cervical.** There is a sudden change of the cervical lordosis at the C5/C6 interspace, with an associated increased interspinous space (arrow) (acute cervical kyphosis sign, divergent spinous process sign). **Comment:** Altered cervical patterns of lordosis may occur as a result of patient positioning, muscle spasm, or posterior ligamentous injury. The "arcual kyphosis" is usually associated with muscle spasm, while the acute cervical kyphosis sign indicates localized intersegmental posterior ligamentous damage.

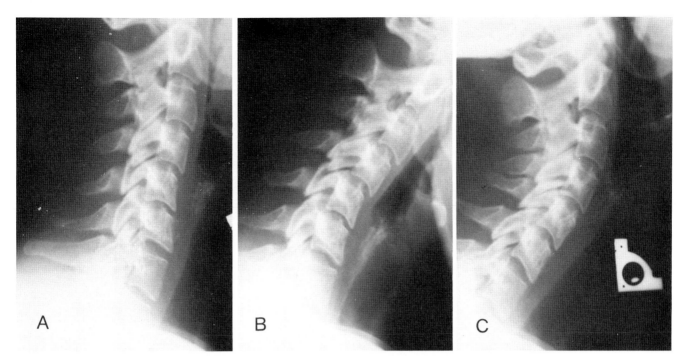

A   B   C

Figure 9.46. STRESS EVALUATION IN LIGAMENTOUS INSTABIL-ITY. A. Neutral Lateral Cervical. Anterolisthesis of C4 is accompanied by a widened interspinous space. **B. Lateral Cervical Flexion.** There is an increase in the anterolisthesis of C4 in the flexion attitude. **C. Lateral Cervical Extension.** A reduction of the anterolisthesis is noted in the extension position. *Comment:* Radiologi-cal signs of ligamentous instability may be minimal or absent on neutral lateral cervical films. Flexion and extension radiographs are necessary to demonstrate the presence of intersegmental ligamentous instability which otherwise may be overlooked. (Courtesy of Kenneth E. Yochum, DC, St. Louis, Missouri)

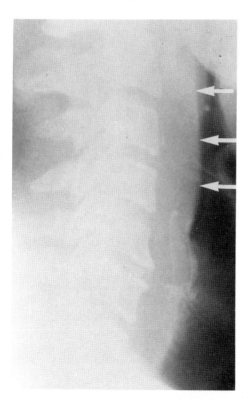

Figure 9.47. POST-TRAUMATIC RETROPHARYNGEAL HEMOR-RHAGE: CERVICAL SPINE. An abnormally increased retropharyngeal interspace (RPI) from C2 to C4 has occurred in the absence of fracture following a whiplash injury (arrows). (Courtesy of Norman W. Kettner, DC, DACBR, St. Louis, Missouri)

this radiolucent cleft will not be seen in the neutral lateral film; therefore, the extension view is essential to its demonstration. If complete avulsion of the disc and rupture of the anterior longitudinal ligament is present, a "lucent cleft" is thought unlikely, in view of the associated local hemorrhage which would fill the cleft with blood. (25) Demonstration of a "lucent cleft" sign is a direct contraindication to osseous manipulation, due to ligamentous instability at the affected level.

The "lucent cleft" sign should not be confused with the "vacuum phenomenon" seen in degenerative changes of the discs. The vacuum phenomenon has a ragged appearance; it is much longer than the lucent cleft sign and is not confined solely to the region adjacent to the anterior end plate. The additional signs of disc space narrowing, hypertrophic degenerative bony changes, and subchondral sclerosis help the observer to recognize the degenerative "vacuum phenomenon," thus avoiding confusion with the post-traumatic "lucent cleft" sign. Lastly, the "lucent cleft" sign is more common in the cervical region, whereas, "vacuum phenomenon" is typically seen in the lumbar region.

Dislocations of the Cervical Spine

Atlanto-Occipital Dislocation. This is a rare and usually fatal injury. Most dislocations occur in an anterior direction and can be detected by a specific measurement method. (Fig. 9.49) (See Chapter 3)

Bilateral Interfacetal Dislocation (BID). Bilateral interfacetal dislocation is the result of a severe hyperflexion injury and is most often found affecting C4 through C7.

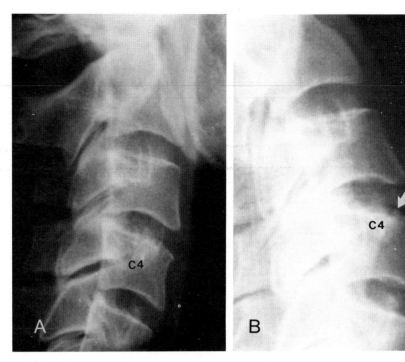

Figure 9.48. VACUUM CLEFT SIGN. A. Neutral Lateral Cervical. Observe closely the discal area adjacent to the anterosuperior corner of the C4 vertebral end plate. No abnormality is seen. **B. Lateral Cervical Extension.** In the same area a radiolucent linear shadow has appeared due to a focal accumulation of nitrogen within an annular tear of the disc ("vacuum cleft" sign) (arrow). ***Comment:***

The formation of this vacuum cleft sign is usually only identified on the extension radiograph. This is a subtle and often overlooked sign of a traumatic intervertebral disc injury which is primarily seen in instances of whiplash. (Courtesy of Donald M. Kuppe, DC, Denver, Colorado)

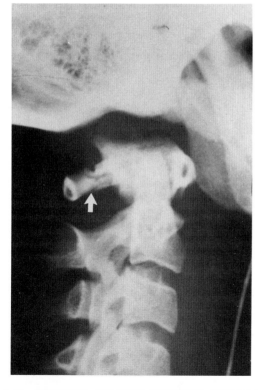

Figure 9.49. ANTERIOR ATLANTO-OCCIPITAL DISLOCATION: CERVICAL SPINE. Complete anterior dislocation of the occipital condyles upon the atlas has occurred. These injuries are frequently fatal and may be associated with posterior arch fractures of C1 (arrow). (Courtesy of Steven B. Wasserman, DC, Long Beach, California)

This injury primarily involves the soft tissues rather than fracture of the skeletal structures. (Fig. 9.50A and B) Those soft tissue structures which are torn are the posterior longitudinal ligament, the posterior ligamentous complex, the annulus fibrosus, and, occasionally, the anterior longitudinal ligament. Anatomically, the superior facets are seen to lie fully anterior to the inferior facets on the lateral radiograph.

In a complete bilateral interfacetal dislocation the facets come to lie within the intervertebral foramina. The body of the dislocated segment is usually displaced anteriorly a distance greater than one-half of the anteroposterior diameter of the body below. (26) If the dislocation is incomplete, oblique radiographs will establish the bilaterality of the lesion.

Chip fractures from the tip of the articulating processes are often found in association with bilateral interfacetal dislocation. Bilateral interfacetal dislocation is an unstable lesion which has a high incidence of cord injuries. Surgical arthrodesis is the usual mode of treatment. (Fig. 9.50B)

Unilateral Interfacetal Dislocation (UID). Unilateral interfacetal dislocation is one of the few injuries caused by a flexion/rotation force. The rotational injury occurs around one of the interfacetal joints, causing it to dislocate into the intervertebral foramen. (Fig. 9.51A–C) In this position the dislocated articular mass is mechanically locked out of place.

On the lateral radiograph, unilateral interfacetal dislocation is characterized by forward displacement of the dislocated segment upon the vertebra below. Alteration in the superimposition of the articular pillars on the lateral view represents a subtle sign of unilateral interfacetal

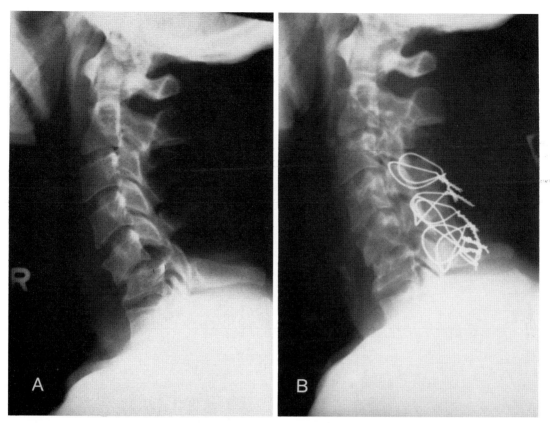

Figure 9.50. BILATERAL INTERFACETAL DISLOCATION.   A. Lateral Cervical. Notice the displacement of the superior anterior articular pillar of C5 in conjunction with an acute deflection deformity of the vertebral body.   **B. Lateral Cervical.** Postsurgical reduction and wire arthrodesis of the previous interfacetal dislocation.   ***Comment:*** A bilateral interfacetal dislocation frequently remains locked, requiring surgical reduction and fusion. Observe the acute widening of the C5/C6 interspinous space.

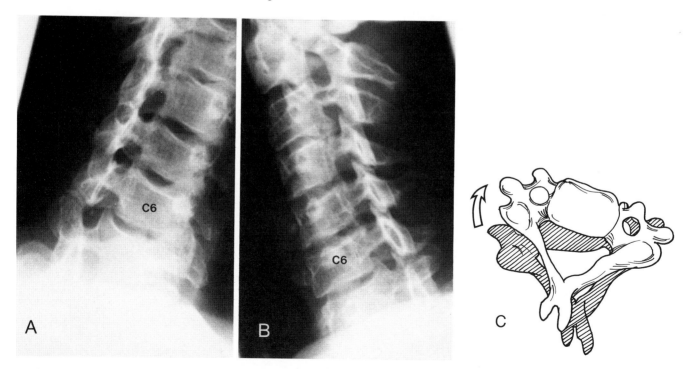

Figure 9.51. UNILATERAL INTERFACETAL DISLOCATION: C6. A. Cervical Oblique. Observe the altered contour to the C6 IVF, with anterior displacement of the articular pillar and vertebral body.   **B. Opposite Cervical Oblique.** No abnormality is visible, with a normally shaped intervertebral foramen, articular pillar, and vertebral body alignment.   **C. Schematic Diagram.** Unilateral interfacetal dislocation occurs in an anterior direction, following a severe rotational trauma.   ***Comment:*** Unilateral interfacetal dislocations are frequently overlooked and are best visualized on oblique radiographs.

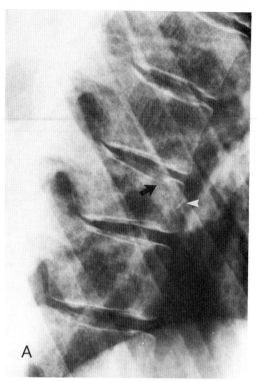

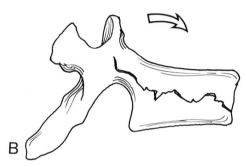

A

B

Figure 9.52. ISOLATED COMPRESSION FRACTURE: THORACIC SPINE. A. Lateral Thoracic. Focal depression of the superior end plate (arrow) of the T10 vertebral body, with a displaced anterior fracture fragment (arrowhead), is identified. A characteristic trapezoidal vertebral shape has been formed due to anterior compression of the superior vertebral end plate. **B. Schematic Diagram.** The usual precipitating force is an anterior compression injury focusing the compressive forces to the anterior aspect of the vertebral body. (Courtesy of Richard M. Nuzzi, DC, Denver, Colorado)

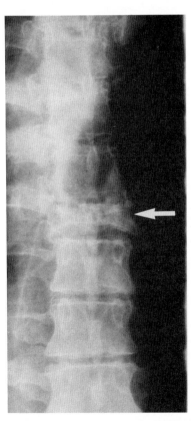

Figure 9.53. COMPRESSION FRACTURE: ANTEROPOSTERIOR RADIOLOGICAL FEATURES. The most notable features are a decrease in vertebral height, with approximation of the vertebral end plates, and associated lateral displacement of the vertebral body margins (arrow). (Courtesy of Lawrence P. Rosenbaum, MA, DC, MD, Linköping, Sweden)

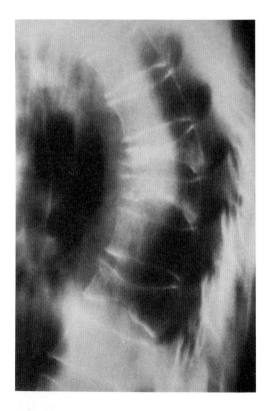

Figure 9.54. MULTIPLE COMPRESSION FRACTURES COMPLICATING OSTEOPOROSIS. Multiple compression fractures are present within the midthoracic spine, as evidenced by decreased anterior body height and biconcave deformities of the vertebral end plates. **Comment:** Thoracic wedge compression fractures are a frequent complication of osteoporosis and may accentuate the kyphotic curvature.

446

dislocation. Frontal radiographs reveal upward rotation of the spinous process of the dislocated segment. Oblique projections are necessary to identify the dislocated facet joint.

FRACTURES AND DISLOCATIONS OF THE THORACIC SPINE

Compression Fracture

Most compression fractures of the thoracic spine occur from T9 through T12 and follow an acute flexion injury. Compression fractures between the T4 and T8 segments occasionally occur in association with injuries related to convulsions or electric shock therapy as a result of violent contractions of the thoracic and abdominal muscles. Most compression fractures in the thoracic spine are wedge shaped, with few having any associated neurological deficit. (Fig. 9.52A and B, 9.53, 9.54) The presence of a paraspinal mass (edema) may be an indirect clue to the presence of a fracture. Additional views (swimmer's lateral) and tomography may be necessary in order to demonstrate fractures of the upper thoracic spine.

Radiographic signs of compression fracture are covered under "Fractures and Dislocations of the Lumbar Spine."

Fracture Dislocation

Fracture dislocation of the thoracic spine occurs most often in the T4–T7 area. Fractures of the lamina, facets,

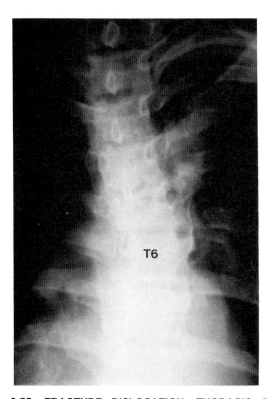

Figure 9.55. FRACTURE DISLOCATION: THORACIC SPINE. There has been a compression deformity of the T5 vertebral body, in combination with a lateral dislocation of the fractured segment. **Comment:** Fracture dislocations of this variety are frequently associated with severe trauma and complicating paralysis.

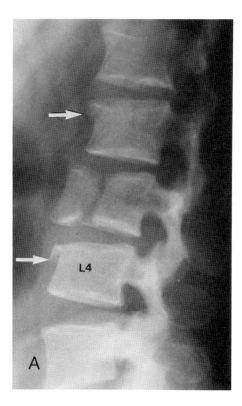

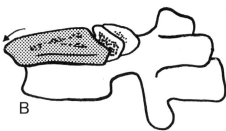

Figure 9.56. COMPRESSION FRACTURE: STEP DEFECT. A. Lateral Lumbar Spine. Step defects (arrows) are present at the anterosuperior corners of the L2 and L4 vertebral bodies, along with a minimal decrease in the anterior vertebral body height. There is an unusual vertical fracture line through the vertebral body of L3. **B. Schematic Diagram: Step Defect. Comment:** The recognition of this step defect may be the only sign of an acute vertebral body fracture. With time, this fracture fragment will be remodeled and will no longer be visible. (Reprinted with permission: Yochum TR, et al: Compression fractures of L2 and L4; an L3 vertical vertebral body fracture. *ACA J Chiro, Radiology Corner*, August 1982)

Table 9.9.
Radiological/Pathological Correlation in Compression Fractures

Radiological	Pathological
Step defect	Cortical offset
Wedge deformity	Anterior impaction
Linear zone of condensation	Impaction, callus
End plate displacement	Impaction, disruption
Paraspinal swelling, psoas obliteration	Bleeding, edema
Abnormal small bowel gas	Reflex adynamic ileus

or vertebral bodies are often associated, (Fig. 9.55) and paralysis is a frequent complication. A great majority of these patients have been in severe automobile accidents.

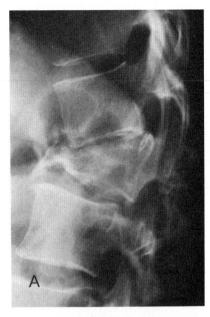

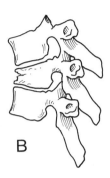

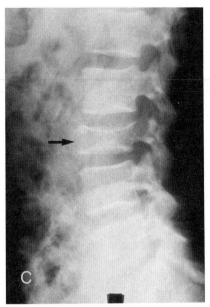

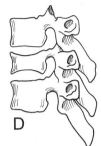

Figure 9.57. TRAUMATIC VERSUS PATHOLOGICAL VERTEBRAL BODY COMPRESSION FRACTURES. A. Lateral Thoracolumbar: Traumatic Compression Fracture. A characteristic trapezoidal configuration of the vertebral body is identified. **B. Schematic Diagram: Traumatic Compression Fracture. C. Pathological Compression Fracture.** Observe the uniform collapse of the L3 vertebral body (arrow). A subtle loss of bone density due to multiple myeloma accompanies this deformity. **D. Schematic Diagram: Pathological**

Compression Fracture. *Comment:* In all compression fractures of the spine the posterior aspect of the vertebral body must be assessed. A decrease in this posterior dimension signifies underlying bone pathology, a radiographic sign which is not found in traumatic benign compression fractures. The most common causes for pathological fractures of this nature are metastatic carcinoma and multiple myeloma.

FRACTURES AND DISLOCATIONS OF THE LUMBAR SPINE

Compression Fractures

Compression fractures of the lumbar spine are the result of a combination of truncal flexion and axial compression. (27) The extent of the vertebral compression and degree of comminution are dependent upon the severity of the force applied and the relative strength of the vertebra. (14) In the aging and geriatric patient with osteoporosis compression fractures are quite common. The most common segmental levels to develop compression fractures are T12, L1 and L2.

Radiographs of optimum quality are necessary in order to adequately demonstrate the subtle and obvious fractures, and, occasionally, tomograms may be necessary. Lateral radiographs best demonstrate the fracture. Many of the compression fractures are work-related injuries, with the first lumbar and twelfth thoracic vertebral bodies being the most common sites for injury. The disruption of the cortical vertebral end plate causes acute symptoms of only 10 days' to 2 weeks' duration, as long as no dislocations accompany the fracture. (28)

Radiographic Signs of Vertebral Compression Fracture. Radiographic signs of vertebral compression fracture include a step defect, wedge deformity, linear zone of condensation, displaced end plate, paraspinal edema, and abdominal ileus. (Table 9.9)

The Step Defect. (Fig. 9.56A and B) Since the anterior aspect of the vertebral body is under the greatest stress, the first bony injury to occur is a buckling of the anterior cortex, usually near the superior vertebral end plate. This sign is best seen on the lateral view as a sharp step off of the anterosuperior vertebral margin along the smooth concave edge of the vertebral body. In subtle compression fractures the "step" defect may be the only radiographic sign of fracture. Anatomically, the actual step off deformity represents the anteriorly displaced corner of the superior vertebral cortex. As the superior end plate is compressed in flexion, a sliding forward of the vertebral end plate occurs, creating this roentgen sign.

Wedge Deformity. (Fig. 9.57A–D) In most compression fractures an anterior depression of the vertebral body occurs, creating a triangular wedge shape. The posterior vertebral height remains uncompromised, differentiating a traumatic fracture from a pathological fracture. This wedging may create angular kyphosis in the adjacent area. It has been estimated that a 30 percent or greater loss in anterior height is required before the deformity is readily apparent on conventional lateral radiographs of the spine. (29)

Linear White Band of Condensation (Zone of Impaction). Occasionally, a band of radiopacity may be seen just below the vertebral end plate which has been fractured. The radiopaque band represents the early site of bone impaction following a forceful flexion injury where the bones are driven together. (Fig. 9.58A and B) Callus formation adds to the density of the radiopaque band later, in the healing stage of the fracture injury. This radiographic sign is striking when present; however, it is an unreliable sign, since it is not present as often as might be expected. Its presence, however, denotes a fracture of recent origin (less than 2 months' duration).

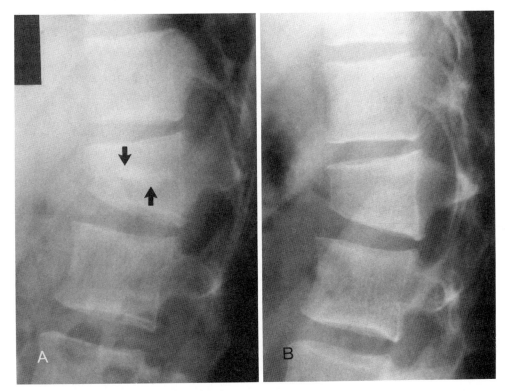

Figure 9.58. COMPRESSION FRACTURE WITH A ZONE OF IMPACTION. A. Lateral Thoracolumbar Spine. A linear radiopaque band extends through the midportion of the L1 vertebral body (arrows). This represents the area of trabecular impaction, resulting in a trapezoid deformity of the vertebral body. **B. Lateral Thoracolumbar Projection: 3 Years Later.** Absence of the zone of impaction signifies a resolved compression fracture; however, the trapezoid deformity of the vertebral body remains permanent.

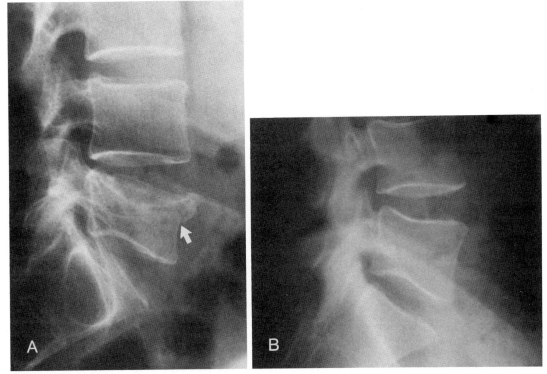

Figure 9.59. DEPRESSED END PLATE FRACTURE VERSUS NUCLEAR IMPRESSION DEFORMITY. A. Compression Fracture: Lateral Lumbar. Significant depression of the superior end plate of the L5 vertebral body, along with a "step" defect (arrow) at the anterosuperior corner, are characteristic signs of acute injury.

B. Nuclear Impression Deformity: Lateral Lumbar Spine. The broad-based, smooth indentation on the inferior surface of the L5 vertebral end plate is characteristic of a nuclear impression (notochordal persistence), and no acute disruption of the vertebral end plate is demonstrated.

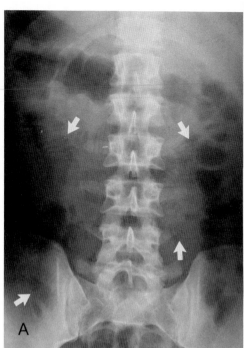

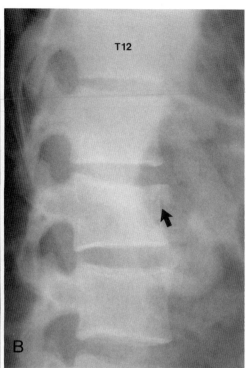

Figure 9.60. ABDOMINAL ILEUS ASSOCIATED WITH VERTEBRAL COMPRESSION FRACTURE. A. AP Lumbar Spine. An excessive amount of small bowel gas is seen (arrows), along with distention of its lumen. **B. Lateral Lumbar Spine.** A wedge type compression fracture, along with a "step" defect (arrow), is present at the superior vertebral end plate of L2. ***Comment:*** The paralytic form of abdominal ileus is often seen following severe trauma and, when present, indicates a likelihood of associated fracture.

Disruption in the Vertebral End Plate. A sharp disruption in the fractured vertebral end plate may be seen with spinal compression fracture. (Fig. 9.59A and B) This may be difficult to perceive on plain films and tomography provides the definitive means to identification. The edges of the disruption are often jagged and irregular.

Paraspinal Edema. In cases of extensive trauma unilateral or bilateral paraspinal masses may occur which represent hemorrhage. These are best seen in the thoracic spine on the anteroposterior projection but may occur adjacent to the lumbar spine, creating asymmetrical densities or bulges in the psoas margins.

Abdominal Ileus. This may occur with severe spinal trauma and is a warning sign to the observer that the trauma has been severe and the likelihood of fracture is great. Abdominal ileus is seen radiographically as excessive amounts of small or large bowel gas in a slightly distended lumen. (Fig. 9.60A and B) It occurs as a result of disturbance to the visceral autonomic nerves or ganglia from paraspinal soft tissue injury, edema, or hematoma.

Determining an Old Versus a New Compression Fracture

Since the wedge shape deformity of the vertebral body persists after the compression fracture heals, additional roentgen signs are necessary to evaluate the time status of a compression fracture. (Table 9.10) The presence of a "step" defect and the white band of condensation are signs of an active or current fracture (less than 2 months old). These two roentgen signs will vanish once the frac-

Table 9.10.
Radiological Criteria for Determining Old and New Compression Fractures of the Spine

	Old	New
Shape	Wedge	Wedge
Step defect	Absent	Present
Band of condensation	Absent	Present
Bone scan	Negative/Positive	Positive

ture totally heals, which may be as long as 3 months in the adult spine.

When the question of presence or recent origin of the fracture arises, a radionuclide bone scan may be helpful. Such scans are positive (hot) with recent fractures undergoing active repair. (29) These scans may stay positive (hot or warm) for as long as 18 months to 2 years following injury. (29) This complicates the evaluation of a patient who has been injured previously (within 2 years). A bone scan may not prove helpful in this type of presentation.

Burst Fractures

These fractures are produced by an explosion of the vertebral body which may occur following a violent axial compression load to the vertebral body, creating a burst fracture. Posterior displaced bone fragments may cause ventral cord or cauda equinal pressure which is best demonstrated by computed tomography.

On the frontal radiograph a vertical fracture line is

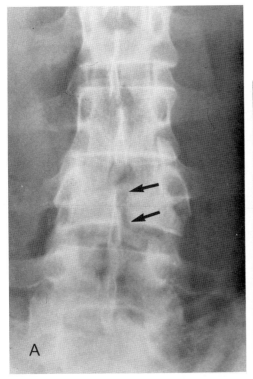
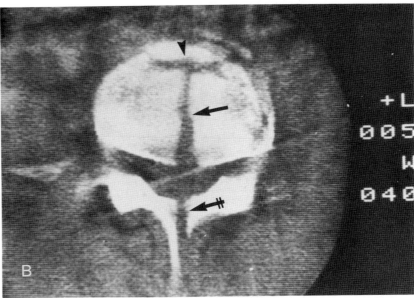

Figure 9.61. BURST FRACTURE: LUMBAR SPINE. A. AP Lumbar Spine. There is a vertical fracture line through the vertebral body of L4 (arrows). **B. Computed Tomogram: L4.** The vertical fracture line in the body of L4 is observed (arrow). A transverse anterior vertebral body fracture (arrowhead), and a fracture through the lamina (crossed arrow) are well demonstrated on this computed tomogram. (Courtesy of Gary L. Whitehead, DC, Las Vegas, Nevada)

often seen, a point which helps differentiate the simple wedge compression fracture from the burst fracture. (Fig. 9.61A and B) Central depression of the superior and inferior end plates occurs with comminution of the vertebral body and is best seen on the lateral film.

Kummel's Disease

Kummel was the first to describe delayed post-traumatic vertebral collapse. (30) Kummel originally described a rarefying process in the vertebral bodies of an injured patient occurring months after an episode of spinal trauma which was clinically inadequate to account for the findings. (28)

The existence of this condition is controversial. In the more recent literature (the last 50 years) few cases have been reported. Schinz et al (31) doubt the existence of Kummel's disease and believe that fractures of the spine are seldom occult and should be diagnosable at the time of injury with good quality radiographs, an opinion which we the authors share.

Fractures of the Neural Arch

Transverse Process Fractures. Transverse process fractures are the second most common fractures of the lumbar spine, with compression fracture being the most common. (31) They occur usually secondary to a severe hyperextension and lateral flexion blow to the lumbar spine from avulsion of the paraspinal muscles. The most common segments to suffer transverse process fractures are L2 and L3. (Fig. 9.62) They are often multiple, and the fracture line is usually obliquely or vertically oriented. Radiographically, the transverse process fracture line appears as a jagged radiolucent separation, usually occurring close to its point of origin from the vertebra. (Fig. 9.63) Frequently, the separated fragment is displaced inferiorly. If the fracture line is horizontal, close inspection for a transverse or chance fracture should be performed. Occasionally loss of the psoas shadow may occur secondary to hemorrhage.

Fractures of the fifth lumbar transverse process are frequently found in association with pelvic fractures, particularly fractures of the sacral ala or disruption of the sacroiliac joint. (14) A confusing appearance simulating fracture of the transverse processes includes congenital transverse process nonunion, especially at L1 and at the psoas margin where it crosses the transverse tip. Occasionally, a fat plane or intestinal gas may be superimposed over the transverse process, mimicking a fracture line. Oblique or tilt views may be necessary to rule out fracture.

Renal damage may occur in association with transverse process fractures of the lumbar spine. A urinalysis searching for hematuria is mandatory in patients with transverse process fractures.

Pars Interarticularis Fractures. Fractures of the pars interarticularis are uncommon. (32) The mechanism of injury is violent hyperextension of the lumbar spine, usually producing the pars fracture at the L4 or L5 level. (Fig. 9.64) The fracture line is seen as a jagged radiolucency which is usually vertically oriented and is best seen on oblique radiographs ("collar" sign).

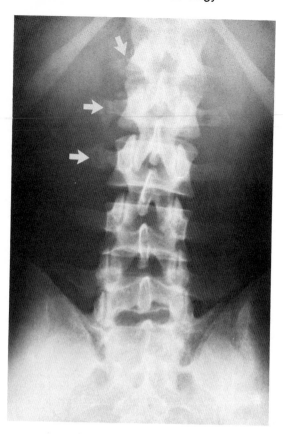

Figure 9.62. MULTIPLE TRANSVERSE PROCESS FRACTURES: LUMBAR SPINE. Healing transverse process fractures are noted involving the left transverse processes of L1, L2, and L3 (arrows). Callus formation is noted adjacent to the fracture line at the L2 and L3 level.

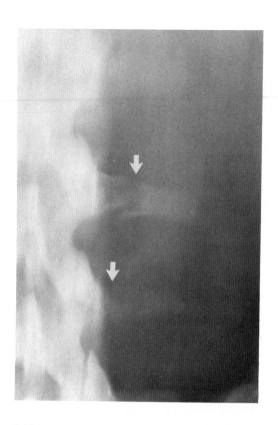

Figure 9.63. TRANSVERSE PROCESS FRACTURES: LUMBAR SPINE, AP TOMOGRAM. Irregular fracture lines are seen at the base of the L3 and L4 transverse processes (arrows). A significant number of patients with transverse process fractures may have hematuria, a sign of renal damage. (Courtesy of Deborah E. Springer, DC and George E. Springer, DC, Denver, Colorado)

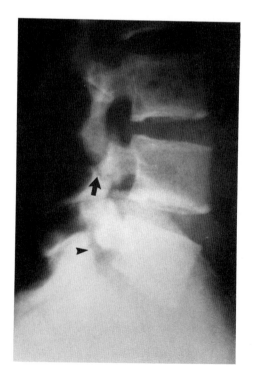

Figure 9.64. UNILATERAL FRACTURE OF THE PARS INTERARTICULARIS: L4. The jagged radiolucent fracture line of the L4 pars is demonstrated (arrow). A bilateral spondylolysis of the pars interarticularis is present at the L5 vertebra (arrowhead). *Comment:* Fractures of the pars interarticularis are uncommon and usually follow violent hyperextension of the lumbar spine, as was the case in this 16-year-old male patient, who was "clipped" while playing football. It is of particular interest to note that the force required to fracture the pars at L4 had no effect on the position of the L5 vertebra, which had bilateral spondylolysis present prior to the trauma. For further discussion concerning displacement in spondylolisthesis, see Chapter 5. (Courtesy of Barton W. DuKett, DC, Bigelow, Arkansas)

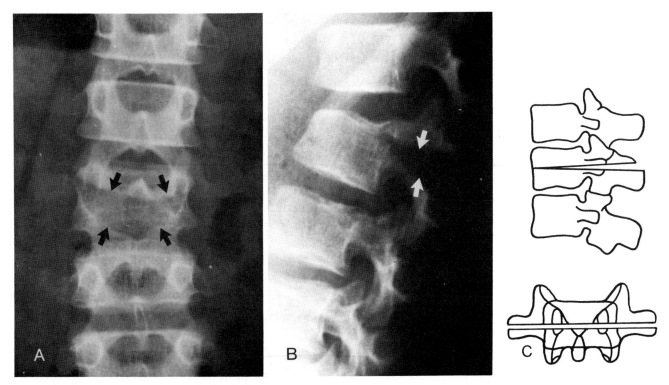

Figure 9.65. CHANCE OR LAP SEATBELT FRACTURE. A. AP Lumbar Spine. There is a clear transverse fracture through the pedicles, pars interarticularis, lamina, and spinous process of the L3 vertebra (arrows). **B. Lateral Lumbar Spine.** There is superior angulation of the superior portion of the fractured vertebra, creating a wide radiolucent gap between the two fracture segments (arrows). This has been referred to as the "empty" vertebra. **C. Schematic Diagram. *Comment:*** The chance or lap seatbelt fracture represents an injury caused by the seatbelt acting as a fulcrum over which the vertebral body and neural arch is split transversely into two parts in severe motor vehicle accidents. This has also been referred to as a "fulcrum" fracture.

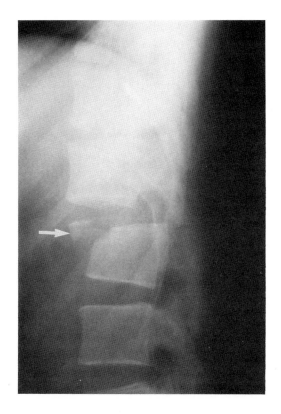

Figure 9.66. FRACTURE DISLOCATION AT THE THORACOLUMBAR JUNCTION. A complete dislocation of T12 upon L1 with an associated teardrop avulsion fracture at the anterosuperior corner of L1 (arrow) is noted. This injury resulted in severance of the spinal cord and paralysis. (Courtesy of David P. Thomas, MD, Melbourne, Australia)

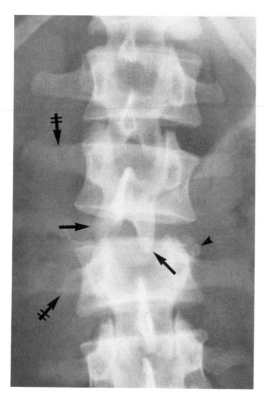

Figure 9.67. FACET DISLOCATION: LUMBAR SPINE. Note the inferior facet dislocations affecting the L2 vertebra (arrows). Associated fractures of the superior vertebral end plate of L3 (arrowhead) and unilateral transverse processes of L2 and L3 (crossed arrows) are present.

Acute fractures of the pars interarticularis should not be confused with spondylolysis of the pars, which is usually the result of a stress fracture. (33) Acute fractures are invariably unilateral, while spondylolysis is usually bilateral. The acute fractures frequently heal without residual defects.

Chance or Lap Seat-Belt Fracture:

In 1948 Chance (34) described a peculiar fracture of the vertebra consisting of "horizontal splitting of the spine and neural arch, ending in an upward curve which usually reaches the upper surface of the body just in front of the neural foramen."

With the advent of the lap seat belt in the 1950's and 1960's, the Chance fracture has been found with increasing frequency as a result of injuries sustained while wearing it. (35) This fracture has also been referred to as a "fulcrum" fracture of the lumbar spine. (14)

This injury is produced by the seat belt acting as a fulcrum over which the vertebral body and neural arch is split transversely into two parts. Often, severe abrasions can be seen on the lower anterior abdominal wall, outlining the position of the seat belt at the time of impact. Internal visceral damage may also occur, such as rupture of the spleen or pancreas and tears of the small bowel and mesentery. Neurological deficit occurs in 15 percent of cases. (36) The most common location for the transverse Chance fracture is in the upper lumbar spine (L1–L3). (36)

Radiographic detection of the Chance fracture is often represented by two appearances on the frontal radiograph: 1) a clear transverse fracture through the osseous elements; and 2) rupture of the soft tissue structures and angulation of the superior portion of the fractured vertebra. (Fig. 9.65A and B) This leaves a wide radiolucent gap between the two fractured segments which has been referred to as the "empty" vertebra. (28) Often, a break in the oval cortex of the pedicles or a split in the spinous process can be seen. (Fig. 9.65C) The lateral radiograph usually demonstrates the radiolucent split through the spinous process, lamina, pedicle, and the upper corner of the posterior aspect of the vertebral body. (Fig. 9.65B) This appearance is characteristic of the Chance or lap seat-belt fracture.

Fracture Dislocation

The vast majority of the fracture dislocations of the lumbar spine occur in the thoracolumbar area following a violent flexion injury. Avulsion fractures (teardrop) are commonly found associated with dislocations of the lumbar spine. (Fig. 9.66) Complete luxation with lateral shift of the spine may create cord or cauda equina paralysis. Most dislocations are anterior in position, without lateral displacement. Shearing injuries to the soft tissue and osseous structures of the neural arch, along with discal rupture and disintegration, may also be found with dislocations of the lumbar spine. (Fig. 9.67)

Fractures of the Pelvis

SACRAL FRACTURES

Sacral fractures usually occur as a result of a fall upon the buttocks or following a direct trauma. There are two types—horizontal and vertical.

Horizontal (Transverse) Fractures. These are the most common type of sacral fractures. The most common location is at the level of the third and fourth sacral tubercle, which is near the lower end of the sacroiliac joint. (Fig. 9.68) The fracture line is frequently difficult to identify due to overlying gas and feces. Often, a cleansing enema of the lower bowel and rectum before the radiological examination facilitates its demonstration. The lateral radiograph is usually required to demonstrate the fracture. (Fig. 9.69) Often, the lower segment of the sacrum may be displaced or angled forward. (1) (Fig. 9.70)

A horizontal fracture of the upper sacrum, affecting the first or second sacral segments, may occur from falls from a height. It is usually associated with suicidal attempts by jumping ("suicidal jumper's" fracture). (2)

Vertical Fractures. These usually occur as a result of indirect trauma to the pelvis. They are visible in the frontal radiograph but not the lateral view. The cephalic tilt view or tomography may be necessary in order to demonstrate the vertical fracture line, which usually runs nearly the entire length of the sacrum. (1) (Fig. 9.71) The normally symmetrical transverse sacral foraminal lines should be carefully scrutinized for detection of the fracture line.

Isolated fractures of the sacrum are uncommon, and a

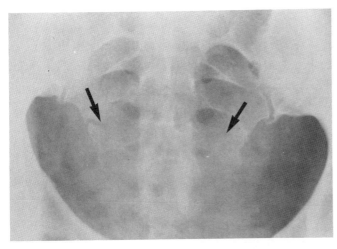

Figure 9.68. HORIZONTAL SACRAL FRACTURE. A radiolucent fracture line is seen just inferior to the fourth sacral foramina (arrows). *Comment:* Horizontal fractures are the most common type of sacral fracture. Their most common location is near the lower end of the sacroiliac joints, around the level of the third and fourth sacral tubercle.

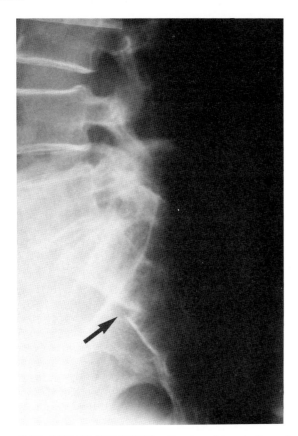

Figure 9.69. SACRAL FRACTURE. Fracture through the anterior surface of the second sacral segment creates an acute offset of its anterior cortical surface (arrow).

diligent search for an associated fracture of the pelvic ring or symphysis pubis is often beneficial.

Coccygeal Fractures

Most fractures of the coccyx are transversely oriented, similar to those of the sacrum. Seldom are they seen on the frontal radiograph; the lateral film best demonstrates this type of fracture. The fracture line is usually oblique in presentation, and slight anterior displacement of the distal coccyx is quite common. (Fig. 9.72) Developmental variation in the position of the distal coccygeal segment may provide some concern to the inexperienced observer.

FRACTURES OF THE ILIUM

Iliac Wing Fractures

The first description of an iliac wing fracture was by Duverney, and this fracture bears his name. (3) They are usually caused by direct force from a lateral direction, causing a splitting of the iliac wing. The fracture line is best seen on oblique views as a single radiolucency (Fig. 9.73A and B) or may appear as a stellate radiation. There is very little separation of the fracture fragments because of the surrounding large muscle attachments. This is a stable fracture.

Malgaigne Fracture

A Malgaigne fracture of the pelvis results from a double vertical shearing injury to the pelvis. (4) It is by far the most common fracture, involving one hemipelvis, and represents approximately one-third of all pelvic fractures. (5) It is defined as an ipsilateral double vertical fracture of the superior pubic ramus and the ischiopubic ramus, with fracture or dislocation of the sacroiliac joint. (Fig. 9.74A and B) Superior or posterior displacement of the entire hemipelvis may occur, with fracture of the fifth

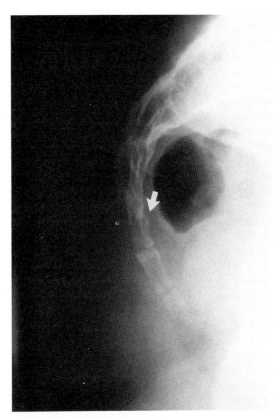

Figure 9.70. FRACTURED SACRUM. There is a fracture of the distal sacrum, with slight anterior displacement of the fracture fragment (arrow). (Courtesy of Philip C. Lening, DC, Golden, Colorado)

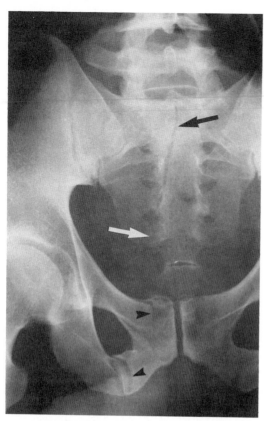

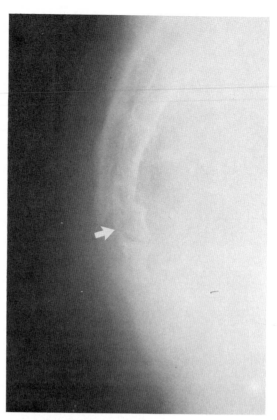

Figure 9.71. VERTICAL FRACTURE OF THE SACRUM. A radiolucent vertical fracture extends through the entire height of the sacrum (arrows). Fractures of the superior and inferior pubic rami are also noted (arrowheads).

Figure 9.72. COCCYX FRACTURE. There is an oblique fracture through the distal surface of the coccyx, with minimal anterior displacement (arrow).

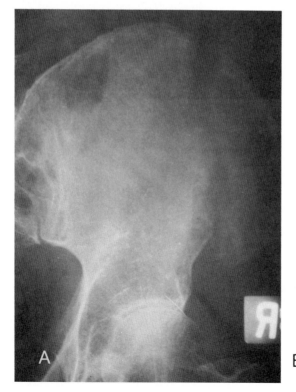

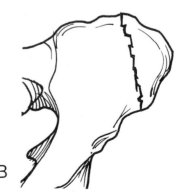

Figure 9.73. DUVERNY'S FRACTURE OF THE ILIAC WING. A. AP Pelvis. There is a large radiolucent fracture line visualized through the lateral surface of the iliac wing (Duverny's fracture). **B. Schematic Diagram: Duverny's Fracture.**

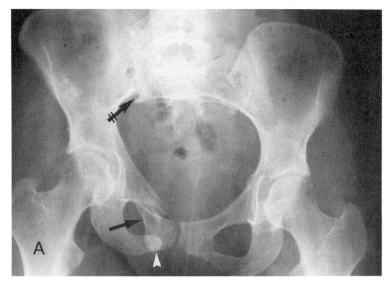

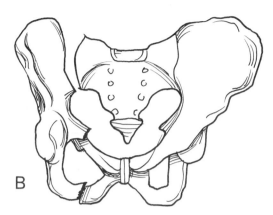

Figure 9.74. MALGAIGNE FRACTURE OF THE PELVIS. **A. AP Pelvis.** Observe the unilateral superior pubic ramus fracture (arrow), inferior pubic ramus fracture (arrowhead), and fracture dislocation through the ipsilateral sacroiliac joint (crossed arrow). This patient has an old, healed Malgaigne fracture. (Courtesy of Joseph W. Howe, DC, DACBR, Los Angeles, California) **B. Schematic Diagram: Malgaigne Fracture.**

lumbar transverse process. This is an unstable fracture, since it has a high morbidity and mortality rate. Rupture of the diaphragm and bowel may complicate the injury.

Bucket-Handle Fracture

The bucket-handle fracture represents a fracture through the superior pubic ramus and ischiopubic junction on the side opposite the oblique force of impact to the pelvis. A fracture or dislocation of the sacroiliac joint on the side of impact is part of the injury. (6) (Fig. 9.75A–C) This fracture is usually the result of an automobile or auto/pedestrian accident. The pubic component of the fracture is usually displaced inward and superiorly. Associated injuries to the abdominal viscera, head, and thorax may be present.

Acetabular Fractures

Approximately 20 percent of all pelvic fractures in adults involve the acetabulum. (7) Most occur in automobile or auto/pedestrian accidents. Almost all acetabular fractures are due to indirect injury, i.e., injury to the foot, knee, or greater trochanter of the femur. This type of fracture is related to the position of the femur at the time of trauma.

A helpful soft tissue sign of fracture of the acetabulum is to search for signs of capsular distension. The fat plane overlying the obturator internus muscle should be observed for displacement or asymmetry. A positive obturator internus sign may indicate a hematoma beneath or within the obturator internus.

There are four basic types of acetabular fractures:

Posterior Rim Fracture (Dashboard Fracture). This type of fracture usually occurs after a blow to the knee while the leg is in flexion and adduction. Often, there is a posterior dislocation of the hip. This fracture also represents one-third of all acetabular fractures. (3)

Simple Posterior Column Fracture. This is an uncommon fracture. On the frontal view the ilioischial line is displaced medially and separated from the teardrop. It is best seen on an external oblique projection.

Central Acetabular Fracture (Explosion Fracture). This type of fracture is the most common acetabular fracture. It divides the innominate bone into superior and inferior halves. In the transverse type, the fracture line bisects the ischial spine. (Fig. 9.76)

In the oblique variety the fracture extends posterosuperiorly to the sacrosciatic notch. This fracture is difficult to diagnose, and a positive obturator internus sign may be the only roentgen finding. If the fracture is severe, there may be central dislocation of the femoral head.

Simple Anterior Column Fracture. The fracture may terminate anywhere along the pubis or ischiopubic junction. On the frontal view there is a loss of continuity of the iliopubic line and medial displacement of the teardrop. This fracture is best visualized on an internal oblique view.

Avulsion Fractures

An avulsion fracture of the ilium is described as a separation of a bony fragment, usually a tuberosity or bony process (apophysis or epiphysis) from a bone. These fractures most commonly occur in athletes, usually prior to fusion of the involved growth center, and are mediated by severe, uncontrolled muscular contractions. They are particularly common in sprinters, long jumpers, gymnasts, hurdlers, and cheerleaders. (4) These fractures might be considered the adolescent equivalent of muscle pulls in mature athletes. (5)

Avulsion fractures of the ilium include: (Fig. 9.77)

Anterosuperior Iliac Spine (ASIS). This involves avulsion by the sartorius muscle. It appears radiographically as a displacement of a bony fragment from the anterosuperior iliac spine which is curvilinear. (Fig. 9.78A and B) Pain is classically relieved by hip flexion.

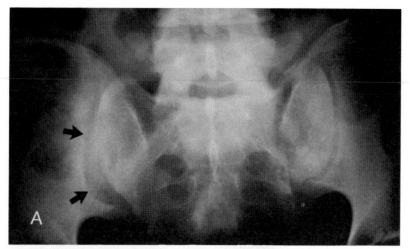

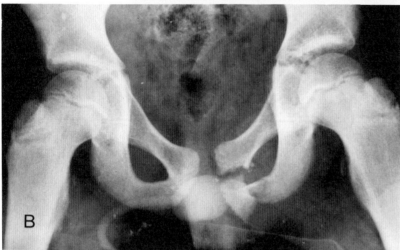

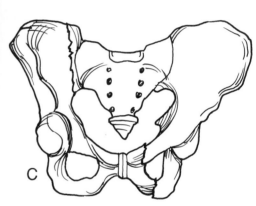

Figure 9.75. BUCKET-HANDLE FRACTURE OF THE PELVIS. A. AP Sacrum. Diastasis of the sacroiliac joint is present (arrows). **B. AP Pelvis.** A contralateral fracture of the pubic ring. **C. Schematic Diagram.** Bucket-handle fracture of the pelvis.

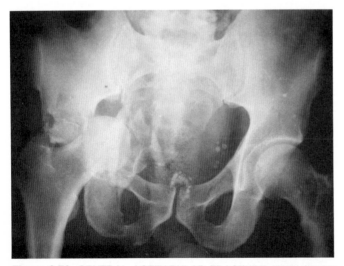

Figure 9.76. CENTRAL ACETABULAR FRACTURE (EXPLOSION FRACTURE). Complete dissolution and bony fragmentation of the acetabulum is noted, as the femoral head has been driven through its roof. The bony fragments are also seen, and an associated fracture through the ipsilateral ischium is present. **Comment:** Central acetabular fractures ("explosion" fractures) are the most common acetabular fracture and divide the innominate bone into superior and inferior halves.

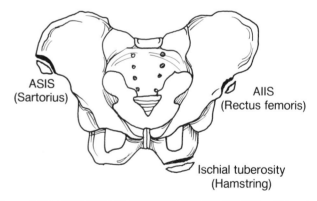

Figure 9.77. AVULSION FRACTURES OF THE PELVIS. This schematic diagram demonstrates the three most common areas of avulsion fractures of the pelvis.

Anteroinferior Iliac Spine (AIIS). This represents avulsion by the rectus femoris muscle. It appears radiographically as a downward displacement of a fragment of bone away from the anteroinferior iliac spine. (Fig. 9.79A and B) Active flexion of the hip in these patients is painfully limited. This is a common fracture in rugby, soccer, or football players.

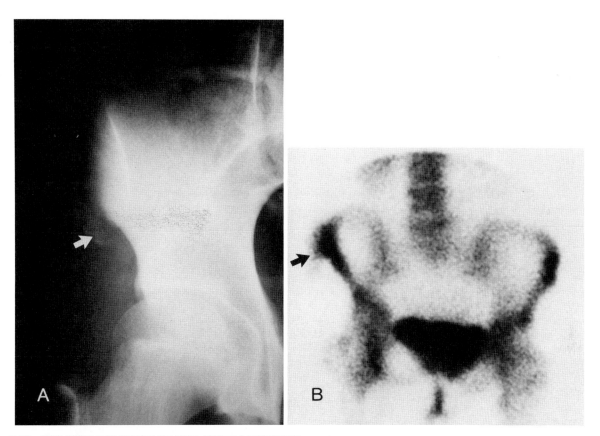

Figure 9.78. AVULSION FRACTURE OF THE ANTEROSUPERIOR ILIAC SPINE. **A. AP Pelvis and Hip.** Avulsion of the anterosuperior iliac spine (ASIS) has occurred, leaving a bony fragment in the adjacent soft tissues (arrow). **B. Bone Scan.** There is a large area of increased radionuclide uptake present in the area of the focal avulsion of the ASIS (arrow). The large semicircular black area near the pubic rami represents the distended urinary bladder.

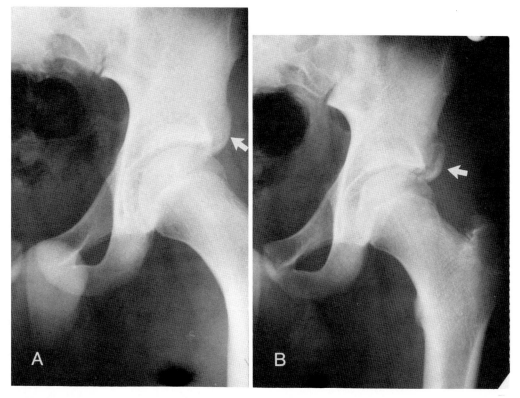

Figure 9.79. AVULSION FRACTURE OF THE ANTEROINFERIOR ILIAC SPINE. **A. AP Hip.** Normal anterosuperior iliac spine (ASIS) (arrow). **B. AP Hip.** An avulsion fracture of the anteroinferior iliac spine (AIIS) is noted (arrow).

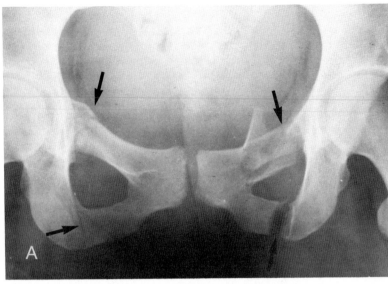

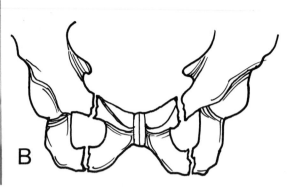

Figure 9.80. STRADDLE FRACTURE OF THE PELVIS. A. AP Pelvis. Double vertical fractures are present involving both the supe-rior pubic rami and the ischiopubic junctions bilaterally (arrows). **B. Schematic Diagram: Straddle Fracture.**

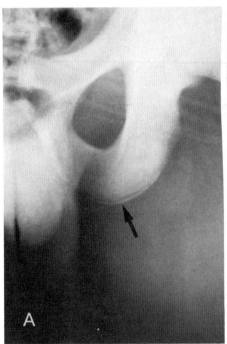

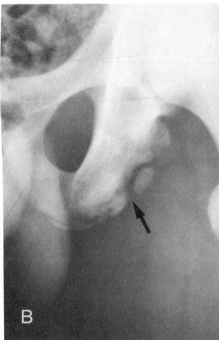

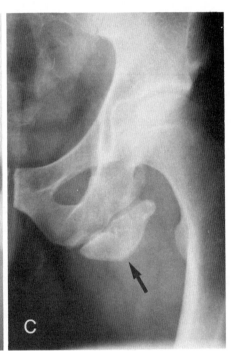

Figure 9.81. AVULSION FRACTURE OF THE ISCHIAL TUBEROS-ITY. A. AP Hip. The normal secondary growth center for the ischial apophysis is noted (arrow). **B. AP Hip.** Fragmentation of the ischial apophysis is observed (arrow). **C. AP Hip.** There is a large bony ossicle noted inferior to the ischial tuberosity, representing the residual overgrowth of the ischial apophysis (arrow) (Rider's bone).

FRACTURES OF THE PUBIS AND ISCHIUM

Straddle Fractures

The straddle fracture or comminuted fracture of the pubic arches is the most common type of unstable fracture of the pelvis. (5,7) This double vertical fracture involves both superior pubic rami and ischiopubic junctions bilat-erally. (Fig. 9.80A and B) The central fracture fragment is usually displaced posterosuperiorly, placing pressure upon the ventral surface of the bladder. Twenty percent of these patients have bladder rupture and urethral tear which may require diagnosis via urethrography and cys-tography. (8)

Avulsion Fractures

Symphysis Pubis. Severe injuries of the major ad-ductor muscles cause a tearing of bone from the superior or inferior pubic rami near the pubic articulation. This injury is common in soccer players.

Ischial Tuberosity (Rider's Bone). This type of frac-ture represents an avulsion of the secondary growth cen-ter (apophysis) for the ischial tuberosity as a result of a forceful contraction of the hamstring group of muscles. (Fig. 9.81A–C) With healing, an unexplained overgrowth of the avulsed apophysis occurs, often leaving a wide radiolucent gap between the avulsed fragment and the parent ischium. This overgrowth may be the effect of hyperemia upon the ischial apophysis. Occasionally, the avulsed ischial apophysis may assume a size larger than the parent ischium. This large overgrowth should not be confused with an extraosseous neoplasm. Usually, the patient's history of a previous severe hamstring injury and the fact that the lesion is asymptomatic secures the proper diagnosis. These fractures are seen most commonly in cheerleaders and hurdlers. The residual bony fragment has been called "rider's bone," as a result of a high percentage of these lesions occurring in horseback riders from chronic stress.

DISLOCATIONS OF THE PELVIS

Sprung Pelvis

The sprung pelvis is a severe injury representing complete separation of the symphysis pubis and one or both of the sacroiliac joints. (Fig. 9.82A and B) It is often stated that the pelvis is opened like a book, with one or both innominates displaced laterally. (4) Because of this analogy, this particular injury is sometimes known as an "open book" or "sprung" pelvis. (9) Severe pelvic basin visceral damage may occur, such as rupture of the urethra.

Pubic Diastasis

This injury represents a shearing separation of the pubic articulation. (Fig. 9.83) The normal distance between the pubic bones should not exceed 8 mm in non-pregnant adults or 10 mm in children. (10) Often, unilateral dislocation of the sacroiliac joint may occur and is frequently overlooked.

ASSOCIATED SOFT TISSUE INJURIES

All fractures of the pelvis may be serious injuries, because of the often associated soft tissue injury.

Common soft tissue complications of pelvic injury include:

Vascular Injuries. Intrapelvic hemorrhage is the most common complication, due to laceration of large blood vessels. Ecchymosis of the scrotum (or labia), inguinal area, and buttocks should make you suspect hemorrhage.

Bladder and Urethral Injuries. The complications are usually due to pubic bone fractures. The incidence is between 10 and 40 percent, depending upon whether the pubic bone fracture is unilateral or bilateral and if one or

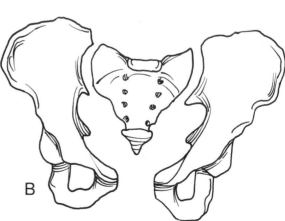

Figure 9.83. PUBIC DIASTASIS. Observe the gross separation of the pubic articulation. A contrast examination was performed to rule out trauma to the bladder and urethra, since this is a common finding accompanying this type of injury. The radiopaque density within the pelvic basin is the contrast-filled bladder.

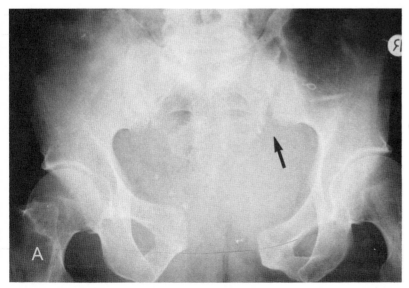

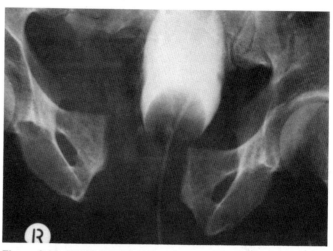

Figure 9.82. SPRUNG PELVIS.   A. AP Pelvis. Severe separation of the pubic articulation and right sacroiliac joint (arrow) characterize the radiographic presentation of a "sprung" pelvis.   **B. Schematic Diagram: "Sprung" Pelvis.**

both pubic rami have been broken. One of the more common injuries is a laceration or complete rupture of the urethra, bladder, and ureters at the trigone, which leads to serosanguineous fluid accumulation within the lower peritoneal cavity. Bruising in the perineum, retention of urine and, especially, fresh blood at the tip of the urethra, are important signs of urinary tract injury in patients who have had pelvic trauma.

Bowel Injuries. This complication usually involves the rectum (laceration or obstruction).

Diaphragm Injuries. The diaphragm is quite often traumatically ruptured in patients with pelvic injury. A radiograph of the chest is a must in all patients who have had pelvic trauma. The left diaphragm is most commonly ruptured, due to the protective effect of the liver on the right side.

Fractures and Dislocations of the Hip

FRACTURE OF THE PROXIMAL FEMUR

General Considerations

Fractures around the proximal femur are relatively uncommon in young to middle-aged patients, with a sharp increase in the geriatric patient. (1) Severe forces are necessary to fracture the proximal femur in the young and middle years, while only moderate to minimal trauma may induce a fracture in the osteoporotic bone of the elderly. Certain predisposing factors may allow fractures to occur, such as the presence of Paget's disease, fibrous dysplasia, benign or malignant bone tumors, osteoporosis, osteomalacia, and radiation-induced osteonecrosis.

The overall incidence of all types of fractures of the proximal femur shows a 2 to 1 female-to-male ratio. (2) A 5 to 1 female predominance exists with intracapsular fractures. (2) The average age is approximately 70 years. (3) It has been estimated that 10 percent of white females and 5 percent of white males will sustain a fracture of the proximal femur by the age of 80 years. (4) The incidence by the age of 90 years increases to 20 percent for women

and 10 percent for men. (4) Many elderly patients with fractures of the proximal femur die within 6 months of the original injury. This occurs secondary to pulmonary or cardiac complications. Therefore, fractures of the proximal femur and their attendant sinister complications are of such proportions that they represent a major health hazard to the elderly and constitute a significant public health issue because of their frequency, morbidity, and cost. (3)

A complete roentgen examination of the hip joint should include an anteroposterior (AP) full pelvis, AP hip spot (involved side), and an oblique or frog-leg projection. A specialized projection such as a groin lateral taken with a horizontal beam and grid cassette may be helpful, particularly with subtle dislocations.

Types of Hip Fractures

The types of hip fractures are divided into intracapsular and extracapsular, as determined by the relationship of the fracture line to the joint capsule. (Fig. 9.84) (Table 9.11)

Intracapsular Fracture. Any fracture involving the femoral head or neck proximal to the trochanters is classified as being intracapsular. These are then named according to the fracture location: 1) subcapital (involving the junction of the femoral head and neck; 2) midcervical (through the midportion of the femoral neck); and 3) basicervical (traversing the base of the femoral neck and its junction with the trochanters).

Most femoral neck fractures are subcapital; midcervical and basicervical fractures are uncommon. (5,6) Subcapital

Table 9.11.
Classification of Fractures of the Proximal Femur

Intracapsular
Subcapital
Midcervical
Basicervical
Extracapsular
Intertrochanteric
Subtrochanteric
Trochanteric

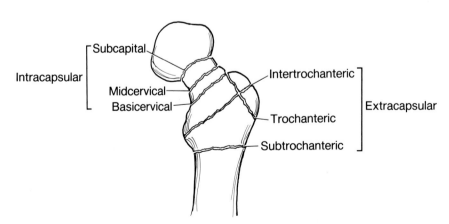

Figure 9.84. PROXIMAL FEMUR FRACTURE CLASSIFICATION. This schematic diagram demonstrates the various types of intrascapular and extracapsular fractures of the proximal femur.

Figure 9.85. SUBCAPITAL FRACTURES.   A. Angular Manifestation. An acute angle at the lateral margin of the femoral neck (arrow) has occurred secondary to a subcapital fracture. Sharp attenuation of the medial cortex (arrowhead) signifies offset of the femoral head and neck.   **B. Impaction Presentation.** A thin radiopacity extends medially from the lateral surface of the femoral neck (arrows), representing the zone of impaction in a subcapital fracture of the femur.

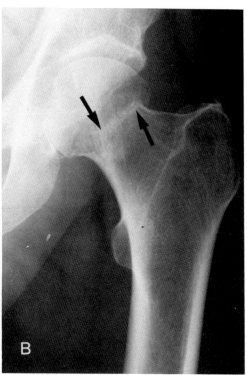

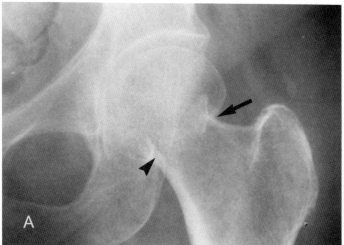

fractures may be impacted, displaced, complete, or incomplete. (3) (Fig. 9.85A and B) In the absence of displacement the fracture line may be difficult to visualize. The most common site is from the junction of the head and neck, superiorly, spiraling anteriorly and inferiorly to the anteromedial aspect of the femoral neck. The much less common midcervical and basicervical fractures are seen as complete transverse fractures involving both the medial and lateral cortices, with a variable degree of displacement. (3) Pathological fractures of the femoral neck are uncommon; when present, they occur in a basicervical location. (3) Nonunion occurs in as high as 25 percent of displaced intracapsular fractures. (3) (Fig. 9.86)

The incidence of avascular necrosis as a complication to femoral neck fractures varies from 8 percent to as high as 30 percent, depending upon early detection and degree of displacement. (7) The major blood supply of the femoral head arises from branches of the medial and lateral femoral circumflex arteries which form a vascular ring around the femoral neck. The branches pass under the capsule and are at risk in intracapsular fracture or dislocation of the hip; therefore, intracapsular fractures are predisposing factors to the development of avascular necrosis. The radiographic changes may appear as early as 3–5 months and as late as 2–3 years after the fracture. (2,7) The average time of appearance of initial radiographic change is 1 year following the injury. (1)

Extracapsular Fracture.   This type of fracture occurs outside of the joint capsule and includes intertrochanteric, subtrochanteric, and avulsion fractures of the greater or lesser trochanters. Avascular necrosis and nonunion are uncommon complications in extracapsular fractures.

The intertrochanteric fractures are usually comminuted, with the greater or lesser trochanter, or both, forming separate fragments. (Fig. 9.87, 9.88A and B) The

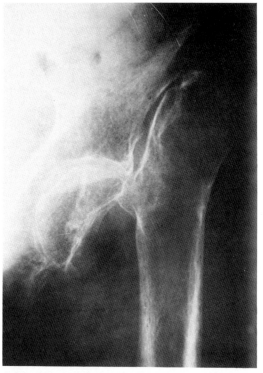

Figure 9.86. OLD SUBCAPITAL FRACTURE OF THE HIP WITH NONUNION.   Nonunion of the fracture site is recognized by the sclerotic margins, the superior displacement of the femoral shaft, and the formation of a pseudarthrosis on the lateral surface of the ilium. (Courtesy of David J. Byrnes, DC, Coffs Harbor, New South Wales, Australia)

oblique fracture line usually splits the trochanters, separating the femur into two components. The proximal component consists of the head and neck, and the distal

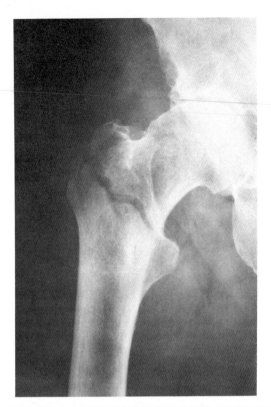

Figure 9.87. INTERTROCHANTERIC FRACTURE OF THE PROXIMAL FEMUR. An oblique fracture line extends from the greater trochanter to the lesser trochanter. This fracture line is extracapsular in location. (Courtesy of Philip S. Bolton, DC, Sydney, Australia)

component includes the shaft and the remainder of the trochanter.

The subtrochanteric fracture is found in the area two inches below the lesser trochanter. This is an uncommon type of fracture of the proximal femur. Mid-diaphyseal fractures follow severe trauma and are prone to malalignment unless treated appropriately. (Fig. 9.89) Pathological fractures of the proximal femur often occur in the subtrochanteric region. Paget's disease and metastatic lesions in the proximal femur may be predisposing factors to the development of a subtrochanteric fracture; thus, the presence of a subtrochanteric fracture should be a signal to the observer to look closely for roentgen signs of adjacent bone disease.

Isolated avulsion fractures of the greater trochanters occur most often in the elderly as a result of a fall. Lesser trochanter avulsions usually occur in children or the adolescent athlete. Most adult lesser trochanter avulsions occur as pathological fractures secondary to a metastatic lesion.

DISLOCATIONS OF THE HIP

Most dislocations of the hip are the result of severe trauma, usually in motor vehicle accidents. Hip dislocations represent 5 percent of all dislocations. (8) They are classified as anterior or posterior, with posterior being the most common type (85%).

Posterior Hip Dislocation

Posterior dislocations occur with the hip in flexion and

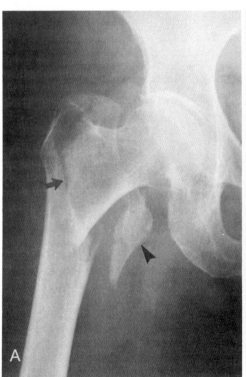

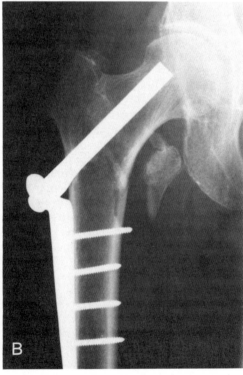

Figure 9.88. COMMINUTED INTERTROCHANTERIC FRACTURE OF THE PROXIMAL FEMUR. **A. AP Hip.** A fracture line from the greater trochanter extends inferiorly (arrow), with displacement of the femoral neck upon the shaft. There is an associated avulsion fracture of the lesser trochanter (arrowhead). **B. AP Hip: Surgical Pinning.** There has been restitution of the normal angle by means of an orthopedic metallic fixation device. The lesser trochanter has not reunited to the femoral shaft.

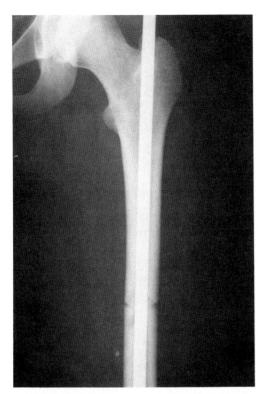

Figure 9.89. MID-DIAPHYSEAL FRACTURE OF THE FEMUR WITH PLACEMENT OF AN INTRAMEDULLARY ROD. Good alignment of a previous mid-diaphyseal fracture of the femur has been obtained by the placement of an intramedullary rod.

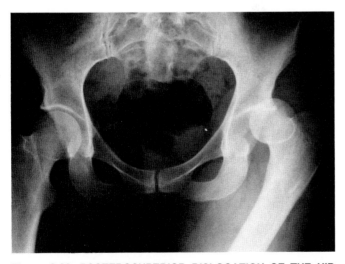

Figure 9.90. POSTEROSUPERIOR DISLOCATION OF THE HIP. Posterosuperior dislocation of the hip is present and represents the most common form of hip dislocation.

usually follow a blow to the knee such as occurs in a dashboard injury. Abduction of the thigh at the time of impact not only induces a posterior dislocation but may result in a fracture of the posterior lip of the acetabulum. This fracture should not be confused with the os acetabuli, a normal variant. Posterior hip dislocation is usually complete, with the entire femoral head out of the acetabulum. (Fig. 9.90)

Anterior Hip Dislocation

Anterior dislocations are caused by forced abduction and extension of the femur. The femoral head usually lies caudal and medial to the acetabulum and near the obturator foramen. (Fig. 9.91)

Complications of Dislocations of the Hip

The most common complication is sciatic nerve paralysis, which occurs in 10–15 percent of cases of posterior dislocation of the hip. (9) This paralysis usually occurs secondary to pressure by the femoral head or displaced acetabular fragments. Myositis ossificans and avascular necrosis of the femoral head occur in 10 percent of cases. (8,9) Post-traumatic degenerative arthritis may occur as a sequella to the previous dislocation.

SLIPPED FEMORAL CAPITAL EPIPHYSIS

General Considerations

Slipped femoral capital epiphysis (SFCE, adolescent coxa vara, epiphyseal coxa vara, epiphyseolisthesis) occurs during the adolescent rapid growth period (10–15 years) and is the result of a slipping of the neck on the femoral head as the head remains in the acetabulum. There is upward displacement, external rotation, and adduction of the neck on the head. The result is a varus deformity, adduction, and external rotation of the femur.

The diagnosis of slipped capital femoral epiphysis requires clinical suspicion. The onset of a limp accompanied by hip pain referred to the knee in an obese adolescent describes the classic presentation. Males are more commonly affected than females, with the peak incidence in males occurring at age 13 and in females at age 12. Blacks are more commonly affected than whites. The left hip is more often involved than the right, and both hips are involved in 20–30 percent of cases. (10) Bilateral involvement is more common in females. Simultaneous bilateral slips are rare, but in cases progressing to bilateral involvement, the second slip usually follows the first within one year. (10) (Fig. 9.92)

Slipped femoral capital epiphysis can be considered a

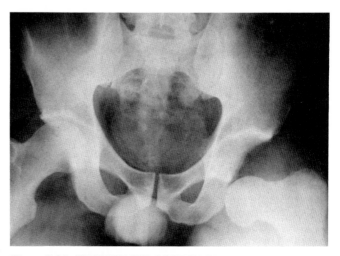

Figure 9.91. ANTERIOR DISLOCATION OF THE HIP. The femoral head lies caudal and medial to the acetabulum, the characteristic position in anterior dislocation of the hip.

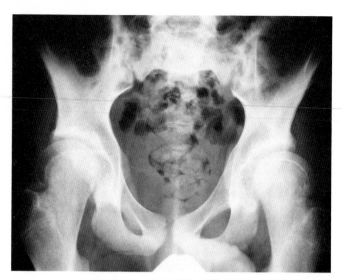

Figure 9.92. BILATERAL SLIPPED FEMORAL CAPITAL EPI-PHYSIS. There is lateral displacement of both femoral capital epiphyses. **Comment:** Slipped femoral capital epiphysis (SFCE) is bilateral in 20–30 percent of cases and affects males more commonly than females, the peak incidence in males occurring at age 13 and at age 12 for females. When unilateral, the left hip is more often involved than the right.

special form of the Type I Salter-Harris epiphyseal fracture, a displacement without visible fracture of either the epiphysis or the metaphysis. Because of the anatomy of the proximal femur, the upper femoral epiphysis is subject to shearing stress, and this may be a predisposing factor to the development of slipped femoral capital epiphysis. About 50 percent of patients have a history of significant injury antecedent to the discovery of slipped femoral capital epiphysis. (10) In such cases it may be the result of trauma and represents an actual traumatic fracture through the growth plate. In some cases it occurs in a normal child without a history of injury. In many cases the exact etiology of the slipped epiphysis is unknown. Many of the children with slipped femoral capital epiphysis tend to be overweight, and slipped femoral capital epiphysis is associated with Fröhlich's type of obesity. Fröhlich's syndrome (adiposogenital dystrophy) is characterized by marked obesity and hypodevelopment of the gonads and is considered a form of hypopituitarism. Slipped femoral capital epiphysis is also associated with renal osteodystrophy and rickets.

Most children with slipped femoral capital epiphysis present with hip, knee, or thigh pain, and a limp. Pain in the thigh and knee is a more common initial presentation than pain in the hip; therefore, a proper orthopedic examination of the hip should be performed in all young patients with knee pain. Irritation of the genu branch of the obturator nerve may explain the knee pain before hip pain in slipped femoral capital epiphysis. Tenderness around the hip exists, with limitation of motion, particularly abduction and internal rotation. The lower extremity gradually develops an adduction and external rotation deformity, with a shortening of leg length. When the slippage is extreme, the gluteus medius is rendered inadequate, and the Trendelenburg test is positive. Bilateral

severe slippage results in a highly characteristic bilateral gluteus medius gait termed a "waddling gait" and is marked by listing of the trunk toward the affected side with each step. (10)

Radiological Features

Radiographic evaluation must include both anteroposterior and frog-leg (oblique) views bilaterally. It is difficult to detect an early or minimal slipped epiphysis on an anteroposterior view, and in many cases the slippage is only demonstrated on the frog-leg view. It is important to obtain films of the hips in any adolescent with unexplained knee pain.

Posterior medial slippage of the epiphysis is usually present. The slip may be predominantly posterior, which would be visible on the oblique (frog-leg) view, or may be predominantly medial, which would then best be visualized on the anteroposterior view. Usually, a combination of posteromedial slippage is present.

The radiographic alterations are usually clearly depicted when the correct signs are searched for in the proper locations. (Table 9.12) Early radiographic changes on the anteroposterior view include a widened, ill-defined growth plate with slight metaphyseal deossification. The height of the epiphysis on the slipped side will be less than on the normal side. Normally, the caput femoris (the part of the femur which is contained within the acetabulum) includes the medial third of the metaphysis. When slipped femoral capital epiphysis occurs, there will be extrusion laterally of the medial one-third of the metaphysis from the acetabulum. As the femoral head is displaced medially and downward, the lower margin of the epiphysis becomes beak-shaped. The frog-leg view will show the abnormal relationship of the femoral head to the femoral neck due to the medial and downward displacement of the femoral head in relationship to the femoral neck.

A very helpful sign enabling detection of slipped capital femoral epiphysis is the use of Klein's line (see Chapter 3). (11) This line is used on the anteroposterior projection and represents a line drawn along the superior lateral cortex of the femoral neck, which extends through a small portion of the lateral margin of the femoral epiphysis, normally. (Fig. 9.93A and B) In slipped epiphysis the femoral epiphysis on the affected side will lie more medial to this line, so that no intersection with the epiphysis occurs at all. It is helpful to compare this with the opposite, uninvolved side. In subtle cases, the alteration in Klein's line may be the only detectable sign of slipped femoral capital epiphysis on anteroposterior radiographs.

Table 9.12.
Radiological Features of Slipped Femoral Capital Epiphysis

Decreased vertical epiphyseal height
Klein's line abnormal
Wide, irregular growth plate
Beaked inferior-medial epiphysis
Increased teardrop distance
Medial buttressing on the femoral neck
Frayed metaphyseal margin

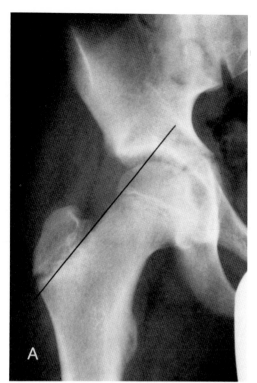

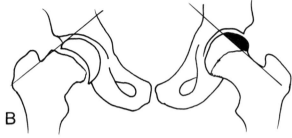

Figure 9.93. SLIPPED FEMORAL CAPITAL EPIPHYSIS: KLEIN'S LINE. A. AP Hip. Normal Klein's line. **B. Schematic Diagram.** Abnormal Klein's line associated with slipped femoral capital epiphysis (SFCE). ***Comment:*** Klein's line is used on the anteroposterior projection of the hip joint and represents the line drawn along the superior lateral cortex of the femoral neck, which extends through a small portion of the lateral margin of the femoral epiphysis, normally. In slipped epiphysis, the femoral epiphysis on the affected side will align more medially to this line so that no intersection with the epiphysis occurs. It is helpful to compare this with the opposite, uninvolved side. In subtle cases this alteration in Klein's line may be the only sign of slipped femoral capital epiphysis on the anteroposterior radiograph.

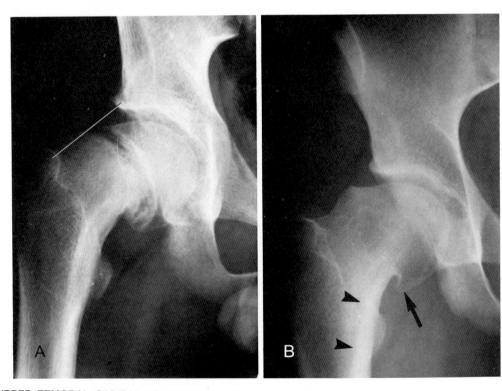

Figure 9.94. SLIPPED FEMORAL CAPITAL EPIPHYSIS. A. AP Hip. There is a significant posteromedial slip of the femoral capital epiphysis, with an alteration in Klein's line. **B. AP Hip.** A 2-year follow-up radiograph after an intramedullary metallic fixation device was placed within the slipped femoral epiphysis demonstrates premature fusion of the growth plate. Early osteophytic formation is present at the anteromedial aspect of the femoral head (arrow). Cortical buttressing (arrowheads) is noted in the area of the femoral neck and the medial aspect of the proximal shaft of the femur. This is a stress response.

(11) (Fig. 9.94A and B) There is an occasional widening of the medial joint space due to intra-articular effusion. In addition, cases which have had a chronic history with no therapy frequently exhibit a layer of periosteal new bone along the medial surface of the femoral neck (buttressing).

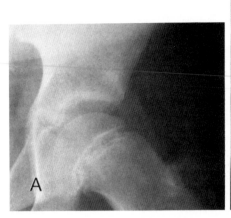
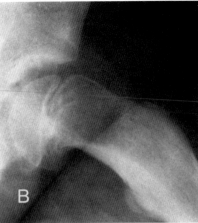
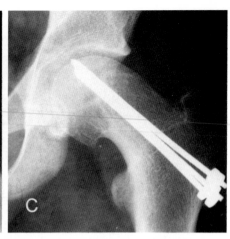

Figure 9.95. TREATMENT FOR SLIPPED FEMORAL CAPITAL EPIPHYSIS. A. AP Hip. B. Frog-Leg Hip. Medial displacement of the femoral capital epiphysis alters the normal relationship of the lateral edge of the femoral epiphysis to Klein's line. The oblique frog-leg projection augments the visualization of the posteromedial epi-physeal slip. **C. Postsurgical Radiograph: AP Hip.** Three threaded metallic pins have been passed through the femoral neck into the area of the epiphysis to prevent further slippage. The metallic fixation has precipitated premature fusion of the growth plate.

Complications

The usual treatment for slipped femoral capital epiphysis is to prevent further slip by fixation of the femoral epiphysis in relationship to the femoral neck by mechanical means, usually some form of threaded pins. Multiple pins are used in order to obtain several points of fixation. The pins are usually removed after growth plate fusion has occurred. (Fig. 9.95A–C)

Following surgical treatment, radiographic follow-up examinations are required until the epiphyseal plate has closed. The opposite and presumed normal hip should also be examined, since bilateral involvement occurs in 20–30 percent of patients, and since this may not happen until weeks or even months after the original slipped epiphysis has occurred.

Complications of slipped femoral capital epiphysis include coxa vara deformity, femoral neck broadening and shortening, avascular necrosis of the femoral head, acute cartilage necrosis (chondrolysis), and degenerative joint disease (osteoarthritis) of the hip. (12) Degenerative joint disease is the most frequent complication. Avascular necrosis or osteonecrosis is an uncommon complication; however, it is more likely to occur if there is operative reduction (forceable manipulation) of the slipped femoral capital epiphysis or if wedge osteotomies of the femoral neck are performed as a corrective procedure (35 percent of cases). (12) For this reason, the displaced slipped femoral capital epiphysis is usually pinned in situ and, if necessary, corrective operative procedures are carried out at a later date. With in situ fixation utilizing pins, the incidence of avascular necrosis is as low as 1.5 percent in some studies. (11,12)

Fractures and Dislocations of the Knee

FRACTURES OF THE KNEE

All bones contributing to the formation of the knee joint may be fractured. (Table 9.13)

Distal Femur

Supracondylar Fractures. These fractures occur in the area of the femur, distal to the shaft and between the condyles. They present as transverse or oblique fractures and are often comminuted. (1) The fracture usually extends into the joint space, limiting the patient's ability to extend the knee. The supracondylar fracture is occasionally associated with fractures or fracture/dislocations of the hip. (2) Supracondylar fractures occur following severe impaction forces on the femur and may also occur with fractures of the tibial shaft. When this occurs, the knee is left isolated from the remainder of the extremity and has been called the "floating knee." (3)

Fractures of the Femoral Condyles. These fractures are intra-articular and are either confined to one or include both condyles. (2) These fractures may be "T" or "Y" shaped and, with separation, the joint frequently becomes deformed. Fractures confined to one condyle are usually obliquely oriented. (Fig. 9.96) A fracture of the condylar articular surface may displace a small osteochondral fragment, resulting in an intra-articular loose body.

Fractures of the Proximal Tibia

Fracture of the Tibial Plateau (Bumper or Fender Fracture). This type of fracture occurs secondary to a forceable thrust of the femoral condyles (which are stronger than the tibial plateau) down upon the tibial plateau. (Fig. 9.97) It is called the "bumper" or "fender" fracture because the tibial plateau is at the approximate height of a car bumper. Since only 25 percent of lateral tibial plateau fractures are due to traffic/pedestrian acci-

Table 9.13.
Sites of Fracture at the Knee

Femur	Patella	Tibia	Fibula
Supracondylar	Waist	Plateau	Styloid
Intercondylar		Condyle	Head
Condylar		Tuberosity	
		Eminences	

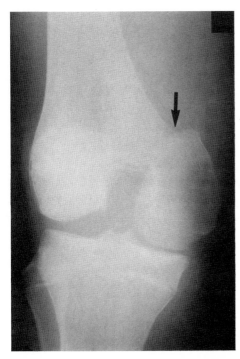

Figure 9.96. FRACTURE OF THE FEMORAL CONDYLE: DISTAL FEMUR. There is a complete fracture affecting the upper margin of the medial condyle of the distal femur (arrow). A large separation between the medial condyle and the remainder of the femur is present.

dents where the knee is struck by an automobile, the fracture is somewhat misnamed. (4,5)

Over half of the patients who sustain a fracture of the tibial plateau are 50 years of age or older. (4) Approximately 5–10 percent of tibial plateau fractures are confined to the medial tibial plateau, another 10–15 percent involve both plateaus, and the remaining 80 percent will be limited to the lateral tibial plateau. (4)

The lateral tibial plateau fracture is quite common and is frequently found in elderly patients with osteoporosis. The radiographic appearance is that of depression of the lateral tibial joint surface, with or without a vertical radiolucent split of the joint margin. The fracture line in undisplaced fractures may be obliquely oriented, and it is often difficult to visualize on the routine anteroposterior and lateral views of the knee. Oblique views are frequently necessary to demonstrate the fracture. (6) Occasionally, tomography may be necessary to establish the size, number, and degree of depression of the fracture fragments. (6) (Fig. 9.98A and B)

Ligamentous injuries occur in 10–12 percent of tibial plateau fractures and occur as a result of severe valgus stress. (4) The medial or lateral collateral ligaments, or the anterior or posterior cruciate ligaments, may be torn. Stress radiographs may be necessary to establish the diagnosis radiographically. After these fractures heal, follow-up radiographic evaluation will demonstrate degenerative osteoarthritis in 20 percent of cases. (4)

Avulsion Fracture of the Anterior Tibial Spine. This fracture occurs at the site of origin of the anterior cruciate ligament. (7) The mechanism of injury is

hyperextension of the knee, with internal rotation of the tibia. They are most often found in children, and over half of these injuries occur in a fall from a bicycle. (7) The radiographic appearance varies with the degree of displacement. Undisplaced fractures consist of a horizontal fracture line at the base of the anterior portion of the tibial spine. Those associated with displacement may allow inversion of the fracture fragment and are usually easier to demonstrate radiographically. (4)

Trampoline Fracture. Fractures of the proximal tibia occur in young children (2–10 years) who jump on a trampoline with another person, if the second person is heavier. As the heavier person jumps, the trampoline mat recoils upward from its stretched downward position. If the smaller child lands on the upward-moving mat at the time its elasticity is reversed by recoil and the springs are shortening to their unstretched length, there is significant upward impaction force applied to the descending child's leg. The force applied at just the right time and angle of impact may be sufficient to cause fractures through the proximal tibial metaphysis. (8)

Avulsion Fracture of the Tibial Tuberosity. This type of fracture usually occurs in association with a comminuted or subcondylar fracture of the proximal end of the tibia. (9) An isolated avulsion fracture of the tibial tuberosity allows for proximal displacement of the fractured fragment and, often, an associated rupture of the infrapatellar tendon. (9) (Fig. 9.99A and B) This injury often takes place during athletic activities where the knee is flexed and the quadriceps tendon contracted and firmly resisting further flexion. (9)

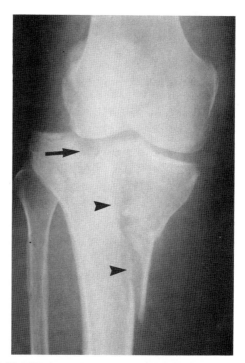

Figure 9.97. TIBIAL PLATEAU FRACTURE (BUMPER OR FENDER FRACTURE): KNEE. The lateral tibial plateau has been depressed, and a radiolucent fracture line is present (arrow). An oblique fracture through the metaphysis below the medial tibial plateau (arrowheads) has allowed caudal displacement of a portion of the medial surface of the tibial plateau.

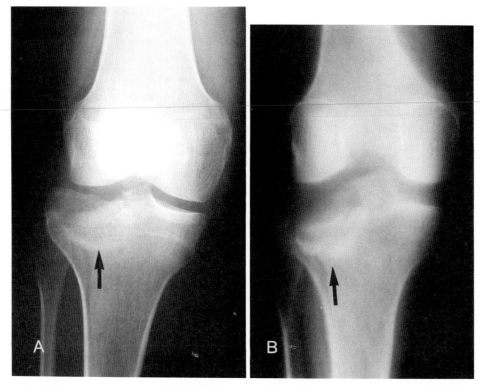

Figure 9.98. BUMPER OR FENDER FRACTURE: A CLASSIC PRESENTATION. A. AP Knee. A characteristic depression of the lateral tibial plateau is noted. Impaction of the lateral tibial plateau is demonstrated by an area of radiopacity (arrow). **B. AP Tomogram: Knee.** Tomographic evaluation of the tibia demonstrates significant caudal displacement of the lateral tibial plateau characteristic of the "bumper" or "fender" tibial plateau fracture. The impaction zone of increased radiopacity is once again demonstrated (arrow).

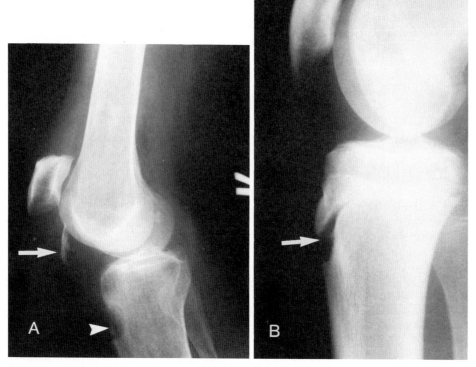

Figure 9.99. AVULSION FRACTURE OF THE TIBIAL TUBEROSITY. A. Lateral Knee. Avulsion of the tibial tuberosity with cephalic displacement is noted (arrow). A radiolucent defect is present in the normal location of the tibial tuberosity (arrowhead). **B. Lateral Knee.** The tibial apophysis during its normal growth may appear to the inexperienced observer to represent an avulsion fracture. The radiolucent area below the tibial growth center represents the cartilaginous plate (arrow). This should not be confused with a fracture or Osgood-Schlatter's disease.

Segond's Fracture. This fracture occurs at the margin of the lateral tibial condyle and represents an avulsion fracture of the bony insertion of the tensor fascia lata (iliotibial band). (10) The significance of the lesion rests in its differential diagnosis from an avulsion fracture of the tip of the proximal fibula.

Fractures of the Proximal Fibula

Isolated fractures of the proximal fibula are very rare and are usually found associated with ligamentous injuries of the knee, fractures of the lateral tibial plateau or ankle; (4) therefore, these associated injuries must be excluded when a fracture of the proximal fibula is noted.

Proximal fibular fractures can present as an impaction, comminuted fracture of the head of the fibula, or avulsion of the proximal pole or styloid process of the fibula. The avulsion injury occurs at the site of attachment of the biceps femoris muscle or lateral collateral ligament. (4) This type of injury may be associated with damage to the common peroneal nerve. (11) The association of ruptures of the lateral capsular and ligamentous structures and peroneal nerve injuries resulting from adduction stresses at the knee has been called the "lateral compartment" syndrome of the knee and "ligamentous peroneal nerve" syndrome. (12)

Lipohemarthrosis

Fractures which enter the joint often create a soft tissue radiological sign of a fat/fluid level secondary to lipohemarthrosis. With an intra-articular fracture, marrow fat may extrude into the joint fluid, along with blood (hemarthrosis). (13) The fat floats upon the superior surface of the blood and synovial joint fluid, creating a fat/fluid level in the suprapatellar bursa (FBI sign—F = fat, B = blood, I = interface). (14)

A horizontal-beam lateral radiograph of the knee is necessary to demonstrate the subtle fat/fluid level. (4) (Fig. 9.100A–C) The presence of lipohemarthrosis is a helpful radiological sign when the clinician is confronted with an injured patient and apparently normal radiographs. Its presence behooves the observer to look closer for an intra-articular fracture.

The knee is the most common joint to be involved; the shoulder is the second most common site. The most likely site for an easily overlooked fracture in association with the presence of lipohemarthrosis is the lateral tibial plateau. (4)

Fractures of the Patella

The patella, because of its superficial position and location within the substance of the quadriceps tendon (which subjects it to the forces of the quadriceps muscle) is susceptible to fracture from both direct and indirect trauma. Fractures of the patella are described by the direction of the fracture. The most common fracture is transverse, or slightly oblique, and involves the midpor-

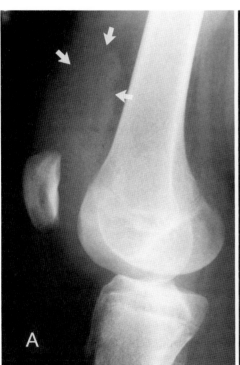
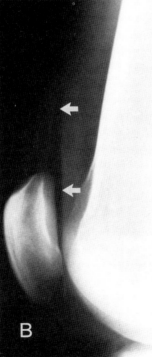
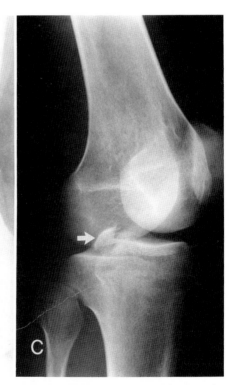

Figure 9.100. LIPOHEMARTHROSIS: AVULSION FRACTURE OF THE TIBIAL EMINENCE. A. Routine Lateral Knee. Observe the anterior displacement of the patella and significant suprapatellar effusion (arrows) in this patient following trauma. No evidence of a fat/blood interface ("FBI" sign) is noted. **B. Cross-Table Lateral: Knee.** A fat/blood interface ("FBI" sign) is noted, with the radiolucent area (arrows) representing the fat and the radiopacity below it representing the sanguinous fluid. **C. Oblique Knee.** Same patient as in B, demonstrating a tibial eminence avulsion fracture (arrow). **Comment:** In order to demonstrate the FBI sign (F=fat, B=blood, I=interface), a cross-table lateral projection is necessary. The patient in Figure A may well have an FBI sign; however, this is a routine lateral film and not a cross-table lateral. The presence of the FBI sign suggests that an intra-articular fracture has occurred, allowing marrow fat to extrude into the joint fluid, along with blood, creating a hemarthrosis.

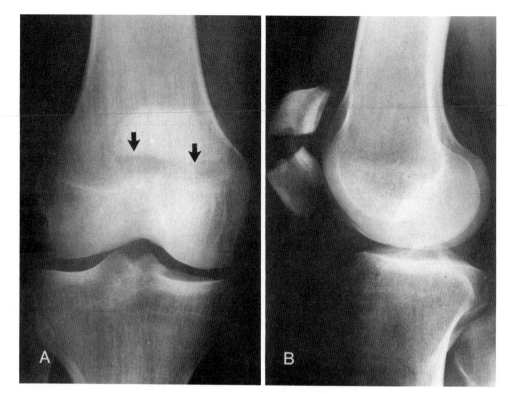

Figure 9.101. PATELLA FRACTURE OF THE KNEE. A. AP Knee. There is a large transverse radiolucent fracture through the patella. This has created a significant radiolucent gap between the superior and inferior pole of the patella (arrows). **B. Lateral Knee.** A transverse fracture of the patella has occurred.

tion of the patella. (15) Transverse patellar fractures represent 60 percent of all types, with comminuted (stellate) accounting for 25 percent and vertical fracture for approximately 15 percent. (15)

Radiographically, the anteroposterior and lateral films will show most patellar fractures. The skyline or tangential view of the patella is the projection which best shows the vertical fracture. The transverse fracture is seen as a radiolucent line, usually through the midportion of the patella. (Fig. 9.101A and B) The stellate or comminuted fracture of the patella presents as a multidirectional radiolucency leaving the patella in fragments. (Fig. 9.102A and B)

The differential diagnosis of patellar fractures is primarily a congenital alteration in the form of a bipartite or tripartite patella. (See Chapter 2) These separated ossicles always occur on the superolateral pole, a rare site for an isolated avulsion fracture. A bilateral presentation is common (80% of cases) and helps confirm the congenital origin. The radiographic appearance of the ossicles are well defined, but this appearance is uncommon with patellar fractures. (Fig. 9.103A and B)

DISLOCATIONS OF THE KNEE

Patellar Dislocation

The patella may dislocate either laterally or around its horizontal or vertical axis. (4) Lateral dislocation is by far the most common type. Lateral patellar dislocation occurs with sudden changes in direction, often while running, as frequently occurs in sports activities. (16) Many times,

the patellar dislocation is transient and has been reduced at the time of injury by an attendant or the patient.

There is a high incidence of osteochondral fractures associated with patellar dislocation, and these have been called "flake" fractures. (17) (Fig. 9.104A–C) These occur as the medial facet of the patella impacts the lateral femoral condyle during the dislocation. These small bony fragments are best seen on the skyline or tangential view of the patella and, if not removed, could be a predisposing factor to the development of degenerative joint disease.

Femorotibial Joint Dislocation

This type of joint dislocation is either anterior or posterior in presentation. (Fig. 9.105) It usually follows severe injury to the knee such as that found in a fall from a significant height or an automobile accident. In either the anterior or posterior dislocation the cruciate ligaments are often torn, along with injuries to the popliteal artery and peroneal nerve. Common tears of the collateral ligaments can be demonstrated by stress radiography. (Fig. 9.106A–C)

Proximal Tibiofibular Joint Dislocation

Dislocation of the proximal tibiofibular joint is classified as anterior, posterior, or superior and is based on the displacement of the head of the fibula. (18) This is an unusual injury, but the anterolateral dislocation is by far the most common. (18) The typical mechanisms of injury are either a fall (landing in the sitting position with the leg flexed beneath the body) or a twisting injury. (4) It is commonly found as a result of participation in various

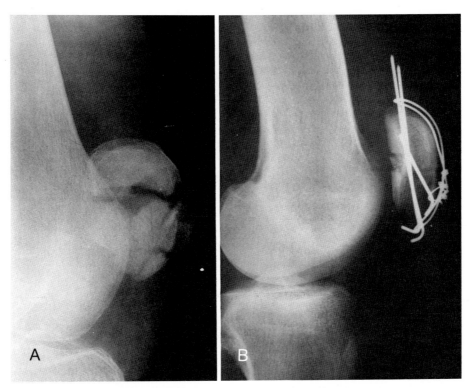

Figure 9.102. COMMINUTED FRACTURE OF THE PATELLA.   A. Oblique Knee. There is a comminuted fracture of the patella, creating a stellate appearance with multiple fragments.

B. Lateral Knee. Surgical fixation is often the treatment of choice in patients with comminuted patellar fractures.

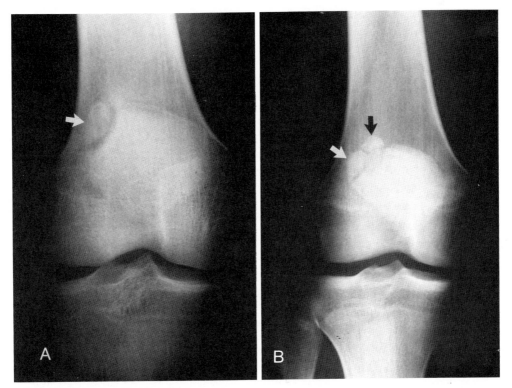

Figure 9.103. NORMAL VARIANT OF THE PATELLA SIMULATING FRACTURE.   A. AP Knee: Bipartite Patella. Occasionally, the patella will exhibit a bony ossicle, representing nonunion of an ossification center (arrow).   **B. AP Knee: Tripartite Patella.** Two bony ossicles (arrows) represent congenital nonunion of the ossification centers.   ***Comment:*** Bipartite and tripartite patellae always occur on the superolateral margins, a rare site for fracture. Most patellar fractures occur in a transverse fashion through the waist. (Courtesy of Kenneth E. Yochum, DC, St. Louis, Missouri)

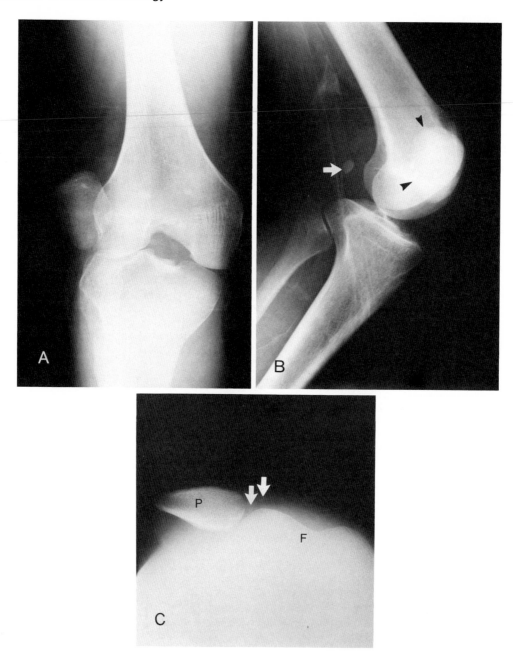

Figure 9.104. DISLOCATION OF THE PATELLA.   A. AP Knee. There is complete *lateral displacement of the patella*.   **B. Lateral Knee.** The *patella is seen superimposed upon the distal femoral condyles* as a result of *gross lateral displacement (arrowheads)*. A fabella is noted in the posterior popliteal fossa (arrow) and should not be confused with an avulsion fragment.   **C. Tangential Knee.** *Complete lateral displacement of the patella (P)* is observed, with *"flake" fractures present adjacent to the lateral condyle* of the distal femur (F) (arrows).

sports and is particularly frequent in parachutists.

The key radiographic appearance is anterior displacement of the head of the fibula. This is best seen on the lateral radiograph. On the frontal view the head of the fibula is seen almost in its entirety, with very little overlap of the lateral tibial condyle. (2) Normally, there is overlap of the tibial condyle at the head of the fibula in the anteroposterior projection.

EPIPHYSEAL INJURIES

Fractures in the area of the knee in children prior to epiphyseal closure may involve the distal femoral or the proximal tibial epiphyses. These lesions may present as any one of the five types of Salter-Harris epiphyseal injuries. (Fig. 9.107)

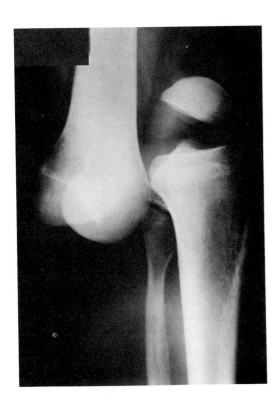

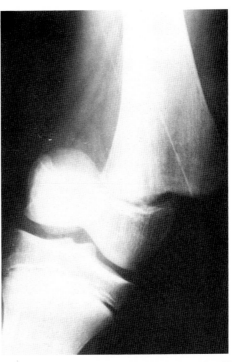

Figure 9.105. FEMOROTIBIAL LUXATION. There is complete dislocation of the femorotibial articulation without fracture. This patient suffered permanent peroneal nerve damage from this injury. (Courtesy of Geoffrey G. Rymer, DC, Sydney, Australia)

Figure 9.107. SALTER-HARRIS FRACTURE OF THE KNEE: TYPE I. There is complete medial displacement of the distal femur on its distal epiphysis.

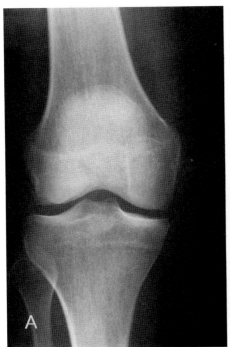

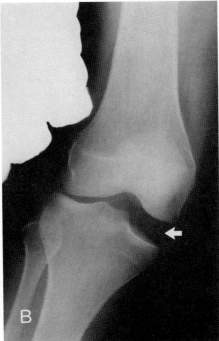

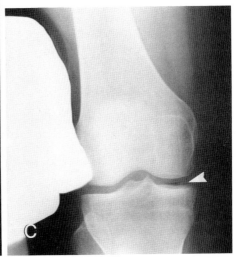

Figure 9.106. STRESS STUDIES OF THE KNEE: LIGAMENTOUS INSTABILITY. A. AP Knee. A routine AP projection of the knee demonstrates no malalignment or instability. **B. AP Knee: Valgus Stress Position.** In the valgus position there is significant widening of the medial joint compartments (arrow), suggesting medial ligamentous instability. This was not appreciated on the original un-stressed AP radiograph (Fig. A). **C. AP Knee: Stress Radiograph.** There is no evidence of malalignment of the medial joint compartment under valgus stress. Observe the normal vacuum phenomenon (arrowhead) present in the medial joint compartment. This is a commonly observed, normal finding with joints under traction.

Fractures and Dislocations of the Ankle

The routine radiographic evaluation of the ankle consists of three views—anteroposterior, lateral, and medial oblique. The medial oblique projection is taken with 35 to 45 degrees of internal rotation of the foot. Special projections (i.e., tomography and stress views) may be helpful in demonstrating subtle fractures or dislocations. The stress views are valuable to confirm ligamentous injuries. (1) They should also be obtained bilaterally whenever there is a question of an increase in width of either the medial or lateral clear space on the radiograph. (1) The views should be obtained with adduction or abduction of the heel and inversion or eversion of the foot, depending upon which ligament is suspect. (2)

FRACTURES OF THE ANKLE

Medial Malleolus Fracture

The medial malleolus is the most distal portion of the tibia. (Fig. 9.108) The fracture is usually transverse or oblique in its orientation. This is due to angular forces generated by movement of the talus against the medial malleoli. Fractures of the medial malleolus distal to the corner formed in the ankle mortise within the plafond are

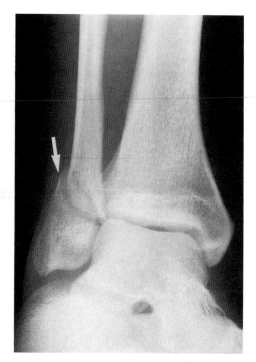

Figure 9.109. DISTAL FIBULA FRACTURE. The most common fracture of the lateral malleolus is an oblique fracture extending upward (arrow). This fracture is best seen on the medial oblique projection.

more stable than those that arise either within the plafond or at the medial corner of the plafond. (3) The plafond is defined as the distal tibial joint surface and is a French term meaning "ceiling." (3) The medial malleolus fracture is best seen on the anteroposterior radiograph as a radiolucent line with adjacent soft tissue swelling.

Lateral Malleolus Fracture

The most distal portion of the fibula is the lateral malleolus. The most common fracture of the lateral malleolus is an oblique or spiral fracture extending from the inferior and anterior margin upward and backward to the posterior margin of the shaft of the distal fibula. (3) (Fig. 9.109) This fracture occurs as a result of outward or external rotation of the foot and is best observed on the medial oblique projection as a radiolucent oblique line with adjacent soft tissue swelling. A variety of small avulsion fractures occur around the tips of either the medial or lateral malleolus. These occur as a result of pull mediated by the medial or lateral collateral ligaments.

Bimalleolar Fracture

Bimalleolar fracture represents a fracture through both the medial and lateral malleolus. The fracture on one side is transverse, because of tensile forces, and the opposite fracture is oblique or spiral. (2) (Fig. 9.110, 9.111) Diffuse soft tissue swelling over the malleoli is often present, alerting the observer to look close for fracture.

Trimalleolar Fracture

Trimalleolar fractures affect the posterior lip of the tibia (sometimes called the third malleolus), in addition to the medial and lateral malleoli. (4) Trimalleolar frac-

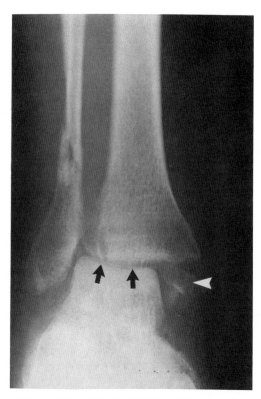

Figure 9.108. MEDIAL MALLEOLUS FRACTURE AND ASSOCIATED DISTAL FIBULA FRACTURE. There is a medial malleolus fracture observed (arrowhead) and an oblique fracture of the distal fibula, along with lateral displacement of the talus. The linear subchondral radiolucency in the talar dome (arrows) is a radiographic sign for an intact blood supply to the talus (Hawkin's sign), which represents the unlikelihood of complicating avascular necrosis.

tures are often found with tibiotalar dislocation. Most are due to external rotation of the foot and are therefore laterally and posteriorly displaced. (4) Fracture of the third

malleolus is best seen on the lateral radiograph, with the fracture fragment being displaced posteriorly and/or superiorly.

Fredrick Cotton, in 1915, described a form of trimalleolar fracture and, in some texts, it is referred to as "Cotton's" fracture. (5) This, however, is incorrect, since Henderson was the first to truly describe the trimalleolar fracture and coin the term. (6) Therefore, the eponym "Cotton's" fracture used in relation to trimalleolar fracture is clearly inappropriate.

Pott's Fracture

Pott's fracture, as classically described, is a partial dislocation of the ankle, with fracture of the fibula within 6–7 cm above the lateral malleolus and rupture of the distal tibiofibular ligaments of the ankle. (7) (Fig. 9.112) Sir Percival Pott described this fracture in 1768 and ascribed the injury to "leaping or jumping." The term "Pott's fracture" has been used erroneously to describe a number of fractures, such as the bimalleolar or trimalleolar fractures. Since neither malleoli are fractured, the term "Pott's fracture" should be avoided.

Dupuytren's Fracture

Dupuytren's fracture was described by Dupuytren based on a single clinical case in 1816 in which a patient who had sustained a fracture of the distal fibula also presented with a widened ankle mortise and medial displacement of the tibia. (8) Dupuytren's fracture, as classically described, is a fracture of the distal fibula (lateral malleolus) with rupture of the distal tibiofibular ligaments, diastasis of the syndesmosis, lateral dislocation of

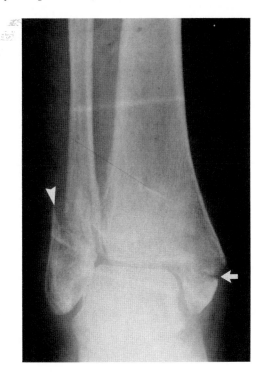

Figure 9.110. BIMALLEOLAR FRACTURE: ANKLE. A characteristic transverse fracture through the medial malleolus (arrow), along with a spiral fracture of the lateral malleolus (arrowhead).

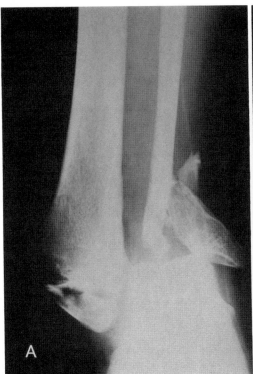 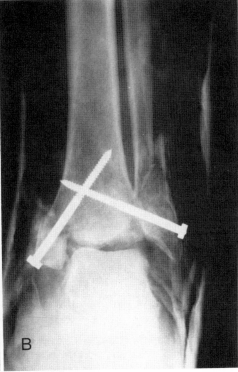

Figure 9.111. BIMALLEOLAR FRACTURE DISLOCATION: ANKLE. A. AP Radiograph. Observe the gross lateral displacement of the talus, with bimalleolar fractures. **B. AP Ankle: Postsurgical Reduction.** Two surgical metallic screws have been placed through the bimalleolar fractures, with good alignment resulting. **Comment:** Fracture dislocation of this magnitude is invariably associated with permanent ligamentous instability of the ankle mortise joint.

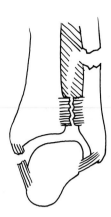

Figure 9.112. POTT'S FRACTURE: SCHEMATIC DIAGRAM, AN-KLE. This fracture is defined as a fracture through the distal fibula, 6–7 cm above the lateral malleolus, accompanied by rupture of the distal tibiofibular ligaments of the ankle.

the talus, and displacement of the foot upward and outward. (8) Unfortunately, Dupuytren's fracture is used to describe several varieties of bimalleolar fractures and, because of its similarity to Pott's fracture, it has created some confusion within the literature. It should only be used as classically described by Dupuytren. (8)

Maisonneuve's Fracture

In 1840 Maisonneuve described a fracture of the proximal shaft of the fibula which bears his name. (9) (Fig. 9.113) This fracture is caused by an inversion and external rotation force applied to the ankle, which forces the talus laterally against the fibula, initially producing rupture of the inferior tibiofibular syndesmosis. As the force is maintained, the fibula, freed from the tibia, continues to be displaced laterally and posteriorly. The superior tibiofibular joint, remaining intact, secures the proximal fibula so that the long lever of the fibula produces a fracture of the fibula in its proximal third.

Maisonneuve's fracture may be easily overlooked because patients rarely complain of pain in the region of the proximal fibula when more painful injuries at the ankle exist. A full view of the entire tibia and fibula should be considered in patients where the mechanism of injury to the ankle is as Maisonneuve described. (9)

Tillaux's Fracture

This fracture is described as a fracture of the medial malleolus, a diastasis of the distal tibiofibular syndesmosis, creating an avulsion of the anterior tubercle of the tibia and a fracture of the lateral malleolus 6–7 cm proximal to the distal end of the fibula. (10) This fracture is best seen on anteroposterior radiographs of the ankle.

Toddler's Fracture

Toddler's fracture occurs in children, following a fall, in the age range of 9 months to 3 years. Occasionally, the trauma may be related to the child getting a foot caught between the slats of the crib, with the spiral fracture occurring as the child rolls over. Often, the child will refuse to bear weight on the extremity. Since the baby is unable to verbalize its complaints, the source of the discomfort is a mystery.

Radiographic examination reveals an undisplaced spiral fracture of the tibia which is usually seen only on one projection—either the anteroposterior or lateral view. (3) (Fig. 9.114A and B) Most toddler's fractures are seen on the anteroposterior view and are not demonstrated on the lateral projection. Rarely, the fibula may be fractured as well. (3) The adult form, where the fractured tibia occurs adjacent to the top of high-top boots, is called a "boot-top" fracture. (Fig. 9.115)

DISLOCATIONS OF THE ANKLE

Since subluxations and dislocations of the ankle joint associated with malleolar fractures have already been discussed, it remains only to consider the displacements that follow extensive ligamentous and capsular damage without fracture. (Fig. 9.111)

The talus may be dislocated at one, two, or all three of its articulations; however, we will consider only those that involve the ankle joint. Dislocation of the talus occurs as an isolated event, in association with fracture of the neck of the talus, or as an element in total extrusion of the talus. (11)

Anterior Dislocation

Isolated dislocation of the ankle may occur in either an anterior or posterior direction. Medial or lateral dislocation is commonly associated with a fracture of the tibia or

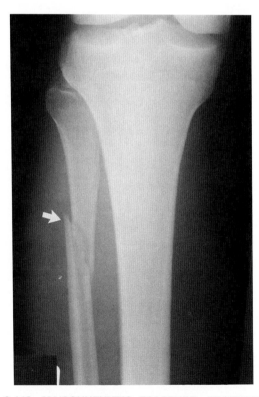

Figure 9.113. MAISONNEUVE'S FRACTURE: PROXIMAL FIB-ULA. An oblique fracture of the proximal fibula (arrow) has occurred secondary to a forceful inversion and external rotation of the ankle. **Comment:** These fractures are often overlooked, due to the severity of the ankle injury, and close inspection of the proximal fibula should be performed in all instances of ankle trauma.

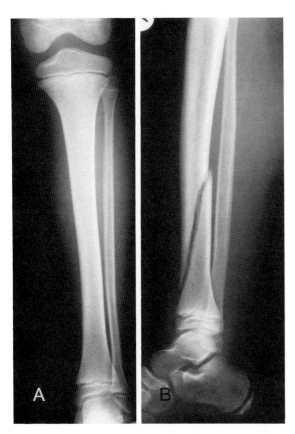

Figure 9.114. TODDLER'S FRACTURE: TIBIA. A. AP Tibia and Fibula. No fracture line is evident. **B. Lateral Tibia and Fibula.** A spiral fracture line is visualized in the distal one-third of the diaphysis of the tibia. *Comment:* This case demonstrates the need for a minimum of AP and lateral radiographs in traumatized patients. The toddler's fracture is often seen in only one of the projections.

fibula. Anterior dislocation follows a force that results in posterior displacement of the tibia on the fixed foot. All ligamentous and capsular attachments from the tibia and fibula to the talus are torn, with the exception, occasionally, of the posterior talofibular ligament. Clinically, the foot is usually slightly dorsiflexed and appears elongated anteriorly. The depressions on either side of the Achilles tendon are obliterated. The talus is prominent anteriorly, and the dorsalis pedis pulse may be absent. (11)

Posterior Dislocation

Posterior dislocation occurs more often than anterior displacement, but both are rare without fracture of the corresponding tibial margin. Posterior dislocation of the talus most often follows a blow to the posterior aspect of the tibia and results in plantar flexion of the ankle with apparent shortening of the foot. Reduction is carried out by exerting traction in the long axis of the limb and lifting the heel forward. Subsequent operative repair of the ligaments is an individual decision. (11)

COMPLICATIONS OF ANKLE FRACTURE

Nonunion

Nonunion is most frequent in fracture of the medial malleolus; it occurs in 10–15 percent of patients treated by closed methods. (11) Nonunion of the lateral or pos-

terior malleolus is rare. (11) Nonunion at the level of the plafond is more commonly symptomatic than that below the plafond. (12)

Traumatic Degenerative Arthritis

Traumatic degenerative arthritis occurs in 20–40 percent of ankle fractures, regardless of the method of treatment. (12,13) Predisposing factors are inaccurate reduction of the mortise, comminution of the plafond, and advanced age. (11)

Ligamentous Instability

Often, fractures and dislocations of the ankle are found with complete or incomplete tears of the supporting ligaments. Ligamentous damage unassociated with fracture often goes ignored and is especially dangerous because it may go unrecognized and untreated, leading to permanent disability of the ankle. In the absence of fracture or obvious dislocation, considerable soft tissue swelling is an indication for stress studies to evaluate for ligamentous damage. (14)

The important ligaments of the ankle joint are the lateral collateral ligament, the medial (deltoid) collateral, and the tibiofibular ligament (tibiofibular syndesmosis). (14) A variety of tears to these ligaments occurs with the numerous types of injuries which can affect the ankle joint. For a more detailed review of the mechanism of injury and types of ligamentous tears, further reading is necessary. (3,11,13,14)

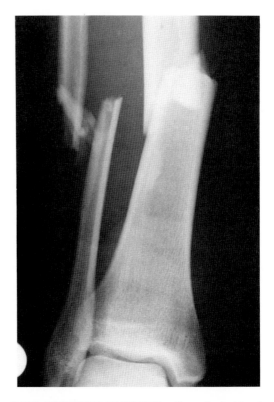

Figure 9.115. BOOT-TOP FRACTURE. Comminuted fractures of the distal tibia and fibula are seen at the level of a skier's boot-top. *Comment:* Fractures of this type may be referred to as "BB," representing both bones. The "BB" fracture can be found in the radius and ulna or in the tibia and fibula.

Fractures and Dislocations of the Foot

FRACTURES OF THE FOOT

Trauma to the foot with fractures is quite common, with fractures of the feet accounting for approximately 10 percent of all fractures. (1,2) Bone and joint injuries can occur from direct trauma, from objects falling on the foot, or from movement of the foot against a variety of objects. (1) Indirect injuries occur from avulsion by tendinous and capsular attachments or excessive torsional motion of the joints. (1) Additionally, overuse or unaccustomed activity may result in stress. (1) Fractures of the tarsal bones and fracture/dislocation of the tarsometatarsal joints are frequently found in diabetic neurotrophic arthropathy. (3) The diagnosis is usually obvious because of the history of diabetes mellitus and the associated radiographic signs of neurotrophic arthropathy. (3) Therefore, a tarsal fracture or fracture/dislocation occurring in the absence of trauma should suggest the need to search for evidence of diabetes. (1)

The routine views of the foot are the dorsoplantar, 35-degree medial oblique, and lateral. (3) An axial projection is necessary when calcaneal fracture is the major concern. Occasionally, varying oblique projections and tomography may be needed in order to demonstrate the fracture or dislocation.

Calcaneal Fractures

The calcaneus is the largest tarsal bone and the one most often fractured. (3,4) It has two major functions—to bear weight and to serve as a springboard for locomotion. (1) Approximately 25 percent of calcaneal fractures involve the various processes of the bone and spare the

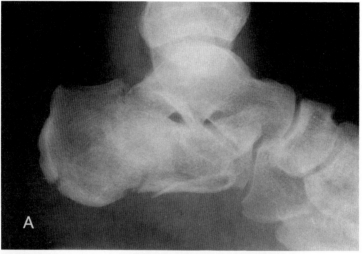

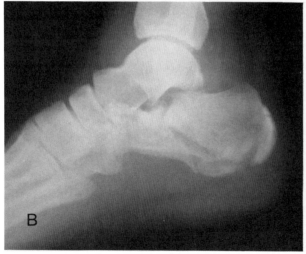

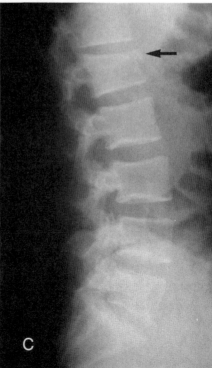

Figure 9.116. COMPRESSION FRACTURES: SUICIDE ATTEMPT. A and B. Right and Left Calcaneus. Both the right and left calcaneus demonstrate comminution fracture secondary to severe forces occurring upon impact with the ground following a suicide jump from a second-story window. **C. Lateral Lumbar Spine.** Observe the associated compression fracture of the superior end plate of the L1 vertebra with a characteristic "step" defect (arrow).

subtalar joint; 75 percent involve the subtalar joint and body of the calcaneus. (5)

There are two basic types of calcaneal fractures—the compressive and the noncompressive (avulsive) type.

Compression Fracture.   This is the result of compression forces generated in crushing injuries as encountered by falling from a height and landing on the feet. (6) Approximately 10 percent of these fractures are bilateral, and 10 percent are associated with vertebral body compression or neural arch fracture of the thoracolumbar spine. (7) (Fig. 9.116A–C) The weight of the body is transmitted through the tibia and talus onto the calcaneus. (1) The resultant fracture is comminuted, and the degree of displacement and comminution is directly related to the magnitude of the forces involved. (1) The fracture usually involves the subtalar joint, with some degree of depression of the posterior facet. Occasionally, a radiolucent fracture line will be seen; however, most cases do not demonstrate such a line. Because of the crushing nature of the injury, it is important to determine Boehler's angle. (8) (Fig. 9.117) (See Chapter 3) Often, an alteration of this angle may be the only sign of fracture.

Boehler's angle is formed by a line drawn from the superior posterior margin of the tuberosity through the tip of the posterior facet. (8) A second line is drawn from the tip of the posterior facet through the superior margin of the anterior process of the calcaneus. The normal angle is 28–40 degrees. (1,8) A Boehler angle of less than 28 degrees indicates depression and probable fracture.

Avulsion Fracture.   Those fractures which spare the subtalar joint are usually of the avulsion type. They involve the anterior process, the sustentaculum tali, the superior portion of the tuberosity, and the medial or lateral surface of the tuberosity. (1) Fractures of the anterior process are the most common form of avulsion fracture of the calcaneus. (9)

A fracture of the superior portion of the tuberosity of the calcaneus is known as a "beak" fracture. (10) The posterior margin of the tuberosity represents the site of insertion of the Achilles tendon, and the "beak" fracture may be the result of avulsion by the Achilles tendon.

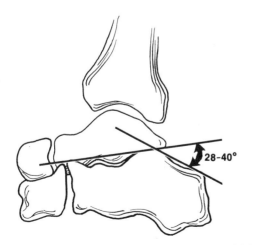

Figure 9.117. BOEHLER'S ANGLE: SCHEMATIC DIAGRAM. A reduction in Boehler's angle to less than 28 degrees is frequently indicative of a calcaneal compression fracture.

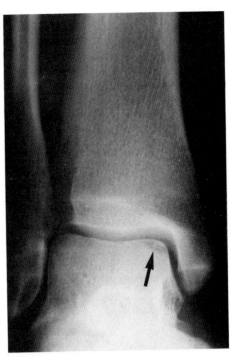

Figure 9.118. OSTEOCHONDRAL FRACTURE OF THE MEDIAL TALAR DOME. A radiolucent defect with a central bone flake is observed in the medial talar dome (arrow). This represents an osteochondral fracture of the articular surface.

Fractures of the Talus

The talus is the second most common tarsal bone to be fractured, following the calcaneus. The most frequent type of fracture is an avulsion, usually on the anterior surface of the talar neck, at the capsular insertion. Fractures are classified according to anatomic site—body, neck, or head. (11)

Talus Body Fractures.   These may be orientated in a transverse or oblique plane. Osteochondral chip fractures of the talar dome occur either at the medial or lateral margins following forceful inversion or eversion injuries, when there is direct contact between the talus and opposing malleolus. (Fig. 9.118)

Talus Neck Fractures.   Avulsions of the anterior surface are the most frequent, followed by vertical fractures. The mechanism of injury in vertical neck fractures is downward force of the anterior tibial lip into the talar neck as it is being forced upward. Usually, these follow an automobile accident and were first described in World War I pilots involved in crash landings where the rudder bar was forced into the sole of the foot (aviator's fracture). (12) (Fig. 9.119) These are the most common fractures to be complicated by avascular necrosis of the talus.

Talus Head Fractures.   These fractures are infrequent and are characterized by the fracture line being well forward of the talar neck.

Complications of Talus Fractures

The main concern with talus fractures is the development of avascular necrosis, which usually involves the body and may occur following a talar neck fracture. (13) This may also complicate talar dislocation. The pattern of

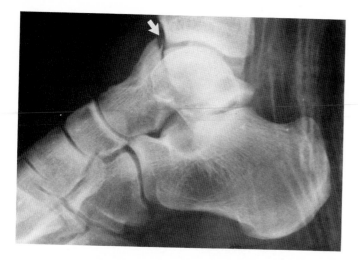

Figure 9.119. AVIATOR'S FRACTURE: NECK OF TALUS. A vertical fracture line extends through the talar neck (arrow). **Comment:** Aviator's fracture of the talus was first described in World War I, when pilots were involved in crash landings where the rudder bar was forced into the sole of the foot.

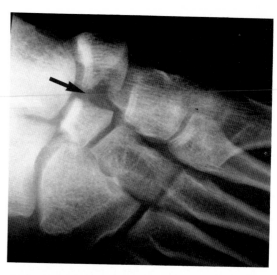

Figure 9.120. FRACTURED TARSAL NAVICULAR. An unusual fracture has occurred through the midportion of the tarsal navicular (arrow), with significant displacement of the medial fragment. **Comment:** Fractures of the tarsal navicular are uncommon.

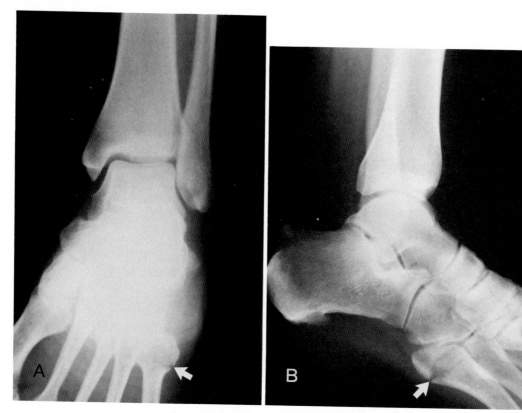

Figure 9.121. JONES' FRACTURE (DANCER'S FRACTURE): BASE OF FIFTH METATARSAL. A. AP Ankle. B. Lateral Ankle. A transverse fracture line is seen at the base of the fifth metatarsal (arrows). **Comment:** The Jones' or "dancer's" fracture is precipitated by an avulsive force exerted from the peroneus brevis tendon when the foot is forcefully inverted and plantar flexed. These fractures are frequently overlooked, since this type of injury causes more noticeable symptoms in the area of the ankle mortise. Close observation of the base of the fifth metatarsal should be performed on every lateral ankle radiograph to rule out a Jones' fracture. This is one of the most frequent injuries of the foot.

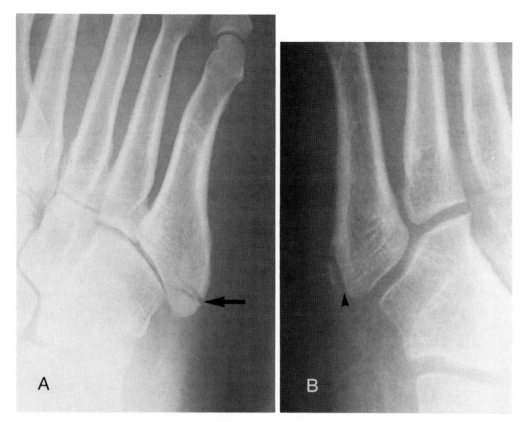

Figure 9.122. JONES' FRACTURE VERSUS NORMAL VARIANT. A. Oblique Foot: Jones' Fracture. Notice the characteristic transverse orientation of the fracture line of the base of the fifth metatarsal (arrow). **B. Oblique Foot: Normal Growth Variation.** The apophysis for the base of the fifth metatarsal is separated by a longitudinally oriented lucent cleft (arrowhead). With skeletal maturation, this radiolucent cleft will eventually ossify and become united to the base of the fifth metatarsal. *Comment:* In the foot of a traumatized young patient recognition of the orientation of the radiolucent cleft will distinguish between transverse fractures of the base of the fifth metatarsal and a normal vertically oriented apophyseal growth.

vascular perfusion to the talar body is such that a neck fracture can significantly compromise its blood supply. Little to no collateral supply exists due to over 60 percent of its external surface being covered by articular cartilage. The main source of blood enters by way of the foramina in the sinus tarsi and tarsal canal. Generally, the more anterior the neck fracture, the greater the likelihood for developing avascular necrosis.

Following a talar fracture, the early formation of a zone of linear lucency beneath the cortex of the dome is a reliable indicator of an intact blood supply with a diminished probability for developing avascular necrosis (Hawkin's sign). (14)

Other Tarsal Fractures

Occasionally, other tarsal bones may fracture.

Navicular Fractures. Avulsion of its dorsal surface is the most frequent type of fracture. Acute eversion may also avulse the medial tuberosity from traction exerted by the tibialis posterior tendon. This infrequent injury must not be confused with the commonly seen accessory ossicle, os tibiale externum. Other navicular fractures are uncommon. (Fig. 9.120)

Cuneiform Fractures. Isolated fractures are rare. More frequently, fractures of the distal aspects of the cuneiforms are associated with tarsometatarsal dislocation (Lisfranc's injury).

Cuboid Fractures. Isolated fractures are unusual. The most common site is at its most lateral margin. Care must be taken not to confuse the accessory ossicles seen adjacent to the cuboid (os peroneum, os versalium) as fractures.

Fractures of the Metatarsals

A dropped heavy object is a frequent cause of metatarsal fracture. The majority involve the shaft or neck. The fracture line may be oblique, spiral, or transverse and requires multiple views for visualization. The second and third metatarsals are the most common skeletal sites for stress fractures to occur.

Jones' Fracture (Dancer's Fracture). The original description by Jones in 1902 of his own fracture incurred while dancing has perpetuated the usage of these synonyms. (15) This is a fracture at the base of the fifth metatarsal due to traction exerted from the peroneus brevis tendon when the foot is forcefully inverted and plantar flexed. (Fig. 9.121A and B) In children there is a longitudinally orientated apophysis adjacent to the fracture region which should not be confused with a fracture. (Fig. 9.122A and B)

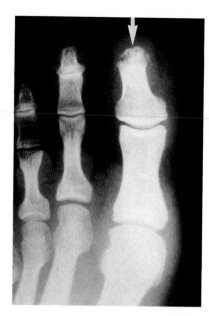

Figure 9.123. CRUSH FRACTURE: DISTAL PHALANX. Comminution of the distal phalanx (arrow) has occurred following a blow from a heavy object.

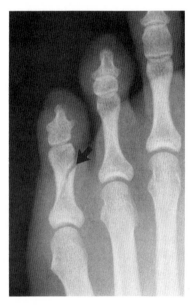

Figure 9.124. BEDROOM FRACTURE: DORSIPLANTAR TOES. An oblique fracture of the shaft of the proximal phalanx of the fifth toe (arrow) has occurred following striking a hard object. (Courtesy of Gaylord H. Hanssen, DC, Doniphan, Nebraska).

Clinically and radiographically, these fractures are frequently overlooked, since pain and swelling from the traumatized lateral tendon sheaths and ankle ligaments misdirect the attention to the ankle mortise. In any patient with ankle/foot trauma, the base of the fifth metatarsal must be carefully scrutinized for this fracture.

Fractures of the Phalanges

In the absence of a clinical history and multiple views of the phalanges, these are easily passed over.

Crush Injuries.   Dropping a heavy object on the toe frequently results in a comminuted phalanx, especially of the distal phalanx. (Fig. 9.123)

Bedroom Fracture.   A direct blow to the toe such as when striking an object with a bare foot, may produce a fracture of any phalanx, especially those of the first and fifth digits. (Fig. 9.124)

Chip Fracture.   Small fractures of the phalangeal articular margins may follow digital hyperextension or, less frequently, hyperflexion forces.

Hallux Rigidus.   A fracture of the hallux phalanx may produce a stiffened, painful first metatarsophalangeal joint. (Fig. 9.125) Radiographically, no articular alteration may be evident initially, but later may demonstrate signs of degenerative arthritis.

DISLOCATIONS OF THE FOOT

Talus Dislocation

The talus is the most common bone in the foot to dislocate. It may dislocate at three joints—the talotibial, talocalcaneal (subtalar), and talonavicular joints. These may occur singularly or together and also can precipitate avascular necrosis of the talus as a complication.

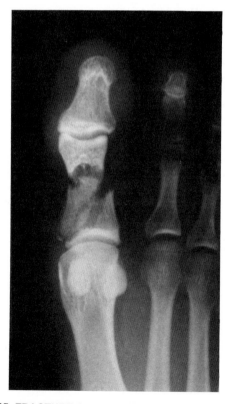

Figure 9.125. FRACTURE OF THE PROXIMAL PHALANX: GREAT TOE. There is a comminuted fracture through the shaft of the proximal phalanx of the great toe, extending immediately distal to the proximal articular surface of the phalanx. **Comment:** This type of fracture may develop into a stiff, painful first metatarsal phalangeal joint (hallux rigidus).

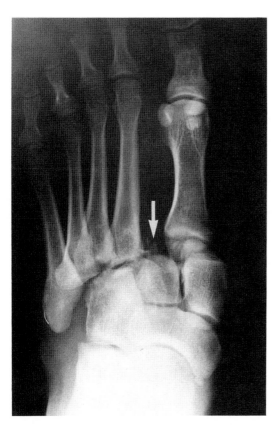

Figure 9.126. TARSOMETATARSAL FRACTURE DISLOCATION (LISFRANC'S DISLOCATION). Displacement of the second through the fifth metatarsal bases has occurred, with associated fractures in the area of diastasis (arrow) between the bases of the first and second metatarsals. The injury usually results from a fall with longitudinal compression or a twisting force through the forefoot. (Courtesy of Gary M. Fieber, DC, Minneapolis, Minnesota)

Other Tarsal Dislocations

Midtarsal Dislocation (Chopart's Dislocation). This is a rare dislocation which separates the foot at the talonavicular and calcaneocuboid joints. (1)

Tarsometatarsal Fracture Dislocation (Lisfranc's Dislocation). The injury has been named after a surgeon in Napoleon's army, not for his description of the injury but because of his method of foot amputation through the same region. (16) The components consist of dorsal dislocation of the metatarsal bases in relation to the opposing tarsals, in combination with fractures at various locations along the site of joint separation. (Fig. 9.126) Additionally, there may be associated lateral displacement of the metatarsals. The most common accompanying fractures are at the base of the second metatarsal and lateral cuboid surface. The injury usually results from a fall, with longitudinal compression or a twisting force through the forefoot.

Phalangeal Dislocations

These are not as frequent as in the hand and are readily recognizable.

Fractures of the Thorax

RIB FRACTURES

General Considerations

Significant force is usually required to produce a fractured rib. They are uncommon injuries of childhood, but with advancing age the incidence gradually increases, after the third decade, as the bones become more rigid and brittle. (1)

Of all fractures, those involving the ribs are the most difficult to observe due to the curvilinear shape of the rib. They usually require multiple oblique views to orient the fracture line to a plane where the x-ray beam can pass directly through the separation. It is not unexpected that a rib fracture will be undetected upon initial examination and appreciated some time later, when enough callus is present, creating a readily observable area of abnormality.

In general, a single AP radiograph is insufficient for the accurate diagnosis of rib fracture and must be supplemented by multiple oblique projections. Often, plain films may be negative, and a bone scan will demonstrate singular or multiple rib fractures. (Fig. 9.127) Occasionally, the bone scan may assist in the evaluation of the traumatized patient, for medicolegal purposes.

Radiological Features of Rib Fractures

A number of features should be searched for to aid in locating a rib fracture. (Fig. 9.128) (Table 9.14)

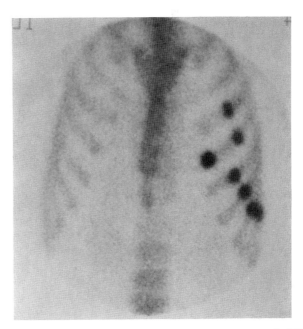

Figure 9.127. RIB FRACTURES: BONE SCAN FEATURES. Multiple focal areas of radioisotopic uptake are present in the anterior ribs. These areas correspond to the sites of rib fractures which were not clearly identifiable on the plain film examination. *Comment:* In view of the difficulty in locating rib fractures, this procedure is particularly useful in medicolegal and equivocal clinical circumstances. (Courtesy of Lawrence A. Cooperstein, MD, Pittsburgh, Pennsylvania)

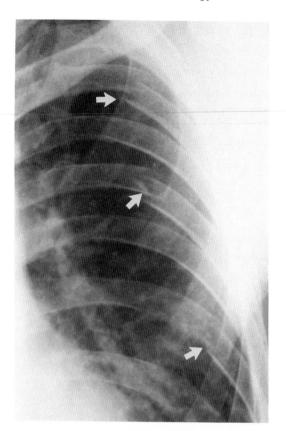

Figure 9.128. RIB FRACTURES: GENERAL FEATURES. Multiple fracture sites are observed (arrows). Rib fractures can be identified by searching for a fracture line, cortical offset, or altered rib angulation and, when multiple, following along the line of injury looking for additional lesions.

Table 9.14.
Radiological Features of Rib Fractures

Radiolucent fracture line
Cortical offset
Altered rib orientation
Pleural deflection
Callus formation
Pleural fluid
Pneumothorax
Subcutaneous emphysema
Diaphragmatic elevation

Fracture Line.   When present, the fracture line will usually cross the rib transversely or obliquely and will be radiolucent. Care must be taken to not misinterpret overlying bronchial air shadows as fracture lines, as evidenced by the lung markings continuing beyond the bony rib margin.

Cortical Offset.   This is a most important feature which is frequently seen without visualizing the fracture line. The superior and inferior cortices will be acutely offset at the fracture site, as evidenced by a sharp "step effect."

Rib Orientation.   A sharp deviation in the contour of a single rib may occur at the fracture site.

Pleural Deflection.   A localized hematoma adjacent to the fracture site may displace the pleura inward, in-

denting into the lung. When the x-ray beam is tangential to the accumulated blood, this will be seen as a radiopaque density which is sharply demarcated, convex toward the lung, and gradually blends beyond the fracture site into its normal position (extrapleural sign).

Other Fractures

When multiple fractures are present, they are usually aligned in a linear fashion at each rib, along the site of the precipitating force. The homolateral costophrenic recess may be blunted due to sanguineous pleural fluid. Other associations include pneumothorax, subcutaneous emphysema, diaphragmatic elevation, and splenic laceration. If callus has begun to form, there will be a localized increase in density and a bulbous expansion at the fracture site. (Fig. 9.129)

Upper Rib (1–3) Fractures

Fractures of the upper three ribs are uncommon, due to the inherent strength and overlying supporting musculature. Therefore, if present, this should suggest severe trauma and other injuries, such as to the trachea, aorta, great vessels, brachial plexus, or spine are likely. (Fig. 9.130)

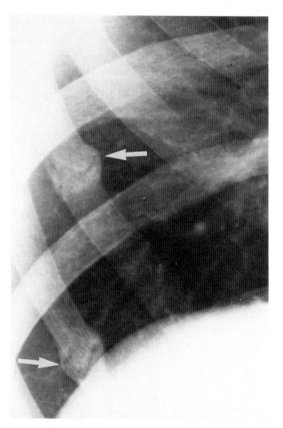

Figure 9.129. HEALING RIB FRACTURES. Two sites of healing rib fractures are identified (arrows). Radiographic features consist of a localized region of increased density, bony expansion of the rib at the fracture site, and visualization of the fracture line. **Comment:** These rib fractures were not apparent on the initial radiographic examination following a chronic episode of coughing. Follow-up radiographs revealed callus formation, which now localizes the previously unrecognized fracture sites.

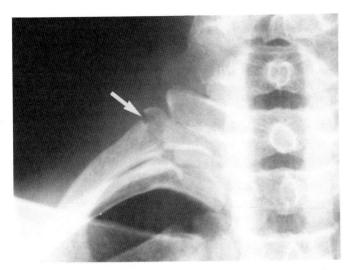

Figure 9.130. FIRST RIB FRACTURE. A single fracture line traverses the first rib, just distal to the costotransverse joint (arrow). *Comment:* Fractures of the upper ribs are frequently associated with severe trauma and additional injuries to the trachea, aorta, great vessels, brachial plexus, or spine.

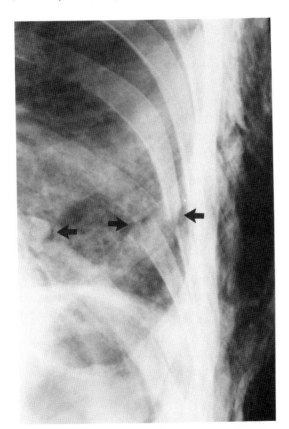

Figure 9.131. MULTIPLE RIB FRACTURES WITH SUBCUTANEOUS EMPHYSEMA. Multiple rib fractures affecting the posterolateral surface (arrows) are associated with subcutaneous emphysema in the overlying soft tissues. Subcutaneous emphysema is a sign of severe pulmonary injury, allowing direct communication between the bronchial tree and the extrathoracic soft tissues.

Middle Rib (4–9) Fractures

These ribs are the most commonly fractured. The fracture site depends on the mechanism of injury but fre-quently is found at the lateral aspect of the rib, where it is easily overlooked. (Fig. 9.131) Fractures of these ribs therefore require multiple views for adequate depiction. Fractures of the mid to lower anterior ribs should stimulate close scrutiny of the spleen and liver for associated injury.

Flail Chest. This is the term used to describe the occurrence of two fractures involving the same rib, thereby causing a section of the rib to lose continuity with the rest of the thoracic wall. Usually, multiple adjacent ribs are affected, which allows the flail segment to move during respiration in an opposite direction (paradoxical motion) and reduces pulmonary gaseous exchange, possibly creating a life-threatening situation.

Golfer's Fracture. When a golfer inadvertently has his swing abruptly halted, such as if the ground is struck rather than the ball, fracture of a rib may occur, usually at its lateral margin.

Passion (Bear Hug) Fracture. Fracture of a rib can occasionally be precipitated when one is the recipient of an overenthusiastic hug.

Lower Rib (10–12) Fractures

These are uncommonly fractured, since they are relatively mobile and yielding; however, if a fracture is observed, associated kidney damage should be evaluated. (Fig. 9.132)

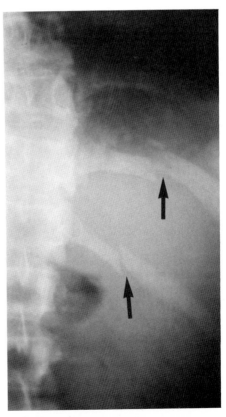

Figure 9.132. LOWER RIB FRACTURES. Fracture lines are seen through both the 11th and 12 ribs (arrows), with minimal displacement. *Comment:* The presence of fractures of the lower ribs warrants careful examination of the urinary system, especially renal function and structure. This should include an intravenous pyelogram and other more sophisticated imaging modalities.

Cough (Post-Tussive) Fracture. In any condition where persistent and/or violent coughing is experienced, stress fractures of the lower anterior ribs may occur. (2) (Fig. 9.129)

Costal Cartilage Injuries. The identification of costal cartilage injuries on plain films is very difficult and generally unrewarding. Nuclear scanning and computerized tomography will assist in their evaluation.

Fractures of the Sternum

Sternal fractures usually follow blunt compressive forces applied to the chest, such as that which occurs in motor vehicle accidents. The most common sites of fracture involve the body or manubriosternal junction and are usually transverse in nature. The best projection is the lateral view, where a fracture line, displacement, and associated hematoma may be observed. (3) (Fig. 9.133) Tomography or computed tomography may be required for optimal visualization of the sternum.

COMPLICATIONS OF THORACIC TRAUMA

Various tissues and organs may suffer damage in association with injuries of the thorax.

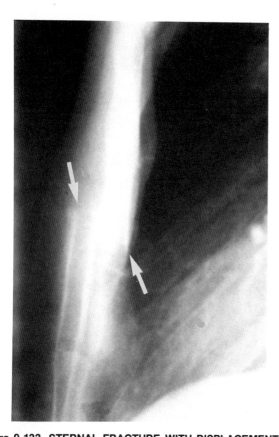

Figure 9.133. STERNAL FRACTURE WITH DISPLACEMENT. A complete fracture through the body of the sternum, with displacement and overlap (arrows) across the fracture site. *Comment:* Sternal injuries are uncommon and usually follow severe blunt trauma to the anterior thorax.

Pleural Complications

Traumatic Pneumothorax. A tear in the pleura reduces the intrapleural negative pressure, which, when lost, allows the lung to collapse.

Hemothorax Complications. Blood may accumulate in the pleural space from ruptured blood vessels. This can be identified by observing blunt costophrenic sulci.

Chylothorax Complications. Lymphatic fluid may accumulate in the same manner as does blood.

Lung Complications

Contusion. An irregular, localized opacity appears shortly after the injury and then gradually resorbs, within 3–10 days.

Pneumonia. This may complicate the immobility of the chest following a rib fracture, due to the inactivation of the normal lung clearing mechanisms.

Other Tissue Complications

Various associated injuries have been reported, including rupture of the spleen, diaphragm, tracheobronchial tree, esophagus, kidney, and heart, as well as formation of aortic aneurysms and lung cysts.

Fractures and Dislocations of the Shoulder Girdle

GENERAL CONSIDERATIONS

Shoulder girdle injuries commonly occur at all ages, although the site of injury varies with age. Fracture of the clavicle is the most common skeletal birth and childhood injury. (Fig. 9.134) Between 20 and 40 years of age, dislocation of the shoulder, acromioclavicular joint separation, and clavicle fractures predominate. In the elderly, shoulder dislocations and surgical neck fractures of the humerus become increasingly more common.

Technologically, the shoulder girdle requires specific projections for proper evaluation. A minimum general survey of the shoulder should include anteroposterior views with internal rotation, external rotation, and abduction ("baby arm"). At least one view should include the upper thoracic cage and lung to the spine. Additional specific projections for the acromioclavicular joint, clavicle, and scapula must be performed, as clinically indicated, for optimum evaluation. A "hotlight" should be routinely used to view the shoulder structures, due to inherent overexposure of thinner body areas such as the distal clavicle and acromioclavicular joint.

FRACTURES OF THE CLAVICLE

Technological Features

The "S" shape and normal overlap with the upper ribcage renders the clavicle a difficult structure to evaluate on straight anteroposterior projections. (Fig. 9.135A and B) The most optimum view is an anteroposterior projection with 15 degrees cephalad tube angulation. Weights (10–15 pounds) may be held to aid in detecting undisplaced fractures. The exposure factors should be approx-

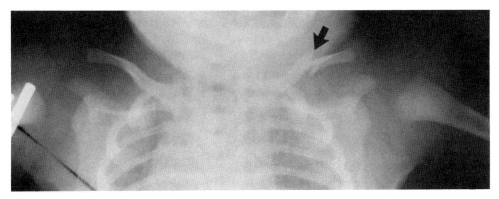

Figure 9.134. BIRTH FRACTURE OF THE CLAVICLE. A midclavicular fracture (arrow) has occurred during the birth process. *Comment:* Fracture of the clavicle is the most common birth fracture.

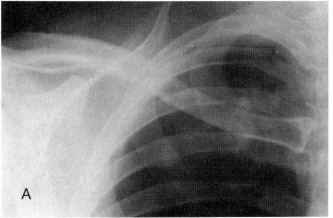

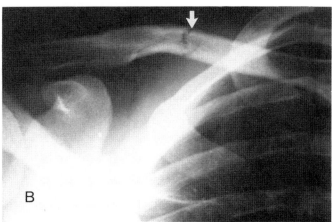

Figure 9.135. CLAVICLE FRACTURE EVALUATION: ANGULATED VERSUS NONANGULATED PROJECTIONS. A. AP Nonangulated Projection. No fracture line is visible. **B. Angulated Projection.** With 15 degrees cephalad tube angulation, the fracture line is clearly evident (arrow). *Comment:* In evaluation of clavicular trauma specific clavicle projections must be obtained to demonstrate fractures, particularly through the midportion of the clavicle. (Courtesy of Kenneth E. Yochum, DC, St. Louis, Missouri).

imately half of that utilized in standard shoulder projections to prevent overexposure.

Radiological Features

Generally, a clavicle fracture follows direct trauma and is the most common bone fractured during birth and in childhood.

Medial Clavicle Fractures. This is the least common site, representing only approximately 5 percent of all clavicle fractures. (1) These are difficult to observe and usually require tomography.

Middle Clavicle Fractures. This is the most common site, representing approximately 80 percent of all clavicle fractures. (1) A force applied to the distal end of the "S" shaped clavicle creates a shearing effect at the middle third, producing the fracture. The fracture is usually complete, with the medial fragment elevated by the action of the sternocleidomastoid muscle and the lateral fragment depressed by the weight of the shoulder and upper extremity. (Fig. 9.136) In addition to malalignment, an overlap at the fracture site is common, with the distal fragment usually lying below the medial fragment. Healing is often associated with extensive callus formation. (Fig. 9.137)

Lateral Clavicle Fractures. These account for approximately 15 percent of all clavicle fractures. (1) There are three varieties: 1) undisplaced; 2) displaced, where the distal fragment moves anterior and inferior; and 3) articular surface extension. (Fig. 9.138)

Whenever a fracture of the lateral third is identified, weightbearing stress views should be obtained to clarify the status of the coracoclavicular ligaments. (2) Notably, fractures which extend into the joint frequently precipitate the onset of degenerative arthritis.

Complications of Clavicle Injuries

Childhood clavicular fractures usually heal without sequelae; however, in adults the incidence of complications increases.

Neurovascular Damage. Associated injury to the underlying neurovascular structures most frequently involves the subclavian artery, less commonly, the vein, and, occasionally, the brachial plexus and sympathetic chain. (3) Compressive effects from the hypertrophic callus can also precipitate pressure-related neurovascular disturbances. (1,4)

Nonunion. A failure to unite the fracture requires

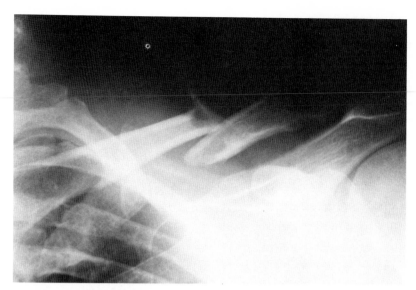

Figure 9.136. CLASSIC MIDCLAVICULAR FRACTURE.   A fracture through the midportion of the clavicle has resulted in superior dis-placement of the medial portion and inferior displacement of the lateral portion.

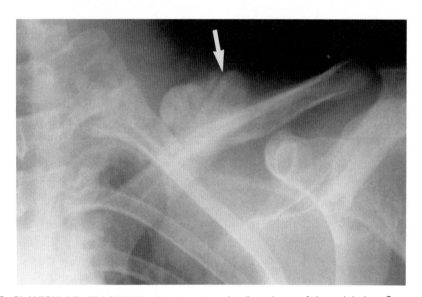

Figure 9.137. HEALING CLAVICULAR FRACTURE.   Exuberant callus formation (arrow) is identified adjacent to a midclavicular fracture. This degree of callus formation is a frequent finding in the healing phase of these injuries. **Comment:** Callus formation of this extent may lead to significant cosmetic disfiguration and compromise of the thoracic outlet.

surgical fixation. The key signs of nonunion are located at the fracture margins, where sclerosis, rounding, and a smooth contour will be visible.

Malunion.   In the presence of fragment overlap and massive callus formation, a cosmetic deformity may result. Correction requires osteotomy, realignment, and fixation.

Degenerative Arthritis.   Painful degenerative arthritis frequently follows intra-articular fractures of the clavicle. This is evidenced by loss of joint space, sclerosis, and osteophyte formation.

Post-Traumatic Osteolysis.   A peculiar bone response to clavicular injury is resorption of the distal segment, usually 1–3 mm, but never more than 2–3 cm. The initiating injury may be relatively minor, often lacking the severity of that required to cause a fracture or dislocation. It first becomes radiologically visible 2–3 months after injury. The precise mechanism is uncertain, although synovial hypertrophy suggests inflammatory osteoclastic activity. (5) Pain is mild to moderate, while the disorder takes a self-limiting course over a number of months.

The earliest radiographic sign in the development of osteolysis is a cystic rarefaction of the clavicular subarticular cortex, followed by cortical dissolution. (5,6) The joint appears wide and the clavicular surface is frayed and irregular or cup-shaped. (Fig. 9.139A and B) With healing, there are varying degrees of bony reconstitution to complete restoration of structure to a permanently tapered distal clavicle and increased joint space.

FRACTURES OF THE SCAPULA

Severe trauma is usually needed to fracture the scapula. Isolated scapular fractures are infrequent, with approximately 80 percent demonstrating other injuries. (7) Routine shoulder views usually adequately demonstrate the scapula; however, special projections may be required for a more thorough examination.

Coracoid View. This view is performed anteroposterior, with 25–40 degrees of cephalad tube tilt.

Axillary Border View. This view is performed anteroposterior, with 25–40 degrees of cephalad tube tilt.

Lateral View. This view is performed posteroanterior, with the patient rotated 35 degrees. It produces a tangential depiction of the scapula body and acromion.

Axillary View. This view is performed superior-inferior, with the cassette in the axilla and the arm abducted. It demonstrates the glenoid, acromion, and coracoid process.

Radiological Features of Scapula Fractures

The majority of fractures involve the scapular body and neck (80%). (7) (Fig. 9.140) When the coracoid or acromion fractures, it is usually in the midportion at the narrowest dimension. An avulsion corresponding to the triceps insertion is often seen at the inferior glenoid rim in association with anterior humeral dislocations (Bankart lesion). (8)

FRACTURES OF THE HUMERUS

Most humeral fractures can be identified on standard anteroposterior views in internal and external rotation.

Radiological Features

Fractures of the mid to proximal humerus occur in five

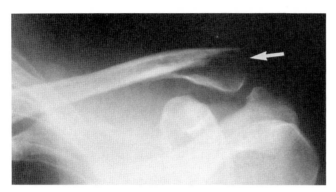

Figure 9.138. FRACTURE OF THE DISTAL CLAVICLE. A fracture line through the distal surface of the clavicle is identified (arrow). *Comment:* Fractures in this location are frequently overlooked due to technical overexposure and require bright light illumination for clear identification. These fractures frequently predispose to degenerative arthritis of the acromioclavicular articulation.

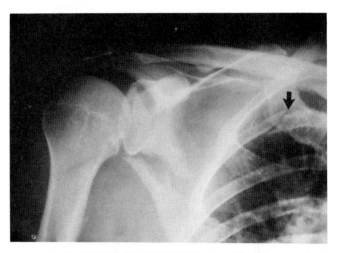

Figure 9.140. SCAPULAR FRACTURE. An oblique fracture line in the subglenoid axillary border of the scapula is visible. An associated rib fracture (arrow) is also seen. *Comment:* The body and neck are the most common sites of scapular fractures. (Courtesy of Gail J. Keilman, DC, Minneapolis, Minnesota)

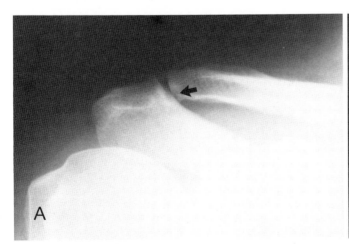

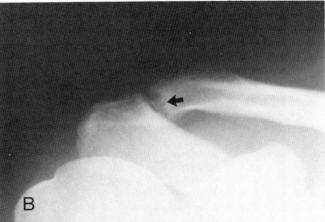

Figure 9.139. POST-TRAUMATIC OSTEOLYSIS OF THE CLAVICLE. A. AP Acromioclavicular Joint. Two months following trauma to the shoulder, a cystic rarefaction (arrow) is present at the inferior aspect of the distal articular surface of the clavicle. **B. AP Acromioclavicular Joint.** There has been extension of the area of rarefaction in the distal clavicle involving the entire distal surface

(arrow). Observe the smooth and regular articular margins of the acromial surface, differentiating it from inflammatory joint diseases (rheumatoid arthritis and septic arthritis). *Comment:* This disorder follows a self-limiting course and resolves with varying degrees of reconstitution of the resorbed bone. (Courtesy of Leo J. Bronston, DC, Sparta, Wisconsin)

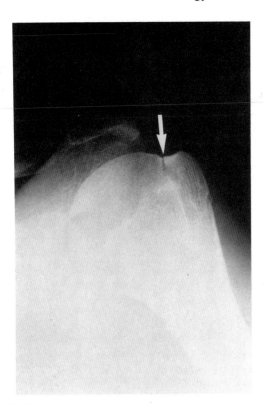

Figure 9.141. FLAP FRACTURE: GREATER TUBEROSITY. The displaced fracture of the greater tuberosity is recognized by the presence of a radiolucent line (arrow). *Comment:* This fracture is best identified in the external rotation view, since the greater tuberosity is brought into profile in this projection.

basic locations—proximal to the anatomical neck, greater tuberosity, lesser tuberosity, surgical neck, and shaft. (9)

Fractures Proximal to the Anatomic Neck. Isolated fractures through the anatomical neck are uncommon and usually occur in combination with other humeral fractures; however, when present, there is a high incidence of developing avascular necrosis of the humeral head. (2)

An impaction fracture on the posterolateral surface of the humeral head is commonly associated with anterior shoulder dislocation. The mechanism is related to the effect of the inferior glenoid rim being forcefully pushed into the articular surface of the humeral head (Hill-Sachs defect, "hatchet" defect). (10) The best routine projection to demonstrate the defect is internal rotation.

Fractures of the Greater Tuberosity (Flap Fracture). Direct trauma or avulsion from the connecting tendons may produce isolated fractures of this structure. (Fig. 9.141) It is not an infrequent fracture accompanying anterior humeral dislocation. (Fig. 9.142) Generally, older patients show a smaller separated fragment than younger individuals.

This fracture is best depicted on the external rotation view. If there has been more than 1 cm displacement of the tuberosity, significant tearing of the rotator cuff tendon has occurred and must be treated by open reduction and the cuff repaired. (4)

Fractures of the Lesser Tuberosity. As an isolated fracture, it is rare.

Fractures of the Surgical Neck. This is the most common site of proximal humerus fractures. (Fig. 9.143, 9.144A and B) The site of the fracture is immediately

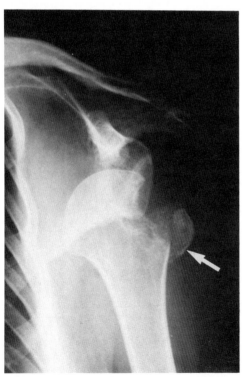

Figure 9.142. FLAP FRACTURE ASSOCIATED WITH ANTERIOR GLENOHUMERAL DISLOCATION. The humeral head is dislocated anteriorly and inferiorly to a subcoracoid position. This is associated with an avulsion fracture of the greater tuberosity of the humerus (flap fracture) (arrow).

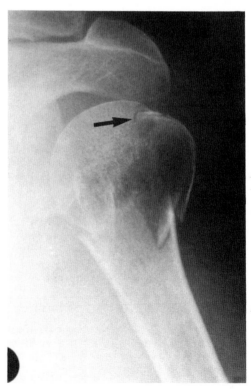

Figure 9.143. SURGICAL NECK FRACTURE: SHOULDER. A transverse comminuted fracture has occurred through the surgical neck of the humerus. There has been extension of the fracture line to involve the greater tuberosity (flap fracture) (arrow).

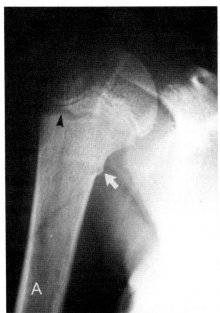
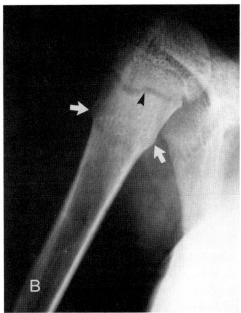

Figure 9.144. TORUS FRACTURE OF THE PROXIMAL HUMERUS.
A. AP Shoulder: External Rotation. A localized bulging of the cortical surface of the medial metaphysis of the proximal humerus is visible (arrow). **B. AP Shoulder: Internal Rotation.** The cortical bulging is seen to involve both the medial and lateral aspects of the proximal humerus (arrows). This is a characteristic finding of a torus fracture. *Comment:* In young patients the normal cartilaginous growth center (arrowheads) should not be misinterpreted as a fracture line. (Courtesy of Gerald A. Fitzgerald, MD, Sydney, Australia)

distal to the tuberosities, at the narrowest point of humeral width. These tend to be comminuted, involving the adjacent tuberosities. Anteromedial displacement of the distal shaft is a frequent accompanying finding due to the action of the pectoralis major muscle. On occasion, injury to the adjacent axillary nerve and artery may complicate the fracture.

Fractures of the Proximal Shaft. Direct trauma is the most common cause for shaft fractures. The relative location of the fracture in relation to muscle insertions determines the type of deformity produced. (4) If the fracture occurs proximal to the pectoralis major attachment, the humeral head will abduct and rotate. Between the pectoralis major and deltoid, the proximal fragment will adduct. Distal to the deltoid, the proximal fragment will abduct.

Complications of Humeral Fractures

Complications of humeral fractures include residual joint stiffness, nonunion, malunion, head avascular necrosis, post-traumatic myositis ossificans, and neurovascular damage.

DISLOCATIONS OF THE SHOULDER GIRDLE

The shoulder joint is by far the most common joint in the body to dislocate, accounting for over 50 percent of all joint dislocations. (4) Of the four joint complexes that comprise the shoulder girdle, dislocations at the glenohumeral joint are the most frequent, being involved in 85 percent of cases. The acromioclavicular joint makes up 12 percent, the sternoclavicular joint 2 percent, and the scapulothoracic joint only 1 percent. (11)

Glenohumeral Joint Dislocations

These are classified further into the direction in which the humeral head has been displaced—anterior, posterior, inferior, and superior.

Anterior Dislocation. This is the most frequent dislocation of the shoulder, making up approximately 95 percent of glenohumeral displacements. (Fig. 9.145) Commonly, associated fractures include impaction of the humeral head in 60 percent of cases (Hill-Sachs defect), fracture of the greater tuberosity in 15 percent of cases, and, less frequently, avulsion of the inferior glenoid rim (Bankart lesion). (12) (Fig. 9.146A and B, 9.147)

According to where the humeral head comes to rest, positional terms are applied—subglenoid, subcoracoid (most common), subclavicular, and, if trapped between two ribs, intrathoracic. Radiological signs include inferior and medial humeral displacement, altered humeral head shape, and the Hill-Sachs and Bankart lesions.

Posterior Dislocation. These are uncommon displacements, making up 2–4 percent of glenohumeral dislocations. They most commonly follow an epileptic convulsion, electric shock (accidental or therapeutic), or direct trauma. These are difficult lesions to identify radiographically.

The key radiographic signs are widening of the joint space more than 6 mm ("rim" sign), (13) double articular surface line ("trough line" sign), (14) lack of humeral head/glenoid fossa overlap, (15) lack of close contact at the anterior joint margin (vacant glenoid sign), cystic appearance of the head ("tennis racquet" appearance), and superior displacement. (4) (Fig. 9.148A and B) Inherent in the displacement is the fact that it is fixed into internal

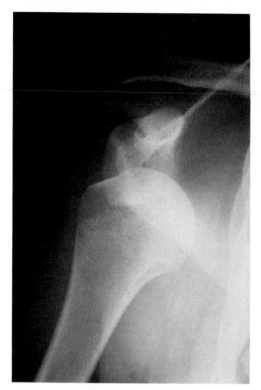

Figure 9.145. SUBCORACOID ANTERIOR DISLOCATION OF THE SHOULDER. The humeral head has been dislocated anteriorly to lay in a subcoracoid position. *Comment:* This is the most common form of shoulder dislocation.

rotation such that no difference in the appearance of the head in the external rotation view is seen.

Inferior Dislocation (Luxatio Erecta). The lesion follows severe hyperabduction trauma such that the humeral neck contacts the acromion, which acts as a fulcrum to lever the humeral head out and displace it inferiorly. The humerus then locks into this hyperabduction position, with the humeral head displaced into a subglenoid position.

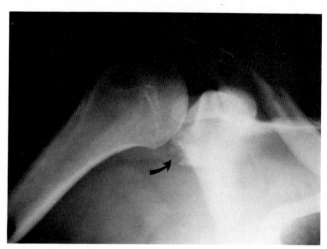

Figure 9.147. BANKART LESION: SCAPULA. An avulsion fracture of the inferior glenoid rim (arrow) at the insertion of the triceps muscle frequently accompanies anterior shoulder dislocations.

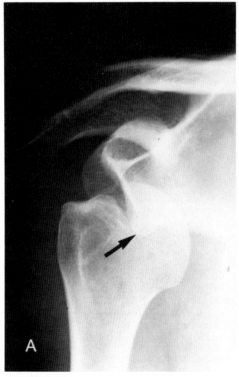

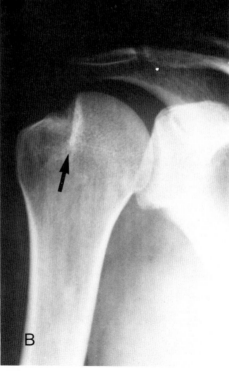

Figure 9.146. HILL-SACHS DEFORMITY ASSOCIATED WITH ANTERIOR HUMERAL DISLOCATION. A. AP Shoulder. An anteroinferior dislocation of the humerus has resulted in an impaction between the inferior glenoid rim and opposing humeral head (arrow). The impaction by the angular surface of the inferior glenoid rim produces the articular defect which has been referred to as the

"hatchet" deformity (Hill-Sachs defect). **B. AP Shoulder: Postreduction Radiograph.** Upon repositioning of the humeral head within the glenoid fossa, the residual effect of compression of the articular surface is clearly identified (arrow). *Comment:* The identification of this Hill-Sachs lesion is a telltale sign of recurrent anterior shoulder dislocation.

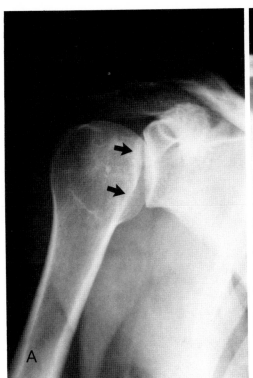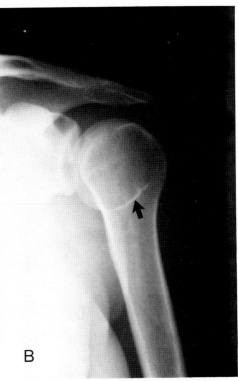

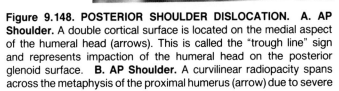

A

B

Figure 9.148. POSTERIOR SHOULDER DISLOCATION. A. AP Shoulder. A double cortical surface is located on the medial aspect of the humeral head (arrows). This is called the "trough line" sign and represents impaction of the humeral head on the posterior glenoid surface. **B. AP Shoulder.** A curvilinear radiopacity spans across the metaphysis of the proximal humerus (arrow) due to severe

internal rotation of the humerus ("tennis racquet" appearance). ***Comment:*** Posterior shoulder dislocations are uncommon, accounting for 2–4 percent of glenohumeral dislocations. They most commonly follow either an epileptic convulsion, an electric shock (accidental or therapeutic), or direct trauma.

Occasionally, the humerus may be only partially subluxed inferiorly (drooping shoulder, hanging shoulder). This is seen in hemarthrosis, joint effusion, stroke, and brachial plexus lesions. (16)

Superior Dislocation. This is a rare type of dislocation requiring considerable force, usually with the elbow flexed and the arm adducted. More commonly experienced is the superior displacement of the humeral head following a tear of the rotator cuff tendon. This reduces the downward holding power of the infraspinatous tendon, allowing the relatively unopposed action of the deltoid to elevate the humerus, which, in longstanding cases, may form a pseudojoint with the undersurface of the clavicle and acromion. If the acromiohumeral distance measures less than 7 mm, this is an indicator of rotator cuff tear. (17,18)

Acromioclavicular Joint Separations

The most optimum radiographic views are anteroposterior projections with 15 degrees of cephalad tilt and with and without 10–15 pounds of weight. These should be done bilaterally, for comparison purposes.

Radiological Features. Three landmarks are assessed on weightbearing and nonweightbearing views to evaluate displacement at the acromioclavicular joint.

1. *Acromioclavicular joint space.* Normally, the space is bilaterally symmetrical, within 2–3 mm of each other, and averages between 2–4 mm in absolute width. (19)

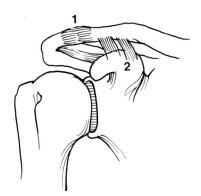

Figure 9.149. LIGAMENTS OF THE ACROMIOCLAVICULAR JOINT. This schematic diagram demonstrates the locations of (1) the acromioclavicular ligaments and (2) the coracoclavicular ligaments.

Table 9.15.
Classification of Acromioclavicular Joint Lesions

| Type | Severity | Ligament Integrity | | X-ray Findings |
		Acromio-clavicular	Coraco-clavicular	
I	Mild	Stretched	Normal	None
II	Moderate	Disrupted	Stretched	Wide joint space Slight clavicle elevation
III	Severe	Disrupted	Disrupted	Wide joint space Severe clavicle elevation

2. *Acromioclavicular joint alignment.* The inferior and superior margins of the clavicle and opposing acromion should be in smooth horizontal alignment.

3. *Coracoclavicular distance.* The distance between the inferior margin of the clavicle and the closest surface of the coracoid is normally 11–13 mm. There should be no more than 5 mm difference in the measurement from right to left. (4,20)

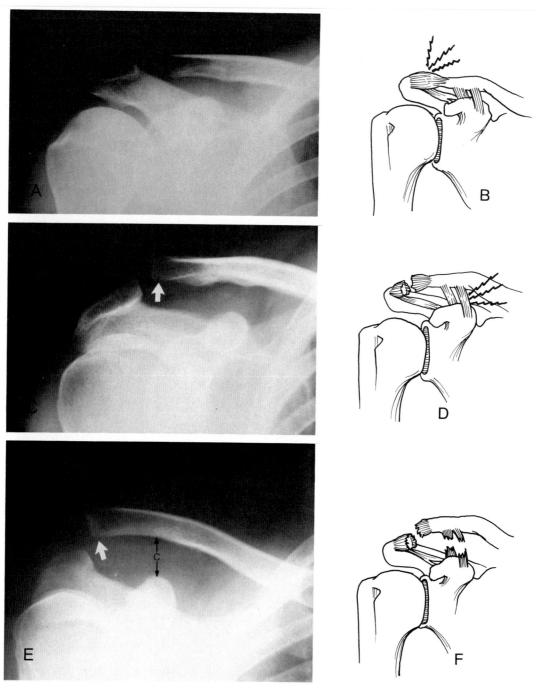

Figure 9.150. CLASSIFICATION OF ACROMIOCLAVICULAR JOINT INJURIES. A. Type I (Mild Sprain): AP Radiograph. B. Type I (Mild Sprain): Schematic Diagram. The acromioclavicular ligament is stretched but not disrupted, and the coracoclavicular ligament is intact. No discernible increase in the joint space or altered alignment is visible. **C. Type II (Moderate Sprain): AP Radiograph (arrow). D. Type II (Moderate Sprain): Schematic Diagram.** The acromioclavicular ligament is torn and the coracoclavicular ligament is stretched but intact. The joint space is widened, and slight elevation of the clavicular head has occurred. **E. Type III (Severe Sprain): AP Radiograph (arrow). F. Type III (Severe Sprain): Schematic Diagram.** Complete disruption of the acromioclavicular and coracoclavicular ligaments has occurred. There is widening of the joint space, distinct elevation of the clavicle, and widening of the coracoclavicular space (C).

Classification of Acromioclavicular Injuries.   (4,19) This is usually based on the degree of injury to the acromioclavicular and coracoclavicular ligaments. (Fig. 9.149) (Table 9.15)

Type I (Mild Sprain).   The acromioclavicular ligament is stretched but not disrupted, and the coracoclavicular ligament is intact. (Fig. 9.150A and B) Even on weight-bearing views, no discernable increase in the joint space or altered alignment is visible. These are treated conservatively.

Type II (Moderate Sprain).   The acromioclavicular ligament is torn, and the coracoclavicular ligaments are stretched but intact. (Fig. 9.150C and D) Radiographically, the joint space is widened, and slight elevation of the clavicle has occurred. These are initially treated conservatively, with a brace, but may require surgery. Old injuries to the coracoclavicular ligament may manifest as ligamentous ossifications.

Type III (Severe Sprain).   Complete disruption of the acromioclavicular and coracoclavicular ligaments has occurred. (Fig. 9.150E and F) Radiographically, there is widening of the joint space, the distal clavicle is distinctively elevated above the acromion, and the coracoclavicular space is widened more than 5 mm from the contralateral side. These usually require joint repair and open fixation.

Sternoclavicular Joint Dislocation

Dislocations of this joint are exceedingly rare and usually follow severe trauma. Anterior displacements are more frequent. Tomography is the technique of choice to demonstrate a sternoclavicular lesion.

Scapulothoracic Joint Dislocation

Severe trauma is required to produce this rare dislocation.

Fractures and Dislocations of the Elbow and Forearm

GENERAL CONSIDERATIONS

Approximately 6 percent of all fractures and dislocations involve the elbow. (1) The frequency of injury at various sites around the elbow differ between adults and children. (2) (Table 9.16) In adults, approximately 50 percent of elbow fractures involve the radial head or neck, 20 percent the olecranon, 10 percent the supracondylar region of the humerus, and 15 percent combinations of fracture/dislocations. Unusual sites of fracture involve the humeral condyles, proximal ulna, capitellum, and coronoid process. In children, the most common fracture site is the supracondylar region of the humerus, accounting for approximately 60 percent of all childhood elbow injuries, the lateral condyle accounts for 15 percent, and separation of the medial epicondyle ossification center accounts for 10 percent. Infrequent other sites include the olecranon, proximal ulna, radial epiphysis, and dislocations.

Table 9.16.
Incidence and Location of Elbow Injuries

| Adults | | Children | |
Location	Incidence	Location	Incidence
Radial head/neck	50%	Supracondylar	60%
Olecranon	20%	Lateral condyle	15%
Supracondylar	10%	Medial epicondyle	10%
Fracture/dislocations	15%		

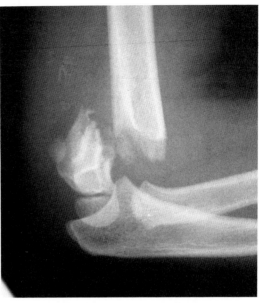

Figure 9.151. SUPRACONDYLAR FRACTURE OF THE HUMERUS.   A complete comminuted fracture is present through the supracondylar region of the humerus. Significant posterior displacement of the distal fragment has also occurred. ***Comment:*** This is the most common fracture of the elbow in children.

Unrecognized elbow fractures frequently produce residual loss of joint mobility and, at times, superimposed degenerative arthritis. The joint and osseous anatomy is complex and requires specific projections for adequate demonstration. A minimum elbow study should include the following views: 1) anteroposterior in full extension; 2) medial oblique; 3) lateral; and 4) axial olecranon projections. In children, confusing growth variations may occasionally be clarified by obtaining similar views of the uninvolved articulation.

Fractures and dislocations of the forearm usually follow significant trauma and are normally readily observable. Standard anteroposterior and lateral projections usually suffice to provide the necessary information required.

FRACTURES OF THE ELBOW

Distal Humerus Fractures

These are normally easily recognized. Notably, up to 95 percent of these fractures extend to disrupt the articular surface. Fractures are classified according to their relationship with the condyles and the shape of the fracture line.

Supracondylar Fractures.   The fracture line extends transversely or obliquely through the distal humerus above the condyles. (Fig. 9.151) This is the most common fracture to occur around the elbow in children (60 percent). Usually, the distal fracture fragment displaces posteriorly.

Intercondylar Fracture. The fracture line extends between the medial and lateral condyles and communicates with the supracondylar region. The resultant fracture line may take on a "T" or "Y" configuration. This type of

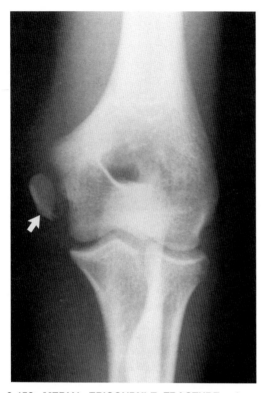

Figure 9.152. MEDIAL EPICONDYLE FRACTURE. An avulsion fracture of the medial epicondyle has occurred (arrow). A similar injury in a developing child or adolescent has been called "Little Leaguer's" elbow, and is usually associated with sports requiring strong throwing motions.

fracture in adults accounts for at least 50 percent of distal humerus fractures. (3)

The transverse fracture line which passes through both humeral condyles is called a transcondylar fracture. A comminuted fracture of the distal humerus, usually with associated ulnar and radial fractures, may occur if an object is struck with the elbow protruding from a car window ("sideswipe" or "baby car" fracture). (1)

Condylar Fracture. A single condyle may be sheared off due to an angular force through the elbow. Fractures may occur along the articular surfaces of the capitellum and trochlea. The convex surface of the capitellum is particularly susceptible to compression and breakage from forces transmitted from the radial head, and they are occasionally found in combination with each other. A small osteochondral fragment may also be sheared off, producing an intra-articular loose body (Kocher's fracture). (1)

Epicondylar Fracture. (Fig. 9.152) These are usually avulsive injuries from traction of the respective common flexor or extensor tendons and collateral ligaments on the medial or lateral epicondyles. Separation of the medial epicondyle is a common injury in sports where strong throwing actions are performed, such as in baseball, especially in adolescents before the apophysis unites to the humerus at between 18 and 19 years of age (little leaguer's elbow). (4)

Fractures of the Proximal Ulna

The two most common sites for fracture are the olecranon and coronoid process.

Olecranon Fracture. (Fig. 9.153A and B) Fractures of the olecranon account for approximately 20 percent of adult elbow fractures, ranking second in frequency to radial neck or head fractures. (2) They may follow direct trauma or an acute flexion avulsion from the triceps insertion. The fracture line is usually best seen on the lateral projection adjacent to the inferior convex surface of the trochlea, but may be proximal or distal to this site. Distraction of the separated fragment may be considerable

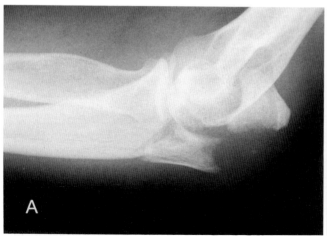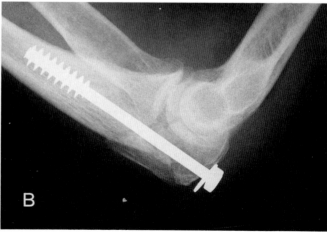

Figure 9.153. OLECRANON FRACTURE WITH REPAIR. A. Lateral Elbow. Two fracture lines have occurred through the olecranon process, with significant proximal retraction of the distal fragment. **B. Lateral Elbow.** A surgical pin has been placed longitudinal through the proximal ulna to realign the fracture fragments. Good appositional realignment has been obtained. **Comment:** Olecranon fractures represent the second most common site for elbow fractures, after the radial head in the adult.

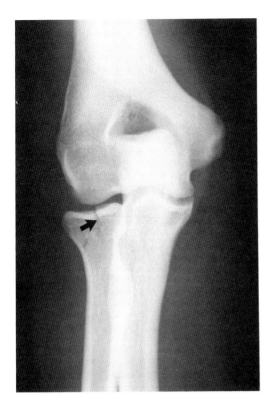

Figure 9.154. CHISEL FRACTURE: RADIAL HEAD. A vertical fracture line extends through the articular surface of the radial head, with minimal offset of the articular contour (arrow).

and requires surgical fixation. Swelling in the adjacent olecranon bursa is a common associated finding.

Coronoid Process Fracture. As an isolated fracture, this type of fracture is uncommon. Usually, it is seen in combination with posterior elbow dislocation. The fractured fragment frequently is small and difficult to identify; therefore, the oblique view provides the best projection, demonstrating the fracture. The precipitating force may be an avulsion from the brachialis muscle or impaction into the trochlea fossa.

Fractures of the Proximal Radius

Fractures of the radial neck and head are the most common fractures of the adult elbow, accounting for approximately 50 percent of all injuries to this region. (2) In children and adolescents, the incidence is significantly less, with a frequency of approximately 15 percent. (5) The majority of proximal radius fractures are due to a fall on an outstretched hand, transmitting a longitudinal axis of force to create impaction of the radial head into the capitellum. An incomplete fracture of the radial head which extends from the center of the articular surface for approximately 10 mm is called a "chisel" fracture. (6) (Fig. 9.154)

Radial Head Fracture. A number of radiological signs must be searched for, since the fracture line may be subtle and easily overlooked.

Fracture Line. A radiolucent line is seen usually orientated vertically and penetrating the articular cortex toward the lateral side of the head. (Fig. 9.155)

Cortical Disruption. At the fracture site, the cortex will be broken.

Cortical Deformity. At the fracture site, a sharp step-off or angulation is common, due to fragment displacement. Depression of the fractured fragment may produce a "double cortical" sign which is seen as a linear opacity paralleling the normal articular cortex. (7) (Fig. 9.156)

Altered Supinator Fat Line. On a normal lateral film, a linear radiolucent line representing the outer fascial plane of the supinator muscle, 1 cm above the anterior radial surface, will be observed. In fractures of the radial head or neck the fat line may be obliterated, blurred, or ventrally displaced by more than 1–2 cm. (8)

Fat Pad Sign. (Fig. 9.157) A useful sign of an intra-articular fracture of the elbow is the clear depiction of displaced humeral capsular fat pads. (9) In the normal elbow a layer of fat ("fat pad") lies between the synovial and fibrous layers of both the anterior and posterior joint capsule. In the lateral projection of the normal elbow the anterior fat pad is seen as an obliquely orientated radiolucency. When acute intracapsular swelling is present from any origin (hemorrhagic, inflammatory, or traumatic), the anterior fat pad is elevated to be orientated horizontally, while the posterior fat pad will now be visible ("fat pad" sign). (10) In joint distensions the elevated fat pads, especially anteriorly, may be obliterated due to hemorrhage or edema; therefore, the posterior fat pad, when visible, is the most reliable sign of intra-articular effusion. In children and adolescents, 90 percent

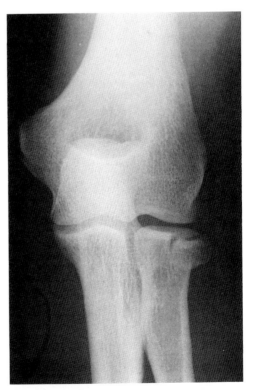

Figure 9.155. DISPLACED RADIAL HEAD FRACTURE. A fracture through the lateral portion of the radial head has occurred, with minimal depression of the articular cortex and lateral displacement of the isolated fragments.

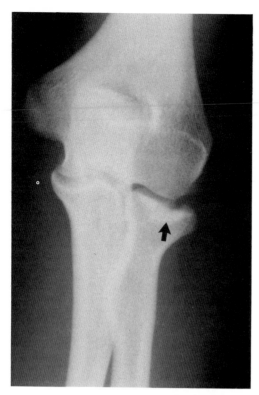

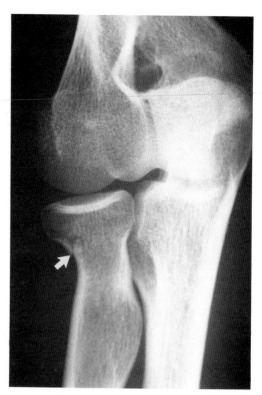

Figure 9.156. RADIAL HEAD FRACTURE: DOUBLE CORTICAL SIGN.   Observe the increased density of the articular cortex of the radial head, with projection of the opacity below the articular surface (arrow). Posteriorly, a fracture line is identified as a linear radiolucency. *Comment:* This "double cortical" sign is the result of an impaction fracture from the capitellum into the radial head, which displaces the cortex distally. Frequently, this is the only sign of a radial head fracture.

Figure 9.158. RADIAL NECK FRACTURE.   A thin fracture line disrupts the medial aspect of the cortex (arrow) and extends laterally towards the elbow.

of posterior fat pad signs will have an associated fracture. (9) In adults the sign is less frequently seen, and its absence does not exclude the presence of a fracture. (10)

Radial Neck Fracture.   The most common fracture is an impaction at the junction of the head and neck. The only sign may be a sharpened angle on the anterior surface, best depicted on the lateral projection. (Fig. 9.157, 9.158) Complete fractures will be readily seen as a transverse lucent line with varying degrees of displacement. A comminuted fracture of the radial head in combination with dislocation of the distal radioulnar joint is called an Essex-Lopresti fracture. (11)

FRACTURES OF THE FOREARM

Forearm fractures may involve the radius or ulna singularly, but, more commonly, they are both effected.

Fractures of Both the Radius and Ulna

As in any bony ring structure such as the pelvis, a fracture in one location is frequently associated with a disruption or another fracture or dislocation somewhere else in the ring. Approximately 60 percent of all forearm

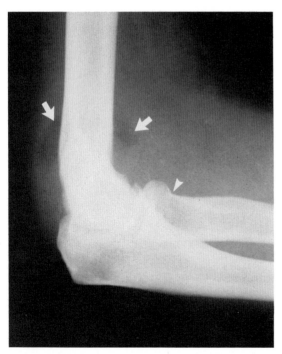

Figure 9.157. FAT PAD SIGN: SUBTLE RADIAL NECK FRACTURE.   Two triangular areas of radiolucency are seen to project away from the distal humeral shaft at the anterior and posterior

aspects (arrows). A subtle fracture of the radial neck is also identified (arrowhead). *Comment:* Whenever both the anterior and posterior fat pads are visible in this projection, a careful search must be performed to rule out a subtle intra-articular fracture. The most common fracture associated with a fat pad sign is a radial head or neck fracture. The posterior fat pad is a more reliable indicator of fracture, since the anterior fat pad may be poorly visualized or present in normal patients.

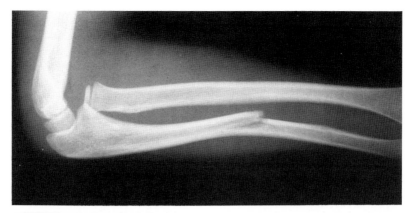

Figure 9.159. NIGHTSTICK FRACTURE: ULNAR FRACTURE. A spiral fracture is evident in the mid diaphysis of the ulna, with anterior angulation at the fracture site. **Comment:** This type of ulnar fracture, when associated with an attempt by the patient to protect the head, has been called a "nightstick" fracture.

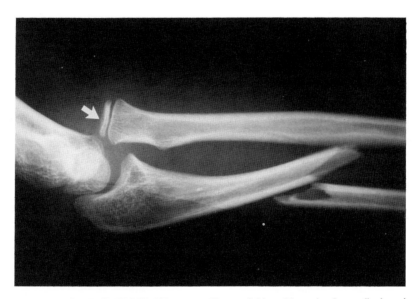

Figure 9.160. MONTEGGIA FRACTURE OF THE FOREARM. A fracture through the proximal one-third of the ulna is present, with associated anterior angulation of the proximal fracture fragment. The radial head has also been displaced anteriorly, with dislocation at the elbow (arrow).

fractures will involve both bones ("B-B" fractures), most commonly in the mid-third of the shaft. (12) Almost all fractures of these bones have associated displacement with angulation and rotation. These almost always require open surgery and fixation.

Isolated Fractures of the Ulna

Two types of fractures of the ulnar shaft have been described—distal and proximal.

Distal Ulnar Shaft Fracture (Nightstick or Parry Fracture). These fractures occur from direct trauma to the forearm, which is raised to protect the head during an assault with a club or hard object. (13) (Fig. 9.159)

Proximal Ulnar Shaft (Monteggia) Fracture. Monteggia in 1814 first described fractures of the proximal ulna with associated anterior dislocation of the proximal radius. (Fig. 9.160) This definition has been widened to include all fractures of the ulnar shaft associated with displacement of the radius in any direction. (14) In children, the ulnar component of this lesion is often a greenstick fracture.

Isolated Fractures of the Radius

The most frequent fracture site is toward the distal shaft of the radius. Other sites are rare. (Fig. 9.161, 9.162)

Distal Radial Shaft (Galeazzi, Piedmont, or Reversed Monteggia) Fracture. (Fig. 9.163) This is a rare but serious traumatic injury of the forearm. It is defined as a fracture of the radius at the junction of the middle and distal thirds, with dislocation of the distal radioulnar joint. (15,16) Despite treatment, they are frequently complicated by nonunion and a tendency to redislocate.

Dislocations of the Elbow

The elbow is the third most common site of dislocation in adults, the shoulder and interphalangeal joints of the fingers being first and second, respectively. In children, it is the most common dislocation. (17,18) They are classified according to the displacement of the radius and ulna relative to the humerus—posterior, posterolateral, anterior, medial, and anteromedial.

Posterior and Posterolateral Dislocations. These are

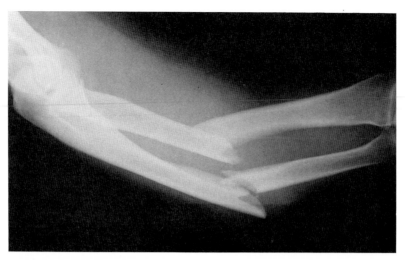

Figure 9.161. RADIUS AND ULNA SHAFT FRACTURES. Oblique comminuted fractures have occurred through the mid-diaphyseal portions of the radius and ulna, with significant angulation and rotational deformity. **Comment:** These are unique fractures that usually follow significant direct trauma to the forearm.

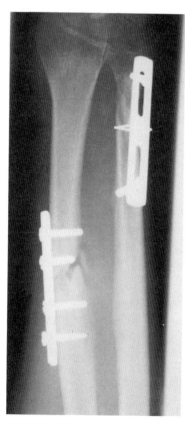

Figure 9.162. SURGICAL FIXATION: RADIUS AND ULNA FRAC-TURES. Metallic plates have been placed across the fracture sites of the radius and ulna to realign the fracture fragments and reduce the amount of residual deformity.

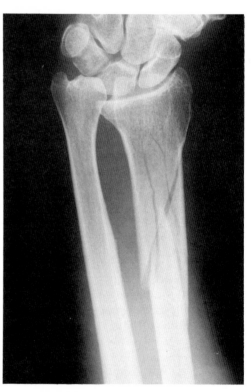

Figure 9.163. GALEAZZI'S FRACTURE. A comminuted fracture of the radius is present at the junction of the middle and distal thirds, with an associated dislocation of the distal radioulnar joint. There has been an overall shortening of the distal radius, which is a common finding in this fracture/dislocation.

the most common dislocations of the elbow, comprising up to 85–90 percent of all such lesions. (17) In practically all elbow dislocations both the radius and ulna will be displaced. More than 50 percent of elbow dislocations will have associated fractures, most commonly of the medial epicondyle and radial head or neck. (19) In chil-dren, an avulsed medial epicondyle may become en-trapped in the joint. A small percentage of posterior dislocations will develop post-traumatic myositis ossifi-cans at the anterior aspect of the joint, usually in the brachialis muscle.

Pulled Elbow. This is a unique, transient disorder which is the result of a sudden pull on the hand of a child between 2–5 years of age by an impatient adult. The child begins to cry immediately, with the forearm held in midpronation. The lesion is due to the radial head slipping out from under the annular ligament, trapping the ligament in the radiohumeral articulation. (20) No radiographic signs of the displacement will be evident. The ligament is easily replaced, often inadvertently, by supinating the hand, producing immediate relief of symptoms.

Fractures and Dislocations of the Wrist

GENERAL CONSIDERATIONS

The wrist is one of the most frequent sites for fractures to occur. Dislocations are less common. Many eponyms have been applied to various fractures and their related deformities to honor those who either first described or most accurately defined the entity.

The osseous and joint anatomy of the wrist is complex and requires specific projections for adequate demonstration. A minimum study of the wrist should include posteroanterior neutral, posteroanterior with ulnar flexion, oblique, and lateral projections. More precise definition of the individual carpal bones and their related soft tissue components requires specialized projections.

FRACTURES OF THE WRIST

Distal Radius Fractures

The distal radius is one of the most common sites of fracture in the wrist. Careful scrutiny of the radius on all projections must be performed to locate frequently overlooked, obscure fracture lines. In the absence of an obvious fracture, close observation on the lateral projection for the pronator quadratus fat line is a useful indicator for the presence or absence of fracture. (Fig. 9.164) Normally, it will be seen as a well-defined linear lucency orientated parallel to the plane of the radius, 2–5 mm from its anterior surface. In almost all cases of distal radius fractures the pronator quadratus fat line will be altered. (1) These alterations include anterior displacement, blurring, irregularity, and obliteration of the line.

Colles' Fracture. (Fig. 9.165A and B) Abraham Colles, in 1814, is credited with the first accurate description of this fracture, which subsequently bears his name. (2) The injury is defined as a fracture of the distal radius approximately 20–35 mm proximal to the articular surface, with posterior angulation of the distal fragment. More than 60 percent will have an accompanying fracture of the ulnar styloid process. (2) The usual mechanism is a fall on an outstretched, extended hand. The physical appearance to the distal forearm and wrist following the fracture has been called the "dinner fork" deformity. The incidence of the fracture increases with age, especially in women, such that by the age of 65 it is 6 times more common in women than in men. (3) Osteoporosis appears to be the underlying influential factor. Complications are common and may be severe. (4)

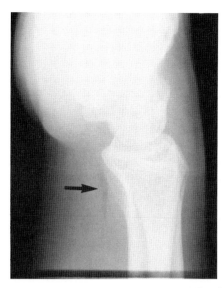

Figure 9.164. NORMAL QUADRATUS FAT LINE. Observe the clearly defined linear radiolucency (arrow) on the anterior aspect of the forearm in relatively close apposition to the distal radius. This fat line represents the outer surface of the pronator quadratus muscle. **Comment:** In the presence of distal radius fractures this fat line may become obliterated, blurred, or displaced away from the radial surface.

The radiological features are distinctive and relatively consistent.

Fracture Line. Usually transverse and comminuted, it is normally readily visible. A variable degree of impaction is apparent on the dorsal surface at the fracture site.

Radial Contour. A sharp cortical overlap is seen at the fracture site, especially visible on the frontal projection due to the proximal migration of the distal fragment.

Radial Length. The overall length of the radius is decreased due to the proximal migration of the distal fragment.

Angulation. The distal fragment is tilted dorsally, as evidenced by the altered angle of the articular surface, which is seen on the lateral projection. Normally, there is 5–15 degrees palmar angulation of the articular surface.

Soft Tissue. The distorted skin contour is apparent. The pronator quadratus fat plane will usually be altered.

Smith's Fracture (Reversed Colles' Fracture). (Fig. 9.166A–C) In 1854 Smith described a fracture of the distal radius with anterior angulation of the distal fragment. (5) The usual mechanism of injury is a direct blow or fall with the wrist being forced into hyperflexion. This mechanism and resultant angular deformity is the direct opposite of a Colles' fracture, and, hence, the synonym "reverse Colles' fracture." Smith's fracture is far less common than Colles' fracture.

Radiologically, the same signs as the Colles' fracture will be visible to varying degrees, except there will be anterior angulation of the distal fragment.

Barton's (Rim) Fracture. (Fig. 9.167A and B) In 1838 Barton described a fracture of the posterior rim of the distal radial articulating surface with associated proximal dislocation of the carpus. (6) A fracture of the anterior

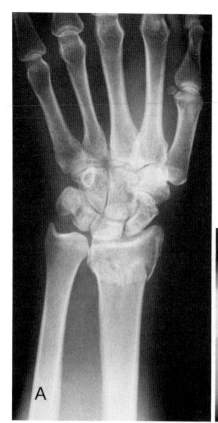

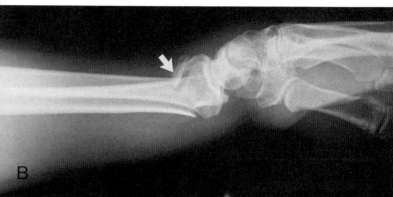

Figure 9.165. COLLES' FRACTURE: DISTAL RADIUS, WITH POSTERIOR ANGULATION.   A. PA Wrist. Visualization of the fracture line is obscured by a zone of impaction, as identified by a transverse linear opacity. However, cortical offset can be identified at the margin of the lateral radius.   **B. Lateral Projection.** The fracture through the distal radius is identified as comminuted in nature, with impaction on the posterior surface (arrow). The articular surface of the distal radius has been angulated in a posterior direction. Observation of the external skin contour reveals the typical "dinner fork" deformity.

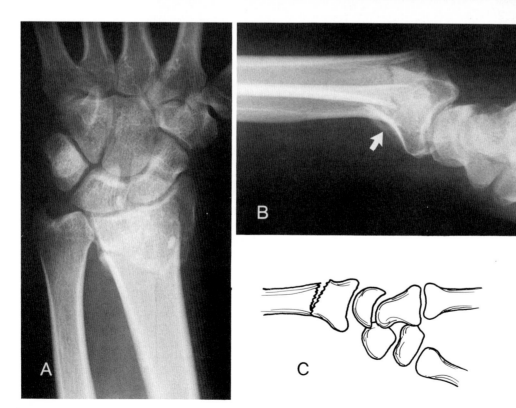

Figure 9.166. SMITH'S FRACTURE.   A. PA Wrist. A transverse fracture line extends through the distal radius, with an associated linear density at the fracture site.   **B. Lateral Wrist.** The fracture line is clearly identified through the distal radius, with impaction at the fracture site on the anterior surface (arrow). Associated anterior angulation of the distal fragment has altered the articular plane in this same direction.   **C. Schematic Diagram.** The combination of a distal radius fracture with anterior angulation of the articular surface characterizes this fracture deformity.

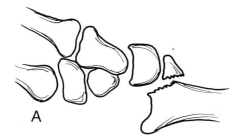
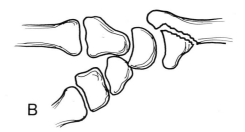

Figure 9.167. RIM FRACTURES OF THE DISTAL RADIUS. A. Schematic Diagram. A fracture of the posterior rim of the distal radial articular surface with associated posterior and proximal dislocation of the entire carpus is called a "Barton" fracture. **B.** A fracture

of the anterior rim of the distal articular surface of the radius with anterior displacement of the entire carpus has been called a "reversed barton" fracture.

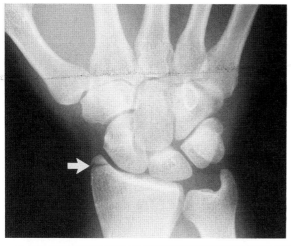

Figure 9.168. CHAUFFEUR'S FRACTURE (HUTCHINSON'S FRACTURE): FRACTURE OF THE RADIAL STYLOID. A small fracture is seen to extend through the distal radial styloid process (arrow). This fracture may be the result of an avulsion or impaction from the adjacent scaphoid.

rim has been called a "reverse Barton's fracture." The usual mechanism is forceful hyperflexion of the wrist to produce the posterior rim fracture.

Radiologically, on the frontal projection the proximal carpal row overlaps the articulating surface of the radius, while on the lateral the posterior rim fracture will be visible, along with the posterior and proximal displacement of the carpals.

Chauffeur's (Backfire, Hutchinson's) Fracture. (Fig. 9.168) These fractures were formerly encountered as a result of a backfire that occurred when attempting to start a car engine with a hand crank, the crank striking the dorsal surface of the wrist. (7) The fracture involves the radial styloid process as an avulsion or radial impaction from the adjacent scaphoid. The fracture line is either transverse or oblique, and, usually, there is no displacement.

Moore's Fracture. Moore in 1880 described, in association with Colles' fracture, a fracture of the ulnar styloid process and dislocation of the distal ulna. (8)

Torus Fracture. (Fig. 9.169A and B) This is the most common fracture of the wrist between 6 and 10 years of age. Typically, the fracture is located 2–4 cm from the

distal growth plate. A torus fracture can occur in any long bone and is the term applied to a buckled cortex following trauma. As such, the key radiological sign is a localized cortical bulge or bump.

Slipped Radial Epiphysis. (Fig. 9.170A and B) This injury is the childhood equivalent of the Colles' fracture. The mechanism involved is a shearing force across the growth plate following a forceful hyperextension injury. The radial epiphysis is usually displaced posteriorly and will almost always have a small, displaced metaphyseal fragment ("corner" sign), classifying it as a Salter-Harris Type II epiphyseal injury. Practically all of these epiphyseal separations are treated successfully by closed reduction, with no effects on growth.

Distal Ulnar Fractures

Ulnar Styloid Process Fracture. (Fig. 9.171) As an isolated fracture, this is an uncommon injury and is usually an avulsion through the ulnar collateral ligament. More frequently, it is found in combination with other fractures and dislocations of the wrist.

Distal Ulnar Shaft (Nightstick) Fracture. (See "Fractures of the Forearm.")

Scaphoid Fractures

The scaphoid is the most common carpal bone to fracture. The usual age of occurrence is between 15 and 40 years of age. Scaphoid fractures are distinctively rare in children. The mechanism of injury is complex, but it essentially consists of various degrees of hyperextension and radial flexion, such as falling on an outstretched hand. These fractures are frequently overlooked and exhibit a significant incidence of complications. The scaphoid is the most common site for *occult* fracture. (9)

Fracture Classification and Incidence. The scaphoid is divided into three regions—the distal pole, waist, and proximal pole. Some add a fourth segment, the tuberosity, which is part of the distal pole. Approximately 70 percent of fractures involve the waist, 20 percent the proximal pole, and 10 percent the distal pole. (9)

Radiological Features. The optimum routine view is the ulnar flexion projection, since it eliminates foreshortening of the scaphoid and may distract the fracture fragments and widen the fracture line. The major radiological sign is identifying the fracture line, which is often difficult. (Fig. 9.172A and B) If no fracture is seen initially,

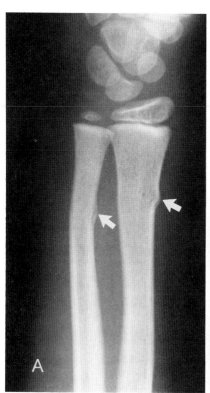

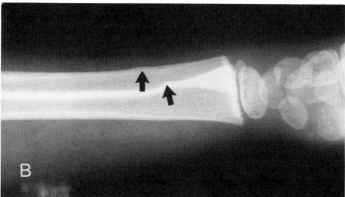

Figure 9.169. TORUS FRACTURE: DISTAL RADIUS AND ULNA. A. PA Wrist. A discrete area of cortical bulging is apparent at the lateral margins of the radius and ulna (arrows). **B. Lateral Wrist.** The cortical bulges are visualized as acute angulations in the posterior cortical contours (arrows). *Comment:* This is the most common fracture of the wrist between the ages of 6 and 10. The bulging of the cortex is due to a buckling of the bone, and is the key radiological sign of this injury.

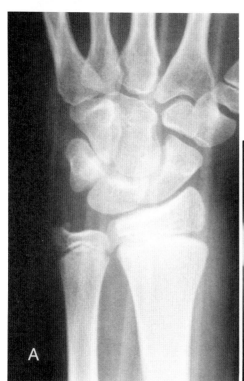

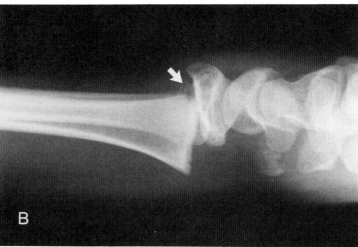

Figure 9.170. SLIPPED RADIAL EPIPHYSIS. A. PA Wrist. There is a subtle separation of the radial growth plate, with ulnar displacement of the distal epiphysis. **B. Lateral Wrist.** The direction of epiphyseal displacement is clearly identified to be posterior in direction. A small displaced metaphyseal fragment from the radius ("corner" sign) (arrow) is also noted. *Comment:* Diagnosis of slipped radial epiphysis requires a minimum of two projections. This injury is the childhood equivalent of the adult Colles' fracture.

yet the clinical picture is suspicious, then precautionary immobilization should be applied and the wrist re-x-rayed in 7–10 days. Bone scans shortly after the fracture event will also help in equivocal circumstances. After this time period, the fracture line widens, due to resorption along the fracture margins (occult fracture). The fracture line is usually transverse or, less commonly, oblique in relation to the long axis of the scaphoid. (Fig. 9.173)

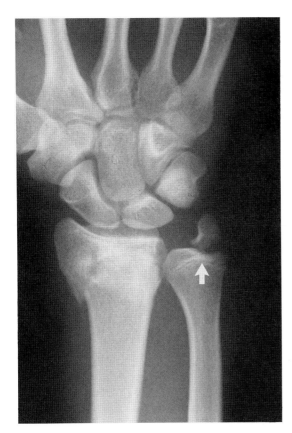

Figure 9.171. ULNAR STYLOID FRACTURE. An avulsion fracture of the ulnar styloid process is clearly visible. The radiolucent line through the distal ulna (arrow) should not be confused with a fracture line, as this represents an unfused epiphyseal growth plate. There is an associated fracture through the distal radius. **Comment:** Isolated ulnar styloid fractures are infrequent. These lesions are usually associated with other fractures of the wrist, especially the distal radius, as is the case here.

A useful soft tissue sign of a subtle scaphoid fracture can be found in alterations to the adjacent scaphoid fat stripe. The normal fat stripe is a linear collection of fat between the radial collateral ligament and tendon sheaths of the extensor pollicus brevis and abductor pollicus longus. In almost 90 percent of fractures involving the radial compartment of the wrist the fat stripe will be displaced laterally or totally obliterated ("navicular fat stripe" sign). (10)

Healing occurs without periosteal callus, the fracture line just gradually disappearing. Healing time varies according to the fracture site. The more distal the fracture,

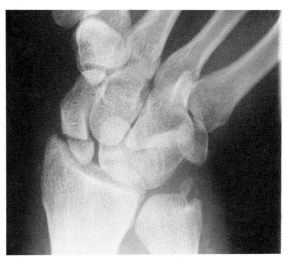

Figure 9.173. PROXIMAL SCAPHOID FRACTURE. An oblique fracture line extends through the proximal portion of the scaphoid. There are associated fractures of the ulnar and radial styloid processes. **Comment:** Fractures of the proximal pole are more likely to result in major complications, such as avascular necrosis, nonunion, and radiocarpal degenerative arthritis.

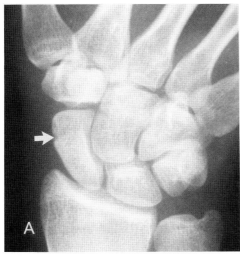

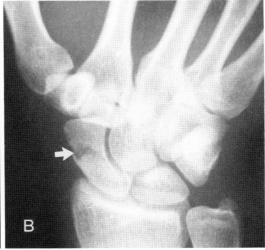

Figure 9.172. OCCULT SCAPHOID FRACTURE. A. PA Wrist: Initial Radiograph. A subtle fracture line is visible through the distal waist region of the scaphoid (arrow). Observe the absence of the navicular fat stripe adjacent to the fracture site. **B. PA Wrist: 3 Weeks Postinjury.** The fracture line is now clearly evident, due to bony resorption at the fracture margins (arrow). **Comment:** The scaphoid is the most common site for occult fracture. Follow-up radiographs, normally within 7 to 10 days of the injury, will usually demonstrate the fracture line as resorption occurs.

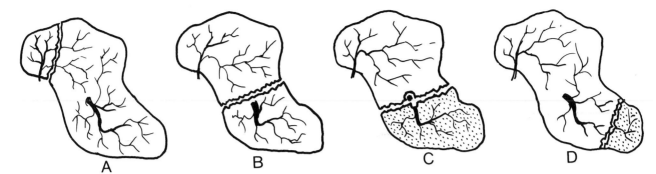

Figure 9.174. SCAPHOID FRACTURE AND BLOOD SUPPLY DISTRIBUTION: SCHEMATIC DIAGRAM.   A. Distal Pole Fracture. B. Distal Waist Fracture.   C. Proximal Waist Fracture.   D. Proximal Pole Fracture.   *Comment:* Fractures distal to the entrance of the main supplying artery have a significantly reduced incidence of avascular necrosis and nonunion. Those fractures proximal to this artery are frequently complicated by these abnormalities. The shaded regions indicate the location for complicating avascular necrosis.

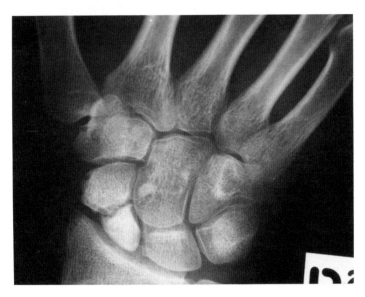

Figure 9.175. SCAPHOID FRACTURE WITH COMPLICATING AVASCULAR NECROSIS.   A wide fracture line can be seen passing through the waist of the scaphoid. The proximal pole is homogene- ously sclerotic, with no evidence of fragmentation. These findings are consistent with an ununited scaphoid fracture with associated avascular necrosis of the proximal pole.

the faster the healing and the less likely the development of complications. The converse applies to those fractures occurring proximally. (Fig. 9.173) The actual time period required for healing ranges between 6 and 20 weeks and will vary with the individual. (4)

Complications.   The major complications consist of avascular necrosis, nonunion, and radiocarpal degenerative arthritis.

Avascular Necrosis.   (Fig. 9.174A–D) This complication is encountered in approximately 10–15 percent of scaphoid fractures. (11) The scaphoid is anatomically predisposed to avascular necrosis following fracture due to the patterns of nutrient blood supply. (Fig. 9.175)

The scaphoid receives a dual blood supply from a small artery which enters and perfuses the distal pole and tuberosity and a larger vessel which enters at the waist and services all of the remaining areas. The entrance site of this larger vessel is variable and may be located more proximally or distally.

In the development of complicating avascular necrosis

the position of the fracture relative to the principal artery is the most crucial factor. If the fracture is distal to the major vessel, then avascular necrosis is unlikely; if proximal, then the probability for avascular necrosis increases significantly. In general, the more proximal the fracture line the greater the probability for avascular necrosis.

Radiological signs of the avascular segment include increased density and fragmentation. The fracture line will appear wider and is often cystic in appearance. All of these signs will take a variable time after the fracture incident to appear, ranging from months to years.

Nonunion.   (Fig. 9.176) Nonunion occurs in approximately 30 percent of fractures involving the waist of the scaphoid. (12) As with avascular necrosis, the major variable that determines the development of nonunion, or even delayed union, is the relationship of the fracture line to the principal artery. If there is delayed diagnosis or inappropriate immobilization, that may also predispose to this complication.

Radiological features of nonunion include widening of

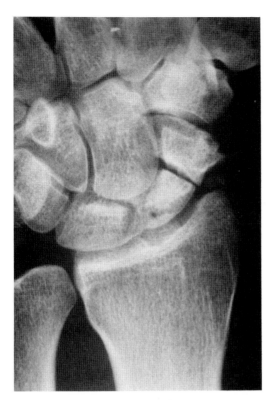

Figure 9.176. SCAPHOID FRACTURE WITH NONUNION. A smooth fracture line traverses the waist of the scaphoid. The opposing margins of the fracture line are sclerotic and well defined. These findings are distinctive for fracture nonunion.

the fracture line, cyst formation, and development of opposing sclerotic surfaces along the fracture line.

Radiocarpal Degenerative Arthritis. (Fig. 9.177) This may follow a healed scaphoid fracture, nonunion or avascular necrosis of the scaphoid, and radius fracture. A decreased radiocarpal joint space, subchondral sclerosis, osteophytes, and subchondral cysts characterize this complication. In the absence of trauma, the presence of these radiocarpal changes should suggest the diagnosis of calcium pyrophosphate dihydrate crystal deposition disease (CPPD).

Fractures of the Triquetrum

This is the second most common carpal bone to fracture. (4) The most common type of fracture is an avulsion from the dorsal surface at the site of attachment of the radiocarpal ligament. (Fig. 9.178) This has been called a Fisher's fracture. (13,14) These fractures usually follow hyperflexion injuries and present with swelling and localized pain on the dorsum of the wrist. Radiologically, they are best identified on the lateral projection as a small, displaced flake of bone.

Fractures of Other Carpal Bones

Fractures of the remaining carpals are unusual and are typically related to a specific type of injury.

Pisiform Fracture. (Fig. 9.179) A direct, impacting blow such as a fall on an outstretched hand is the usual mechanism. The most common fracture is a vertical fracture dividing the bone into approximate halves.

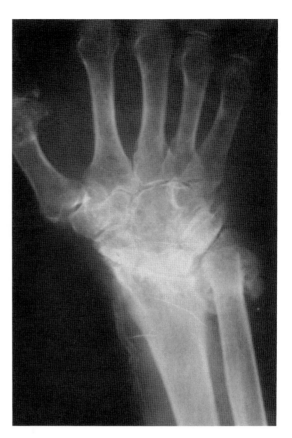

Figure 9.177. SCAPHOID FRACTURE WITH RADIOCARPAL DEGENERATIVE ARTHRITIS. Severe loss of radiocarpal joint space, osteophytes, subchondral sclerosis, and associated cyst formation are visible throughout the carpal and distal radius articulations. Careful scrutiny of the proximal pole of the scaphoid demonstrates its resorption, most likely secondary to mechanical deformation and avascular necrosis. **Comment:** This is a severe form of post-traumatic radiocarpal degenerative arthritis in a retired professional boxer. His opposite hand appeared similar. (Courtesy of Stephen W. Hayman, DC, De Land, Florida)

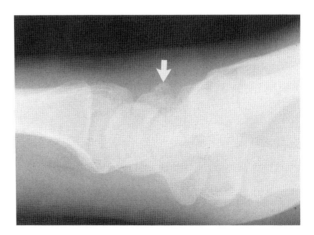

Figure 9.178. AVULSION FRACTURE OF THE TRIQUETRUM (FISHER'S FRACTURE). A small avulsed fragment can be seen displaced posteriorly from the surface of the triquetrum (arrow). Some minimal overlying soft tissue swelling is also appreciated. **Comment:** This fracture is the second most common fracture of the wrist, with the scaphoid being the most common.

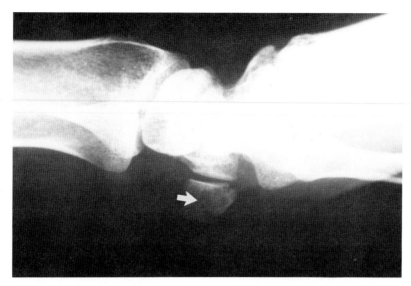

Figure 9.179. PISIFORM FRACTURE.   An oblique fracture line is seen through the midportion of the pisiform (arrow). These fractures usually are the result of a direct blow to the pisiform from falling on a hyperextended hand, which typically divides the pisiform in half. (Courtesy of Klaus W. Weber, MD, Hechingen, West Germany)

Trapezium Fracture.   (Fig. 9.180) These most commonly follow hyperabduction thumb trauma and typically fracture the radial portion of the bone.

Trapezoid Fracture.   This is the least commonly fractured carpal bone.

Capitate Fracture.   The capitate is an uncommon carpal to fracture, and, when it occurs, it is usually associated with scaphoid or perilunate dislocations. (4) The most frequent fracture is transverse, through the waist.

Hamate Fracture.   This bone may fracture in various areas. The hook is a common site of fracture, which occurs as the result of a direct blow such as may occur in club or racquet sports where the butt end strikes directly over the protuberance. (15,16) On the frontal view the circular contour of the hamate may not be seen. (17) A special tangential view with the wrist in hyperextension is usually needed for diagnosis.

Lunate Fracture.   This fracture is uncommon, since it tends to dislocate before it fractures. If a fracture is seen in the lunate, the diagnosis of Kienbock's disease (avascular necrosis) is likely.

DISLOCATIONS OF THE WRIST

Dislocations of the wrist are relatively uncommon but involve predictable locations. The classification of these injuries identifies two patterns: 1) a single bone which dislocates relative to the remaining carpals; and 2) a single bone which remains in normal position, but with the surrounding bones dislocating.

A useful guideline in evaluating the carpal relationship on the posteroanterior projection is to visually inspect the three carpal areas. (18) (Fig. 9.181) Arc 1 is formed by connecting the proximal articular surfaces of the proximal carpal row; arc 2, the distal articular surfaces of the proximal row; and arc 3, the proximal surfaces of the distal carpals (capitate, hamate). These arcs should be smooth and demonstrate proper intercarpal alignment. Disruptions of these arcs indicate a carpal displacement.

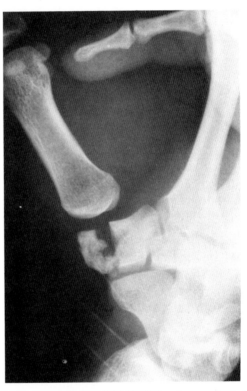

Figure 9.180. TRAPEZIUM FRACTURE.   A comminuted fracture of the lateral portion of the trapezium has occurred. Significant widening of the first metacarpal trapezium articulation is also identified, due to severe ligamentous injury.

Single Carpal Dislocations

Lunate Dislocation.   (Fig. 9.182) This is the most common carpal to dislocate, usually following a hyperextension injury. When the lunate dislocates, it tilts forward and anterior, disrupting its articulation with the capitate but maintaining close approximation with the

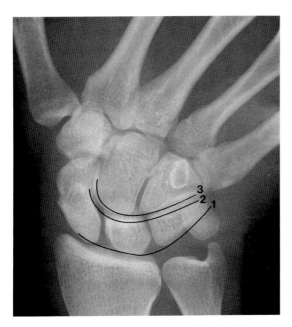

Figure 9.181. THE THREE ARCS OF CARPAL ALIGNMENT. Three curvilinear lines are constructed along the articular margins at the midcarpal and radiocarpal joints. In a normal PA view of the wrist these lines should be smooth and continuous across the connecting joint spaces. *Comment:* Visual inspection of these three arcs is a useful method for detecting carpal displacements.

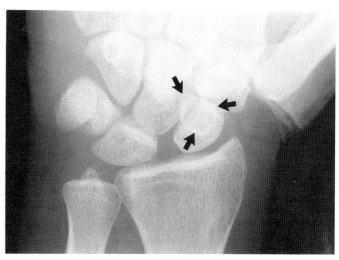

Figure 9.183. SCAPHOID OR ROTATORY SUBLUXATION. The scaphoid is considerably shortened in its longitudinal dimension, with the formation of a rounded cortical contour at its distal margin ("ring" sign) (arrows). A widening of the scapholunate space ("Terry Thomas" sign) has occurred due to disruption of the interconnecting ligament. *Comment:* The scaphoid is the second most common bone to be displaced in the wrist. The combination of the "ring" and "Terry Thomas" signs renders the diagnosis.

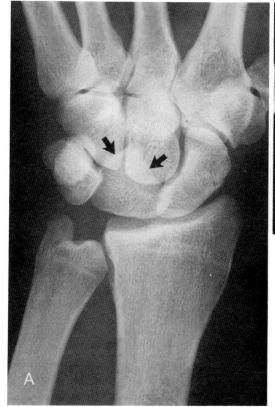

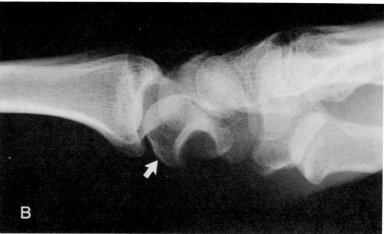

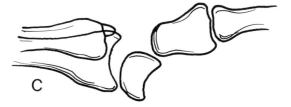

Figure 9.182. LUNATE DISLOCATION. A. PA Wrist. Note the overlap of the distal lunate with the capitate. The triangular shape ("pie" sign) (arrows) is characteristic of anterior dislocation. **B. Lateral Wrist.** The lunate can be seen displaced anteriorly and tilted forward at its superior aspect (arrow). **C. Schematic Diagram.**

Observe the relationships between the radius/lunate and lunate/capitate. *Comment:* Anterior lunate dislocation is the most common carpal displacement. The characteristic findings are well demonstrated with the triangular appearance on the PA film and the anterior forward displacement on the lateral projection.

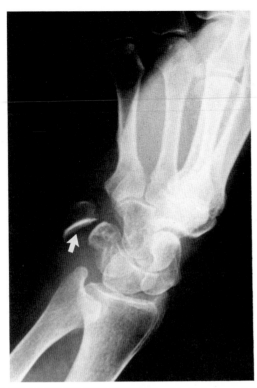

anterior rim of the distal radius. This is best seen on the lateral view. On the posteroanterior view the lunate is altered in shape to appear triangular, with the apex pointing distally ("pie" sign). Inspection of the three carpal arcs will demonstrate disruption of arcs 2 and 3 at the midcarpal joint.

Scaphoid.   (Fig. 9.183) This is the second most common carpal to be displaced. Complete dislocation is infrequent, with lesser degrees of subluxation being more common. As the scaphoid displaces, it moves laterally and rotates anteriorly (rotary subluxation). On the posteroanterior view this will be seen as a small, foreshortened scaphoid which appears circular in shape ("ring" or "signet ring" sign). (19) Additionally, there will be an increase in the space between the scaphoid and lunate of more than 4 mm ("Terry Thomas" sign). (19,20)

Other Carpal Dislocations.   These are distinctively unusual and require the occurrence of severe trauma. (Fig. 9.184)

Multiple Carpal Dislocations

Perilunate Dislocations.   These usually are comprised of dorsal displacements of all the carpal bones except the lunate, which maintains its normal position with the radius. This is best seen on the lateral projection. On the posteroanterior projection the capitate will be seen to overlie the lunate.

Transcaphoid Perilunate Dislocations.   (Fig. 9.185) This is virtually the same injury as the perilunate dislo-

Figure 9.184. PISIFORM DISLOCATION.   Displacement of the pisiform away from the triquetrum is clearly seen (arrow). This is an uncommon site for carpal dislocation.

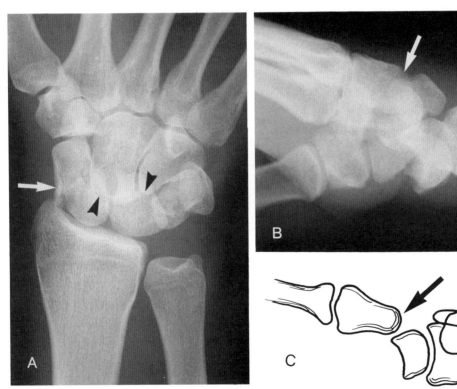

Figure 9.185. TRANS-SCAPHOID FRACTURE AND PERILUNATE DISLOCATION.   A. PA Wrist. A transverse fracture through the waist of the scaphoid (arrow) has occurred in association with posterior dislocation of the distal fragment and distal carpal bones. The superimposed densities of the hamate and capitate (arrowheads) signify this posterior dislocation and proximal migration.   **B. Lateral Wrist.** The posterior displacement of the distal carpal row can be identified, especially the capitate (arrow).   **C. Schematic Diagram: Lateral Projection.** Note the posterior displacement of the capitate in relation to the normally aligned lunate (arrow).   **Comment:** Trans-scaphoid fracture and perilunate dislocations follow severe traumatic injury to the wrist. Characteristically, the fracture is through the midwaist of the scaphoid, with associated posterior displacement of the distal fragment and distal carpal row.

cations, except there is an associated fracture through the waist of the scaphoid. The proximal fragment stays in its normal position with the lunate, while the distal portion displaces from the other carpal bones dorsally.

deQuervain's Fracture Dislocation. Described in 1907 by deQuervain, this consists of anterior dislocation of the lunate, along with the proximal fragment of a fractured scaphoid. (21)

Fractures and Dislocations of the Hand

GENERAL CONSIDERATIONS

The phalanges and metacarpals are the most common sites of skeletal injury in the entire skeleton. (1) Phalangeal fractures are more common than metacarpal fractures. In the majority of cases only a single bone or joint will be affected. Most can be treated conservatively, with only a few requiring open reduction and soft tissue repair or pin fixation.

Radiological examination routinely should have no less than three projections, including posteroanterior, oblique, and lateral views. If a single digit is involved, collimated views in these positions should be done to enhance detail. Examination of the thumb requires specialized projections. Knowledge of the locations and appearances of the many sesamoid bones and nutrient canals will reduce the probability of misdiagnosis.

FRACTURES OF THE HAND

Second to Fifth Metacarpal Fractures

Of all the metacarpals, the fifth is the most commonly fractured, the majority of which occur in the distal half.

Boxer's Fracture. This is a transverse fracture of the neck of the second or third metacarpal, the result of a straight, jabbing type of blow with the fist. (2)

Bar Room Fracture. (Fig. 9.186A and B) This type of fracture is also transverse in nature, involving the neck of the fourth or fifth metacarpals and is the result of a "roundhouse" type of blow characteristic of the inexperienced fighter. (2,3) This exposes the fourth and fifth metacarpal heads to absorption of the force of the delivered blow.

In most metacarpal neck fractures there will be anterior angulation of the metacarpal head, with variable degrees of shortening and rotation of the fracture fragment.

Shaft Fracture. (Fig. 9.187A and B) When present, these usually involve the third and fourth metacarpals, often simultaneously. Dorsal angulation and displacement across the fracture site quite commonly occurs.

Base Fracture. These fractures are rarely seen.

First Metacarpal Fractures

Most thumb metacarpal fractures occur at or near the base. Four distinct patterns are found—Bennett's, Rolando's, transverse, and a Salter-Harris Type II which occurs in adolescents.

Bennett's Fracture. (Fig. 9.188A and B) This injury actually is a fracture/dislocation which was first described by Bennett in 1882. (4,5) This type of fracture is defined as an intra-articular fracture through the base of the first metacarpal, with dorsal and radial displacement of the shaft. A small medial fragment remains closely aligned to the trapezium.

Rolando's (Comminuted Bennett's Fracture). (Fig. 9.189) In 1910 Rolando described a comminuted intra-articular fracture at the base of the first metacarpal. (6) This is a difficult fracture to treat and is the least common of all first metacarpal fractures. (1)

Transverse Fracture. This is the most common fracture of the first metacarpal. (7) (Fig. 9.187A) On occasion,

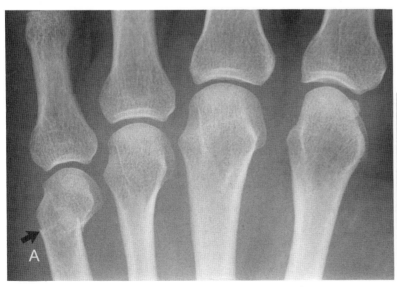

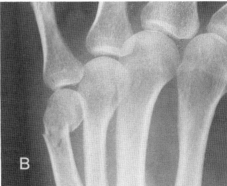

Figure 9.186. BAR ROOM FRACTURE (FIFTH METACARPAL NECK FRACTURE). A. PA Hand. A transverse fracture is seen at the junction of the fifth metacarpal head and shaft (arrow). Some slight radial displacement of the head is also present. **B. PA Oblique Hand.** The oblique view reveals the significant anterior displacement of the metacarpal head, common in these injuries. *Comment:* These metacarpal head fractures are common following a direct blow to the metacarpal phalangeal joints, particularly on the ulnar side of the hand.

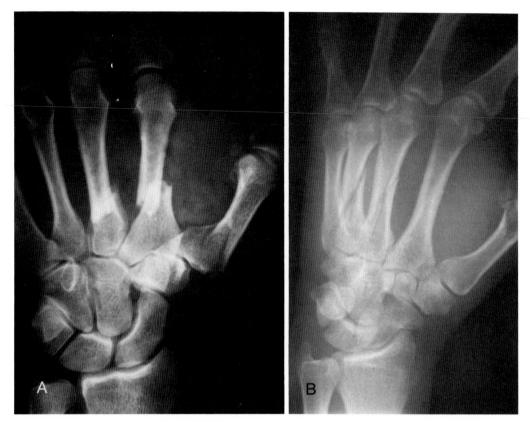

Figure 9.187. METACARPAL SHAFT FRACTURES. A. PA Hand. Transverse fractures are visualized through the first, second, and third metacarpal shafts. There has been a considerable degree of displacement and overlap, particularly at the second and third met- acarpals. **B. Oblique Hand.** Multiple oblique fractures are seen extending through the shafts of the third and fourth metacarpals, as well as the proximal phalanx of the fifth digit. (Courtesy of James R. Brandt, DC, FACO, Coon Rapids, Minnesota)

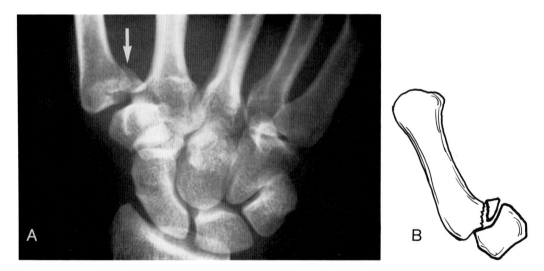

Figure 9.188. BENNETT'S FRACTURE. A. Oblique Wrist. An oblique intra-articular fracture is present (arrow), extending through the base of the first metacarpal, with associated posterior and radial displacement of the adjacent shaft. **B. Schematic Diagram.**

the fracture line may be oblique, but it remains extra-articular.

Phalangeal Fractures

Fractures of the phalanges are collectively more com- mon than metacarpal fractures. Distal phalangeal frac- tures are the most common, comprising 50 percent of all phalangeal fractures, while 15 percent affect the proximal phalanges, and 10 percent the middle phalanges. (8)

Fractures of the Distal Phalanges. The middle finger

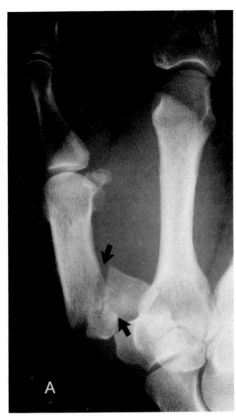

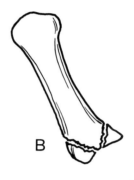

Figure 9.189. ROLANDO'S FRACTURE (COMMINUTED BEN-NETT'S FRACTURE). A. PA Thumb. A comminuted intra-articular fracture (arrows) is evident at the base of the first metacarpal which is associated with posterior and radial displacement of the distal metacarpal shaft. **B. Schematic Diagram.**

is the most common site of fracture. (8) Four types of fracture occur—transverse, longitudinal, comminuted, and chip.

Transverse fractures occur toward the base. (Fig. 9.190A and B) Longitudinal fractures may split the phalanx in half and extend all the way to the joint. Comminuted fractures are the most common and are usually limited to the distal tuft. Chip fractures involve the posterior or anterior corners at the phalangeal base. A posterior chip fracture inactivates extension of the distal interphalangeal joint and produces a flexion deformity ("mallet" or "baseball" finger). (Fig. 9.191A and B)

Fractures of the Middle Phalanges. Most fractures occur in the distal shaft. Another common fracture is one which occurs on the anterior surface, at the base of the phalanx, and is called a "volar plate" fracture. (Fig. 9.192)

Fractures of the Proximal Phalanges. Most fractures involve the middle and proximal shafts. (Fig. 9.193) These infrequently continue into the adjacent joint.

Turret Exostosis. This represents a bony protuberance, usually on the ulnar and dorsal aspects of the base of the proximal or middle phalanx. (9) The exostosis represents organization of a traumatic subperiosteal hemorrhage. The hematoma first appears as a soft tissue mass and then ossifies. It produces a painful lump on the dorsal aspect of the fingers and may interfere with flexion. Often, a healed scar of a previous laceration may be

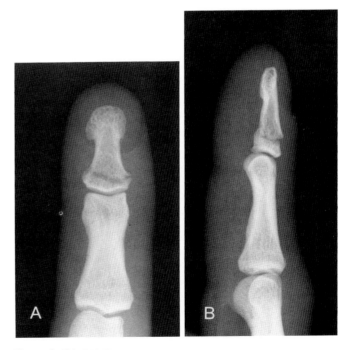

Figure 9.190. DISTAL PHALANX FRACTURE. A. PA Distal Phalanx. A transverse fracture is present through the base of the distal phalanx. **B. Lateral Distal Phalanx.** There is little displacement across the fracture line.

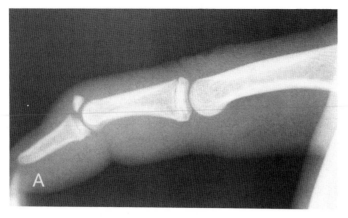

Figure 9.191. POSTERIOR CHIP FRACTURE OF THE DISTAL PHALANX ("MALLET" FINGER OR "BASEBALL" FINGER). A. Lateral Finger. A posterior chip fracture at the base of the distal phalanx is clearly seen. Also, observe the inability to extend the distal interphalangeal joint. B. Schematic Diagram. *Comment:* These posterior chip fractures are usually secondary to sudden forced flexion of the articulation, with resultant avulsion of the attachment of the extensor tendon.

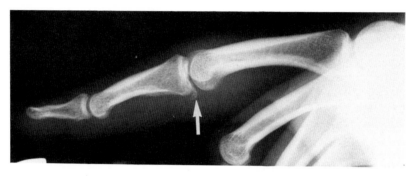

Figure 9.192. VOLAR PLATE FRACTURE. A small chip fracture is seen at the anterior aspect of the distal phalanx (arrow). Because of the small fragment, these fractures are frequently overlooked and may require specific oblique films for identification.

identified in the overlying skin. Recurrence rate following surgical removal is high. It may radiographically simulate a sessile osteochondroma, with the clinical history being the key to the differential diagnosis.

DISLOCATIONS OF THE HAND

Metacarpophalangeal Joint Dislocation

Dislocations are usually readily apparent. (Fig. 9.194) The index and little fingers are most common to dislocate. This type of dislocation is classified by two subgroups—simple and complex. Simple dislocations are easily reducible; complex dislocations have an entrapped, avulsed volar plate within the joint and require open reduction. A diagnostic sign of a complex dislocation is the presence of a sesamoid bone within a widened joint space. (10)

At the first metacarpophalangeal joint a tear or complete rupture of the ulnar collateral ligament results in an instability which has been called "gamekeeper's" thumb. (Fig. 9.195A and B) Campbell in 1955 noted the common occurrence of the injury in English gamekeepers who killed rabbits by breaking their necks between their thumb and forefinger. (11) The term has subsequently lingered in the literature to describe any injury associated with ulnar collateral ligament instability. A more modern mechanism of injury occurs from incorrect placement of a ski pole, producing abduction and extension of the thumb as the skier's momentum carries him downhill.

Radiographic examinations are usually negative, unless an abduction stress view is taken where a widening of the ulnar joint compartment and radial shaft of the proximal phalanx will be apparent. (1) Occasionally, a small fragment from the radial margin of the base of the proximal phalanx will be avulsed. Partial tears and sprains are treated with immobilization, complete tears with open repair, and avulsion fractures by pinning.

Interphalangeal Dislocations

The majority of interphalangeal dislocations follow acute hyperextension and result in posterior displacement of the phalanx. (Fig. 9.196) Anterior dislocations are rare. Usually, only one joint of the same digit will be dislocated and, infrequently, two joints. (Fig. 9.197) In association with the dislocation there frequently is a small volar plate fracture which may become entrapped in the joint and prevent closed reduction.

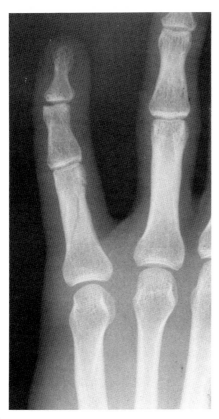

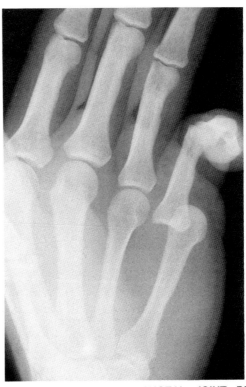

Figure 9.193. PROXIMAL PHALANGEAL FRACTURE. A spiral fracture is visible in the proximal phalanx of the fifth digit. No significant displacement or intra-articular extension is seen.

Figure 9.194. METACARPOPHALANGEAL JOINT DISLOCATION. Complete dislocation of the fifth metacarpal phalangeal joint has occurred, with posterior displacement of the proximal phalanx.

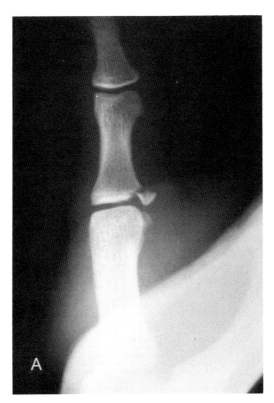

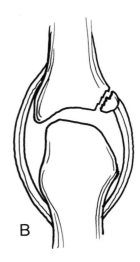

Figure 9.195. GAMEKEEPER'S THUMB. A. PA Thumb. A small avulsed triangular fragment is evident at the ulnar side at the base of the proximal phalanx. **B. Schematic Diagram.** The avulsion of the phalangeal base is secondary to severe abduction at the first metacarpal phalangeal joint. **Comment:** Gamekeeper's thumb does not always have an associated fractured phalangeal base. Frequently, on plain films no abnormality will be seen. Specific abduction stress views will, however, demonstrate ligamentous instability.

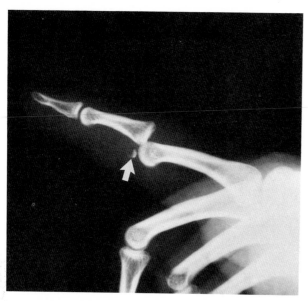

Figure 9.196. INTERPHALANGEAL JOINT DISLOCATION. A characteristic posterior displacement of the middle phalanx has occurred, with an associated volar plate fracture (arrow). *Comment:* These interphalangeal joint dislocations are the most common encountered.

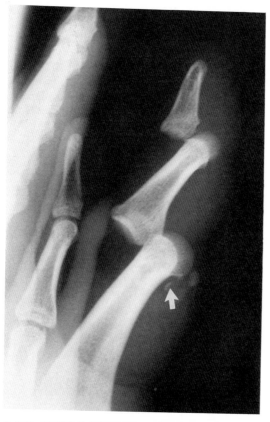

Figure 9.197. DOUBLE INTERPHALANGEAL JOINT DISLOCATION. Posterior dislocation has occurred at both the distal and proximal interphalangeal joints. There is an associated small volar plate fracture, with the fragment adjacent to the anterior aspect of the metacarpal head (arrow). *Comment:* Double interphalangeal joint dislocations are exceedingly rare. (Courtesy of Gerald A. Fitzgerald, MD, Sydney, Australia)

Stress Fractures

GENERAL CONSIDERATIONS

Stress fractures can occur in normal or abnormal bone which is subjected to an undue amount of repeated stress. Following a brief period of swelling, radiographs usually demonstrate the lesion.

Definitions

Fatigue Fracture. Fatigue fractures occur secondary to an abnormal amount of stress or torque applied to a bone with normal integrity.

Insufficiency Fracture. Insufficiency fractures occur with normal stress placed upon a bone which has an underlying weakness or pathological process present. The cause of insufficiency fractures are diverse and include Paget's disease, osteoporosis, osteomalacia or rickets, osteopetrosis, fibrous dysplasia, and osteogenesis imperfecta. (1)

Etiology of Stress Fractures

The major cause of stress fractures is an abnormal degree of repetitive trauma. This often is related to increased physical exertion as is found in sports activities. Stress fractures may also occur due to an altered muscular imbalance placed upon the skeletal structures. Stress may follow certain surgical procedures such as bunionectomy (metatarsals), (2) in the pubic rami following hip replacement, (3) or in knee surgery. (4)

Common Sites for Stress Fractures

The metatarsals are a very common site, with the middle and distal portions of the shaft of the second and third metatarsals being most frequently affected. (4) (Fig. 9.198A–C, 9.199A–C) The proximal tibia is also a common location, with a high incidence in joggers, marchers, and ballet dancers. (5) (Fig. 9.200A and B) Stress fracture of the calcaneus is found in military recruits and long-distance runners. (6) (Fig. 9.201) The proximal or distal metaphyses of the fibula are not uncommon sites for stress fractures, usually being found in runners and ballet dancers. (7) The distal portion is affected more often than the proximal aspect. (Fig. 9.202)

The pars interarticularis of the lower lumbar spine (L4, L5) is the most common site for stress fracture of the entire skeleton. It may be found with or without spondylolisthesis. (8) (Fig. 9.203) Stress fractures of the second and third metatarsals may complicate Morton's syndrome. (9) This syndrome is defined as a congenitally short first metatarsal, with a broad base to the second metatarsal. This congenital malformation creates unusual stress to the neck of the second and third metatarsals. (See Chapter 2) Other sites and their associated activities are outlined. (Fig. 9.204A and B, 9.205A and B) (Table 9.17)

CLINICAL FEATURES

The clinical findings of stress fractures are characteristic. Pain which is related to activity and is relieved by rest is typical. Soft tissue swelling with localized tenderness over the area of stress fracture is observed. Almost

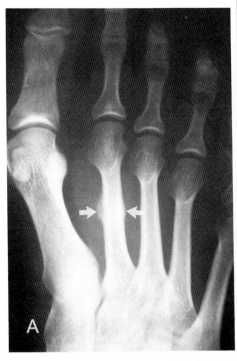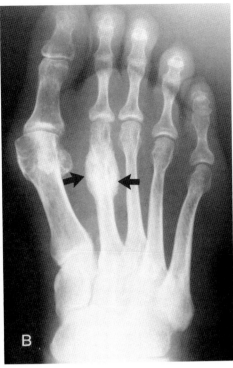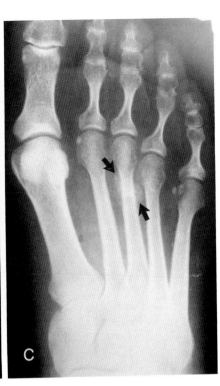

Figure 9.198. STRESS FRACTURE: METATARSALS. A. Dorsiplantar Foot. A thin layer of periosteal bone formation is present adjacent to the midshaft of the second metatarsal (arrows). This is frequently the first radiographic manifestation of stress fracture in this location. **B. Dorsiplantar Foot.** A thick layer of solid periosteal new bone is present adjacent to the distal metatarsal shaft (arrows). This represents a longstanding stress fracture with significant callus formation. **C. Dorsiplantar Foot.** A cloudy, veil-like density is seen adjacent to the distal third metatarsal (arrows). This represents periosteal callus formation due to the presence of a stress fracture. **Comment:** The earliest manifestations of stress fractures are often subtle and consist primarily of periosteal callus formation at the fracture site. It is very unusual to see the fracture line in these injuries in the earliest phases.

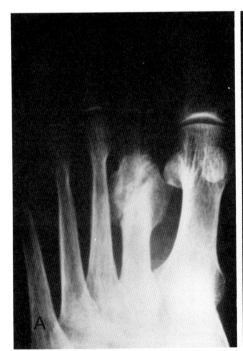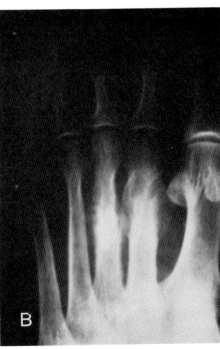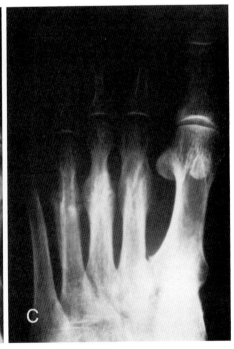

Figure 9.199. METATARSAL STRESS FRACTURES: SERIAL PROGRESSION. A. Dorsiplantar View: Initial Film. An oblique radiolucent fracture line is seen through the second metatarsal shaft. This is surrounded by extensive proliferative callus formation. **B. Dorsiplantar View: 2 Months After Initial Film.** A second stress fracture is visualized in the shaft of the third metatarsal adjacent to the original fracture site. Residual callus formation is noted surrounding the initial stress fracture. **C. Dorsiplantar View: 6 Months After Initial Film.** A third stress fracture is observed in the shaft of the third metatarsal. **Comment:** The serial progression of the stress fractures in this case is somewhat unique, since the patient was a 60-year-old energetic gardener who refused to quit the extensive stooping involved in her gardening. The stress related to that position created the serial stress fractures over a period of 6 months. (Courtesy of Donald B. Tomkins, DC, DACBR, Canistota, South Dakota. Special thanks to James F. Winterstein, DC, DACBR, Chicago, Illinois for his help in obtaining this case)

519

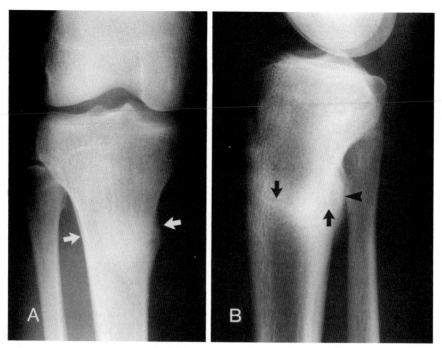

Figure 9.200. STRESS FRACTURE: PROXIMAL TIBIA. A. AP Knee. Observe the exuberant callus formation surrounding the proximal diaphysis of the tibia (arrows). **B. Lateral Knee.** A horizontal radiolucent fracture line is demonstrated through the area of stress fracture (arrows). Extensive callus formation is noted on the posterior surface of the tibia adjacent to the fracture line (arrowhead). *Comment:* The proximal tibia is a common location for stress fractures, which are found in joggers, marchers, and ballet dancers.

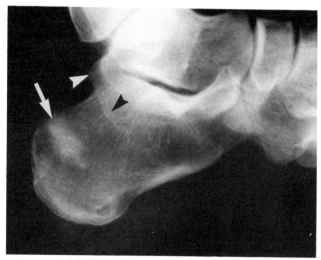

Figure 9.201. STRESS FRACTURE: CALCANEUS. A dense radiopaque band is present in the posterosuperior portion of the calcaneus (arrow). This is a typical location for stress fracture affecting the calcaneus. Of incidental note is vascular calcification in the posterior tibial artery (arrowheads).

any bone can be affected, with the bones of the lower extremity being more frequently involved. More than one site can be present, with serial radiographs showing fractures at various stages. (Fig. 9.199A–C)

RADIOLOGICAL FEATURES

The initial radiographic examination may fail to reveal the fracture line. This is influenced by the location of the

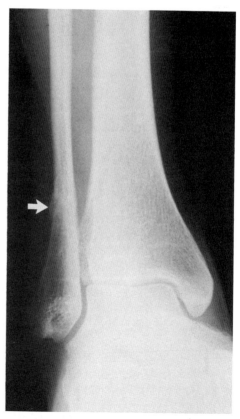

Figure 9.202. STRESS FRACTURE: DISTAL FIBULA. Periosteal new bone formation, along with a radiolucent fracture line, is seen in the distal diaphysis of the fibula (arrow). *Comment:* Stress fractures of the fibula are most commonly found in ballet dancers and joggers. (Courtesy of Philip C. Huyler, DC, Nassau, Bahamas)

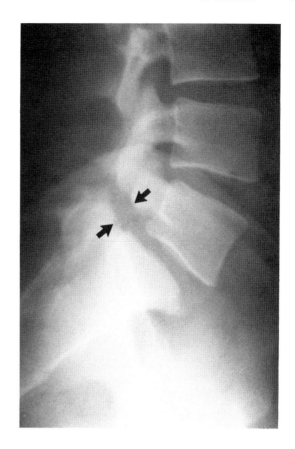

Figure 9.203. STRESS FRACTURE: LUMBAR PARS INTERARTIC-ULARIS. Spondylolysis of the pars interarticularis of L5 is observed (arrows). A 10 percent spondylolisthesis of L5 upon the sacrum is noted. **Comment:** The majority of pars interarticularis defects seen in the lumbar spine are the result of stress fracture.

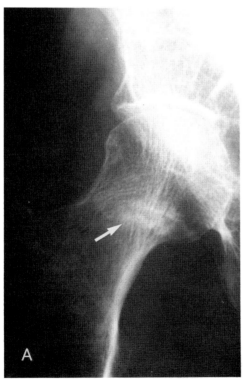

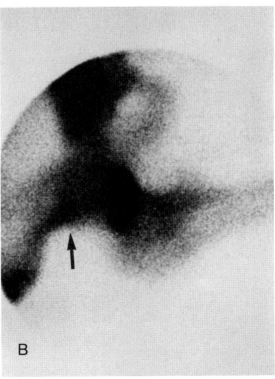

Figure 9.204. STRESS FRACTURE: PROXIMAL FEMUR. A. AP Hip. The stress fracture can be appreciated by the radiopaque transverse band which is present in the area of the femoral neck (arrow). **B. Bone Scan.** There is a focal area of increased radio-nuclide uptake in the area of the stress fracture of the femoral neck (arrow). **Comment:** Stress fractures of the femoral neck are a frequent complication of osteoporosis and are also found in marathon runners.

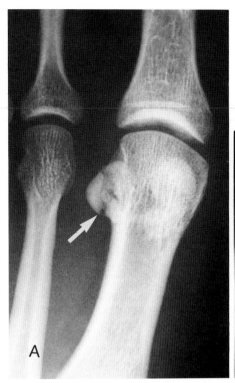

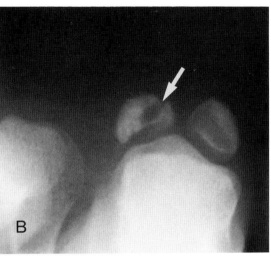

Figure 9.205. STRESS FRACTURE: SESAMOID BONE OF THE GREAT TOE. A. Dorsiplantar View: Great Toe. There is fragmentation and radiopacity noted within the lateral sesamoid bone on the plantar surface of the great toe (arrow). **B. Axial Metatarsal Head View.** A stress fracture with radiopacity and fragmentation of the sesamoid bone is observed (arrow). **Comment:** This stress fracture occurred in a female marathon runner who experienced severe plantar foot pain while training. (Courtesy of Gary M. Guebert, DC, DACBR, St. Louis, Missouri)

fracture and the interval between the time of injury and that of the radiographic examination. Tomography may be helpful in demonstrating the fracture line; however, the definitive means of detection is the bone scan. Whenever there is any doubt, a bone scan should be given consideration. (1)

Roentgen Signs of Stress Fractures

Periosteal Response. The most frequently seen and reliable roentgen sign of stress fracture is periosteal and endosteal cortical thickening. (Table 9.18) The degree of new bone formation can be extreme and usually assumes a *solid* pattern of periosteal response. This cortical thickening is localized to the area of stress fracture, creating an eccentric protuberance of the cortex.

Fracture Line. Frequently, the exuberant periosteal new bone will obscure the radiolucent fracture line within the cortex. At other times, the fracture is too thin to be depicted on the radiograph. Tomography often will demonstrate the fracture line through the dense sclerosis, when plain films do not.

Transverse Opaque Bands. When the stress fracture is viewed *en face*, the periosteal callus forms a linear, transverse, radiopaque band. The margins of this density are hazy and poorly defined, which differentiates it from a growth arrest line. The calcaneus is a characteristic site to visualize such a dense radiopaque line traversing vertically through the bone. (Fig. 9.201)

DIFFERENTIAL DIAGNOSIS

Osteomyelitis

Since osteomyelitis may create a significant periosteal response, an early infectious focus can resemble a stress fracture. The lack of bone destruction adjacent to the periosteal callus is the key roentgen sign, since infectious lesions will produce lytic bone destruction.

Osteosarcoma

Early lesions of osteosarcoma may be confused with stress fractures. Both produce periosteal response, with stress fracture assuming a *solid* pattern and osteosarcoma creating a *spiculated* pattern. Bone destruction will be seen with osteosarcoma, a roentgen sign not present with stress fractures. Often, tomography will demonstrate a linear radiolucent fracture line, securing the diagnosis of stress fracture.

Osteoid Osteoma

The radiographic appearance of osteoid osteoma and stress fracture are very similar. The key roentgen sign which allows differential diagnosis is usually seen on tomographic views and overpenetrated plain films. This sign is the oval radiolucent nidus of osteoid osteoma versus the linear radiolucent fracture line in stress fractures.

Table 9.17
Activity-Related Sites for Stress Fractures

Bone	Location	Activity
Calcaneus	Posterior, plantar portion	Jumping, parachuting, marching, prolonged standing
Clavicle	Outer one third	Persistent tic, radical neck surgery
Femur		
(a) Shaft	Distal one third	Ballet, long distance running
(b) Neck	Midcervical, subcapital	Ballet, marching, long distance running, gymnastics
Fibula	Distal shaft	Long distance running
	Proximal shaft	Jumping, parachuting
Hamate	Hook	Equipment holding (tennis, golf, baseball)
Humerus	Distal shaft	Throwing sports
Metatarsals		
(a) First	Base	Marching, ground stomping
(b) Second	Distal and midshaft	Marching, ground stomping, ballet
(c) Third	Distal metaphysis	Morton's syndrome
(d) Fifth	Shaft, base	Running on banked track fields
Navicular (Tarsal)	Distal one half	Ground stomping, marching, long distance running
Patella	Proximal pole	Hurdling
Pelvis	Obturator ring	Stooping, bowling, gymnastics
Phalanx	Tuft	Guitar players
Ribs		
(a) First	Posterior	Pack carrier, chronic dyspnea
(b) 7–9	Posterolateral	Coughing, golf
Scapula	Coracoid process	Trap shooting
	Inferior glenoid lip	Baseball players
Sesamoids	First metatarsal	Standing, jumping, running
Spine		
(a) Lower cervical	Spinous process	Clay shoveling
(b) Upper thoracic	Spinous process	Clay shoveling
(c) Lower lumbar	Pars interarticularis	Ballet, gymnasts, polevaulters, football players, cricket bowlers, weight lifters, divers
Tibial Shaft	Mid and distal	Long distance running, ballet
	Proximal	Jumping, parachuting, basketball players
Ulna	Coronoid process	Throwing sports
	Olecranon	Throwing sports
	Shaft	Pitchfork work, wheelchair

Adapted From: Rowe LJ: Metatarsal stress fracture.
ACA Council, Roentgen Brief, September 1982.

Growth Arrest Lines

These present as discrete radiopaque lines through the metaphysis of the bone. The radiopaque line of stress fracture is broader, with a hazy, ill-defined margin to its edge. Additionally, growth arrest lines are usually found in other bones as bilateral, symmetrical, well-defined radiopaque bands.

Table 9.18.
Radiological Features of Stress Fractures

Localized solid periosteal/endosteal new bone
Subtle or absent fracture line
Narrow, poorly-defined, opaque band
Positive bone scan

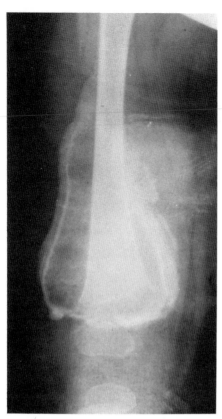

Figure 9.206. BATTERED CHILD SYNDROME: THIGH Extensive hemorrhage has lifted the periosteum, creating large, wavy periosteal new bone formation. No fractures are identified on this femoral radiograph.

The Battered Child Syndrome

A devastating syndrome in children has emerged within the past half century which involves repeated abusive trauma. Caffey in 1946 was the first to describe multiple fractures in the long bones of patients who were suffering from subdural hematomas. (1)

The term "battered child syndrome" was offered by Kempe and others in 1962, which created an enormous public reaction. (2) These children are frequently under 2 years of age when exposed to this trauma, and usually under 6 years of age when brought for medical attention. Usually, those who inflict the injuries are the parents or guardians.

The hallmark of this syndrome is clinial and radiological evidence of repeated injury. (3) Clinically, multiple bruises or burns of varying degrees of severity are the usual findings. The key to the radiographic diagnosis is the demonstration of multiple fractures at varying stages of healing. (1,3) Quite often, a fresh fracture may be seen next to a callused, deformed bone. The classical radio-

Table 9.19.
Radiological Features of the Battered Child Syndrome

Fractures in different stages of healing
Multiple closely approximated fractures
Metaphyseal corner fractures
Epiphyseal displacements
Exuberant periosteal new bone

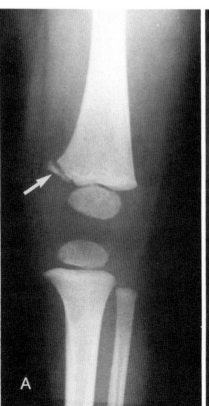

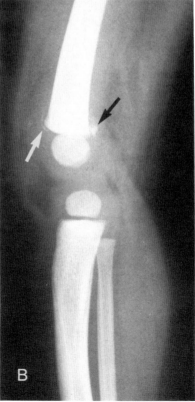

Figure 9.207. BATTERED CHILD SYNDROME: A CHARACTERISTIC FRACTURE FRAGMENT. A. AP Knee. A characteristic corner fracture is observed affecting the medial aspect of the metaphysis of the distal femur (arrow). **B. Lateral Knee.** Multiple fracture fragments of the distal metaphysis of the femur are identified (arrows).

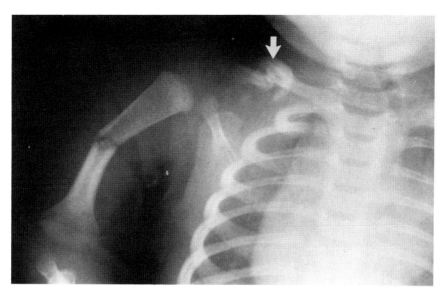

Figure 9.208. BATTERED CHILD SYNDROME: MULTIPLE FRAC-TURES OF THE SHOULDER. A recent fracture of the mid-dia-physis of the humerus is observed. A fracture of older origin is present in the distal aspect of the clavicle, with exuberant callus formation (arrow). *Comment:* The key to the radiographic diagnosis of battered child syndrome is the demonstration of multiple fractures at varying stages of healing, as is seen in this case. The classic radiographic signs are fractures in the corners of the metaphyses, with or without associated epiphyseal displacement, and exuberant periosteal new bone formation along the diaphyses and metadia-physes of the long bones.

graphic signs are fractures of the corners of the meta-physes, with or without associated epiphyseal displace-ment, and exuberant periosteal new bone formation along the diaphyses and metadiaphyses of the long bones. (3) (Fig. 9.206) (Table 9.19) Corner fractures around the knee and the medial aspect of the metaphysis of the distal femur are characteristic. (Fig. 9.207A and B)

Other common sites involving occurrence of this syn-drome are the ribs, skull, clavicle, and scapula. Spinal fractures are uncommon. Since many of these children are severely shaken while held by their arms, bilateral humeral fractures are also common. (Fig. 9.208) Addition-ally, as the limb is shaken, the periosteum is pulled from the shaft where it is loosely attached and shears off portions of the metaphysis where it is tightly attached. (3) This creates significant solid periosteal new bone for-mation which appears wavy and dense.

Other conditions such as infantile cortical hyperostosis, congenital syphilis, scurvy, and osteogenesis imperfecta may be considered in the differential diagnosis. In general, they are readily excluded by clinical and radiographic signs.

"In infants who are victims of abuse, fractures of the thoracic and lumbar spinous processes are likely to be the result of violent shaking. Although initial radiographs appear normal, subsequent studies may reveal extensive ossification within the adjacent soft tissues. These ab-normalities are subtle and easily overlooked, in part ex-plaining the rarity of such reports in the literature. The authors recommend that lateral views of the vertebral column should be obtained whenever infant abuse is sus-pected." (4)

Post-Traumatic Myositis Ossificans

GENERAL CONSIDERATIONS

Traumatic myositis ossificans (myositis ossificans post-traumatica, ossifying hematoma, traumatic ossifying myositis, or heterotopic post-traumatic bone formation) represents a heterotopic bone formation in the soft tissues. The process occurs most often in muscle but may also occur in fascia, tendons, joint capsules, and ligaments. Most occur following any local injury sufficient to cause bruising of the muscle or a frank hemorrhage within it. The most common sites are the brachialis anterior (elbow) (Fig. 9.209A and B), quadriceps femoris (thigh) (Fig. 9.210), adductor muscles of the thigh, and medial collat-eral ligament of the knee (Pellegrini-Stieda disease) (Fig. 9.211), and in cases of rupture of the coracoclavicular ligament of the shoulder. (1) Other lesser known sites are the deltoid in foot soldiers, due to the trauma caused by carrying a rifle. The constant pressure of the saddle against the adductors in riders may cause ossification in the adductor magnus and is known as Prussian's disease or, erroneously, as a "saddle tumor." (1) (Fig. 9.212) Bed-ridden and wheelchair-confined patients frequently pro-duce heterotopic bone at areas of gravitational stress, most commonly found at the ischial tuberosities. (Fig. 9.213)

PATHOLOGICAL FEATURES

The process can be divided into three stages—pseu-dosarcoma, differentiation, and maturation.

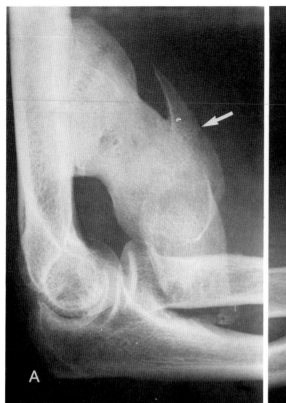

Figure 9.209. POST-TRAUMATIC MYOSITIS OSSIFICANS: EL-BOW. A and B. Bilateral Lateral Elbows. The large ossified masses present anterior to the distal humerus represent post-traumatic myositis ossificans (arrows). The brachialis anterior is the most common muscle involved in the area of the elbow.

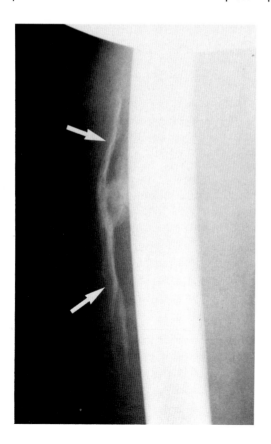

Stage One: Pseudosarcoma

The sequence of events begins with a traumatic incident in which tissue is crushed or torn. Blunt trauma is common. The precise stimulus that causes metaplastic formation of bone instead of normal repair and scar formation is unknown. Following crushing of the muscle, there is extensive damage and cell death. Holes appear in the sarcolemmal sheath and fluid accumulates. The sarcolemmal nuclei proliferate, the sarcolemma disappears, and the fluid diffuses into the tissues. Phagocytes invade and remove the fibers, enlarging the holes. The capillary bed dilates, as in fracture, producing the clinical symptoms of heat, swelling, and tenderness ("charley horse"). Since the damage is greatest in the center of the traumatized area, these tissues may totally liquefy or be replaced by sheets of nonspecific cells. The breakdown of cellular material in the traumatized area induces a transient inflammatory infiltrate ("myositis").

Unless further trauma is added by injudicious massage, excessive stretching, surgery, or other activity, the stage

Figure 9.210. POST-TRAUMATIC MYOSITIS OSSIFICANS: ANTERIOR THIGH. There is a wavy, ossific density present in the anterior thigh involving the quadriceps femoris (arrows). (Courtesy of Mark J. Lieffring, DC, Cloquet, Minnesota)

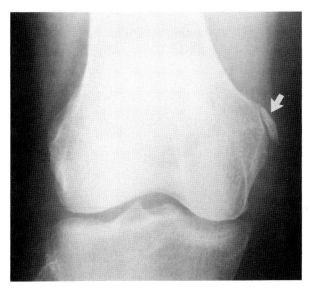

Figure 9.211. MEDIAL COLLATERAL LIGAMENT OSSIFICATION. There is ossification in the area of the medial collateral ligament following avulsion (arrow). This has been referred to as Pellegrini-Stieda disease.

and the least differentiated are at the periphery. (Fig. 9.214)

Stage Three: Maturation

As the lesion matures, it shrinks in size, and the periphery becomes heavier and more developed, as is the case with fracture callus. It develops a "periosteum" that separates it from the surrounding tissue, although muscle fibers are frequently attached to the peripheral portion. The inner central area may become entirely cystic, showing removal of liquefied debris, or it may become demarcated as in an infarct and never become replaced. Eventually, the activity subsides and the lesion becomes stable.

Once the periosteum develops, it is easier to remove the lesion surgically. Surgical removal of immature lesions is contraindicated because of the high incidence of recurrence, often with involvement of a larger area than that included in the original lesion. Some ossifications completely disappear, and the smaller ones regress because of osteoclastic resorption within the muscle belly. There is complete restoration of muscle contour, but muscle function is never totally normal. (2)

of degeneration lasts approximately 15 days. It is followed by a phase of activity with extensive proliferation of all mesenchymal cell types. Identifiable osteoid formation is minimal at this stage. A biopsy during this 2-to-4-week period can lead to an erroneous diagnosis of neoplasia. It is a period of indecision for the clinician, radiologist, and pathologist. The clinical history of blunt trauma at the appropriate time is essential in reaching a proper diagnosis.

During the initial 6-to-7-week period the lesion has identifiable zones only if excised in its entirety. The center of the lesion is necrotic, surrounded by zones with less tissue damage.

Stage Two: Differentiation

During the second and third months following injury, the mesenchymal cells differentiate into fibroblasts, osteoblasts, chondroblasts, and so forth. Giant cells are numerous and remove the necrotic debris. Fibrous tissue formation and some primitive osteoid deposition occur. Blood supply to the center of the lesion is precarious. Most of the necrotic cells undergo liquefactive necrosis and resorption, which may leave a cyst filled with fluid, or the area may fill with sheets of nonspecific cells.

Near the periphery of the lesion, where the damage is least, repair is more prompt and complete, leading to mineralization. The matrix will proceed to ossification, with the best developed, mature trabecular bone at the periphery and progressively less differentiated zones in the central portion. This characteristic zoning of the myositis ossificans, with the most mature tissue at the periphery, distinguishes it from neoplasms of bone in which the best differentiated portions are in the center of the lesion

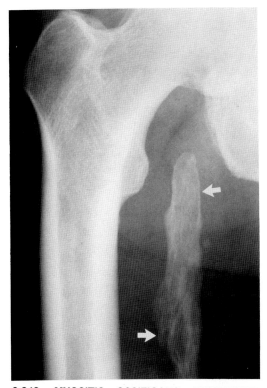

Figure 9.212. MYOSITIS OSSIFICANS: PRUSSIAN'S DISEASE. There is a large, well-organized ossifying hematoma present in the adductor magnus muscle (arrows). Observe the dense cortical margin, with a relatively radiolucent center. ***Comment:*** This has been referred to as "Prussian's disease" and is the result of the constant pressure of the saddle against the adductor muscles, which was found frequently in Prussian soldiers who were horseback riders.

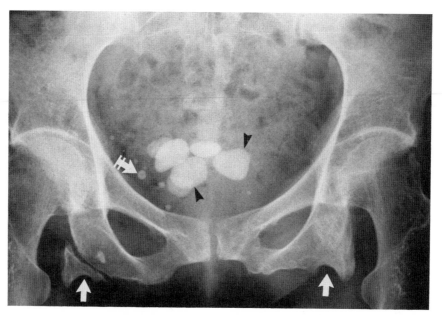

Figure 9.213. POST-TRAUMATIC MYOSITIS OSSIFICANS: THE NONAMBULATORY PATIENT. There are ossifying hematomas below both ischial tuberosities (arrows). These represent sites of myositis ossificans post-traumatica in a nonambulatory patient restricted to a wheelchair. It occurred as a result of constant mechanical pressure on the soft tissues. Because of the lack of activity and urinary stasis, multiple bladder calculi have developed (arrowheads). These may be differentiated from phleboliths by the lack of a radiolucent center (crossed arrow).

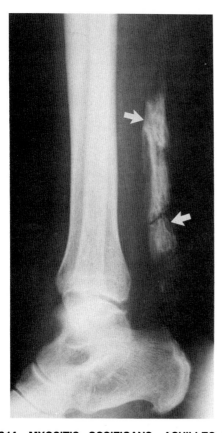

Figure 9.214. MYOSITIS OSSIFICANS: ACHILLES TENDON. There is ossification of a large hematoma present within the Achilles tendon (arrows). This is sometimes associated with rupture of the tendon.

Table 9.20.
Radiological Features of Post-Traumatic Myositis Ossificans

EARLY FEATURES
Hazy soft tissue mass
Cloudy ossification
LATER FEATURES
Round or linear
Smooth, dense, outer border
Relatively lucent center
No connection with adjacent bone

RADIOLOGICAL FEATURES

The ossifying hematoma may be visible radiographically within 3–4 weeks after the initial injury. (1,3) Initially, the roentgen appearance is a fine, lacy radiopacity, which is followed later by a cloudy ossification within a well-defined mass. Its size depends upon the degree of initial trauma and the overall size of the hematoma. Eventually, sequential studies demonstrate a bony mass which is very radiopaque in its peripheral margins, with the center of the lesion appearing relatively radiolucent. (Fig. 9.214) The bony mass usually measures 4–5 cm but may be as large as 25 cm on occasion. The soft tissue osseous mass distinctively has no direct connection with the closest bone. (Table 9.20)

Radiological diagnosis is essential, since biopsy of this mass in its early stages may show what would appear to be a sarcomatous change centrally. A radiological sign important in making the distinction between this and a bone neoplasm is the characteristic lucent zone (cleavage

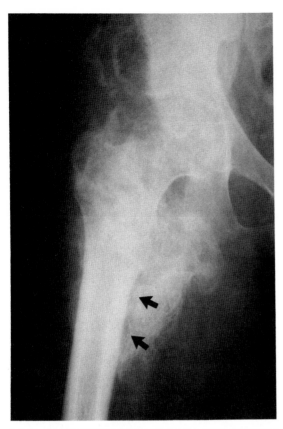

Figure 9.215. PSEUDOSARCOMA APPEARANCE OF MYOSITIS OSSIFICANS POST-TRAUMATICA. A large soft tissue mass is present adjacent to the proximal femur. Observe the dense peripheral cortical rim, with a more radiolucent center, which suggests myositis ossificans rather than sarcoma. A clearly defined margin between the soft tissue mass and the cortex of the femur aids in the differential diagnosis (arrows).

plane) between the calcified mass and the subadjacent cortex. (4,5) The mass is usually located adjacent to the diaphysis of a tubular bone, but the cortex of the bone is intact. Other important confirmatory properties are a dense periphery with a more lucent center and decrease in volume with time. (Fig. 9.215) Increased uptake of bone-seeking radionuclide may be noted.

DIFFERENTIAL DIAGNOSIS

Extraskeletal sarcoma may be difficult to differentiate from myositis ossificans. This condition is rare and tends to occur in older adults. Synovioma, in one-third of cases, may calcify and can be located remote from the joint due to its association with tendon sheaths; therefore, this tumor must be given consideration when evaluating a calcified soft tissue mass. A parosteal sarcoma may have a similar appearance, but no lucent zone between it and the diaphysis should be visible. Other soft tissue calcifications such as tumoral calcinosis may present as a densely calcified mass but have an amorphous calcific rather than maturely ossific nature. (6)

Summary Tables

The following tables are a summary of the named and eponymic fractures (Tables 9.21–9.33), the named radiological signs in association with trauma (Table 9.34), and the most common fracture sites (Table 9.35).

Table 9.21.
Named and Eponymic Fractures General Terms

AVULSION	Separated bone fragment from a muscle, tendon, or ligament.
BUTTERFLY FRAGMENT	Isolated triangular-shaped cortical fragment in a comminuted fracture.
BANANA-LIKE FRACTURE	Transverse pathological fracture through a bone affected with Paget's disease.
CHIP (CORNER) FRACTURE	A small bone fragment originating from a joint margin.
CLOSED FRACTURE	Fracture does not penetrate the skin.
COMMINUTED FRACTURE	Two or more bony fragments.
DIASTATIC FRACTURE	Separation of a partly movable joint.
IMPACTION FRACTURE	Trabecular telescoping.
(a) Depressed	Inward bulging of the outer cortex.
(b) Compression	Decreased bone size due to trabecular telescoping.
INCOMPLETE FRACTURE	Fracture only extends partially across the bone.
(a) Greenstick	Buckled trabeculae.
(b) Torus	Buckled trabeculae with a cortical bulge.
INFRACTION FRACTURE	A small impaction fracture.
INSUFFICIENCY FRACTURE	Stress fracture through diseased bone.
OBLIQUE FRACTURE	Fracture line at 45 degrees to the long axis.
OCCULT FRACTURE	A subtle, unidentifiable fracture, usually seen on followup x-rays 7–10 days after trauma.
OPEN FRACTURE	Fracture penetrates the skin.
PATHOLOGICAL FRACTURE	Fracture through diseased bone.
POST-TRAUMATIC ARTHRITIS	Secondary degenerative joint disease due to altered joint mechanics following trauma
PSEUDARTHROSIS	Residual motion between fracture fragments, creating a false joint.
PSEUDOFRACTURE	An incomplete pathological fracture-like defect.
SALTER-HARRIS CLASSIFICATION	Growth plate injuries.
SPIRAL FRACTURE	Fracture line bends circumferentially and longitudinally along the bone.
STRESS (FATIGUE) FRACTURE	Microfracture due to repetitive stress.
THURSTON-HOLLAND FRAGMENT	Metaphyseal fragment in a Salter-Harris Type II epiphyseal injury.
TRANSVERSE FRACTURE	Fracture line at 90 degrees to the long axis.

Table 9.22
Named and Eponymic Fractures of the Skull and Facial Bones

BLOWOUT FRACTURE	Fracture through the infraorbital plate.
DIASTATIC FRACTURE	Fracture with separation of a suture.
GROWING FRACTURE	Widening of the sutural space due to leptomeningeal cyst.
LEFORT I–III FRACTURE	Facial bone fracture/separations.
PING PONG FRACTURE	A depressed skull fracture in a child.
STELLATE FRACTURE	A depressed skull fracture where multiple fracture lines radiate from its center.
TRIPOD FRACTURE	Three fractures through the zygomatic arch, orbital and maxillary processes.

Table 9.23.
Named and Eponymic Fractures of the Cervical Spine

BURSTING FRACTURE OF THE ATLAS	Synonym for Jefferson's fracture.
BURST FRACTURE OF THE BODY	Comminuted vertebral body fracture.
CARROT STICK FRACTURE	Fracture through the ankylosed discovertebral junction in ankylosing spondylitis.
CLAY SHOVELER'S FRACTURE	Avulsion of a lower cervical segment spinous process.
COALMINER'S FRACTURE	Synonym for clay shoveler's fracture.
HANGMAN'S FRACTURE (HANGEE'S FRACTURE)	Bipedicular fracture of the axis.
JEFFERSON'S FRACTURE	Fractured anterior and posterior arch of the atlas.
PILLAR FRACTURE	Fractured articular pillar.
TEARDROP FRACTURE	A displaced, triangular fragment from the anteroinferior body corner.
TRAUMATIC SPONDYLO-LISTHESIS	Synonym for hangman's fracture.
WEDGE FRACTURE	Compressed anterior vertebral body fracture.

Table 9.24.
Named and Eponymic Fractures of the Lumbar Spine

CHANCE FRACTURE (SEATBELT FRACTURE)	Horizontal fracture through a single body and posterior arch.
FULCRUM FRACTURE	Synonym for a Chance fracture.

Table 9.25.
Named and Eponymic Fractures of the Pelvis

BUCKET HANDLE FRACTURE	Superior and inferior pubic ramus fracture with a fracture or separation of the contralateral sacroiliac joint.
DASHBOARD FRACTURE	Posterior acetabular rim fracture.
DUVERNEY'S FRACTURE	Iliac wing fracture.
EXPLOSION FRACTURE	Central acetabular fracture.
MALGAIGNE'S FRACTURE	Superior and inferior pubic ramus fracture with a fracture near or separation of the ipsilateral sacroiliac joint.
OPEN BOOK FRACTURE	Synonym for a sprung pelvis.
PRUSSIAN'S DISEASE	Myositis ossificans of the adductor muscles from horseback riding.
RIDER'S BONE	Avulsion of the secondary growth center of the ischium which subsequently does not unite and dramatically enlarges.
SPRUNG PELVIS	Separation of the pubic symphysis and both sacroiliac joints.
STRADDLE FRACTURE	Bilateral superior pubic rami and ischiopubic fractures.
SUICIDAL JUMPER'S FRACTURE	Horizontal fracture through the first or second sacral segments associated with falls from a height.

Table 9.26.
Named and Eponymic Fractures of the Knee

BUMPER (FENDER) FRACTURE	Medial or lateral tibial plateau fracture from a severe varus/valgus stress.
FLAKE FRACTURE	Osteochondral fragment separated from the medial facet of the femoral surface of the patella following dislocation.
FLOATING KNEE	Supracondylar femur fracture in combination with proximal tibia fracture.
LIPOHEMOAR-THROSIS	Fat and blood in a joint due to an intra-articular fracture.
SEGOND'S FRACTURE	Avulsion of the lateral tibia at the insertion of the tensor fascia lata.
TRAMPOLINE FRACTURE	Proximal tibial metaphysis in children (2–10).

Table 9.27.
Named and Eponymic Fractures of the Ankle

B-B FRACTURE	Both bones of the leg or forearm are fractured simultaneously (tibia and fibula; radius and ulna).
BIMALLEOLAR FRACTURE	Medial and lateral malleolar fractures.
BOOT-TOP FRACTURE (SKIER'S FRACTURE)	Distal diaphyseal/metaphyseal spiral fracture of the tibia and fibula in an adult.
COTTON'S FRACTURE	Erroneous synonym for trimalleolar fractures.
DUPUYTREN'S FRACTURE	Distal fibula fracture 6–7 cm above the malleolus, disrupted distal tibiofibular ligament, diastasis, lateral talus dislocation, up and out foot displacement.
MAISSONEUVE FRACTURE	Proximal fibula fracture due to an inversion and external rotation injury of the ankle.
POTT'S FRACTURE	Distal fibula fracture 6–7 cm above the malleolus with disruption of the distal tibiofibular ligament.
TILLAUX'S FRACTURE	Fractures of the medial malleolus, anterior tibial tubercle, and lateral malleolus 6–7 cm from its tip with diastasis of the distal tibiofibular joint.
TODDLER'S FRACTURE	Distal diaphyseal/metaphyseal spiral fracture of the tibia in an infant.

Table 9.28.
Named and Eponymic Fractures of the Foot

AVIATOR'S ASTRALGUS	Synonym for aviator's fracture.
AVIATOR'S FRACTURE	Fracture through the neck of the talus.
BEAK FRACTURE	Avulsion of the posterior calcaneal tubercle.
BEDROOM FRACTURE	Phalangeal fracture from striking an object.
CHOPART'S DISLOCATION	Dislocation between the talonavicular and calcaneonavicular joint.
DANCER'S FRACTURE	Synonym for Jones' fracture.
JONES' FRACTURE	Avulsion fracture of the styloid of the fifth metatarsal base.
LISFRANC FRACTURE/DISLOCATION	Dorsal dislocation of the metatarsal bases with associated fractures.
MARCH FRACTURE	Stress fracture of the second and third metatarsals.

Table 9.29.
Named and Eponymic Fractures of the Thorax

COUGH FRACTURE	Stress fracture of a rib due to repetitive coughing episodes.
FLAIL CHEST	Two fractures of the same rib which isolates a fragment, allowing paradoxical motion during respiration.
GOLFER'S FRACTURE	Lateral rib fracture incurred from striking the ground rather than the ball.
HUG FRACTURE	Synonym for passion fracture.
PASSION FRACTURE	Rib fracture following an overenthusiastic hug.

Table 9.30.
Named and Eponymic Fractures of the Shoulder

BANKART LESION	Avulsion of the triceps insertion of a small fragment from the inferior glenoid rim.
DROOPING SHOULDER	Inferior subluxation of the humeral head due to hemarthrosis, infection, effusion, stroke, and brachial plexus lesions.
FLAP FRACTURE	Avulsion fracture of the greater tuberosity of the humerus.
HATCHET DEFECT	Synonym for Hill-Sachs defect.
HILL-SACHS DEFECT	An impaction fracture at the posterosuperior surface of the humeral head from the inferior glenoid rim following recurrent anterior shoulder dislocation.
SEPARATED SHOULDER	Acromioclavicular joint dislocation.
SUBLUXIO ERECTA	Inferior dislocation of the humerus with the humerus fixed in abduction.

Table 9.31.
Named and Eponymic Fractures of the Elbow and Forearm

BABY CAR FRACTURE	Synonym for sideswipe fracture.
CHISEL FRACTURE	Vertical fracture of the radial head extending 10 mm from the articular surface.
ESSEX-LOPRESTI FRACTURE	Radial head comminuted fracture with distal radioulnar dislocation.
GALEAZZI FRACTURE	Fracture of the junction of the distal and middle third of the radial shaft and dislocation of the inferior radioulnar joint.
KOCHER'S FRACTURE	Osteochondral fracture of the capitellum.
LITTLE LEAGUER'S ELBOW	Avulsion of the medial epicondyle.
MONTEGGIA FRACTURE	Fracture of the proximal ulnar shaft with dislocation of the radial head.
NIGHTSTICK FRACTURE	Fracture of the ulnar shaft when the arm is raised to protect the head from a blow.
PARRY FRACTURE	Synonym for nightstick fracture.
PIEDMONT FRACTURE	Synonym for Galeazzi fracture.
PULLED ELBOW	Radial head pulled out from under the annular ligament.
REVERSE MONTEGGIA FRACTURE	Synonym for Galeazzi fracture.
SIDESWIPE FRACTURE	Fracture of the distal humerus, radius, and ulna when an elbow protruding from a car window is struck by an object.
TRAFFIC FRACTURE	Synonym for sideswipe fracture.

Table 9.32.
Named and Eponymic Fractures of the Wrist

BARTON'S FRACTURE	Posterior rim fracture of the distal radius.
CHAUFFEUR'S FRACTURE	Fracture of the radial styloid.
COLLES' FRACTURE	Fracture of the radius within 20–35 mm of the joint and posterior angulation of the distal fragment.
DE QUERVAIN'S FRACTURE/ DISLOCATION	Anterior dislocation of the lunate, along with the proximal fragment of a fractured scaphoid.
FISHER'S FRACTURE	Dorsal avulsion of the triquetrum.
MOORE'S FRACTURE	Colles' fracture in conjunction with fractured ulnar styloid process and ulnar dislocation.
REVERSE BARTON'S FRACTURE	Anterior rim fracture of the distal radius.
REVERSE COLLES' FRACTURE	Synonym for Smith's fracture.
RIM FRACTURE	Synonym for Barton's fracture.
SMITH'S FRACTURE	Fracture of the radius within 20–35 mm of the joint and anterior angulation of the distal fragment.

Table 9.33.
Named and Eponymic Fractures of the Hand

BAR ROOM FRACTURE	Fourth or fifth metacarpal neck fracture with anterior displacement of the head.
BENNETT'S FRACTURE	Intra-articular fracture through the base of the first metacarpal, with dorsal and radial displacement of the shaft.
BOXER'S FRACTURE	Second or third metacarpal neck fracture with anterior displacement of the head.
GAMEKEEPER'S FRACTURE	Disruption of the ulnar collateral ligament at the first metacarpophalangeal joint.
ROLANDO'S FRACTURE	Comminuted intra-articular fracture at the base of the first metacarpal.
VOLAR PLATE FRACTURE	Fractured anterior articular margin at the base of the middle phalanx.

Table 9.34.
Named Radiological Signs in Association With Trauma

Sign	View	Region	Definition
Acute Kyphosis Sign	Lateral	Cervical	Kyphotic angulation localized to one level indicates damage to the posterior spinal ligaments and potential vertebral instability following a hyperflexion injury.
Collar Sign	Oblique	Lumbar	Lucent defect through the pars interarticularis simulating a collar on the scottie dog.
Corner Sign	Any	Any	Small metaphyseal fractures, especially found in multiple locations, suggesting "battered child" syndrome.
Corner Sign	Lateral	Wrist	Metaphyseal fragment of the radius associated with slipped epiphysis.
Divergent Spinous Process Sign	Lateral	Cervical	Due to cervical kyphosis, the spinous processes are divergently orientated to each other as a result of posterior ligamentous damage.
Double Cortical Sign	AP	Elbow	Double cortex to the articulating surface of the radial head due to a depressed fracture.
Double Spinous Sign	AP	Cervical	Double contour to a lower cervical spinous due to a clay shoveler's fracture.
Empty Vertebra Sign	AP	Lumbar	A split in the pedicle creates an open space due to the presence of a Chance fracture.
Extrapleural Sign	Tangential	Thorax	Opaque, convex, well-defined soft tissue density arising adjacent to a rib. A sign of rib disease or traumatic injury such as a hematoma following fracture or metastases.
FBI Sign	Cross-Table	Knee	F = fat; B = blood; I = interface. Usually seen in the knee as a sign of intra-articular fracture.
Fat Pad Sign	Lateral	Elbow	Visualization of posterior fat pad seen in intra-articular fractures, most commonly the radial head.
Half Moon Sign	AP	Shoulder	Lack of the normal semilunar overlap density of the humerus and scapula due to posterior shoulder dislocation.
Hawkin's Sign	AP	Ankle	The presence of a linear subcortical zone of radiolucency in the talar dome following fracture of the talus. This is a good sign of an intact blood supply and a decreased likelihood for avascular necrosis.
Lucent Cleft Sign	Extension	Cervical	Small linear radiolucency adjacent to the anteroinferior end plate, representing a region of avulsion of some annular fibers.
Navicular Fat Stripe Sign	PA	Wrist	Obliteration of displacement of the navicular fat stripe due to fracture of the radial styloid, scaphoid, or trapezium.
Pie Sign	PA	Wrist	Triangular shape of the lunate due to anterior lunate dislocation.
Pronator Quadratus Fat Line Sign	Lateral	Wrist	Obliteration or displacement of the pronator quadratus fat line due to fracture of the distal radius.
Rim Sign	AP	Shoulder	Widened glenohumeral joint space greater than 6 mm in posterior humeral dislocation.
Ring Sign	PA	Wrist	Circular configuration of the scaphoid due to dislocation.
Signet Ring Sign	PA	Wrist	Synonym for ring sign.
Supinator Fat Line Sign	Lateral	Elbow	Obliteration or displacement of the supinator fat line due to fracture of the proximal radius.
Terry Thomas Sign	PA	Wrist	Widened scapholunate space more than 4 mm due to scapholunate disassociation with ligament rupture.
Trough Line Sign	AP	Shoulder	Double cortical contour to the superomedial humeral head is visible due to compression fracture associated with posterior shoulder dislocation.
Vacant Glenoid Sign	AP	Shoulder	Absent humeral head in anterior compartment of the joint due to posterior humeral dislocation.
Vertebral Body Step Defect	Lateral	Cervical Thoracic Lumbar	Sharp offset of the cortex due to compression fracture.

Table 9.35.
Most Common Fracture Sites

GENERAL		**ANKLE**	
Nonunion	Clavicle, ulna, tibia	Tibia	Medial malleolus
Compression	Vertebral bodies	Fibula	Lateral malleolus
Post-traumatic arthritis	Hip, knee, ankle	Talus	Dome margins
SKULL AND FACIAL BONES		Dislocation	Posterior
Skull: Linear Fracture	Cranial vault	**FOOT**	
Depressions	Parietal, temporal	Tarsal	Calcaneus
Facial	Tripod	Calcaneus	Compression
Mandible	Body	Talus	Neck
CERVICAL SPINE		Metatarsals	Base of the fifth
Atlas	Posterior arch		metatarsal
Axis	Base of the odontoid	**SHOULDER GIRDLE**	
	(Type II)	Clavicle	Mid third
Body	C5–C7	Scapula	Body, neck
Pillar	C6	Humerus	Surgical neck
Spinous	C7	Dislocation	Anterior
Transverse Process	C7	**ELBOW**	
Lamina	C5, C6	Child	Supracondylar
Facet Dislocation	C4–C7	Adult	Radial head/neck
THORACIC SPINE		Humerus	Supracondylar
Body	T9–T12	Ulna	Olecranon
LUMBAR SPINE		Radius	Head/neck
Chance Fracture	L1–L3	Dislocation	Posterior
Body Fracture	L1, L2	**WRIST**	
TVP Fracture	L2–L3	Carpal	Scaphoid
Pars Fracture	L4, L5	Scaphoid	Waist
PELVIS		Radius	Colles' fracture
Hemipelvis	Malgaigne's fracture	Ulna	Styloid process
Acetabulum	Central fracture	Dislocation	Lunate
Avulsions	ASIS, AIIS	**HAND**	
HIP		Metacarpal	4th, 5th metacarpal
Proximal Femur	Subcapital		necks
Hip Dislocation	Posterior	Phalanges	Distal phalanx
KNEE		Thumb	Transverse
Femur	Supracondylar	Dislocation	Posterior
Tibia	Lateral plateau		
Fibula	Styloid process		
Patella	Transverse		

REFERENCES

Types of Fractures
1. Felson B: *Roentgenology of Fractures and Dislocations,* New York, Grune & Stratton, 1978.
2. Rogers LF: *Radiology of Skeletal Trauma,* vol 1 and 2, New York, Churchill Livingstone, 1982.
3. Steinbach HL, Kolb FO, Giljillan R: A mechanism for the production of pseudofractures in osteomalacia (Milkman's syndrome). *Radiology* 62:388, 1954.
4. Salter RB, Harris WR: Injuries involving the epiphyseal plate. *J Bone Joint Surg (Am)* 45:587, 1963.
5. Holland CT: Radiographical note on injuries to distal epiphyses of radius and ulna. *Proc R Soc Med* 22:23, 1929.
6. Juhl JH: *Paul and Juhl's Essentials of Roentgen Interpretation,* ed 4, Philadelphia, Harper & Row, 1981.
7. Cruess RL, Dumont J: Current concepts, fracture healing. *Can J Surg* 18:403, 1975.
8. Schenk R, Willenegger H: On the morphological findings in primary fracture healing. *Symp Biol Hung* 7:75, 1967.
9. Stevens DB: Postoperative orthopedic infections. *J Bone Joint Surg (Am)* 46:96, 1964.

Fractures of the Skull and Facial Bones
1. Bell RS, Loop JW: The utility and futility of radiographic skull examination for trauma. *N Engl J Med* 284:236, 1971.
2. Taveras JM, Wood EH: *Diagnostic Neuroradiology,* ed 2, Baltimore, Williams & Wilkins, 1976.

3. Rogers LF: *Radiology of Skeletal Trauma,* vol 1 and 2, New York, Churchill Livingstone, 1982.
4. Genieser NB, Becker MH: Head trauma in children. *Radiol Clin North Am* 12:333, 1945.
5. Carlson GO, Haverling M, Molin C: Isolated fracture of the base of the skull within the sella region. *Acta Radiol* 14:662, 1973.
6. Reynolds DF: Traumatic effusion of the sphenoid sinus. *Clin Radiol* 12:171, 1961.
7. Grossart KWM, Samuel E: Traumatic diastasis of cranial sutures. *Clin Radiol* 12:164, 1961.
8. Felson B: *Roentgenology of Fractures and Dislocations,* New York, Grune & Stratton, 1978.
9. North JW: On the importance of intracranial air. *Br J Surg* 58:826, 1971.
10. Mallew RW: Fractures of the nasofrontal complex. *Otolaryngol Clin North Am* 29:335, 1969.
11. Smith B, Regan WF Jr: Blow-out fracture of the orbit. *Am J Ophthalmol* 44:733, 1957.
12. Milauskas AT, Fueger GF: Serious ocular complications associated with blowout fracture of the orbit. *Am J Ophthalmol* 62:670, 1966.
13. LeFort R: Etude experimentale sur les fractures de la machoire superieure. *Rev Chir* 23:208, 1901.
14. Henny FA: Fractures of the jaw. *Semin Roentgenol* 6:397, 1971.
15. Melmed EP, Loonin AJ: Fractures of the mandible: A review of 909 cases. *Plast Reconstr Surg* 56:323, 1975.

Fractures and Dislocations of the Spine
1. Gehrig R, Michaelis LS: Statistics of acute paraplegia and tetraplegia on a national scale. *Paraplegia* 6:93, 1968.

2. Stauffer ES, Kaufer H: Fractures and dislocations of the spine. In Rockwood CA Jr, Green DP: *Fractures,* vol 2, Philadelphia, JB Lippincott, 1975.
3. Riggins RS, Kraus JF: The risk of neurological damage with fractures of the vertebrae. *J Trauma* 17:126, 1977.
4. Castellano V, Bocconi FL: Injuries of the cervical spine with spinal cord involvement (myelic fractures): Statistical considerations. *Bull Hosp Joint Dis* 31:188, 1970.
5. Jefferson G: Fracture of the atlas vertebra. Report of four cases, and a review of those previously recorded. *Br J Surg* 7:407, 1920.
6. Sherk K, Nicholson JT: Fractures of the atlas. *J Bone Joint Surg (Am)* 52:1017, 1970.
7. Sinbert SE, Berman MS: Fracture of the posterior arch of the atlas. *JAMA* 114:1996, 1940.
8. Yochum TR, Rowe LJ: Arthritides of the upper cervical complex. *ACA J Chiro,* January 1981.
9. Elliott JM, Rogers LF, Wissinger JP, et al: The hangman's fracture. *Radiology* 104:303, 1972.
10. Cornish BL: Traumatic spondylolisthesis of the axis. *J Bone Joint Surg (Br)* 50:31, 1968.
11. Garger WN, Fischer RG, Halfmann HW: Vertebrectomy and fusion for "teardrop fracture" of the cervical spine: Case report. *J Trauma* 9:887, 1969.
12. Anderson LD, D'Alonzo RT: Fractures of the odontoid process of the axis. *J Bone Joint Surg (Am)* 56:1663, 1974.
13. Schatzker J: Fractures of the dens (odontoid process): An analysis of thirty-seven cases. *J Bone Joint Surg (Br)* 53:392, 1971.
14. Rogers LF: *Radiology of Skeletal Trauma,* vol 1 and 2, New York, Churchill Livingstone, 1982.
15. Miller MD, Gehweiler JA, Marintez S, et al: Significant new observations on cervical spine trauma. *AJR* 130:659, 1978.
16. Smith GR, Beckly DE, Abel MS: Articular mass fracture: A neglected cause of post-traumatic? *Clin Radiol* 27:335, 1976.
17. Vines FS: The significance of "occult" fractures of the cervical spine. *AJR* 107:493, 1969.
18. Harris JH Jr: Acute injuries of the spine. *Semin Roentgenol* 13:53, 1978.
19. Cancelmo JJ Jr: Clay shoveler's fracture: A helpful diagnostic sign. *AJR* 115:540, 1972.
20. Scher AT: The value of the anteroposterior radiograph in "hidden" fractures and dislocations of the lower cervical spine—A case report. *S Afr Med J* 55:221, 1979.
21. Abel MS: Occult traumatic lesions of the cervical spine. *Crit Rev Clin Radiol and Nucl Med* 7:469, 1975.
22. Davis AG: Injuries of the cervical spine. *JAMA* 127 (3):149, 1945.
23. Fineman S, Borrelli FJ, Rubinstein BM, et al: The cervical spine: Transformation of the normal lordotic pattern into a linear pattern in the neutral posture. *J Bone Joint Surg (Am)* 45:1179, 1963.
24. Scher AT: Ligamentous injury to the cervical spine—two radiological signs. *S Afr Med J* 53:802, 1978.
25. Reymond RD, Wheeler PS, Peravic M, et al: The lucent cleft, a new radiographic sign of cervical disc injury or disease. *Clin Radiol* 23:188, 1972.
26. Beatson TR: Fractures and dislocations of the cervical spine. *J Bone Joint Surg (Br)* 45:21, 1963.
27. Roaf R: A study of the mechanics of spinal injuries. *J Bone Joint Surg (Br)* 42:810, 1960.
28. Gehweiler JA, Osborne RL Jr, Becker RF: *The Radiology of Vertebral Trauma,* Philadelphia, WB Saunders, 1980.
29. Dibos PE, Wagner HN Jr: *Atlas of Nuclear Medicine—Bone,* Philadelphia, WB Saunders, 1978.
30. Kummel H: Über die traumatischen erkrankungen der wirbelsäule. *Deutsch Med Wchnschr* 21:180, 1895.
31. Schinz HR, et al: *Roentgen Diagnostics,* ed 2, vol 2, New York, Grune & Stratton, 1967.
32. Melamed A: Fracture of pars interarticularis of lumbar vertebra. *AJR* 94:584, 1965.
33. Wiltse LL, Widell EH, Jackson DW: Fatigue fracture: The basic lesion in isthmus spondylolisthesis. *J Bone Joint Surg (Am)* 57:17, 1975.
34. Chance GQ: Note on type of flexion fracture of spine. *Br J Radiol* 21:452, 1948.
35. Dehner JR: Seatbelt injuries of the spine and abdomen. *AJR* 111:833, 1971.
36. Rogers LF: The roentgenographic appearance of transverse or Chance fractures of the spine: The seat belt fracture. *AJR* 111:844, 1971.

Fractures and Dislocations of the Pelvis
1. Furey WW: Fractures of the pelvis with special reference to associated fractures of the sacrum. *AJR* 47:89, 1942.
2. Roy-Camille R, Saillant G, Gagna G, et al: Transverse fracture of the upper sacrum—Suicidal jumpers fracture. *Spine* 10:838, 1985.
3. Duverney JG: *Traite des Maladies de Os,* vol 1, Paris, DeBure l'Aine, 1751.
4. Malgaigne JF: *Treatise on Fractures,* Philadelphia, JB Lippincott, 1959.
5. Rogers LF: *Radiology of Skeletal Trauma,* vol 1 and 2, New York, Churchill Livingstone, 1982.
6. Dunn AW, Morris HD: Fractures and dislocations of the pelvis. *J Bone Joint Surg (Am)* 50:1639, 1968.
7. Lansinger O: Fractures of the acetabulum. *Acta Orthop Scan* 165:1, 1977.

8. Conolly WB, Hedberg EA: Observations on fractures of the pelvis. *J Trauma* 9:104, 1969.
9. Trunkey DD, Chapman MW, Lim RC, et al: Management of pelvic fractures in blunt trauma injury. *J Trauma* 14:912, 1974.
10. Muecke EC, Currarino G: Congenital widening of the pubic symphysis. *AJR* 103:179, 1968.

Fractures and Dislocations of the Hip
1. Stevens L, Freeman PA, Nordin BEC, et al: The incidence of osteoporosis in patients with femoral neck fracture. *J Bone Joint Surg (Br)* 44:520, 1962.
2. Barnes R, Brown JT, Garden RS, et al: Subcapital fractures of the femur. A prospective review. *J Bone Joint Surg (Br)* 58:2, 1976.
3. Rogers LF: *Radiology of Skeletal Trauma,* vol 1 and 2, New York, Churchill Livingstone, 1982.
4. Alffram PA: An epidemiologic study of cervical and trochanteric fractures of the femur in an urban population. Analysis of 1,664 cases with special reference to etiologic factors. *Acta Orthop Scand* 65:11, 1964.
5. Klenerman L, Marcuson RW: Intracapsular fractures of the neck of the femur. *J Bone Joint Surg (Br)* 52:514, 1970.
6. Brown JT, Abrami G: Transcervical femoral fracture. *J Bone Joint Surg (Br)* 46:648, 1964.
7. Baylis AP, Davidson JK: Traumatic osteonecrosis of the femoral head following intracapsular fracture. Incidence and earliest radiological features. *Clin Radiol* 28:407, 1977.
8. Epstein HC: Traumatic dislocations of the hip. *Clin Orthop* 92:116, 1973.
9. Hunter GA: Posterior dislocation and fracture—dislocation of the hip. A review of fifty-seven patients. *J Bone Joint Surg (Br)* 51:38, 1969.
10. Ratliff HHC: Traumatic separation of the upper femoral epiphysis in young children. *J Bone Joint Surg (Br)* 50:757, 1969.
11. Klein A, et al: Roentgenographic features of slipped capital femoral epiphysis. *AJR* 66:361, 1951.
12. Rowe LJ, Nook BC: Avascular necrosis as a complication to previous slipped femoral capital epiphysis. *ACA J Chiro, Radiology Case Report,* May, 1985.

Fractures and Dislocations of the Knee
1. Neer CS, Shelton ML: Supracondylar fracture of the adult femur. A study of one hundred and ten cases. *J Bone Joint Surg (Am)* 49:591, 1967.
2. Seinsheimer F: Fractures of the distal femur. *Clin Orthop* 153:169, 1980.
3. Blake R, McBryde A: The floating knee: Ipsilateral fractures of the tibia and femur. *South Med J* 68:13, 1975.
4. Rogers LF: *Radiology of Skeletal Trauma,* vol 1 and 2, New York, Churchill Livingstone, 1982.
5. Reibel DB, Wade PA: Fractures of the condyles of the tibia. *J Trauma* 2:337, 1962.
6. Newberg AH, Greenstein R: Radiographic evaluation of tibial plateau fracture. *Radiology* 126:319, 1978.
7. Roberts JM, Lovel WW: Fractures of the intercondylar eminence of the tibia. *J Bone Joint Surg (Am)* 52:827, 1970.
8. Boyer RS, Jaffe RB, Nixon GW, et al: Trampoline fracture of the proximal tibia in children. *AJR* 146:83, 1986.
9. Hand WL, et al: Avulsion fractures of the tibial tubercle. *J Bone Joint Surg (Am)* 53:1579, 1971.
10. Schultz RJ: *The Language of Fractures,* Baltimore, Williams & Wilkins, 1976.
11. Platt H: On the peripheral nerve complications of certain fractures. *J Bone Joint Surg (Am)* 10:403, 1928.
12. Towne LC, et al: Lateral compartment syndrome of the knee. *Clin Orthop* 76:160, 1971.
13. Saxon HM: Lipohemarthrosis. *Br J Radiol* 35:122, 1962.
14. Wenzel WW: The FBI sign. *Rocky Mount Med J* 69:71, 1972.
15. Bostrom A: Longitudinal fractures of the patella. *Reconstr Surg Traumatol* 14:136, 1974.
16. Scheller F, Martenson L: Traumatic dislocation of the patella. *Acta Radiol Suppl* 336:5, 1974.
17. Rogers LF, Hendrix RW: Sports-related knee injuries. *Contemp Diag Radiol* 11:1, 1979.
18. Ogden JA: Subluxation and dislocation of the proximal tibiofibular joint. *J Bone Joint Surg (Am)* 56:145, 1974.

Fractures and Dislocations of the Ankle
1. Edeiken J, Cotler JM: Ankle injury. The need for stress films. *JAMA* 240:1182, 1978.
2. Kleiger B: Mechanisms of ankle injury. *Orthop Clin North Am* 5:127, 1974.
3. Rogers LF: *Radiology of Skeletal Trauma,* vol 1 and 2, New York, Churchill Livingstone, 1982.
4. McDaniel WJ, Wilson FC: Trimalleolar fractures of the ankle. *Clin Orthop* 122:37, 1977.
5. Cotton FJ: A new type of ankle fracture. *JAMA* 64:318, 1915.
6. Henderson MS: Trimalleolar fracture of the ankle. *Surg Clin North Am* 12:867, 1932.
7. Pott P: *Some Few General Remarks on Fractures and Dislocations,* London, Hawes Clarke & Collins, 1768.
8. Dupuytren G: Of fractures of the lower extremity of the fibula, and luxations of the foot. [Reprinted in] *Medical Classics* 4:151, 1939.
9. Maisonneuve JG: Recherches sur la fracture du perone. *Arch Gen de Med* 7:165, 1840.

10. Protas JM, Kornblatt BA: Fractures of the lateral margin of the distal tibia, the Tillaux fracture. *Radiology* 138:55, 1981.
11. Rockwood CA, Green DP: *Fractures*, Philadelphia, JB Lippincott, 1975.
12. Burwell HN, Charnley AD: The treatment of displaced fractures at the ankle by rigid internal fixation and early joint movement. *J Bone Joint Surg (Br)* 47:634, 1965.
13. Klossner O: Late results of operative and nonoperative treatment of severe ankle fractures. *Acta Chir Scand [Suppl]* 293:1, 1962.
14. Edeiken J, Cotler JM: Ankle. In Felson B: *Roentgenology of Fractures and Dislocations*, New York, Grune & Stratton, 1978.

Fractures and Dislocations of the Foot
1. Rogers LF: *Radiology of Skeletal Trauma*, vol 1 and 2, New York, Churchill Livingstone, New York, 1982.
2. Zatkin HR: Trauma to the foot. *Semin Roentgenol* 5:419, 1970.
3. Kraft E, Spyropoulos E, Finby N: Neurogenic disorders of the foot in diabetes mellitus. *AJR* 124:17, 1975.
4. Rockwood CA, Green DP: *Fractures*, Philadelphia, JB Lippincott, 1975.
5. Essex-Lopresti P: The mechanism, reduction technique, and results in fractures of the os calcis. *Br J Surg* 39:395, 1952.
6. Caue EF: Fractures of the os calcis—The problem in general. *Clin Orthop* 30:64, 1963.
7. Rowe CR, Sakellarides T, Freeman PA, et al: Fractures of the os calcis. *JAMA* 184:98, 1963.
8. Boehler L: Diagnosis, pathology, and treatment of fractures of the os calcis. *J Bone Joint Surg (Am)* 13:75, 1931.
9. Dachtler HW: Fractures of the anterior superior portion of the os calcis due to indirect violence. *AJR* 25:629, 1931.
10. Thomas HM: Calcaneal fracture in childhood. *Br J Surg* 56:664, 1969.
11. Pennal GF: Fractures of the talus. *Clin Orthop* 30:53, 1963.
12. Coltart WD: Aviator's astragalus. *J Bone Joint Surg (Br)* 34:545, 1952.
13. Canale ST, Kelly FB Jr: Fractures of the neck of the talus. *J Bone Joint Surg (Am)* 60:143, 1978.
14. Hawkins LG: Fractures of the neck of the talus. *J Bone Joint Surg (Am)* 52:991, 1970.
15. Jones R: Fracture of the base of fifth metatarsal bone by indirect violence. *Ann Surg* 35:697, 1902.
16. Foster SC, Foster RR: Lisfranc's tarsometatarsal fracture dislocation. *Radiology* 120:79, 1976.

Fractures of the Thorax
1. Reynolds J, Davis JT: Injuries of the chest wall, pleura, lungs, bronchi, and esophagus. *Radiol Clin North Am* 4:383, 1966.
2. Rogers LF: *Radiology of Skeletal Trauma*, vol 1 and 2, New York, Churchill Livingstone, 1982.
3. Kattan KR: Trauma of the bony thorax. *Semin Roentgenol* 13:69, 1978.

Fractures and Dislocations of the Shoulder Girdle
1. Pavlov H, Freiberger RH: *Roentgenology of Fractures and Dislocations. Shoulder*. Edited by B. Felson, New York, Grune & Stratton, 1978.
2. Heppenstall RB: Fractures and dislocations of the distal clavicle. *Orthop Clin North Am* 6:477, 1975.
3. Yates OW: Complications of fractures of the clavicle. *Injury* 7:189, 1975.
4. Rockwood CA, Green DP: *Fractures*, Philadelphia, JB Lippincott, 1975.
5. Levine HL, Pais MJ, Schwartz EE: Post-traumatic osteolysis of the distal clavicle, with emphasis on early radiologic changes. *AJR* 127:781, 1976.
6. Madsen B: Osteolysis of the acromial end of the clavicle following trauma. *Br J Radiol* 36:822, 1963.
7. Imatani RJ: Fractures of the scapula: A review of 53 fractures. *J Trauma* 15:473, 1975.
8. Bankart ASB: Recurrent or habitual dislocation of the shoulder joint. *Br Med J* 1:1132, 1923.
9. Neer CS II: Displaced proximal humeral fractures. Part I. Classification and evaluation. *J Bone Joint Surg (Am)* 52:1077, 1970.
10. Hill HA, Sachs MD: The grooved defect of the humeral head—A frequent unrecognized complication of dislocations of the shoulder joint. *Radiology* 35:690, 1940.
11. Rowe CR: An atlas of anatomy and treatment of mid clavicular fractures. *Clin Orthop* 58:29, 1968.
12. Rockwood CA, Green DP: *Fractures*, Philadelphia, JB Lippincott, 1975.
13. Arndt JH, Sears AD: Posterior dislocation of the shoulder. *AJR* 94:639, 1965.
14. Cisternino S, Rogers LF, Stufflebaum BC, et al: The trough line: A radiographic sign of posterior shoulder dislocation. *AJR* 130:951, 1978.
15. Nobel W: Posterior traumatic dislocation of shoulder. *J Bone Joint Surg (Am)* 44:523, 1962.
16. Lev-Toaf AS, Karasick D, Rao VM: Drooping shoulder—Nontraumatic causes of glenohumeral subluxation. *Skel Radiol* 12:34, 1984.
17. Alexander C: The acromiohumeral distance in health and disease. *Proc Coll Radiol Aust* 3:102, 1959.
18. Petersson CJ, Redlund-Johnell I: Joint space in normal glenohumeral radiographs. *Acta Orthop Scand* 54:274, 1983.
19. Allman FL Jr: Fractures and ligamentous injuries of the clavicle and its articulation. *J Bone Joint Surg (Am)* 49:774, 1963.
20. Prolass JJ, Stampfli FW, Osmer JC: Coracoid process fracture diagnosis in acromioclavicular separation. *Radiology* 116:61, 1975.

Fractures and Dislocations of the Elbow and Forearm
1. Rockwood CA, Green DP: *Fractures*, Philadelphia, JB Lippincott, 1975.
2. Conn J Jr, Wade PA: Injuries of the elbow. A ten year review. *J Trauma* 1:248, 1961.
3. Knight RA: Fractures of the humeral condyles in adults. *South Med J* 48:1165, 1955.
4. Brogdon BG, Crow NE: Little leaguer's elbow. *AJR* 83:671, 1960.
5. Rogers LF: *Radiology of Skeletal Trauma*, vol 1 and 2, New York, Churchill Livingstone, 1982.
6. Schultz RJ: *The Language of Fractures*, Baltimore, Williams & Wilkins, 1976.
7. Nelson S: Some important diagnostic and technical fundamentals in the radiology of trauma, with particular emphasis on skeletal trauma. *Radiol Clin North Am* 4:241, 1966.
8. Rogers SL, MacEwan DW: Changes due to trauma in the fat plane overlying the supinator muscle: A radiologic sign. *Radiology* 128:643, 1969.
9. Norell HG: Roentgenologic visualization of the extracapsular fat. Its importance in the diagnosis of traumatic injuries to the elbow. *Acta Radiol* 42:205, 1954.
10. Hunter RD: Swollen elbow following trauma. *JAMA* 230:1573, 1974.
11. Essex-Lopresti P: Fractures of the radial head with distal radioulnar dislocation. *J Bone Joint Surg (Br)* 33:244, 1951.
12. Smith H, Sage FP: Medullary fixation of forearm fractures. *J Bone Joint Surg (Am)* 39:91, 1957.
13. DuToit FP, Grabe RP: Isolated fractures of the shaft of the ulna. *S Afr Med J* 56:21, 1979.
14. Bado JL: The Monteggia lesion. *Clin Orthop* 50:71, 1967.
15. Reckling FW, Pellier LF: Ricardo Galeazzi and Galeazzi's fracture. *Surgery* 58:453, 1965.
16. Hughston JC: Fracture of the distal radial shaft. *J Bone Joint Surg (Am)* 39:249, 1957.
17. Linscheid RL, Wheeler DK: Elbow dislocations. *JAMA* 194:1171, 1965.
18. Asher MA: Dislocations of the upper extremity in children. *Orthop Clin North Am* 7:583, 1976.
19. Neviager JS, Wickstrom JK: Dislocation of the elbow. A retrospective study of 115 patients. *South Med J* 70:172, 1977.
20. Salter RB, Zaltz C: Anatomic investigations of the mechanisms of injury and pathologic anatomy of the "pulled elbow" in young children. *Clin Orthop* 77:134, 1971.

Fractures and Dislocations of the Wrist
1. MacEwan DW: Changes due to trauma in the fat plane overlying the pronator quadratus muscle. A radiologic sign. *Radiology* 82:879, 1964.
2. Colles A: On the fracture of the carpal extremity of the radius. *Edinb Med Surg J* 10:182, 1814.
3. Alfram P, Bauer GCH: Epidemiology of fractures of the forearm. *J Bone Joint Surg (Am)* 44:105, 1962.
4. Rockwood CA, Green DP: *Fractures*, Philadelphia, JB Lippincott, 1975.
5. Smith RW: *A Treatise on Fractures in the Vicinity of Joints, and on Certain Forms of Accidental and Congenital Dislocations*, Dublin, Hodges & Smith, 1854.
6. Barton JR: Views and treatment of an important injury to the wrist. *Med Examiner* 1:365, 1838.
7. Edwards HC: Mechanism and treatment of backfire fracture. *J Bone Joint Surg (Am)* 8:701, 1926.
8. Moore EM: Three cases illustrating luxation of the ulna in connection with Colles' fracture. *Med Record* 17:305, 1880.
9. Mazet R Jr, Hohl M: Fractures of the carpal navicular. *J Bone Joint Surg (Am)* 45:82, 1963.
10. Terry DW Jr, Ramin JE: The navicular fat stripe. A useful roentgen feature for evaluating wrist trauma. *AJR* 124:25, 1975.
11. Graham J, Wood SK: Aseptic necrosis of bone following trauma. In Davidson JK (ed): *Aseptic Necrosis of Bone*, Amsterdam, Excerpta Medica, 1976.
12. Rogers LF: *Radiology of Skeletal Trauma*, vol 1 and 2, New York, Churchill Livingstone, 1982.
13. Kohler A, Zimmer EA: *Borderlands of the Normal and Early Pathologic in Skeletal Roentgenology*, ed 3, New York, Grune & Stratton, 1968.
14. Bartone NF, Grieco RV: Fractures of the triquetrum. *J Bone Joint Surg (Am)* 38:353, 1956.
15. Bowen TL: Injuries of the hamate bone. *Hand* 4:235, 1973.
16. Carter PR, Eaton RG, Littler JW: Ununited fracture of the hook of the hamate. *J Bone Joint Surg (Am)* 59:583, 1977.
17. Norman A, Nelson J, Green S: Fractures of the hook of the hamate: Radiographic signs. *Radiology* 154:49, 1985.
18. Gilula LA: Carpal injuries: Analytic approach and case exercises. *AJR* 133:503, 1979.
19. Hudson TM, Caragol WJ, Kaye JJ: Isolated rotatory subluxation of the carpal navicular. *AJR* 126:601, 1976.
20. Frankel VH: The Terry Thomas sign. (Letter). *Clin Orthop Rel Res* 129:321, 1977.
21. deQuervain F: *Spezielle Chirurgische Diagnostik für Studierende und Aertze*, Leipzig, FCW Vogel, 1907.

Fractures and Dislocations of the Hand
1. Rockwood CA, Green DP: *Fractures*, Philadelphia, JB Lippincott, 1975.

2. Brown PS: Management of phalangeal and metacarpal fractures. *Surg Clin North Am* 53:1393, 1973.
3. Terrett AGJ, Molyneux TP: Hit or miss? The impact of three cases. *J Aust Chiro Assoc* 14 (4):153, 1984.
4. Bennett EH: Fractures of the metacarpal bones. *Dublin J Med Sci* 73:72, 1882.
5. Rowe LJ: Bennett's fracture. A case study. *ACA Council Roent, Roentgen Brief,* November 1983.
6. Rolando S: Fracture de la base due premier metacarpein et principalement sur une variete non encore decrite. *Presse Med* 33:303, 1910.
7. Gedda KO: Studies on Bennett's fracture. Anatomy, roentgenology, and therapy. *Acta Chir Scand* 193:1, 1954.
8. Butt WB: Fractures of the hand. *Can Med Assoc J* 86:371, 1962.
9. Wissinger HA, McClain EJ, Boyes JH: Turrett exostosis: Ossifying hematoma of the phalanges. *J Bone Joint Surg (Am)* 48:105, 1966.
10. Green DP, Terry GC: Complex dislocation of the metacarpophalangeal joint. *J Bone Joint Surg (Am)* 55:1480, 1972.
11. Campbell CS: Gamekeeper's thumb. *J Bone Joint Surg (Br)* 37:148, 1955.

Stress Fractures

1. Daffner RH: Stress fractures: Current concepts. *Skel Radiol* 2:221, 1978.
2. Michetti ML: March fracture following a McBride bunionectomy. *J Am Podiatry Assoc* 60:286, 1970.
3. Resnick D, Guerra J Jr: Stress fractures of the inferior pubic ramus following hip surgery. *Radiology* 137:335, 1980.
4. Drez D Jr, Young JC, Johnston RD, et al: Metatarsal stress fractures. *Am J Sports Med* 8:123, 1980.
5. Burrows HJ: Fatigue infraction of the middle of the tibia in ballet dancers. *J Bone Joint Surg (Br)* 38:83, 1956.

6. Winfield AC, Dennis JM: Stress fractures of the calcaneus. *Radiology* 72:415, 1959.
7. Symeonides PP: High stress fracture of the fibula. *J Bone Joint Surg (Br)* 62:192, 1980.
8. Wiltse LL, Widell EH Jr, Jackson DW: Fatigue fracture: The basic lesion in isthmic spondylolisthesis. *J Bone Joint Surg (Am)* 57:17, 1975.
9. Morton D: *The Human Feet*, New York, Columbia University Press, 1948.

The Battered Child Syndrome

1. Caffey J: Multiple fractures in the long bones of infants suffering from chronic subdural hematoma. *AJR* 56:163, 1946.
2. Kempe CH, Silverman FN, Steele BF, et al: The battered-child syndrome. *JAMA* 181:17, 1962.
3. Kogutt MS, Swischuk LE, Fagan CJ: Patterns of injury and significance of uncommon fractures in the battered-child syndrome. *AJR* 121:143, 1974.
4. Kleinman PK, Zito JL: Avulsion of the spinous processes caused by infant abuse. *Radiology* 151:389, 1984.

Post-Traumatic Myositis Ossificans

1. Thompson HC, Garcia A: Myositis ossificans. *Clin Orthop* 50:129, 1967.
2. Thorndike A: Myositis ossificans traumatica. *J Bone Joint Surg (Am)* 22:315, 1940.
3. Ackerman LV: Extra-osseous localized nonneoplastic bone and cartilage formation (so-called myositis ossificans). *J Bone Joint Surg (Am)* 40:279, 1958.
4. Yochum TR, et al: Post-traumatic myositis ossificans. *ACA J Chiro, Radiology Corner*, July 1982.
5. Goldman AB: Myositis ossificans circumscripta, a benign lesion with a malignant differential diagnosis. *AJR* 126:32, 1976.
6. Norman A, Dorfman HD: Juxtacortical circumscribed myositis ossificans: Evolution and radiographic features. *Radiology* 96:301, 1970.

Index

Page numbers in **boldface** indicate main discussions; those followed by *t* and *f* indicate tables and figures, respectively. Page numbers followed by *leg* indicate pages on which the concept cited is discussed only in the figure legend.

ABC's
 of joint evaluation, 542–43
 of radiographic evaluation, 1070–71
abdomen
 anteroposterior projection positioning,
  90, 90*f*–91*f*
 artifacts in, 39, 41, 1085*f*, 1103*f*–4*f*
 evaluation
  in obese patient, 90
  in tall patient, 90
 film placement for interpretation, 1069
 garment artifact in, 1085*f*, 1103*f*–4*f*
 KUB projection positioning, 90, 90*f*–91*f*
 kVp for, 2*t*
 MRI, xxviii*f*
 normal anatomy, 91*f*
 soft tissues, demonstration, 30, 32, 34
 upper, demonstration, 86
abdominal aorta, MRI, xxviii*f*
abdominal aortic aneurysm, 1022, 1022*f*–23*f*
abdominal ileus, with compression
  fracture(s), 450, 450*f*
abduction, definition of, 6
abscess. *See also* Brodie's abscess; psoas
  abscess
 in coccidioidomycosis, 958
 in tubercular spondylitis, 941*f*, 942–43
accessory bones, 155*f*
accessory ossicle, 158*f*, 159*f*, 160*f*
 description, 98
 radiological features, 98
accessory transverse process sign, **1126**
 condition(s) associated with, 1126
acetabular angle
 landmarks, 203, 219*t*
 measurement, **203,** 203*f*
 normal, 203*t*, 219*t*
 significance, 203, 219*t*
acetabular depth
 landmarks, 201, 219*t*
 measurement, **201,** 201*f*
 normal, 201*t*, 219*t*
 significance, 201, 219*t*
acetabular dysplasia, 202, 203
acetabular fracture(s), **457,** 458*f*
 central, 457, 458*f*
 explosion. *See* acetabular fracture(s),
  central
 posterior rim fracture, 457
 simple anterior column fracture, 457
 simple posterior column fracture, 457
acetabulum
 demonstration, 45, 46
 Paget's disease, malignant degeneration,
  864*f*
 triradiate cartilage, 153*f*

Achilles tendon
 demonstration, 63
 myositis ossificans, 528*f*
achondroplasia, 113, 331*t*, **355–58,** 356*f*,
  357*f*, 358*f*, 376, 1127*f*
 clinical features, 356, 404*t*
 with congenital central stenosis, 304
 homozygous, 356
 neurological complications, 357–59
 pathological features, 356
 radiological features, 356
acid phosphatase, 345
 normal laboratory value, 350*t*
 with metastatic bone tumors, 700
aclasis, definition of, 793
acromegaly, 209, 211, **1052–55**
 capsule summary, 1055
acromioclavicular joint
 alignment, 496
 anteroposterior projection positioning,
  70, 70*f*
 degenerative joint disease, 571*f*, 572
 demonstration, 67
 injuries, classification, 495*t*, 496*f*, 497
 kVp for, 2*t*
 ligaments, 495*f*
 normal anatomy, 70*f*
 rheumatoid arthritis, 607
 separations, **495–97**
  classification, 495*t*
  radiological features, 495–96
acromioclavicular joint space, 495
 abnormal, 212*f*
 landmarks, 212, 221*t*
 measurement, **212,** 212*f*
 normal, 212*t*, 212*f*, 221*t*
 significance, 212, 221*t*
acromiohumeral joint space
 landmarks, 211, 221*t*
 measurement, **211,** 211*f*
 normal, 211*t*, 221*t*
 significance, 211, 221*t*
acro-osteolysis, 401, 401*f*, 648*f*–50*f*
acrosclerosis. *See also* scleroderma
 definition of, 647*t*
acrosyndactyly, 134
Actinomyces bovis, 958
Actinomyces israelii, 958
actinomycosis, **958**
acute anterior cervical cord syndrome, 438,
  439*leg*
acute kyphosis sign, 442, 442*f*, 533*t*
adamantinoma, **779–80**
 positions in bone, 333*t*
 site of origin, 855*t*
 sites of involvement, 332*t*, 779, 779*f*

adduction, definition of, 6
adductor magnus, post-traumatic myositis
  ossificans in, 525, 527*f*
adductor muscles, of thigh, post-traumatic
  myositis ossificans in, 525
adiposogenital dystrophy, 466
age
 and skeletal abnormalities, 330
 and thoracic kyphosis, 185
A/G ratio, 351
 in multiple myeloma, 731
alar ligament, instability, 180
Albers-Schönberg's disease. *See*
  osteopetrosis
alcoholism, osteonecrosis in, 978
alkaline phosphatase, 345
 with metastatic bone tumors, 700
 normal laboratory value, 350*t*
Allopurinol, 662
ameloblastoma. *See* adamantinoma
Amipaque. *See* metrizamide
amphiarthroses, definition of, 7
amyloidosis, in multiple myeloma, 732
anatomy, 6–7
Andersson lesion, 620, **623,** 625*f*, 625*t*
androgen, in bone metabolism, 329
anemia, 961. *See also* sickle cell anemia
 chronic hemolytic. *See* thalassemia major
 in multiple myeloma, 730, 731
 in osteopetrosis, 390, 393*leg*
 in Paget's disease, 861
aneurysmal bone cyst, 330, 334*f*, 338*f*, 341*f*,
  706, 781, 784, 824, 825, **849–53**
 age distribution, 849
 age of maximum incidence, 855*t*
 blown out appearance, 851, 851*f*
 capsule summary, 853
 clinical features, 849–50
 incidence, 849
 location, 332*t*, 849–50, 850*f*, 856*t*
 pathological features, 850–51
 periosteal buttress, 851, 851*f*
 positions in bone, 333*t*
 primary, 850
 prognosis, 852–53
 radiological features, 851–52
 secondary, 850, 851
 sex distribution, 849
 signs and symptoms, 849
 site of origin, 855*t*
 soapbubble pattern, 851, 851*f*
 spine, 852
 treatment, 852–53
aneurysms, **1020–24.** *See also specific*
  anatomic entity
 etiology, 1020, 1020*t*

computed tomography—*continued*
  window level, 276
  window width, 276
computed tomography metrizamide
    myelography, 286, 287*f*
  in diagnosis of disc disease, 300–302
  in disc disease, 292
  of herniated nucleus pulposus, 296
congenital anomalies, 96. *See also specific
    anomaly*
congenital block vertebra. *See* block
    vertebra, congenital
congenital dislocated hip. *See* congenital hip
    dysplasia
congenital hip dysplasia, 127, 127*f*, 132, 206
  acetabular angle in, 203
  longstanding, 127, 128*f*
congestive heart failure, in scoliosis, 233
conjoined nerve root, 298, 299*f*
  CT, 301*f*
conjunctivitis, in Reiter's syndrome, 637
Conradi-Hunermann syndrome, 362, 363,
    364*f*
contrast examinations, 318–21
contrast media, 147*f*, 148*f*. *See also specific
    medium*
  artifact caused by, 1117*f*, 1118*f*
  in scoliosis assessment, 236
control console, in CT and MRI, definition
    of, 274
coracoclavicular distance, 496
coracoclavicular ligaments, 495*f*, 497
cord compression syndrome, 96
corduroy cloth appearance, 798, 799*f*, 800*f*,
    801*f*, 802*f*, 885*f*, 1034*f*
corduroy cloth vertebra, **1127**, 1128*f*
  condition(s) associated with, 1127
corner fracture. *See also* fracture(s), chip
  in battered child syndrome, 524*f*, 525
  definition of, 529*t*
corner sign, 505, 506*f*, 533*t*, 1046
corner vertebra, **1127–28**
coronoid process, detection, 73
cor pulmonale, 233
cortex, of bone, 7, 328–29
  pencil thin, 335, 338*f*
cortical destruction, in bone lesions, 337,
    338*f*
cortical expansion, in bone lesions, 337,
    338*f*
cortical hyperostosis. *See* infantile cortical
    hyperostosis
cortical integrity, with bone lesions, 333–37,
    338*f*
cortical saucerization, in Ewing's sarcoma,
    762, 763*f*
cortical thickening, in bone lesions, 337,
    338*f*
cortical thickness, 7
cortical thinning, with bone lesions, 333–37,
    338*f*
cortical white line, 936, 937*f*, 948, 950*f*
corticosteroid therapy, osteonecrosis in, 978
Corynebacterium infection, 926
costal cartilage injuries, 488
costal joint, arthrosis, 555*f*
costochondral calcification, 146*f*
Cotton's fracture. *See* trimalleolar fracture
cottonwool appearance, 305*f*, 858*f*, 859*f*, 872
cotton wool calcification, 837
cough fracture, 486*f*, 488, 531*t*
coxa magna, 997*f*, 998
coxa plana, 997*f*, 998

coxarthrosis. *See* hip joint, degenerative
    joint disease
coxa valga, **128–29**, 206, 376
  adolescent, **128–29**, 129*f*, 206, 206*f*, 207,
    999. *See also* slipped femoral capital
    epiphysis
  epiphyseal. *See* slipped femoral capital
    epiphysis
  in fibrous dysplasia, 894
CPPD. *See* calcium pyrophosphate
    dihydrate crystal deposition disease;
    pyrophosphate arthropathy
craniovertebral region, anomalies of, **96–98**
cranium, bones of, 6*t*
C-reactive protein, 345
  normal laboratory value, 350*t*
creeping substitution, 996, 1010
crescent sign, 837, 981, 981*f*, 985, **996**, 996*f*,
    997*f*, 1000, 1015
CREST syndrome. *See also* scleroderma
  definition of, 647*t*
cretinism, 113, 366, **1055**, 1133*f*
Crohn's disease, 615
  and enteropathic arthritis, 626, 627*f*
Crookes' tube, xxv
CRT. *See* cathode ray tubes
CT numbers, definition of, 276
CT scan. *See* computed tomography
cuboid bone
  demonstration, 57, 58
  fracture(s), 483
cumulus cloud appearance, 747, 749*f*
cuneiform(s)
  demonstration, 57
  fracture(s), 483
  third, demonstration, 58
cup and saucer deformity. *See* pencil in cup
    deformity
Cupid's bow contour, 115, 118*f*, 122*f*, 124*f*,
    1128, 1128*f*
cupped vertebra, **1128**. *See also* H vertebra
  condition(s) associated with, 1128
curlers, artifacts caused by, 1104*f*
cursor, definition of, 275
Cushing's disease, **1056–59**
cystic fibrosis, and thoracic kyphosis, 185
cystic tuberculosis, 951, 952*f*
cysts. *See also* aneurysmal bone cyst;
    Baker's cyst; simple bone cyst
  in ankylosing spondylitis, 622
  epidermoid inclusion, 830*leg*
  phalangeal, in tuberous sclerosis, 403,
    403*f*
  in rheumatoid arthritis, 605, 606, 607*f*,
    608
  subarticular degenerative, 342
  subchondral, 549*f*, 550, 563, 566*f*
    in hemophilia, 970
    in hip joint, 563–65, 566*f*
    mimicking neoplasm, 350*f*
    in osteonecrosis, 981

dagger sign, 620, 622*f*, 625*t*
dancer's fracture. *See* Jones' fracture
dashboard fracture, 530*t*. *See also* acetabular
    fracture(s), posterior rim fracture
Davis series, 21
  in whiplash syndrome, 441
degenerative arthritis, 211
  after clavicular injury, 490
  differential diagnosis, 545
  radiocarpal, 509, 509*f*
  scoliosis with, 234*f*, 235

degenerative disc disease, xxviii*f*, **676–77**
  demonstration on MRI, 287, 287*f*, 561*f*
  diagnostic imaging, 292–302
  pathology, 291–92
degenerative joint disease, 114, 331*t*, 349*f*,
    546–73, 600, 617*t*. *See also*
    degenerative arthritis; *specific joint*
  acromioclavicular joint space in, 212
  age of onset, 540*t*
  articular deformity in, 550
  asymmetrical distribution, 548
  capsule summary, 573
  clinical features, **546–47**
  with CPPD, 666
  differential diagnosis, 652*t*
  intra-articular loose bodies in, 550
  joint subluxation in, 550
  nomenclature, 546, 546*t*
  nonuniform loss in joint space, 548, 563,
    565*f*
  osteophytes in, 547, 548
  pathogenetic development, 547, 547*f*
  pathological features, **547–48**
  primary, 546
  radiological features, 548*f*, **548–73**, 549*f*
  radiological-pathological correlation, 548*f*
  relative frequency, 540*t*
  scoliosis caused by, 233, 233*f*
  secondary, 546
  skeletal distribution, 546–47, 546*f*
  in slipped femoral capital epiphysis, 468
  spinal distribution of, 550–51, 550*f*
  subchondral bone cysts, 550
  subchondral sclerosis in, 549–50
  target sites of involvement, 550–73. *See
    also specific anatomical area*
dental fillings, artifacts caused by, 1118*f*
dentures, swallowed, radiographic
    appearance, 1107*f*
de Quervain's disease, 679
de Quervain's fracture/dislocation, 513, 532*t*
dermal inclusion tumor. *See* adamantinoma
diabetes
  and diffuse idiopathic skeletal
    hyperostosis, 577
  maternal, and congenital anomalies, 127
  misdiagnosis, in ochronosis, 682
  neurotrophic arthropathy in, 583, 586*f*,
    589*f*
  septic arthritis in, 937, 937*f*
  vascular calcification in, 926*f*
diaphragm
  injury, with pelvic fracture(s), 462
  radiographic appearance, 1114*f*
diaphyseal aclasis. *See* hereditary multiple
    exostosis
diaphysis, 6, 7, 328*f*, 328
  lesion in, 334*f*, 762, 762*f*
  proximal, demonstration, 45, 46
diarthroses, definition of, 7
diastasis, 419
diastematomyelia, 113, 121, 121*f*
Diaz's disease, 994*t*, **1015**
diffuse idiopathic skeletal hyperostosis,
    149*leg*, 304, 562*f*, 562*leg*, **575–81**, 582,
    614, 617*t*
  age of onset, 540*t*
  anterior lucency in, 576*f*
  candle flame, 579*f*–80*f*
  capsule summary, 581
  clinical features, 576–77, 576*t*
  diagnostic criteria, 578–79
  differential diagnosis, 580

Lofgren's syndrome, 686
long bones, 6–7
    components, 6
    fibrosarcoma in, 766
    long lesion in, 333, 336f
    in multiple myeloma, 733–35, 737f–38f
    osteosarcoma in, 744
    in progressive diaphyseal dysplasia, 399,
        399f, 400f
    pseudarthrosis, in neurofibromatosis,
        904–5
    in sickle cell anemia, 964
    in systemic lupus erythematosus, 645
    in thalassemia, 968
longitudinal ligament. See anterior
        longitudinal ligament
longus colli, in hydroxyapatite deposition
        disease, 674, 675f
long vertebra, 947, 951t, 1130, 1131f
    condition(s) associated with, 1130
loose bodies
    in degenerative joint disease, 567, 568f
    intra-articular, in degenerative joint
        disease, 550, 550f
    in knee, with osteonecrosis, 988
    osteochondral. See
        synoviochondrometaplasia
    radiographic appearance, 589f
    in synoviochondrometaplasia, 591–93,
        592f
Looser's lines, 418, 858. See also
        pseudofracture(s)
lordoscoliosis, definition of, 227
lover's heels, 637, 639
low back pain, 187, 189
    evaluation, 322leg
    with herniated nucleus pulposus, 294
    incidence, 273
    in spondylolisthesis, 255, 268
    in stenosis, surgical therapy, 308–10
lower extremities
    bones of, 6t
    fracture(s), in osteogenesis imperfecta,
        381, 382f
    in infantile cortical hyperostosis, 372,
        374f
    lines and angles of, 219t, 220t
    measurements, 200–210
    in melorheostosis, 385, 386f
    in osteopetrosis, 393f
lozenge-shaped vertebra, 1130
    condition(s) associated with, 1130
LPO. See left posterior oblique position
lucent cleft sign, 442–43, 444f, 533t
lumbar curve, definition of, 227
lumbar gravity line, 191, 191f
    landmarks, 191, 217t
    normal values, 217t
    significance, 191, 217t
lumbar instability
    degenerative
        evaluation, 192, 192f
        measurement, 194, 194f
    flexion/extension evaluation, 192, 192f
    lateral bending, measurement, 194, 194f
    van Akkerveeken's measurement of, 192,
        192f
lumbar intervertebral disc angles
    landmarks, 187, 217t
    measurement, 187, 187f
    normal values, 187t
    significance, 187, 217t
lumbar lordosis, 195

in ankylosing spondylitis, 620
    landmarks, 187, 217t
    measurement, 187, 187f
    normal values, 217t
    significance, 187, 217t
lumbar rib, 150f
lumbar spine. See also spine
    in achondroplasia, 358f, 359f
    anomalies, 112–25
    anteroposterior angulated view, in
        spondylolysis and spondylolisthesis,
        255
    anteroposterior lumbopelvic projection
        positioning, 30, 30f, 31f
    anteroposterior lumbosacral spot
        positioning, 36, 36f–37f
    anteroposterior nonangulated view, in
        spondylolysis and spondylolisthesis,
        255
    apophyseal articulations, in degenerative
        joint disease, 555–56, 557f
    avulsion fracture(s), 454
    bone island in, 812leg, 815f
    bones of, 6t
    bulging disc in, imaging, 293
    carcinoma in, 324f
    central stenosis, 305
    common artifacts, 6t
    compression fracture, 480f
        step defect, 447f
    compression fracture(s), 448–50
        radiographic signs of, 448–50
    CT axial image at L4/L5, 286f
    degenerative joint disease, 549f, 555–58
    demonstration, 44, 90
    diffuse idiopathic skeletal hyperostosis,
        579f, 580
    disc herniation, 189
        posterolateral, 194, 194f
    discography, 288f
    in Ewing's sarcoma, 761, 762f
    facet arthrosis, 555–56, 557f
    facet dislocation, 454, 454f
    fibrosarcoma in, 766f
    fibrous dysplasia, 899f
    flexion/extension
        landmarks, 193, 218t
        normal measurements, 193
        significance, 193, 218t
    foraminal stenosis, 308
    fracture(s), 416f, 448–54
        named and eponymic, 530t
    fracture dislocation, 454
    giant cell tumor in, 785f
    growth variants, 150f
    hard to see areas, 1071t
    hemangioma, 800f, 801f, 802f
    herniated nucleus pulposus, imaging,
        294–96
    kVp for, 2t
    L4/L5 degeneration, 199
    L4 level, computed tomogram, xxviif
    L5/S1 degeneration, 199
    L5 vertebra
        demonstration, 36, 38
        trapezoidal shape, 151f
    lateral, 4f
    lateral bending, normal measurements,
        194
    lateral bending instability
        landmarks, 194, 218t
        normal values, 218t
        significance, 194, 218t

lateral hemivertebra, 113, 115f, 116f
lateral lumbosacral projection positioning,
        32, 32f, 33f
lateral lumbosacral spot positioning, 38,
        38f
lateral recess stenosis, 309f
lateral view, xxvif
    in spondylolysis and spondylolisthesis,
        255–57
lines and angles of, 217t, 218t
measurements, 186–99
metastatic disease in, 705f, 711f, 714f,
        715f, 717f
Metrizamide myelography, xxvif
    in Morquio's syndrome, 378, 378f
MRI, xxviiif, 283–85, 284f
    in multiple myeloma, 733f, 736f
    neural arch, fracture(s), 451–54
    neurofibromatosis, 904f, 906f
    neurotrophic arthropathy, 586f
    normal anatomy, 33, 33f, 35, 35f, 37f, 38f
    oblique projections, 34, 34f, 35f
    ossification, in fibrodysplasia ossificans
        progressiva, 369, 370t–71f
    in osteogenesis imperfecta, 382, 384f
    osteoid osteoma, 820f
    in osteopetrosis, 394f, 395f
    in osteopoikilosis, 396, 398f
    osteoporosis, in multiple myeloma, 732,
        733f
    Paget's disease in, 858f, 861f, 862f, 878f,
        879f, 880f, 884f, 885f
        malignant degeneration, 867f
    pedicle
        agenesis, 109, 116, 119f
        congenital absence of, 119f
    plain film radiography, 322f
    plasmacytoma, 742f
    posterior venous cleft in, 150f
    schematic axial view, 286f
    segmental instability, prediction, 199
    specimen radiograph, 31f, 33f, 35f
    step defect in, 150f
    stress fracture, 523t
    transverse process
        agenesis, 162t
        anomalous malformation, 151f
        congenital nonunion, 451
        fracture(s), 451, 452f
        length, landmarks, 199, 218t
        length, significance, 199, 218t
        length measurement, 199, 199f
        trauma, named radiological signs, 533t
    ventral hemivertebra, 113, 115f
lumbar vertebra, normal, axial view of,
        291f
lumbosacral angle
    landmarks, 189, 217t
    measurement, 189, 189f
    normal values, 189t, 217t
    significance, 189, 217t
lumbosacral articulation, on CT, xxviif
lumbosacral curve, definition of, 227
lumbosacral disc angle
    landmarks, 189, 217t
    measurement, 189, 189f
    normal values, 217t
    significance, 189, 217t
lumbosacral lordosis angle
    landmarks, 188, 217t
    measurement, 188, 188f
    normal values, 188t, 217t
    significance, 188, 217t

osteoblastoma—*continued*
  pathological features, 824
  radiological features, 824–25, 824*t*
  sex distribution, 822
  signs and symptoms, 822–23
  site of origin, 855*t*
  skeletal sites. *See* osteoblastoma, location
  treatment, 825
osteochondral loose bodies. *See*
    synoviochondrometaplasia
osteochondritis dessicans, 157*leg*, **1009–14**
  capsule summary, 1014
  clinical features, 1009
  of knee, vs. spontaneous osteonecrosis,
    986, 986*t*
  location, 1009, 1009*t*, 1009*f*, 1010–14
  pathological features, 1009–10
  radiological features, 1010*t*, 1010–14
  sites of involvement. *See* osteochondritis
    dessicans, location
osteochondrodystrophy. *See* Hurler's syndrome
osteochondroma, 343*f*, 795*f*
  cartilagenous cap, 788, 789*f*
  cauliflower, 789*f*–90*f*, 795*f*–96*f*
  fracture, 789, 790*f*
  incidence, 786
  location, 332*t*, 856*t*
  malignant degeneration, 746, 757*f*, 788
    features suggesting, 788*t*
    propensity for, 911*t*
  multiple, 786, 787*f*, 794*f*–95*f*
  positions in bone, 333*t*
  pressure erosion from, 796*f*
  prognosis, 790
  radiological features, 792*t*
  sessile, 789–90, 791*f*, 794*f*
  site of origin, 855*t*
  skeletal sites. *See* osteochondroma,
    location
  solitary, **786–92**, 787*f*
    age distribution, 787
    capsule summary, 792
    clinical features, 787
    incidence, 786
    location, 787
    malignant degeneration, 788
    pathological features, 787–88
    radiological features, 788–90
    sex distribution, 787
    treatment, 790
  vs. supracondylar process, 132
osteochondromatosis. *See*
    synoviochondrometaplasia
  multiple. *See* hereditary multiple
    exostosis
osteoclast activating factor, 732
osteogenesis imperfecta, 128, 137*leg*,
  380–82, 381*f*–85*f*, 518, 1037
  bowing deformities in, 381, 382*f*
  clinical features, 381, 405*t*
  congenita, 381
  fracture in, 381, 382*f*
  radiological features, 381–82, 407*t*
  tarda, 381
osteoid osteoma, 262, 262*f*, 331*t*, **816–22**
  age distribution, 816
  age of maximum incidence, 855*t*
  vs. bone island, 814–15
  cancellous, 818
  capsule summary, 822
  clinical features, 816
  cortical, 818
  differential diagnosis, 818, 820–21, 930

en-bloc excision, 821*f*
  in hard-to-see area, 820*f*
  incidence, 816
  location, 332*t*, 816, 817*f*, 818, 856*t*
  nidus, 816, 818, 818*f*
  pain in, 816, 817*leg*, 931*leg*
  pathological features, 816–18
  positions in bone, 333*t*
  prognosis, 821–22, 822
  radiological features, 818–21, 821*t*
  scoliosis due to, 233*f*
  sex distribution, 816
  signs and symptoms, 816
  skeletal sites. *See* osteoid osteoma,
    location
  spinal, 818, 820*leg*
  vs. stress fracture, 522
  subperiosteal, 818
  treatment, 821–22
osteoid seams, 1041, 1045
osteology, 6–7
osteolysis
  acral, 1059, 1060*f*
  post-traumatic, after clavicular injury, 490
osteoma, 344*f*, **807–10**. *See also* osteoid
    osteoma
  giant, 807, 807*f*
  ivory, 807*f*, 808*f*, 809*f*
  radiographic appearance, 807, 808*f*–10*f*
  radiological features, 810*t*
  skeletal distribution, 807, 807*f*
osteomalacia, 172–73, 418, 518, **1041–42**,
  1043*f*–44*f*
  and basilar impression, 98
  capsule summary, 1042
  clinical features, 1041
  definition of, 1041
  deformity in, 1042, 1044*f*
  etiology, 1041, 1041*t*
  in neurofibromatosis, 905
  pathological features, 1041–42
  radiological features, 1042
osteomyelitis, 330, 346*f*, 420. *See also* Garré's
    sclerosing osteomyelitis; mycotic
    osteomyelitis; nonsuppurative
    osteomyelitis; suppurative
    osteomyelitis; syphilitic osteomyelitis
  as fracture complication, 424*f*, 425
  historic considerations, 921
  in sickle cell anemia, 964, 964*t*
  vs. stress fracture, 522
osteonecrosis, **978–93**
  in alcoholism, 978
  in Caisson disease, 978
  capsule summary, 983
  causes, 978
  clinical features, 978–79, 995
  in collagen disease, 979
  with corticosteroid therapy, 978
  disorders associated with, 979*t*
  epiphyseal infarction, 979, 980*t*
  in Gaucher's disease, 979
  in gout, 979
  in hemoglobinopathy, 979
  metaphyseal/diaphyseal infarction, 980
  in pancreatitis, 979
  pathological features, 979–80
  primary, 994
  with radiation, 979
  radiological features, 980–83
  secondary, 994
  skeletal distribution, 978, 979*f*
  in slipped femoral capital epiphysis, 468

spontaneous, 978. *See also* femoral head
  and neck, spontaneous
  osteonecrosis; knee, spontaneous
  osteonecrosis
  clinical features, 978
  steroid-induced, **1056–59**
  in systemic lupus erythematosus, 644*f*,
    645
  in trauma, 978
osteopathia condensans disseminata. *See*
    osteopoikilosis
osteopathia striata, 386, **389**, 389*f*
  clinical features, 389, 405*t*
  radiological features, 389, 407*t*
osteopenia
  definition of, 1031
  effect on radiographs, 5
  generalized, in neoplastic disorders, 1038
osteopetrosis, **389–91**, 390*f*–96*f*, 518, 1126*f*,
  1133*f*
  clinical features, 389–90, 405*t*
  laboratory findings, 390
  pathological features, 390
  radiological features, 390–91, 407*t*
  spondylolisthesis in, 252*f*
  spondylolysis with, 249
osteopetrosis generalisata. *See* osteopetrosis
osteophytes, 547–48, 554*f*, 556–61, 562*f*,
  563, 571
  in ankylosing spondylitis, 622
  claw, 558, 559*f*
  in CPPD, 668
  definition of, 543
  lumbar spine, 559*f*
  traction, 559*f*. *See also* traction spurs
osteopoikilosis, 386, **396**, 397*f*–98*f*, 812, 813*f*
  clinical features, 396, 406*t*
  pathological features, 396
  radiological features, 396, 407*t*
osteoporosis, 331, 335, 518, **1031–41**, 1130*f*
  in childhood leukemia, 974–76
  conditions associated with, 1032*t*
  in congenital disorders, 1037
  of Cushing's disease, 1056
  definition of, 1031
  disuse, 1039, 1040*f*
  extremity manifestations, 1038*f*
  fracture(s) in, 1033, 1036, 1037*f*
  generalized, 1031, **1031–38**. *See also*
    osteoporosis, senile
    capsule summary, 1038
    clinical features, 1032
    pathological features, 1032
    radiological features, 1032–33
    sites of involvement, 1033–37
  iatrogenic, 1056
  immobilization, 1039
  incidence, 1032
  in juvenile rheumatoid arthritis, 612, 614
  localized, 1031
  in metabolic and endocrine disorders,
    1037–38
  multiple compression fractures with, 446*f*
  in multiple myeloma, 732, 733*f*
  in nutritional disorders, 1037
  postmenopausal, 1031–38. *See also*
    osteoporosis, generalized
  post-traumatic. *See* reflex sympathetic
    dystrophy syndrome
  regional, 1031, **1038–41**
    capsule summary, 1041
  regional migratory, 1040
  in rheumatoid arthritis, 605

senile, 1031–38, 1056. *See also*
  osteoporosis, generalized
  effect on radiographs, 5
  in sickle cell anemia, 964
  and spondylolysis, 246
  and thoracic kyphosis, 185
  transient regional, 1039–40
  in vascular disorders, 1037
osteoporosis circumscripta, 869, 874f, 872,
  876f
osteopsathyrosis idiopathica. *See*
  osteogenesis imperfecta
osteosarcoma, 330, 331t, 344f, 346f, 347f,
  743
  age of maximum incidence, 855t
  central, **743–50**
    age distribution, 744
    capsule summary, 750
    clinical features, 744
    incidence, 743
    laboratory findings, 745
    location, 744–45, 744f
    metastasis, 746, 746f–47f
    pathological features, 745–46
    prognosis, 747
    sex distribution, 744
    signs and symptoms, 744
    treatment, 747
  extraosseous, **754**
  vs. hemangioma, 804*leg*
  ivory, 745f, 746f, 747, 748f
  juxtacortical. *See* sarcoma, parosteal
  location, 332t, 856t
  lytic vs. sclerotic, radiographic
    appearance, 747, 748f
  metastatic, 746f–47f
    hypertrophic osteoarthropathy
      secondary to, 658f
  multicentric, **750,** 750f, 751f
  parosteal. *See* sarcoma, parosteal
  periosteal, 355f
  periosteal response in, 747, 748f–49f
  positions in bone, 333t
  radiological features, 746–47
  relative incidence, 700t
  sclerotic appearance, 746, 746f
  secondary, **753,** 754f
  site of origin, 855t
  vs. stress fracture, 522
  surface. *See* sarcoma, parosteal
osteosarcomatosis. *See* osteosarcoma,
  multicentric
osteosclerosis. *See* osteopetrosis
osteosclerosis generalisata. *See* osteopetrosis
osteosi eberneizzante monomelica. *See*
  melorheostosis
os tibiale externum, 158f
os trigonum, 157f, 158f
ovarian shield, 1084f, 1096f
  radiographic appearance, 1119f
overhanging margin sign, 662f, 663, 663f,
  664
owl's eyes appearance, 115, 118f

pacemaker, radiographic appearance, 1094f
pad sign, 732
Paget, James, 856
Paget's coxopathy, 861
Paget's disease, 172–73, 205, 330, 417f, 418,
  518, 707, 710, 716f, **856–86,** 1131f–32f
  age distribution, 857
  alkaline phosphatase levels in, 345,
    867–68

anemia in, 861
avulsion fracture in, 875, 883
and basilar impression, 98
basilar invagination in, 172f, 305, 305f,
  857–58, 859f
within block vertebra, 884f
candle flame appearance, 874, 883f
capsule summary, 886
central stenosis in, 305
clinical features, 857–68
complications, 857–64, 858t
cortical integrity in, 338f
cottonwool appearance. *See* cottonwool
  appearance
deformity in, 857, 859f
differential diagnosis, 875, 884f–85f,
  891*leg*, 892, 897
etiology, 857, 857t
expansile manifestations, 857, 858f
fracture(s) in, 858, 863
vs. hemangioma, 798, 802f
high output cardiac failure in, 862
incidence, 856–57
joint degeneration in, 861, 862f
laboratory findings, 867–68
location, 865–67, 868f
malignant degeneration, 753, 754f, 862–65
  age distribution, 863
  incidence, 863
  pathological findings, 863
  prognosis, 864
  propensity for, 911t
  radiological findings, 863–64
  sex distribution, 863
  signs and symptoms, 863
  site distribution, 863
  treatment, 864
and metastatic disease, 870
with multiple myeloma, 739f
named radiographic signs, 875t
with osteoblastic metastasis, 717f
vs. osteoblastic metastatic carcinoma, 707,
  710, 720f, 875, 884f
and osteosarcoma, 744–45
pathological features, 868–70
pathological fracture(s) in, 858
polyostotic, 872–73, 877f, 878f
prognosis, 875–78
pseudofractures in, 858–61
radiological features, 870–75, 875t
Schmorl's nodes with, 114
sex distribution, 857
signs and symptoms, 857
skull in, 305f
spinal stenosis in, 312f, 861, 862f
spondylolysis with, 249
stages of, 869–70, 874t
subarticular extension, 865, 873, 874f, 882f
subtrochanteric fracture in, 464
treatment, 875–78
ureteric colic in, 862
vertebral manifestations, 305f
V-shaped lytic defect, 874, 883f
Paget's sarcoma, multifocal involvement,
  866f
pain. *See also* low back pain
  in ankylosing spondylitis, 615
  in Brodie's abscess, 817*leg*, 930, 931*leg*
  in chondrosarcoma, 754
  in metastatic bone tumors, 700
  in multiple myeloma, 730
  in osteoid osteoma, 816, 817*leg*, 931*leg*
  in osteosarcoma, 744

in slipped femoral capital epiphysis, 466
spinal-related
  incidence, 273
  radiological approaches, 273–74
in spondyloepiphyseal dysplasia, 368*leg*
in spondylolysis and spondylolisthesis,
  253, 269
paintbrush metaphyses, 1045f, 1046
palato-occipital line. *See* Chamberlain's line
pancake vertebra, 1033
Pancoast's tumor, 701*leg*
pancreatitis, osteonecrosis with, 979
panda bear appearance, 287f
Panner's disease, 994t, **1016–17,** 1016f
pannus, 596, 596f, 616, 629
pantopaque, 285
  excretion, 1117*leg*
paracondylar process
  AP open mouth projection, 97f
  AP tomogram, 97f
  description, 97
  radiological features, 97
paracondyloid anomalies, 96
paraglenoid sulci, normal variants, 152f
paralellogram of Kopitz, 204
paramastoid anomalies, 96
paranasal sinuses
  normal anatomy, 11, 11f, 12, 12f
  radiographic positioning for, 11, 11f
  Water's projection, 12, 12f
paraodontoid notches, 140f
paraspinal edema, with compression
  fracture(s), 450
parasyndesmophytes, 634
parathormone, in bone metabolism, 329
paravertebral bony confines, on CT, xxviif
paravertebral musculature, on CT, xxviif
parietal bone, fracture, 426f
parietal foramina, 136f
parosteal sarcoma. *See* sarcoma, parosteal
parotid gland, carcinoma, 704*leg*
Parry fracture. *See* nightstick fracture
pars interarticularis
  defect in, 150f, 244. *See also*
    spondylolisthesis; spondylolysis
  AP detection of, 255, 256f
  in Eskimos, 244
  and stress, 262, 264f, 265f
  at unusual levels, 246, 248f
  demonstration, 34
  fracture(s), 246, 248, 251*leg*, 451–54,
    452f
  stress fracture, 518, 521f
  thin, 151f
partial volume averaging, 279
part position, definition of, 2
passion fracture, 487, 531t
patella
  bipartite, 129, 130f, 472, 473f
  bones of, 6t
  degenerative enthesopathy, 569f
  demonstration, 48, 49, 53
  diffuse idiopathic skeletal hyperostosis,
    580, 581f
  epiphyseal disorders, 994t
  fracture(s), 130*leg*, 471–72, 472f–73f
  giant, 872f
  in hemophilia, 972
  neoplastic disease, 781
  osteochondritis dessicans, 1013
  stress fracture, 523t
  tripartite, 472, 473f
  tumors, 836